Progressive Brain Disorders
in Childhood

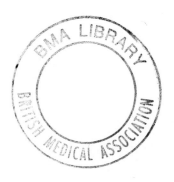

Progressive Brain Disorders in Childhood

Juan M. Pascual

Departments of Neurology and Neurotherapeutics, Physiology and Pediatrics and
Eugene McDermott Center for Human Growth & Development/ Center for Human Genetics,
The University of Texas Southwestern Medical Center, Dallas

Children's Medical Center Dallas

Parkland Memorial Hospital

Department of Biological Sciences, The University of Texas at Dallas

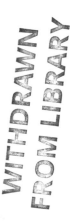

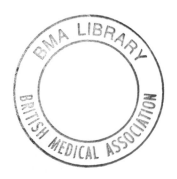

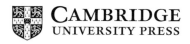

CAMBRIDGE
UNIVERSITY PRESS

CAMBRIDGE
UNIVERSITY PRESS

University Printing House, Cambridge CB2 8BS, United Kingdom

One Liberty Plaza, 20th Floor, New York, NY 10006, USA

477 Williamstown Road, Port Melbourne, VIC 3207, Australia

4843/24, 2nd Floor, Ansari Road, Daryaganj, Delhi – 110002, India

79 Anson Road, #06–04/06, Singapore 079906

Cambridge University Press is part of the University of Cambridge.

It furthers the University's mission by disseminating knowledge
in the pursuit of education, learning, and research at the highest
international levels of excellence.

www.cambridge.org
Information on this title: www.cambridge.org/9781107042056
10.1017/9781107323704

© Juan M. Pascual 2017

First published 2017

Printed in the United Kingdom by Clays, St Ives plc.

A catalogue record for this publication is available from the British Library.

Library of Congress Cataloging in-Publication Data
Names: Pascual, Juan M., author.
Title: Progressive brain disorders in childhood / Juan Pascual.
Description: Cambridge, United Kingdom ; New York, NY : University
Printing House, 2017. | Includes bibliographical references and index.
Identifiers: LCCN 2016047642| ISBN 9781107042056 (hardback : alk. paper) |
ISBN 9781107686106 (pbk. : alk. paper)
Subjects: | MESH: Brain Diseases | Child
Classification: LCC RJ496.B7 | NLM WS 340 | DDC 618.928–dc23 LC record
available at https://lccn.loc.gov/2016047642

ISBN 978-1-107-04205-6 Hardback

To Albertina and Albertina Manuela

The human understanding from its own peculiar nature willingly supposes a greater order and regularity in things than it finds, and though there are many things in nature which are unique and full of disparities, it invents parallels and correspondences and non-existing connections.

Francis Bacon, The New Organon Or True Directions Concerning The Interpretation Of Nature, Aphorism XLV (2000), p. 42. Cambridge University Press, Cambridge, UK.

Contents

ix

Preface

Neurobiology and the practice of neurology have reached overlap and interdependence. Yet, the bounds of neuroscience are broader, providing neurologists with an ever-growing variety of concepts and techniques. Whereas clinical neurology is an applied science, neuroscience is tasked with the explanation of phenomena that span many orders of magnitude: from cells to nervous systems and their interactions with the environment. This awesome diversity accounts for uneven scientific progress. How neural cells arise, work, and die is progressively better understood such that the next great scientific frontier is posited by the higher order question of what purpose do cells and ensembles of cells serve in the context of the brain and of the organism. In other words, *what* causes them to develop certain properties rather than others and *why* are they ultimately needed? Despite justified enthusiasm in many subfields of neurobiology, it seems that these and many other fundamental uncertainties still remain unmitigated. For example, in spite of the well-known importance of neural activation for perception and movement, why is most of the brain's metabolic activity carried out in disregard of external events? Or why do individual cerebral nuclei not adhere to a simple evolutionary plan to preserve the function of brain structures across all organisms that interact with the environment in similar fashion? Or why do neural stem cells grown under the appropriate conditions self-organize into brain organoids? We simply do not know. An unsettling perspective into these unknowns is that function (and biological purpose) comprises more than we can observe, thus remaining hidden. This too has repercussions in neurology: We set out to alleviate human disease, but still ignore much of what disease does to the complete organism, or even how most of the brain functions in a diseased state. We are thus limited to the observable, the commonly describable as seen with our tools and perspectives. Sometimes, as Wittgenstein noted, the brighter the light that is projected against an object, the longer the shadow that is cast.

This book teaches what can be observed in the course of the formidable interplay between brain disease and the developing individual. In the process, we will learn what can be treated, prevented, or at least anticipated. Physicians are compelled to treat affected individuals, but also to contribute new knowledge, ever mediating the obsolescence of their own scientific context. In the spirit of this principle, and in contrast with other texts, this book makes no attempt to fill explanatory gaps. To the contrary, voids in knowledge have been highlighted and presented as unmet opportunities for investigation. It is hoped that, at the very least, the identification of obscure areas should help researchers working on therapies devise strategies that circumvent obstacles for which investigation must be temporarily postponed. The book makes no emphasis on the historical developments of individual diseases, as I have found them generally uninformative for our purpose, and so I have focused solely on useful facts rather than on the uneven paths that led to them. References have been kept to a minimum. All cases described have been taken from the cited literature or from my clinic records without substantive modification.

This text has several limitations. First, the perceived dichotomy between mind and brain in health and disease is not within its scope, but I hope to remediate this deficiency in a future occasion. Second, it has not been possible to credit all relevant sources of information, which I hope other authors will patiently understand. Next, the book betrays my own deficiencies and areas of insufficient knowledge, but I will gladly try to rectify them if they are pointed out to me. In the interim, I will accept any allegations of conducting my own education in public, as Hegel accused Schelling of doing. Lastly, and unfortunately, the practice of diagnosing and caring for neurodegenerative disorders in young persons lacks excitement by today's societal standards. I lack the power to change this perception, which is prevalent even among physicians. Indeed, when considering the medical training and resources devoted to this endeavor it does seem that "out of the crooked timber of mankind few straight things are ever made."[1] Nevertheless, I hope that the plight of the many individuals afflicted by these diseases will become at least imaginable after reading the text.

A word on terminology: Common designations, such as "developmental delay" or "mental retardation," are implied or used by force of habit, but with some regret: A "delay" implies subsequent progress along a path, and perhaps eventual arrival, but disturbed development ("developmental delay") usually fails to arrive at the expected destination, or even to follow the normal path, just as it is usually unclear what is "retarded" in the mind of many disabled affected individuals. The term "plasticity" (another favorite) carries a beneficial connotation, but has also been used with caution here, as both adaptive and maladaptive phenomena can result from a "plastic" brain. I have also refrained from referring to "disease modifying" therapies to signify interventions that alter the overall course of a disorder because any treatment that changes any aspect of a disease is a modifier of such a disease. "Seizure disorders" have been referred to by the more economic word epilepsy. Casuistic, classifications, and diagnostic criteria have been restrained to a minimum in keeping with the frontispiece, as they rarely reflect the more complex reality. Common forms of a disease are termed as such or referred by the term canonical rather than "classic," as there is little "classicism" in the study of disorders that have been known for less than a century in most cases. In sum, the usage of words of ordinary language is given priority over clinicians' unnecessary tendency to change the use of terms that are established in common dictionaries.

I wish to thank my family for time lost and not regained in what at times seemed comparable to Sisyphus' task. My production team and editor at Cambridge University Press, Nick Dunton, have been all than an author can ask for and much more. My colleagues have shared clinical demands while I was reading and writing. To them, I owe gratitude and much enlightenment. It is through discussions with them that my own ideas have taken shape. The two generations of affected individuals and families that I have cared for constitute the essence and fabric of this book. Their resilience and loyalty to the selfless cause of scientific understanding for its own sake is a testimony to the heights of the human condition.

---

[1] Immanuel Kant, *Toward Perpetual Peace and Other Writings on Politics, Peace, and History*, p. 9. Yale University Press, New Haven, USA, 2006.

Introduction

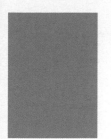

Introduction

Principles of Progressive Brain Disorders in Childhood

Throughout this book, emphasis is made on principles. Several of them are described here.

The Role of Genomics in Neurological Practice. Imminent changes in the approach to disease genomics will simplify the identification of affected individuals and strengthen the observational and mechanistic perspectives adopted in this book. Rather than rendering observation and clinical understanding irrelevant or obsolete, detailed genomic information complements the approach to neurological disorders by circumscribing the origin of disease to specific abnormal protein function. Further, comprehending the impact of mutations on the organism will always rely on empirical description and experimentation. Diagnosing will be greatly simplified for both typical and atypical affected individuals when their complete genome is analyzed as a matter of routine, rendering many ancillary procedures irrelevant. Diseases will thus be identified with increasing accuracy, but most of them will continue to be confronted with insufficient treatments. Therefore, observational and mechanistic research can only be expected to flourish.

Variable Expression of Later-onset Childhood Neurodegenerative Disorders. That late-manifesting diseases deviate from stereotypic forms of presentation is puzzling, especially for canonical single-gene defects for which early (infantile or juvenile) disease forms are well characterized. In general, late-onset disease forms are much more variable in manifestations and also milder in clinical course. It seems reasonable to assume that one gene should impair one biological process and that this should lead to only one form of disease. Yet, the phenomenon of late-onset disease variability may relate to the uncovering, by the primary disease process, of otherwise sub- or pre-clinical forms of dysfunction that differ from the primary disease and which become manifest in conjunction with it. According to this contention, a late-onset disease-causing mutation may have a permissive effect on latent pathology that manifests variably as it unfolds in later life. By extension, this may also account for the early-onset single-gene diseases that are associated with different phenotypes.

Primary and Secondary Injury. That all or much of a phenotype may be due to pathological processes far removed from the original causal defect seems to stand to reason. This may account for the existence of common final pathways of disease, in which two or more primary pathological processes converge into a shared set of biological events. These ultimate events may supplant the original disease mechanism and give rise to most of the observable clinical and biological abnormalities. For example, mutations in disparate, biologically unrelated genes may converge into the same type of abnormality by impairing a single cell structure. This, however, should not uncritically lead to the elevation of the secondary process to the status of centrality. The fact that vulnerable nodes occur in all biological systems does not necessarily imply that these nodes are targets for disease amelioration or reversal, for it is the primary process that may require remediation. In other words, some of the more eloquent nodes may be a source of epiphenomena rather than reporters of central pathogenesis.

Patterns of Neural Regression. Whereas the phenomenology of normal neural development and behavior is relatively well understood, much less is known about the behavioral neurology of neurodegenerative deterioration in children. This is compounded by the naturally evolving set of powers of the developing brain, which are impacted in both unknown global and selective ways by progressive diseases. It is not known whether the familiar diseases that primarily involve neural circuits in the adult operate similarly in the child because the nature and function of such circuits in development remains underinvestigated.

Table 1.1 Patterns and stages of neurobehavioral degradation in childhood

	Intellectual deterioration	Combined intellectual and motor deterioration
Early	Language decline	Extrapyramidal manifestations and language decline
Intermediate	Loss of individuation	Loss of ambulation and individuation
Advanced	Passivity	Inability to sit and indifference

In contrast with the adult, and regardless of disease mechanism, there are two main observable patterns of deterioration in children: a mostly intellectual pattern of decline and a combined motor and intellectual pattern of degeneration.

For unknown reasons, sensory system degeneration, while biologically observable, is largely silent in children, such that it is the motor and intellectual behaviors that define the phenotype. In the intellectual pattern of deterioration, language is generally compromised and constitutes the first sign of disease. Self-awareness of intellectual deterioration is very rare in children, as are memory and comprehension complaints. A second stage of intellectual deterioration is characterized by the loss of individual awareness. The child's aspirations, self-preservation tendencies, and self-consciousness are lost in this phase. Lastly, a third stage is characterized by impassivity to the external and internal environment. In the combined motor and intellectual pattern of deterioration, extrapyramidal manifestations (principally ataxia and dystonia) are usually more disabling than pyramidal tract dysfunction. Motor deterioration proceeds on par with intellectual decline, giving the appearance of global encephalopathy. Later, loss of ambulation tends to coincide with loss of self-individuation. In a third phase, the inability to sit is accompanied by indifference to the environment. In contrast with the adult, the ill child is less prone to reflect on his or her own mortality despite the capacity to do so when confronted with others' illnesses.

Localization in Neurodegenerative Neurology. The developing brain is much less specialized regionally and functionally than the adult nervous system. In children, the extent or size of an injury is more important than its location (Figure 1.1). Therefore, there are usually few practical gains from attempting to localize lesions or pathological processes. Even highly circumscribed lesions such as focal strokes tend to be silent or cause defects that would be unexpected in an adult. Many acquired focal lesions recover rapidly and leave no sequelae. Similarly, the ability to predict later life residual deficits is very limited. The main predictor of future neural performance is the size of residual unaffected brain volume rather than site of injury or neural circuit affected. Similar observations were made by Soviet scientists on adult soldiers who suffered two sequential brain injuries: Whereas the clinical consequences of the first injury could be predicted on a functional anatomical basis, impairment due to the second injury depended not on its location but on its size.

Infections, Injuries, Immunizations, and Other Potential Precipitant Factors. Many childhood degenerative disorders follow or temporally associate with seemingly unrelated injuries or otherwise inconsequential pathological processes. For example, Leigh syndrome often manifests some time after a trivial respiratory or gastrointestinal infant illness. This has given rise to debate, as the causal role of several common interventions such as vaccinations has been called into question in relation to numerous severe neurological disorders. The source of this argument against causation is rooted in a particularly strict conception of the notion of causation in which a cause must always act via a known all-or-nothing mechanism. However, it seems likely that a single – and otherwise innocent – event could set in motion a dormant disease mechanism when acting at the appropriate time, and that the absence or prevention of such an event would allow the pathological mechanism to remain quiescent or unprovoked. If this counterfactual argument is accepted, there seems to be little reason to negate causation. In this paradigm, causation is a probabilistic – rather than a mechanistic – event acting through unclear mechanisms, and one that is not well reflected in the law or in common medical practice. The debate will thus likely continue.

Early Diagnosis and Early Treatment. A common argument is that early treatment of a severe disease

5

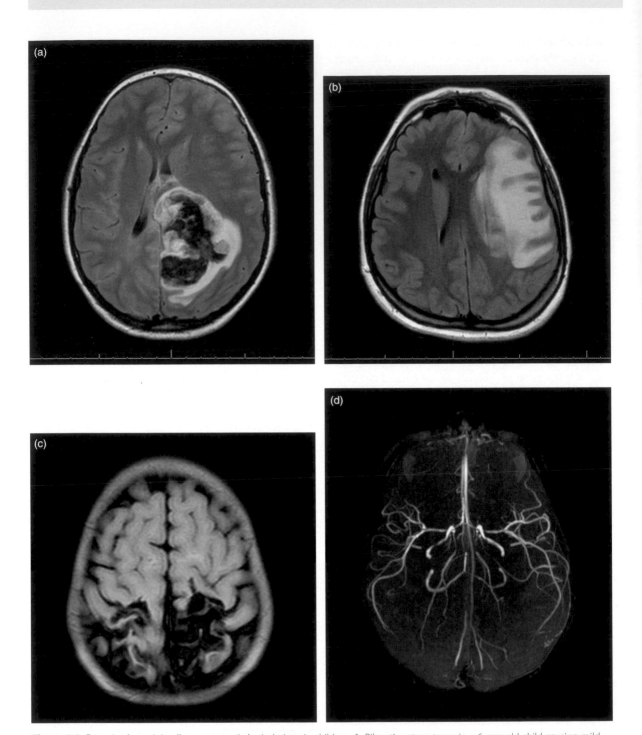

Figure 1.1 Extensive but minimally symptomatic brain lesions in children. A. Pilocytic astrocytoma in a 6-year-old child causing mild headaches. B. Tumefactive multiple sclerosis in an 11-year-old girl associated with right finger numbness. C. Chronic ischemic injury to the hemispheres in a 4-year-old leading to mild leg spasticity. D. Magnetic resonance angiography of the case in C. Severe stenosis of the arteries that irrigate the cerebral hemispheres is noted in the context of widespread cerebral circulatory failure. There is reduced flow through the supraclinoid internal carotid and vertebrobasilar arteries. The superior portion of the basilar artery and the proximal posterior cerebral arteries exhibit particularly reduced flow.

should lead to better outcomes or even to reversal of disease manifestations in contrast with treatments administered in more advanced disease stages. This notion, however, is clouded by the assumption that most treatments modify fundamental disease biological aspects. The reality is that therapy for neurological disorders is often far removed from primary pathological events. If a treatment addresses a secondary (in terms of importance) biological abnormality or a disease manifestation that results from the uncovering of an unrelated premorbid pathological state, then time to treatment may afford little impact on disease course. Given the current widespread uncertainties about what constitute primary and secondary events in the vast majority of neurological disorders, it seems unlikely that early treatments obligatorily afford superior benefit to delayed forms of therapy.

Tolerability of Severe Mutations. Man is prone to deleterious mutations. In a significant fraction of cases, individuals affected by a canonical, well-known disease harbor two or more mutations in unrelated genes, one or more of which may remain silent as a disease modifier. Analogously, some so-called obligatory disease-causing mutations occur in normal subjects. The simplest interpretation of these paradoxes resides in the concept of gene. A functioning gene extends beyond the self-replicating DNA structure that specifies the genetic code to include regulatory elements of genomic and non-genomic nature. This principle was advanced in the mid-twentieth century, when the structure of DNA and the mechanism of inheritance were unknown. Thus, a pathogenic mutation may be viewed as a necessary – but not always sufficient – prerequisite for the expression of a phenotype. The role of the environment, understood as the exposure to the cell's external and internal milieu also needs to be called into question, since most cells of all organisms are exposed to a strictly controlled environment that varies little with lifestyle and other extrinsic factors. It is thus possible that higher order properties that emerge from simpler biological processes such as mutations account for causation and pathogenesis as observed in medical practice.

Evidence-based Medicine and Other Statistical Constructs. The foundational documents of the evidence-based current state that one advantage of this new approach to medicine is that therapeutic interventions can be effectively assessed with little regard for underlying pathophysiological mechanisms. Today, the practice of evidence medicine constitutes a form of reductionist phenomenology devoid of mechanistic insight. In its extreme form, it is a reincarnation of the trial-and-error approach to therapeutic development validated by statistical reasoning. The value of such conceptual construct in neurodegenerative disorders is very limited – if not outright misleading – for several reasons: First, the relative rarity of these diseases render them statistically intractable. Second, important individual variations can be negated by lumping together several disorders with a similar phenotype – such as autistic spectrum disorders – with the intent of achieving a sufficient sample size at the expense of disregarding crucial biological differences. Third, evidence-based medicine assigns a quantitative evidence value to qualitative outcomes that are not easily amenable to numeric ordering. Fourth, this approach is oblivious to individual innovation and therapeutic experimentation, which is how many treatments have been developed.

The chapters that follow have been structured to first provide an overview of normal neurological development as it relates to illness and deterioration. A discussion of the main forms of neurodegenerative mechanisms follows. Next, individual neurodegenerative diseases have been divided by age of onset, understanding that such boundaries are largely arbitrary. Lastly, the phenomenon of regression and behavioral deterioration is analyzed for several non-degenerative conditions, many of which are amenable to effective treatment. The book has been written for continuous reading. However, individual chapters are self-contained and can be read separately. Clinical case reports and text boxes summarizing the main disease features are provided in many cases to facilitate retention of the material. When possible, clinical histories have been given precedence over ancillary diagnostic methods. As reflected in the cases described in the text, today much of the medical literature containing the most thorough medical histories and clinical insights emerges from underdeveloped countries where ancillary investigations are often relegated to a confirmatory role or rendered superfluous by clinical acumen. I try to follow that paradigm in my own medical practice.

Rise and Decline of the Child

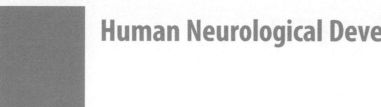

Human Neurological Development

Chapter 2

The Developing Child

Neural and psychologic development allows the child to receive, assimilate, recall, and integrate information during development, and to use that information to adapt to the environment within the constraints of his organism. This definition of psychological growth permits a descriptive outline of the organism's functional maturation, including changes in reflex ability, elaboration of motor activity, development of the special senses, and ultimately achievement of cognition and highly organized behavior. Tests have been devised to relate observed behavior to cognitive abilities. The use of such tests in the evaluation of human intelligence has historic respectability, although the elements that define cognition cannot be easily separated from those that comprise behavior. Numerous normative tables of postnatal motor, sensory, and behavioral milestones have been constructed for human development. A normal from a grossly abnormal performance can be distinguished with ease, but smaller deviations from normal are seldom appreciated in infancy. In fact, many such tables list the average age at which a given function develops but fail to provide the range of normal. In most instances tables have been constructed from a population that is homogeneous with regard to ethnic and socioeconomic background. Even in a homogeneous population, however, there is variation in the development of specific functions, whether simple reflexes or complex behavior.

Even the simplest behaviors manifest a strong developmental dependence. Initially, the fetus responds to reflex stimuli with whole body movements. Only later in gestation, with neurologic maturation, do movements of a single extremity appear or opening and closing of the mouth occur. Reflex movement away from a stimulus precedes movement toward the same stimulus. Thus, avoidance and withdrawal predominate, whereas movements directed toward a stimulus, such as those that occur in the rooting response, develop later. Only gross insults during gestation disrupt the maturation of reflex patterns so that an examination at birth is frequently an unreliable indicator of neurological disease. A general depression of reflexes and of all neural activity or seizures commonly reflects such insults sustained in the perinatal period, and these, too, are not necessarily good prognosticators of future development. Mild forms of perinatal insult disturb the neonatal examination little if at all.

There is significant developmental variability in infancy. For example, some normal infants maintain fragments of tonic neck responses for 6 months after birth, while in others the response disappears within the first months of life. The range of response is even greater for the crossed adductor response, which does not disappear in some normal infants until after 12 months of life. Similarly, the development of certain reflexes evolves over a period of time. For example, the neck righting reflex develops within the first month of life in some, but is not present in all infants until the tenth month of life. The parachute response appears between 5 and 12 months of age in normal infants. When considering the onset of more complicated functions (for example those included in the Denver scale), including the development of language, the discrepancies among normal children become even greater. Some normal children are able to combine two words by 18 months of age, whereas others fail to speak until 36 to 48 months of age. This makes it unreliable to evaluate the effects of an insult on normal development by evaluating single functions.

Retardation of all milestones over a sustained period of time is more reliable when diagnosing a developmental abnormality.

Neonatal insults must be extremely severe to effect delays in the achievement of the diverse developmental milestones that are apparent during the first month of life. For example, even hydranencephalic children (without cerebral hemispheres) may escape detection on casual neurologic examination, although careful scrutiny will usually detect deviations from normal, especially in visual responses. Most insults sustained early in life are, in contrast, usually mild and are unlikely to cause noticeable abnormalities in simple reflex, sensory, and motor functions early in life. Cognitive and complex behavioral dysfunction can only be evaluated fully in more mature life, often years after the cessation of the injury. Further, abnormal neurologic findings during the first three postnatal days might not be representative of the entire neonatal period. In addition, the infant's overall state of reactivity is difficult to reliably evaluate during the first week following birth. Sleep and feeding are also important factors. After awakening, the latency of infant responses gradually decreases until a maximum speed is achieved 40 minutes later. After eating, the speed of reaction diminishes progressively during the ensuing 60 minutes.

The variability of intelligence with age is well known. Psychomotor examination of children from 1 month to 18 years of age has revealed the lack of predictability of infantile developmental or intelligence quotients (IQ) under 2 years of age. When children are reexamined at 8 years of age, only one-fifth maintain any constancy in IQ. Scores on infant intelligence scales cannot be generalized beyond the items tested. Studies on developmental changes in mental performance in children from 2 to 17 years of age have found a lack of stability in serial testing after 2 years of age. One child in seven will display changes of greater than 40 IQ points when using the revised Stanford–Binet Intelligence Scale. Parental aspirations and discipline appear to be of greater importance than other internal or external variables.

In contrast with IQ measurements, the reliability of a clinical examination in estimating future development ment has been recognized. Particularly when conducted after 20 weeks of age, such appraisals correlate well with later intelligence scores. Predictions improve when test scores are combined with a pediatrician's rating, evaluations of social quotient, a perinatal stress evaluation, and an evaluation of parental socioeconomic status. Even in earliest infancy, it is necessary to separate motor from psychic development, such that a lack of predictability in many studies is based on an overemphasis of motor skills, which may not be adequate predictors of later intellectual function in less severely impaired infants.

The ability to enhance specific activities of an infant by positive reinforcement suggests that infants even in the neonatal period are capable of learning. Infants as young as 2 months of age increase motor activity in order to manipulate visual stimulation offered to them. Crying during neonatal life seems to be related to maternal responses as well as instinctive needs. The broad contact stimulation that occurs with cuddling may be a physiologic determinant in reducing crying in the infant. Rapid cessation of crying even in the hydranencephalic child can be achieved in this manner. Even within the same family, the evaluation of early developmental milestones may be influenced by factors that would appear to have no influence on cognitive development. For example, within the same family, the use of sentences occurs earlier in firstborn children and in girls than in boys. Children of lower socioeconomic status tend to walk earlier than those of the upper classes. It would appear, then, that there are significant cultural, socioeconomic, and sexual influences on early motor development.

Chapter 3

Language Development

Symbolic language is a unique human attribute that profoundly influences man's capacity to understand and solve problems. Stages in the development of language begin with the earliest sounds: fussing, crying, and cooing. The second stage is babbling, which often involves sounds not present in the English phonemic system as well as the reduplication of sounds. Because babbling occurs in deaf children, it is not simply imitation, but rather a product of intrinsic cerebral development that is reinforced with age and experience. It bears no phonologic or grammatical relation to later patterns that are determined by environmental contact. After babbling comes a stage of single words, initially imitative with little conception of meaning, but later with an enlarging vocabulary characterized by increased precision in the meaning of each word. After this comes a stage of word combinations and finally one characterized by syntax, in which whole sentences can be constructed with a concept of the relationship between the parts. Babbling in language development is associated with pleasurable reinforcement as a learning process in which the infant begins to link different sensory impressions with motor control.

The elaboration of language, including vocabulary size, the precision of meaning, and the use of syntax, is heavily dependent on cultural determinants. The demands made for verbal precision at home and at school heavily influence the development of language in the infant and child. Language is the most important mechanism by which a culture is transmitted. One can transmit the use of simple skills without the use of language, but to propagate the technology and abstractions on which our society depends requires the use of verbal symbols. Historic information can thus be understood relatively rapidly by the ability to appreciate the experience of others through the use of the spoken or written word. The development of language results in a fundamental discontinuity between the human and other mammalian species. With maturation, language becomes one, if not the principal, tool by which man learns and is tested. Thus, the ability to use language becomes increasingly important in the evaluation of intelligence. Therefore, when evaluating the implications of intelligence testing in man, one must take into consideration many factors that influence the ability to use language, including race, socioeconomic background, family structure, culture, and relationship with the examiner.

Bibliography

Dodge P.R., Prensky A.L., Feigin R.D. (1975). *Nutrition and the Developing Nervous System*, Saint Louis: Mosby.

Assessment of Neural Performance

The Neurological Examination of Newborns, Infants, and Children

In the majority of cases, a complete history and neurological examination will correctly identify the diagnosis or at least the syndrome in the neurologically ill child.

Neurological History

The history is perhaps the most important component of the assessment. The history should identify in chronological order the onset and setting of the symptoms and a description of their frequency, duration, and impact on all aspects of the child's well-being. Most intellectually normal children older than 5 years can communicate much of their own history.

Following the completion of the chief complaint and history of the present illness it is important to start with a review of the pre-conception health of both parents and a history of the pregnancy. The events surrounding the delivery should be documented and include the place of birth, birth weight, length, and head circumference. The family history is also important. This information includes any early and unexpected death in first-degree relatives and any history of spontaneous abortion and the result of any autopsies or metabolic or genetic studies. The history should determine whether any relatives have been evaluated for neurological or psychiatric disorders and whether there are members of the family with unexplained but relevant health problems.

Neurological Examination

Evaluation of a child's language, social skills, and motor skills is also important. The physician should note the child's willingness to participate in the evaluation. Many younger children are more collaborative in their parent's laps or while playing. A brief mental status and cognitive function evaluation might be conducted in this context. Depending on the age and maturity of the child,

the completion of a puzzle, telling a story, or drawing a person may provide an estimate of cognitive capacity. The alertness level of a newborn depends on several factors, including environmental temperature, the time of the last feeding and the gestational age. Premature infants younger than 28 weeks of gestation do not consistently manifest periods of alertness, whereas gentle physical stimulation applied to the older infant arouses the child from sleep followed by a period of alertness. Sleep and waking patterns are well developed at term. When in doubt, sequential assessment of the infant is valuable in assessing neurological function.

The order in which the neurological examination is performed depends on the child's capacities and context. The infant head should be viewed from above. The newborn has two fontanelles: an anterior diamond-shaped fontanelle and a smaller posterior fontanelle. The size of the anterior fontanelle is approximately 2 × 2 cm at birth and the posterior fontanelle may fit the tip of a finger or is closed at birth. Closure of the anterior fontanelle is variable; the average age is 9 months, but it may not close until 18 months of age. The posterior fontanelle normally closes at 1 month of age. Auscultation of the cranium is an important part of the examination. Bruits are best identified over the anterior fontanelle, temporal region, or the orbits. Soft, symmetric bruits are usually normal under 4 years of age. Determination of the head circumference provides an indirect measure of brain growth. If the measurements are abnormal, the parents' head circumferences should be measured and compared.

Tactile reflexes are informative in young infants. These reflexes have a sensory afferent arc and motor efferent arc. Examples include the rooting reflex, Galant or trunk-incurvation reflex, abdominal reflex, grasp reflex, plantar response, and extension of the fingers with gentle dorsal hand stroking. The most important tactile reflexes of the newborn are the suck and swallow reflexes.

Olfactory reflexes in the neonate, using aromatic odors, elicit sucking or withdrawal responses except in sleep. Anosmia may be detected as early as 28 weeks' gestation. Examination of the optic disc and retina is an essential component of the neurological examination. Prior to the examination, a mydriatic agent can be instilled into the eye to dilate the pupils. The optic disc is gray-white in the newborn and blond child. The older child's optic disc is usually pink. Assessment of vision can be accomplished as early as 28 weeks of gestation when the normal premature will blink to a bright light and by 32 weeks of gestation, when eye closure is maintained until the light source is removed. At 37 weeks, a normal premature will turn the head and eyes to a light and by 40 weeks visual fixation and the ability to follow a light or the examiner's face is well developed. Optokinetic nystagmus, tested by a rotating drum or a strip of cloth with broad vertical stripes slowly drawn horizontally in front of the eyes, is present in the alert term newborn and young infant. Visual acuity in term infants is in the range of 20/150 and reaches 20/20 by approximately 6 months of age. The pupils react normally to light by 30–32 weeks of gestation. Full ocular movements may be noted as early as 25 weeks of gestation using the doll's eye maneuver. Premature infants may display mild disconjugate eye movements at rest, with one eye horizontally displaced from the other by 1–2 mm. The corneal response is elicited by lightly touching the cornea with a cotton applicator and observing the degree of eye closure compared to the opposite side. Motor function assessment of the trigeminal nerve consists of observing the masseter, pterygoid, and temporalis muscles during mastication and jaw movements as well as the jaw jerk. Trigeminal sensory function in the premature is best evaluated by stimulating each of the three zones of the face bilaterally and the inside of the nostril and noting asymmetrical grimacing of the face. Taste in the anterior two-thirds of the tongue is supplied by the facial nerve and may be tested in a cooperative child by placing sugar or saline solution on one side of the extended tongue. Screening for hearing loss is an important component of the neurological examination because discovery and treatment of hearing loss during the first 3 months of age is associated with a better prognosis. Normal infants

pause sucking briefly when a loud sound is presented to an ear. A normal infant will habituate to the sound after several rings, but neurologically abnormal infants do not habituate. In addition, a normal hearing infant older than 3 months of age will turn the head to the side of the stimulus. Vestibular function may be assessed by the caloric test. Approximately 5 mL of ice water is introduced into the auditory canal by syringe following examination of the tympanic membrane to ensure that it is intact. The glossopharyngeal nerve can be tested by the presence of a gag response when the posterior pharynx is stimulated. A unilateral lesion of the vagus causes weakness and asymmetry of the ipsilateral soft palate and a hoarse voice or cry due to paralysis of a vocal cord. Bilateral vocal cord paralysis may cause respiratory distress, regurgitation, and pooling of secretions with an immobile, low-lying soft palate. Visualization of the vocal cords is necessary to confirm the diagnosis. The accessory nerve innervates the sternocleidomastoid and trapezius muscles. These muscles may be tested by voluntary forceful rotation of the child's head and neck against the examiner's hand. Examination of the tongue includes its size, mobility, and shape.

Tone is evaluated by assessing the resistance to passive motion at an individual joint. A premature infant is normally hypotonic compared to the term infant. Tone in the premature and infant is measured by the scarf sign where the infant arm is gently pulled across the chest. If the elbow easily reaches beyond the opposite shoulder the child is likely hypotonic. Measurement of the popliteal angle is another reliable maneuver to assess tone. The lower extremity is passively flexed onto the abdomen and the leg extended at the knee. Normal infants have a popliteal angle of 80 degrees. Assessment of power in the newborn is less reliable than the older child. Shoulder girdle strength is determined by suspending the infant by the axilla. A weak child will slip through the examiner's hands. If an infant is unable to grasp the examiner's finger or a suitable object tightly, it is likely that weakness is present. Infants with decreased power in the lower extremities manifest diminished spontaneous movements in the legs and will not support their weight by placing their feet on the examining table when supported by the axilla. Muscle power is graded in the cooperative child as follows: 0, no contraction; 1, trace of contraction; 2, movement with gravity eliminated; 3, movement against gravity; 4, movement against gravity or resistance; 5, normal power. Grade 4 can be further subdivided.

A sensory examination can be difficult in a newborn because of unreproducible responses. With the older child looking away, the examiner touches the foot and then moves upward with cotton or painful stimulus. The normal child will look directly at the stimulated area and a cooperative child may accurately point to the area of stimulation.

Bibliography

Haslam R.H. (2013). Clinical neurological examination of infants and children. *Handb Clin Neurol*. 111:17–25.

Chapter 5

Neuropsychological Assessment of Children

Neuropsychological assessment, whose aim is the early identification of cognitive and behavioral dysfunction, is an important element of regular well-child visits and of the diagnostic evaluations of the child with a progressive neurological disorder. Several tools (neuropsychological tests and developmental assessment scales) are utilized depending on the age and competence of the child.

Intelligence tests for children evaluate skills that are essential to school performance. The Stanford–Binet test is based on verbal performance and covers the ages of two years to 23 years, providing a mental age and an intelligence quotient (IQ).

Wechsler intelligence scales, which are subdivided according to age, are a standard for the quantification of intellectual capacities. These scales consist of a series of standardized questions and answers that determine an individual's potential in different intellectual areas, such as level of information on general topics, interaction with the environment and capacity to solve every-day problems. The Wechsler preschool and primary scale of intelligence (WPPSI) is a version of the Wechsler scales for younger children that allows the assessment of the intelligence of children aged between four and six and a half years of age. It consists of six verbal and five performance subtests. Usually, the application of five subtests of each of the verbal and performance subscales suffices for a reliable analysis. This scale also allows gathering some information on how a child's behavior is organized. The Wechsler Intelligence Scale for Children-III (WISC-III) is the scale most widely used to assess the intelligence of children aged between 6 and 17 years. It provides scores for verbal and performance scales, as well as a full scale IQ score. It includes

different types of tasks, allowing for the observation of the child's strengths and weaknesses. Children with motor difficulty often are penalized in this test, and therefore it should not be used when such a deficit is observed. The WISC-III block design subtest aims at checking the capacity of analysis, synthesis, and planning of visuospatial coordinates and constructive praxis. Individuals are asked to reproduce drawings shown to them using multi-colored blocks. A limit time is established for each model.

When children cannot express themselves verbally, the Raven's progressive matrices and the Columbia mental maturity scale may be used. These tests assess general intelligence and estimate a child's general ability to reason independently of language. The aim of Raven's progressive matrices is to find out the relations between the figures and imagine which of them (of a total of eight) completes the system.

The Boston naming test is one of the most widely used tests to assess language. It is designed to measure object naming from line drawings. It is applied to children aged six years or older with difficulty understanding or producing words or written verbal material.

Other tests are also used, such as the verbal fluency test, comprehension tests (e.g., Token test), and several other text, written, and reading comprehension tests. Some assessments also include the following topics: speech organs, oral habits, and language development.

Bibliography

Costa D.I., Azambuja L.S., Portuguez M.W., Costa J.C. (2004). Neuropsychological assessment in children. *J Pediatr (Rio J)*. 80(2 Suppl):S111–16.

Maturation of the Electroencephalogram in Infancy

Electroencephalogram (EEG) recordings can provide valuable information from premature infants aged 25 weeks of gestation to young adults. This requires that recording conditions be adapted to different situations, not only of age but also of environment, asepsis, and child behavior. The two major determinants of EEG features are level of vigilance and age. Standard EEG examination includes spontaneous sleep until the age of 5 years and hyperventilation and intermittent light (photic) stimulation in older children. The temporal course of EEG changes parallels brain maturation. These EEG changes are particularly rapid in early age and involve both temporal and spatial organization. In premature babies, EEG changes are noticeable approximately every 2 weeks; in infancy every month; and in childhood every year, before reaching the relatively invariant adult pattern between 8 and 12 years of age.

There are three stages of vigilance: awake, active sleep (AS) (precursor of rapid eye movements (REM) in the older child), and quiet sleep (QS) (precursor of slow wave sleep (SWS)). The newborn falls asleep in AS and this persists until the age of 2 to 3 months, REM sleep reaches 50 percent of total sleep, whereas for the adult it is only 20 percent. Each sleep stage lasts around 20 minutes.

Following the first 3 weeks of life, the neonatal EEG organization is replaced by a spatial–temporal organization that is specific to infancy and early childhood: nycthemeral organization changes, with increasingly longer periods of daytime wakefulness and nocturnal sleep such that naps decrease in number and duration. The diffuse, low amplitude theta activity that is characteristic of the infant at birth is replaced by a more regular theta activity, the frequency of which increases from 4 Hz at 3 months to 5 Hz by 5 months and 6–7 Hz by the end of the first year of life. These rhythms that precede the occipital alpha rhythm initially involve centro-

occipital then occipital areas. A visual arrest reaction exists from 3 months of age post term. In infancy and early childhood there is an intermediary stage between wakefulness and the first stage of slow sleep (SS), which is called somnolence; this stage is characterized by hypnagogic hypersynchrony of the background: high-amplitude slow waves (3–4 Hz) that are diffuse and rhythmic with centro-parietal predominance. This pattern is nearly constant between 8 and 12 months in the normal child. The organization of sleep comprises the following stages: a) disappearance of the trace alternant of QS by 3 weeks post term, which is replaced by polymorphous 1 Hz delta waves; b) appearance of sleep spindles by 6 weeks; c) vertex spikes and K complexes characteristic of stage II SS appear by 5–6 months; d) the amount of time spent in the AS stage of sleep decreases from 50 percent at birth to 30 percent by 1 year of age.

From the age of 5 months onwards, the tracing at awakening is comparable to that of somnolence with diffuse hypersynchrony of the background activity.

The normal EEG between 12 and 36 months is characterized by an awake occipital rhythm that increases from rapid theta to low alpha frequency (6–7 Hz in the 2nd year of life, 7–9 Hz in the 3rd year), allowing for significant interindividual variability. Theta rhythms are frequent at that age and diffusely distributed. During somnolence, hypnagogic hypersynchrony while falling asleep decreases progressively from 75 percent between 1 and 2 years to 57 percent between 2 and 3 years. Other patterns may be present during drowsiness, particularly the anterior theta aspect that consists of monomorphous fronto-central rhythms of variable duration (which is present in about 10 percent of children). Bursts of theta slow waves and spikes are frequent upon falling asleep.

The normal EEG from 3 to 5 years of age is characterized by further changes. During wakefulness, the occipital background activity exhibits rising frequency in the alpha band (8–9 Hz), but usually remains intermingled with theta or even delta (1.5–4 Hz) activities that also involve posterior areas. During somnolence, hypnagogic hypersynchrony disappears progressively from 3 years of age. It is replaced by anterior rhythmic high-amplitude theta activity that is rarely mixed with bursts of sharp waves. In sleep, stages I–II are still characterized by high-amplitude vertex spikes or sharp waves and spindles. The occipital predominance of delta slow waves of SS disappears progressively. Stages III and IV of SS, which are characterized by an increasing abundance of delta slow waves, can be seen from 3 years of age. K complexes can be identified that predominate at the vertex, which appear spontaneously or are triggered by auditory stimulation. Awakening reactions are similar to those typical of the younger child.

Between 6 and 12 years, the awake EEG is characterized by an occipital alpha rhythm with increasing frequency, reaching around 11 Hz by 10–11 years of age. Theta rhythms are still present in the occipital areas, reacting to opening of the eyes as does the alpha rhythm, but tend to decrease from the age of 12 years. During sleep, spindle bursts do not last for more than 1 second, their topography evolving from central to frontal areas. In K complexes vertex spikes are intermingled with the spindles. REM sleep comprises low amplitude and desynchronized activity, consisting of theta, alpha, and beta rhythms. Awakening is characterized by a more rapid transition from sleep to wakefulness and a progressive decrease in duration and amplitude of theta waves.

There is little modification from 13 to 20 years. The occipital alpha rhythm continues to have a mean frequency of 10 Hz but with a lower amplitude than at a younger age. Asymmetry of the amplitude never exceeds 20 percent, in favor of the nondominant hemisphere. The slow posterior component decreases in adolescence. Rapid rhythms may be seen in frontal areas. Hyperventilation modifies the tracing in less than 20 percent of cases. Photic driving may be present for rapid frequencies (6–20 Hz). Transition between wakefulness and sleep stage I is, as in adults, characterized by a diffuse desynchronization of the background activity.

Bibliography

Plouin P., Kaminska A., Moutard M.L., Soufflet C. (2013). Developmental aspects of normal EEG. *Handb Clin Neurol.* 111:79–85.

Magnetic Resonance Imaging of the Developing Brain

Magnetic Resonance (MR) imaging is an important diagnostic modality in neurology. As a consequence of the superior contrast resolution of MR imaging, computerized tomography scanning has been largely replaced, except for the visualization of bone structures and brain calcifications that are not well detected by MR imaging or for the emergency setting.

MR Imaging Changes During Brain Development

The infant's age must be taken into account because myelination exhibits a different appearance at various stages of development, especially during the first year of life.

At term (40 weeks), myelination appears hyperintense on sagittal T1-weighted images. The anterior part of the pons is still poorly myelinated. The corpus callosum is still thin and also little myelinated. From the basal ganglia, myelinated white matter tracts can be followed toward the rolandic sulci.

Two weeks after birth at term, on T1-weighted images, myelination is seen in the medulla oblongata, middle cerebellar peduncle, tegmentum pontis, inferior colliculus, decussation of the superior cerebellar peduncles, optic tracts, posterior limb of the internal capsule and ascending tracts toward the rolandic sulci. On T2-weighted images, the tegmentum pontis and mesencephalon appear darker than the ventral pons. Myelin can also be seen in the superior vermis, posterior limb of the internal capsule, basal ganglia, and ascending tracts into the rolandic sulci.

At 2 months, in the posterior fossa, T2-weighted images show that cerebellar myelination has progressed. The bright ring around the dentate nucleus has disappeared, but the peripheral white matter of the cerebellum is still bright. There is still a difference in signal intensity between the basis pontis and the tegmentum pontis. In the mesencephalon, the pyramidal tracts and decussation of the superior cerebellar peduncles can readily be seen.

At 3 months, the myelinated structures can easily be identified on T1-weighted images. The optic tract is well myelinated, as is the optic radiation. The posterior limb of the internal capsule is fully myelinated. Myelin has now spread to the precentral gyrus and will advance dorsally and ventrally to the occipital, frontal, and, finally, the temporal lobes.

At 4 months of age, on T2-weighted series, the pons basis and tegmentum display low signal, as do the middle cerebellar peduncles. The white matter of the cerebellum is well myelinated. At the level of the mesencephalon, the decussation of the superior cerebellar peduncles, the inferior colliculus, the pyramidal tracts and the optic tract display low signal. The posterior limb of the internal capsule also appears dark. A difference is visible between the poorly myelinated white matter in the frontal and temporal regions and the occipital and parietal region, where full myelination has started.

At 5–6 months of age, the genu of the corpus callosum starts to myelinate intensely. On T1-weighted images myelination will soon appear to be complete. At this stage, T2-weighted images provide the most information about maturation of the brain.

At 7–8 months of age, on T2-weighted images, the central parts of the brain are now well myelinated, including the genu of the corpus callosum.

At 12–13 months of age, the adult pattern is visible in all cerebral lobes except the temporal lobe, which is the latest to complete myelination. The T2-weighted series shows that the spread of myelin into the arcuate fibers is still not complete. Completion of myelination on T2 is demonstrable at the end of the 2nd year except for the temporal lobe, which completes myelination at about 4.5 years of age.

Magnetic Resonance Spectroscopy

Proton magnetic resonance spectroscopy, generally known as MR spectroscopy, uses the magnetic properties of protons to interrogate brain metabolism. The protons that contribute to the spectral signal include those present in water, lipids, N-acetylaspartate (NAA), creatine (Cr), choline (Cho), lactic acid and several amino acids. Additional metabolites that can be isolated using special techniques include myoinositol, glutamate, and glutamine. Thus, it is possible to routinely detect the spectral peak that represents the N-acetyl methyl resonance of NAA at 2.02 ppm, the methyl and the methylene resonance of Cr, including free creatine and phosphocreatine, at 3.02 ppm and 3.93 ppm, respectively, and the methyl resonances of choline-containing compounds (Cho) at 3.22 ppm. When techniques using short echo times (15–30 ms) are used, a considerably increased number of resonances with short T2 relaxation times can be visualized. Most obvious is a signal from multiple collapsed resonances of myoinositol at 3.56 ppm. A complex pattern of coupled resonances between 2.1 and 2.5 ppm together with a further group of resonances around 3.8 ppm arise from glutamine and glutamate. The resonances of γ-aminobutyric acid (GABA) overlap with the greater resonances of Cr, glutamate, and NAA. Pyruvate is below the level of detection under normal circumstances but, when elevated, it gives rise to a peak at 2.36 ppm. In case of elevated tissue levels of free lipids, for instance as a result of myelin breakdown or spectral contamination by fat from the skull, broad resonances are seen at 0.9 and 1.3 ppm.

In the mature brain NAA is almost entirely confined to neurons and their axons. NAA is considered to be a neuron and axon-specific marker. In certain diseases, the NAA resonance is diminished, probably signifying neuronal or axonal dysfunction or loss. The Cr peak represents the total amount of creatine and phosphocreatine. Total creatine remains constant under many conditions. For this reason, Cr may be used as internal reference for quantification. Cr is only present intracellularly; therefore, Cr has also been considered a marker for cellular density. A decrease of the creatine peak is seen in creatine metabolism disorders including biosynthetic and cerebral transport defects. Elevated Cho is typical of conditions of high cell density and enhanced membrane turnover, such as brain growth, myelination, demyelination, inflammation and tumor growth. Lactate is usually undetectable in the normal brain. Lactate levels are increased under conditions of enhanced anaerobic glycolysis such as respiratory chain defects, seizures, and ischemia. Elevated lactate may also be characteristic of disorders with increased numbers of macrophages, such as active demyelination and tissue necrosis.

Bibliography

Boddaert N., Brunelle F., Desguerre I. (2013). Clinical and imaging diagnosis for heredodegenerative diseases. *Handb Clin Neurol.* 111:63–78.

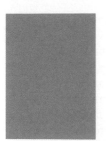

Death and Palliation in Neurodegenerative Disorders

The Declining Child

Neurodegenerative diseases are an important cause of progressive disability and death in childhood. With few exceptions, the ultimate outcome of children with these conditions has not improved in recent decades, whereas the time of death has been significantly postponed in most cases. These diseases represent a very diverse group with an extensive range of incapacitating neurological, neuromuscular, metabolic, and other clinical features. Their unifying features include the progressive and inexorable deterioration, the inevitability of early death and, in most cases, an inherited cause.

Communicating Death Expectations

In most of the degenerative disorders, only supportive care is possible from the time of diagnosis. This negative prospect is usually soon realized by the child's parents. Both the terminal phase of the disease and bereavement start at the time that the inevitability of death is conveyed or noticed. Therefore, it is particularly important how the diagnosis of such conditions is communicated to parents. Even many years later, the time of diagnosis remains a vivid memory for most parents. Many can remain dissatisfied with the way the information was given to them. Most parents value being communicated the diagnosis as soon as possible in an open and sympathetic way. They also welcome early and appropriate information about the disease, its causes, and its progression. The provision of information about self-help groups can be beneficial. Many organizations provide contact, advice, and help over the months and years of illness that are to follow. Often, groups of families, with the prospect of many years of caring for their children, necessitate respite care and the support of children's hospices. The fact that a child has inherited a fatal condition as a result of abnormal genes from one or both parents predisposes some families to feelings of guilt and self-blame. This needs to be kept in mind when communicating the diagnosis and throughout the course of the illness.

Management of Manifestations

Neurodegenerative diseases are rare and, except in specialized centers, medical professionals in general practice or even specialist pediatricians may have little or no direct experience with them. Often, over time, the parents accumulate a great extent of technical knowledge. This can result in a situation when practitioners may be reluctant to venture an opinion on treatment, even when it is appropriate for them to do so. It should be taken into account that children with unusual diseases are also prone to common illnesses and require the same treatment.

Frequently, the assessment of the severity of symptoms in these children is difficult. Age and understanding of the child are always a factor and, in addition, many children suffer from brain damage or reduced intellect as a result of their disease. This shifts the emphasis to careful observation of the child and necessitates special attention to the opinions of the parents, who may be the only source of reliable information relevant to the presence or severity of problematic symptoms.

Pain occurs in some children with progressive neurodegenerative illnesses. It can be difficult to recognize and assess and should be evaluated and relieved as effectively as possible. Causes of pain include muscle spasms, reflux esophagitis, constipation, and joint pains, all of which require treatments appropriate to the cause. It is not often severe, and opioids are seldom required, though they should be used if necessary.

Epilepsy is common in these diseases and may have been a presenting symptom. Control of seizures in such children does not differ from that used in more conventional circumstances, with the use of usually one, or at the most, two anticonvulsants used at full dose rather than smaller doses of a larger number of drugs. Increasing the number of anticonvulsants can risk additional side effects and interactions without improving control. A paradoxical situation can occur where seizures diminish in frequency when the medication is gradually reduced.

The care of pressure areas is not usually a problem in childhood, but the combination of prolonged immobility, deformity, and severe illness which may be encountered in chronic progressive disease increases the risk of pressure wounds. The best management is to prevent their occurrence by strict nursing care. Regular turning, up to hourly, combined with care of the pressure areas can prevent wound formation.

Feeding and nutritional difficulties are particularly common in children with progressive degenerative conditions when they affect the neurological and neuromuscular mechanisms that are required for swallowing. Sometimes, feeding difficulties are simply a result of generalized weakness and consideration should be given to causes that may respond to acceptable treatment. In many children with fatal illnesses, feeding problems are not amenable to treatment. In such cases, realistic eating goals can be set for pleasure and comfort since nutritional goals aimed at the restoration or maintenance of health may be inappropriate. When the child retains the capacity to eat, frequent, small meals are preferred. Temperature, consistency, and flavor are important. Purees are usually easier to swallow than liquids. Nasogastric or nasoduodenal tube feeding is often regarded as distressing. Although this may be true in some cases, it is usually well tolerated by most children. While a nasogastric tube will enable fluids, food, and drugs to be given, it will not alleviate the problems that may be caused by excess secretions and may make them worse. Open or percutaneous gastrostomy techniques are available and should be considered with the family if tube feeding is likely to be necessary for a prolonged amount of time.

Problems with chest infections may become frequent and serious in the child with a neurodegenerative disorder. They are often the final cause of death for many children. Recurrent hospital admissions for treatment of pneumonia are common. Hypoventilation, especially at night, can cause headaches, nausea and drowsiness during the day and restlessness at night. Supplemental oxygen either just at night or during the day may relieve these symptoms.

Bibliography

Goldman A. (ed.) (1998). *Care of the Dying Child*, Oxford: Oxford University Press.

Mechanisms of Neurological Loss of Function

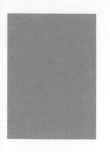

Degeneration in the Central Nervous System

Neural cells degenerate and die when they activate one or more of several mechanisms involved in cellular destruction. Only the most common mechanisms are discussed here.

Mechanisms of Neural Cell Death

Apoptosis

Programmed cell death is an important mechanism of cell loss in neurodegeneration and development. During the development of the nervous system, an excessive number of neurons is produced. This overproduction of neurons is followed by a programmed demise of approximately one half of the original cells. The precisely controlled process is referred to as naturally occurring neuronal death, which is a conserved cellular mechanism in diverse organisms, ranging from invertebrate species such as the nematode, *Caenorhabditis elegans*, and insects to nearly all of the studied vertebrate species. Natural neuronal death is believed to mold the nervous system's cellular structure and function.

Neuronal cells are eliminated by two major waves of programmed cell death, namely, the early death of proliferating precursors and young postmitotic neuroblasts, and the late death of postmitotic neurons. While the mechanism of the selective late death of postmitotic neurons is well explained by the competition among neurons for limiting amount of target-derived trophic factors (the neurotrophic theory), the regulation of the early wave of natural neuronal death is not well understood. There are suggestions that it is linked to cell cycle regulation and the removal of cells with irreparable DNA damage, or that it is regulated by factors such as bone morphogenetic proteins, Wnts (Wingless-related integration site proteins), fibroblast growth factors, and Sonic Hedgehog.

Apoptosis is characterized by cell shrinkage, chromatin condensation, DNA fragmentation, membrane blebbing, and the formation of apoptotic bodies that are rapidly phagocytosed by macrophages. Apoptosis is an energy-dependent process that requires ATP for protein synthesis and signal activation such as apoptosome formation and protein kinase-mediated phosphorylation reactions. An ATP threshold level is required for a cell to undergo apoptosis. When the depletion of ATP is severe, apoptotic cell death is replaced by necrosis.

Apoptosis may be triggered either by extrinsic stimuli through cell surface death receptors, such as TNFα (tumor necrosis factor-α), Fas (apoptosis stimulating fragment), and TRAIL (TNF-related apoptosis inducing ligand) receptors or by intrinsic stimuli via a mitochondrial signaling pathway. In either case, activation of cysteine aspartyl proteases, called caspases results in mitochondrial membrane permeabilization, chromatin condensation, and DNA fragmentation, thereby leading to the destruction of the cell. These events bestow the apoptotic cell a distinct and characteristic morphology that includes the rounding up of the cell so that it appears pyknotic, the condensation of chromatin, the fragmentation of the nucleus, and the shedding of apoptotic bodies, vacuoles containing cytoplasm, and intact organelles.

Necrosis

Necrosis is a nonphysiological, unregulated pathological form of cell death characterized by chromatin clumping and swelling of intracellular organelles in the early stages, and disintegration of cell organelles and membranes in the later stages. During necrosis, the outer cellular membrane is disrupted and the intracellular components are released into the intercellular space, resulting in an inflammatory response. Caspase cascades are not activated and the morphological characteristics of apoptosis are absent. Whereas necrosis is viewed as an accidental form of cell death, certain cells can adopt a programmed necrosis or necroptosis phenotype upon Fas ligand (FasL) or tumor necrosis factor (TNF) stimulation. In this instance, the kinase activity of receptor interacting protein 1 (RIP1), a protein that is recruited at the death inducing signaling complex (DISC) by death receptor activation, which normally is characteristic of apoptosis, mediates necrotic cell death. The function of RIP1 in cell necrosis has been confirmed in studies where the hyperactivation of poly (ADP-ribose) polymerase-1 (PARP-1) in mouse embryonic fibroblasts is mediated by RIP1, TNRF-associated factor 2 (TRAF2), and c-Jun N-terminal kinase (JNK) signaling. Activated JNK induced mitochondrial membrane potential change and release of apoptosis inducing factor that is associated with cell necrosis.

Necrotic death is typically followed by inflammatory reactions. Necrotic cells selectively release factors like HMGB1 (high-mobility group protein 1) and HDGF (hepatoma-derived growth factor) to evoke an inflammatory response and are sensed by NLRP3 (NACHT; NAIP, neuronal apoptosis inhibitor protein), C2TA (MHC class 2 transcription activator), HET-E (incompatibility locus protein from *Podospora anserina*) and TP1 (telomerase-associated protein), LRR (leucine-rich repeat) and PYD (pyrin domains-containing protein 3), a core protein of the inflammasome, resulting in inflammasome activation and the subsequent release of the pro-inflammatory cytokine IL (interleukin) 1β. NLRP3 inflammasome activation is triggered through ATP produced by mitochondria released from damaged cells.

Autophagy

Autophagy, in contrast with apoptosis and necrosis, is a caspase-independent form of cell death in which the cytoplasm is destroyed by lysosomal enzymes. Autophagy is an evolutionarily conserved mechanism that involves catabolic degradation of large protein complexes or intracellular organelles by lysosomes and thereby functions in the elimination of damaged organelles and in cell remodeling during development and differentiation. Autophagy was first described in yeast as a prosurvival mechanism because membrane lipids and proteins are recycled for mitochondrial ATP production when nutrients are reduced. Autophagy can mediate cell death during oxidative damage or starvation.

Autophagy represents a conserved lysosomal degradation pathway that sequesters and degrades cytoplasmic cargo. Autophagy is essential for the survival, differentiation, and development of eukaryotic organisms, and participates in host immunity and homeostatic maintenance. Three distinct autophagy mechanisms have been identified: macroautophagy, chaperone-mediated autophagy, and microautophagy. Macroautophagy (or simply autophagy) is the best characterized of these pathways and begins with the enclosure of a membranous crescent known as a phagophore around specific and non-specific cytoplasmic cargoes to form an autophagosome. In the canonical autophagy pathway, the outer membrane of the autophagosome then fuses with a lysosome to degrade its contents in an autolysosome.

Two ubiquitin-like conjugation systems conserved from yeast to mammals are required for the initiation of autophagy. The Atg (autophagy protein) 5–Atg12–Atg16L1 complex, coupled with microtubule-associated protein light chain 3 (LC3) complexes, is required for formation of the nascent autophagosome. Conjugation of these complexes to the autophagosome membrane helps recruit other autophagy proteins for the maturation of this compartment. Under basal conditions, LC3 is distributed diffusely in the cytoplasm. Upon the induction of autophagy, LC3 is modified, lipidated to LC3-II and localizes to both the inner and outer autophagosome membranes. In mammalian cells, LC3-II is found on mature autophagosomes and is used as one of the standard markers for autophagic activity.

Bibliography

Ghavami S., Shojaei S., Yeganeh B., et al (2014). Autophagy and apoptosis dysfunction in neurodegenerative disorders. *Prog Neurobiol.* 112:24–49.

Nikoletopoulou V., Markaki M., Palikaras K., Tavernarakis N. (2013). Crosstalk between apoptosis, necrosis and autophagy. *Biochim Biophys Acta.* 1833(12):3448–59.

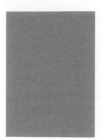

Axonal Degeneration

Mechanisms of Axonal Degeneration

Degeneration of the axon is an important step in the mechanism of degenerative neurological diseases. The axon represents the largest functional entity in many neuronal populations, spanning up to more than one meter in human motor neurons. Whereas dysfunction of the cell soma and its consecutive degeneration in the course of neurological disorders dominates neuropathology, axonal degeneration can also be an important pathological mechanism. Like apoptosis, most forms of axonal degeneration seem to be active self-destructing cellular processes involving a cascade comprising various molecular elements. Different forms of axonal degeneration have been described with regards to localization on the axon and temporal evolution. Although common molecular convergence points probably exist, mechanistic differences are found for each type of axonal degeneration. The most extensively studied form of axonal degeneration is the sequential degeneration following the traumatic lesion of an axon. This includes acute axonal degeneration in the vicinity of the lesion and Wallerian degeneration of the distal part of the axon. The study of axonal degeneration in chronic neurological diseases represents a greater challenge, as this process does not occur simultaneously in all axons of a certain tract and often proceeds over extended time periods.

Acute Axonal Degeneration

Acute axonal degeneration is a rapid axonal disintegration (within several hours) following a traumatic lesion in the central nervous system. It is confined to the adjacent 300–400 µm of the proximal and distal end of the axon and has been described in the spinal cord and the optic nerve. At first, for 10–30 min after a traumatic lesion, the axon remains stable with regard to its macroscopic morphological appearance. On the molecular level, however, a signaling cascade has already been activated, resulting in the fragmentation of the axon. It is initiated by rapid calcium influx into the axon and a consecutive transient rise of the axoplasmic calcium concentration within 40 s after lesion. Application of calcium channel inhibitors at the time of the lesion blocks this rise in cytosolic calcium and almost completely inhibits acute axonal degeneration. Calcium influx leads to an activation of the calcium-sensitive protease calpain, which reaches its maximum 30 min after the lesion. The first changes at the ultrastructural level become visible within the first 30 min after lesion and consist of the condensation and misalignment of neurofilaments followed by the fragmentation of microtubules. Both focal neurofilament compaction and microtubular proteolysis have been associated with calpain activation in other disease models and the ERK (extracellular signal–regulated kinases)/MAPK (mitogen-activated protein kinase) pathways have been suggested as molecular mediators. Therefore, the initial calpain activation might also be responsible for these early ultrastructural changes in acute axonal degeneration. Moreover, the rapid breakdown of the cytoskeleton probably leads to the early impairment of axonal transport. Signs in favor of this assumption are accumulations of organelles, mainly mitochondria and vacuoles, eventually leading to local axonal swellings that can be found early in axons undergoing acute axonal degeneration. Another characteristic ultrastructural feature of acute axonal degeneration is the local activation of autophagy. The number of autophagosomes in the axon significantly increases within the first 6 h after lesion. Pharmacological inhibition of autophagy attenuates acute axonal degeneration but this effect is not as pronounced as after calcium channel blockage. The latter not only inhibits acute axonal degeneration but also reduces autophagy, suggesting that autophagy is a downstream target of calcium influx.

Wallerian Degeneration

Wallerian degeneration is the degradation of axons distal to a lesion site. After a traumatic lesion, the parts of the axon that are not affected by acute axonal degeneration initially stay morphologically stable for the first 24 to 72 h. Then, the distal part of the axon undergoes a progressive fragmentation that resembles the fragmentation typical of acute axonal degeneration and that finally leads to a complete removal of the distal part of the axon. Wallerian degeneration proceeds directionally along the axon with a speed ranging from 0.4 mm/h in cultured primary neurons to 24 mm/h in the mouse sciatic nerve. In the peripheral nervous system, the direction of Wallerian degeneration depends on lesion type. Complete transection of the nerve leads to an anterograde fragmentation proceeding from proximal to distal, whereas a crush lesion results in retrograde fragmentation starting at the far distal end of the axon. Although macrophages and glia participate, especially in the final removal of the axon fragments, the mechanism of Wallerian degeneration seems to be intrinsic to the axon.

The molecular machinery underlying Wallerian degeneration is not well understood, although progress has been made with the help of the WldS mouse. In this mouse mutant, axon stumps distal to the lesion site survive ten times longer than axons in wild-type animals, while the survival of the neuronal cell body is not altered. The mutant protein WldS, which is responsible for the slowing of the degenerative process in WldS mice, is a chimeric gene product consisting of a fragment of the polyubiquitination factor UFD2a/UBE4b and the full-length nicotinamide mononucleotide adenylyltransferase-1 (NMNAT1). NMNAT1 is a key protein of the nicotinamide-adenine dinucleotide (NAD+) salvage pathway in mammals. UBE4b is an E4-type ubiquitin ligase that can add multiubiquitin chains to substrates of the ubiquitin-proteasome degradation pathway. The functionally most important molecular sites of WldS are the ATP-binding site and the NMN+ binding site of NMNAT1 and the valosin-containing protein (VCP)-binding site of UBE4b, as has been shown by knock-out experiments. Both a functional NMNAT1 and a functional UBE4b fragment are required for the neuroprotective action of WldS. This is suggested by the observation that, although disruption of the enzymatic activity of NMNAT1 in transgenic WldS mice results in a strongly reduced neuroprotective phenotype, overexpression of NMNAT1 alone is not sufficient to protect lesioned axons from degeneration in mammalian neurons. Moreover, NMNAT1 functions not only with enzymatic activity, but also as a chaperone.

Chronic Axonal Degeneration

The evolution of axonal degeneration in chronic neurodegenerative diseases is more difficult to study, owing to a limited availability of experimental manipulation procedures. However, various morphological forms of chronic axonal degeneration have been described. The principal type is termed dying back degeneration. This form of degeneration has been described in amyotrophic lateral sclerosis, Lewy body disease, spinocerebellar ataxia, peripheral neuropathies, and toxic neuropathies. It is initiated by a dysfunction of the synapse or a degeneration of the distal regions of the axon. This is followed by a degeneration of the whole axon in a distal-to-proximal direction, finally leading to a fragmentation of the axon morphologically resembling that of Wallerian degeneration. The biochemical mechanisms underlying this form of degeneration are not known, but synaptic pathology, mitochondrial dysfunction and disturbances of axonal transport probably participate. Dying back degeneration is similar to axonal pruning and axosome shedding, a process that is observed in the developmental maturation of the neuromuscular synapse or target selection, e.g., by retinal ganglion cell axons.

Bibliography

Lingor P., Koch J.C., Tönges L., Bähr M. (2012). Axonal degeneration as a therapeutic target in the CNS. *Cell Tissue Res.* 2012; 349(1):289–311.

Yan T., Feng Y., Zhai Q. (2010). Axon degeneration: Mechanisms and implications of a distinct program from cell death. *Neurochem Int.* 56(4):529–34.

Neurodegenerative and Other Progressive Disorders in Childhood

Progressive in Utero Disorders

Chapter 11

Prenatal Inborn Metabolic Errors

There are relatively few signs that indicate fetal neurodegeneration or regression. Among these, decreased fetal movements (usually compared by the mother to a previous normal pregnancy), intrauterine growth retardation and abnormal heart sounds are the most significant. Various techniques allow for the monitoring of only gross fetal development: ultrasonography may illustrate polyhydramnios and enlarged cerebral ventricles and magnetic resonance imaging can detect micro or macrocephaly and agenesis of the corpus callosum.

Progressive prenatal deterioration is often caused by inborn metabolic diseases. More than 700 inborn errors of metabolism are known. Inborn errors of metabolism are caused either by enzyme deficiencies leading to an increase of substrate and lack of product of the affected reaction or by deficiencies of transporters that result in the accumulation of substrates in certain intracellular compartments. As most of the potentially toxic intermediates that accumulate in inborn errors of metabolism are removed by the placenta, they are unlikely to contribute to dysfunction or dysgenesis. In utero, the affected fetus is detoxified by their mother as potentially toxic; water-soluble compounds are released via the placenta to the maternal organism where they are either metabolized or excreted. After birth, the neonate becomes generally more catabolic, which leads to mobilization of endogenous compounds, such as carbohydrates, amino acids, and fatty acids. In inborn errors of metabolism, these cannot be fully metabolized, resulting in toxic byproducts that lead to metabolic decompensation. These diseases are appropriate for newborn screening in the first days of life.

An exception to this principle is hypoplasia of corpus callosum, as is sometimes prenatally observed in nonketotic hyperglycinemia and sulfite oxidase deficiency. Other amino acid synthesis defects can also lead to prenatal symptoms: microcephaly in serine deficiency (detectable by amino acid analysis in fetal cord blood), and brain malformations in glutamine synthetase deficiency. Impaired folate metabolism is involved in a large fraction of neurodevelopmental defects collectively referred to as spina bifida. Defects of glycogen synthesis (typically brancher enzyme deficiency) may cause severe fetal distress. In contrast, defects in energy metabolism in general are frequently associated with congenital malformations, especially of the brain, as many morphological developmental processes are dependent upon energy metabolism. However, mitochondrial disorders in particular rarely manifest during fetal life. In fetal tissues anaerobic glycolysis is the major source of cellular energy, thus explaining why fetal wastage due to respiratory chain disorders is not a major feature of well-established mitochondrial diseases. In contrast, the rapidly increasing energy requirements of the growing neonate can explain the frequent neonatal presentation of these disorders, which are discussed separately.

An intermediate condition is exemplified by defects of mitochondrial beta-oxidation of fatty acids, as they may sometimes be symptomatic prenatally (notably the HELLP syndrome of maternal hemolysis, elevated liver enzymes and low platelet count) and, in this case, organic acid and acylcarnitine analysis in amniotic fluid can be diagnostic. However, it seems unlikely that inborn fetal errors of fatty acid oxidation are the only contributing factor to maternal pre-eclampsia and HELLP syndrome as there is a discrepancy in the incidence of these pregnancy complications (2–7 percent for pre-eclampsia and 0.5 percent for HELLP syndrome) compared with the incidence of inborn errors of fatty acid oxidation (which exhibit a cumulative prevalence of 1 in 10,000 newborns). Additional maternal manifestations of a fetal inborn metabolic disorder of fatty acid oxidation may include pre-eclampsia (which is associated with hypertension, edema, proteinuria), eclampsia (with severe hypertension, encephalopathy, seizures), and acute fatty liver of pregnancy.

Maternal Phenylketonuria

Phenylketonuria is an autosomal recessive genetic disease affecting 1 in 7500 live births. Infantile phenylketonuria is discussed separately. In maternal phenylketonuria, the fetus can sustain damage from impaired maternal phenylalanine metabolism. The offspring born to mothers with phenylketonuria is at risk of malformations when exposed to high concentrations of maternal phenylalanine in utero. Poorly controlled maternal phenylketonuria during pregnancy may result in microcephaly, mental retardation, congenital heart disease, and intrauterine growth retardation.

Treatment with a phenylalanine-restricted diet from before conception or no later than the earliest weeks of the first trimester reduces the risk to the fetus and mostly results in normal offspring. In untreated pregnancies of phenylketonuric mothers with blood phenylalanine levels $\geq$ 1,200 µmol/L (recommended values are 120 to 240 µmol/L), the frequency of these abnormalities increases, approaching 85 percent for microcephaly and mental retardation and 15 percent for congenital heart disease. Tetralogy of Fallot is frequent in maternal phenylketonuria, accounting for 19 percent of those with congenital heart disease when compared with the expected frequency of only 4 percent among all children. As cardiogenesis occurs during the 4th to 10th gestational week, control of maternal phenylketonuria initiated after the 8th week should have no effect in preventing congenital heart disease but might be effective in preventing or ameliorating other teratogenic effects of maternal phenylketonuria.

Microcephaly may be due to globally reduced brain volume or to abnormal regional brain development. Offspring of untreated mothers with phenylketonuria also exhibit compromised brain development in utero, which manifests as microcephaly and mental retardation. Hypoplasia of the corpus callosum is a feature of maternal phenylketonuria and is probably due to inhibition of callosal development during the 8th to 20th week of gestation.

The pathogenesis of maternal phenylketonuria may involve the placental transport of amino acids. Phenylalanine shares active placental transport with other neutral amino acids such that competition may occur. In addition, phenylalanine metabolites such as phenylacetic acid or phenylethylamine may be toxic.

The treatment of phenylketonuria involves a phenylalanine-restricted diet, supplemented by a phenylalanine-free amino acid mixture. The desired target values for blood phenylalanine during pregnancy are lower than in adult phenylketonuria.

Bibliography

Dimauro S., Garone C. (2011). Metabolic disorders of fetal life: glycogenoses and mitochondrial defects of the mitochondrial respiratory chain. *Semin Fetal Neonatal Med.* 16(4):181–89.

Illsinger S., Das A.M. (2010). Impact of selected inborn errors of metabolism on prenatal and neonatal development. *IUBMB Life.* 62(6):403–13.

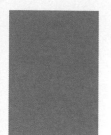

Newborn Disorders

Zellweger Disease

A male newborn, the product of 39 weeks of gestation, was admitted to the intensive care unit soon after birth due to severe hypotonia, poor suck, jaundice, a weak cry, and seizures with onset on the fourth day of life. Birth weight, length, and head circumference were 2068 g (<10th percentile), 49 cm (25–50th percentile) and 32 cm (<10th percentile). The baby had a dysmorphic face with a large bulging fontanelle, prominent forehead, low set ears, small mandible, hypoplasia of the orbital area, cleft palate, and a depressed nasal bridge. His abdomen was distended and hepatomegaly was present (3 cm below the costal margin). His extremities had a single palmar transverse crease on both hands, club feet, and limited extension of the knees. Examination of his level of awareness revealed drowsiness, but he opened his eyes spontaneously. There was persistent horizontal nystagmus. The light reflex was sluggish but isochoric. His facial expression was symmetric but diminished. There was global hypotonia with decreased muscle mass. He could hardly lift his extremities and his overall activity was markedly decreased. Tendon reflexes were decreased. Moro or suck reflexes were not elicited. He also developed intractable ictal apnea with severe oxygen tension desaturation in excess of 10 times per day. He harbored compound heterozygote mutations in the PEX1 gene.

Zellweger Disease

Onset: At birth, with dysmorphic features, seizures, hypotonia, and severely depressed motor activity and arousal.

Additional manifestations: Cataracts, pigmentary retinopathy, optic atrophy, sensorineural deafness, hepatomegaly and stippled calcifications of patellae, femora, and humeri. Death typically ensues in several months.

Disease mechanism: Autosomal recessive defect in peroxysomal biogenesis due to loss of function of the targeting proteins peroxins or their receptors, with systemic metabolic consequences.

Testing: Biochemical testing of plasma or red blood cells.

Treatment: None effective. Dietary lipid supplementation or restriction has been largely ineffective.

Research highlights: Murine models of peroxin deficiency.

Clinical Features

Zellweger syndrome, a relative common peroxysomal disease, includes a spectrum of neonatal and infantile autosomal recessive disorders that arise from defective peroxysomal synthesis and occur in 1 in 50,000 births. The spectrum includes Zellweger disease, neonatal adrenoleukodystrophy, and infantile Refsum disease. Rhizomelic chondrodysplasia punctata is also a peroxysomal biogenesis disorder, but it exhibits sufficiently distinctive limb features (rhizomelia) to be considered separately from this spectrum. A second major class of peroxysomal disorders includes defects in which individual peroxysomal enzymes are deficient. The most common of these disorders affect older individuals and include X-linked adrenoleukodystrophy and Refsum disease. Infantile Refsum disease and X-linked adrenoleukodystrophy are covered separately due to their relative frequency.

Newborns with Zellweger disease are severely ill and exhibit a characteristic facial appearance, with prominent forehead, hypertelorism, epicanthal folds, superior orbital ridge hypoplasia, and depressed nasal bridge. They manifest severe hypotonia, apnea, hepatopathy, and feeding difficulties. Seizures are common. There is pigmentary retinal degeneration and sensorineural deafness. There are also skeletal

Table 13.1 The peroxysomal disorders

Disorders of peroxysomal biogenesis	Single-enzyme peroxysomal defects
Zellweger syndrome	X-linked adrenoleukodystrophy
• Zellweger disease	Refsum disease
• Neonatal adrenoleukodystrophy	
• Infantile Refsum disease	
Rhizomelic chondrodysplasia punctata	

abnormalities (Figure 13.1). They make no developmental gains and usually die within a few months.

Pathology

Defective neuronal migration without inflammation is the hallmark of Zellweger syndrome. Brain weight is often increased. There is typically centrosylvian or parasylvian pachygyria and polymicrogyria (Figure 13.2). The Sylvian fissure may be vertically disposed. The cortex is thickened. Its outer portions contain large neurons that are normally found in deep cortex, whereas neurons usually found in the superficial cortex remain trapped in deep cortex and subcortical white matter. In the cerebellum, Purkinje cells are ectopically found in the white matter and include multiple major dendrites. Some of the elongated cerebral nuclei appear discontinuous and there is palisading of neurons.

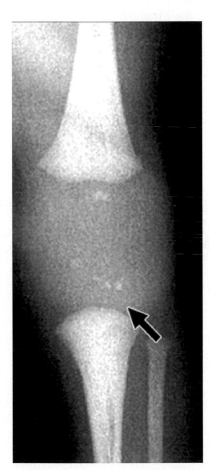

Figure 13.1 One-day-old boy with Zellweger syndrome. Knee radiograph illustrates calcified stippled appearance (arrow) of the patella. Reproduced with permission from Thomas B et al. MRI of Childhood Epilepsy Due to Inborn Errors of Metabolism. *Am J Radiol.* 2010; 194: W367–W374.

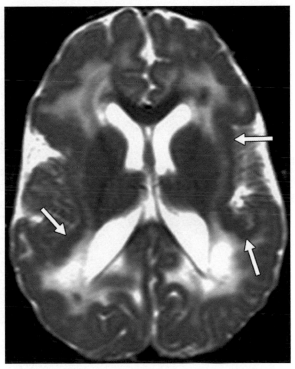

Figure 13.2 11-month-old girl with Zellweger syndrome who presented with hypotonia, seizures, and dysmorphic facial features. Axial T2-weighted MR imaging shows T2 hyperintensity within the periventricular white matter of both frontal and parietal lobes. In addition, there is extensive malformation of cortical development compatible with diffuse polymicrogyria, especially in perisylvian regions (arrows). Reproduced with permission from Ibrahim M et al. Inborn Errors of Metabolism: Combining Clinical and Radiologic Clues to Solve the Mystery. *Am J Radiol.* 2014; 203: W315–W327.

Cerebral macrophages can be prominent and contain abnormal lipid cytosomes. Some neurites display lamellar and lipid profiles. The white matter does not contain inflammatory cells typical of leukodystrophy (lymphocytes or plasma cells). Reactive astrocytosis can be either inconspicuous in the white matter or severe in areas with heterotopia. Astrocytes and oligodendrocytes contain abnormal lipid cytosomes, which probably contain very long chain fatty acids.

Pathophysiology

Peroxysomes are reduced or absent in Zellweger syndrome. As a result, multiple metabolic abnormalities ensue, including defects in very long chain fatty acid oxidation, plasmalogen synthesis, and phytanic acid oxidation. In these disorders, catalase, a peroxysomal enzyme that is used as a disease marker, is found in the cytosol. Excess of very long chain fatty acids and reduction of plasmalogen have been postulated to lead to neuronal migration defects.

Nascent peroxysomes incorporate proteins known as peroxins, which are coded by PEX genes. Peroxins receive target sequences in the endoplasmic reticulum, which specify their fate as peroxysomal proteins. Peroxysomal target sequence 1, which is recognized by the receptor PEX5, is utilized by most proteins that will be harbored in the peroxysomal matrix. PEX1 deficiency constitutes the most common cause of peroxysomal biogenesis disorders. PEX1 interacts with PEX6, which accounts for a smaller percentage of peroxysomal biogenesis disorders (Figures 13.3 and 13.4). In contrast, other PEX mutations are rarer. There is a relatively high frequency of two PEX1 mutations in the general population (the missense Gly843Asp and the frameshift 2097TinsT), a

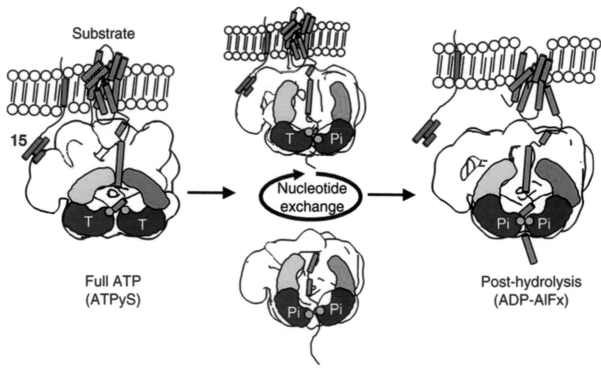

Figure 13.3 Model for Pex1/6 movements during ATP binding and hydrolysis.
The Pex1/6 complex anchors to the peroxisomal membrane via binding of Pex6 N domains to Pex15. Pex1 N domains establish interactions with the substrate. ATP binding to Pex1 D2 and Pex6 D2 (full ATP, ATPγS) elevates substrate-binding loops in the D2 domain, ready to grab the substrate. ATP turnover creates a power stroke that pulls the substrate along the central pore (post hydrolysis, ADP-AIFx). Nucleotide exchange in Pex6 D2 or Pex1 D2 translocates the substrate along the central pore (Pex1/6WBATP, Pex1WBATP/6). One Pex1 and Pex6 protomer are denoted as a simple cartoon representation. Conserved aromatic residues of substrate-binding loops are shown as green dots. Representative tertiary structures of substrate protein (purple) and membrane anchor Pex15 (green) are depicted as cartoon representations. Nucleotide occupancy of each D2 domain is indicated by T for ATP or Pi for the transition state. Reproduced with permission from Ciniawsky S et al . Molecular snapshots of the Pex1/6 AAA+ complex in action. *Nat Commun.* 2015; 6:7331.

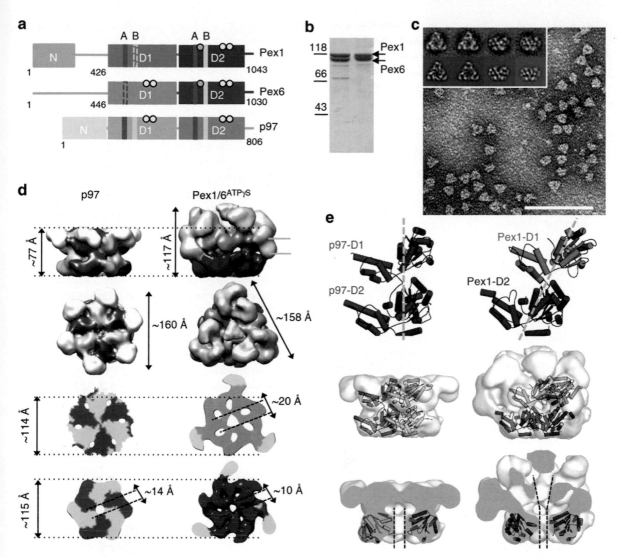

Figure 13.4 Pex1/6 hexamers are trimers of dimers. (a) Schematic domain representation of Pex1/Pex6 protomers compared with p97 (N domain, D1/D2 domain). Conserved motifs and residues of each AAA+ domain are indicated: Walker A (A, magenta bars), Walker B (B, turquoise bars), substrate-binding loops (green dots) and arginine finger residues (yellow dots). Non-canonical Walker A and B motifs are indicated as dotted lines. (b) Coomassie-stained SDS–polyacrylamide gel electrophoresis of purified Pex1/6ATP (5µg, lane 1) or Pex1/6 DWBATP (5µg, lane 2) overexpressed in *E. coli* or *Saccharomyces cerevisiae*. (c) Raw negative stain electron micrograph showing Pex1/6 complexes (40µg/ml) incubated with ATPγS. Representative class averages derived from multivariate statistical analysis show top and side views of the Pex1/6ATPγS complex (inset, upper row) and corresponding reprojections of the final 3D reconstruction in the Euler angle directions assigned to the class averages (lower row). Each class contains an average of 5–10 images. Scale bar, 100nm. (d) Pex1/6ATPγS EM density map as side, top and cross-section views of D1 and D2 rings. Colour code: Pex1 D1 (orange), Pex1 D2 (red), Pex6 D1 (pale blue), Pex6 D2 (blue) and Pex1/6N domains (grey). Equivalent views of p97 filtered to 20Å are shown for comparison. p97 single subunits are coloured alternately light and dark grey. Cross-section viewing planes are indicated by green lines. (e) Cartoon representation of a p97 protomer without N domains and of a Pex1 protomer homology model, seen from the side of the complex. Domain offset between Pex1 D1 and Pex1 D2 is indicated by green dotted lines. Walker A and Walker B motifs are shown as spheres and coloured as in a (upper row). Side view of a p97 dimer fitted as a rigid body into low-pass filtered p97 crystal structure and Pex1/6 heterodimer docked to Pex1/6ATPγS 3D map (middle row). Cut-open side views of the low-pass filtered p97 crystal structure with p97 D2 placed into the EM density map and of Pex1/6ATPγS map with fitted Pex1 D2 and Pex6 D2 homology models. Black dotted lines indicate the central channel (lower row). Reproduced with permission from Ciniawsky S et al. Molecular snapshots of the Pex1/6 AAA+ complex in action. *Nat Commun*. 2015; 6:7331.

phenomenon that accounts for most Zellweger syndrome cases. Individuals homozygous for Gly843Asp exhibit milder phenotypes; those homozygous for 2097insT manifest Zellweger disease and those heterozygous for Gly843Asp and 2097TinsT display intermediate severity.

Diagnosis

Several metabolites situated upstream peroxysomal metabolism accumulate in plasma. Among these, very long chain fatty acids, 3α,7α,12α-trihydroxy-cholestanoic acid and pristanic and phytanic acids are elevated, whereas the ratio pristanic:phytanic acid is preserved. Red blood cell plasmalogen is diminished. Fibroblast catalase assay reveals cytoplasmic localization with excess cytosolic very long chain fatty acids and diminished plasmalogen synthesis.

Several peroxisomal disorders are associated with distinct bile acid abnormalities and each disorder has a characteristic pattern of abnormal bile acids that accumulate, which is often used for diagnostic purposes.

Treatment

There is no effective therapy. Dietary treatments have focused on supplementing deficiency plasma substrates or on the reduction of the dietary consumption of excess metabolites. Both approaches have proven minimally efficacious or ineffective. They have included administration of lipids, and of cholic and deoxycholic acid, and restriction of dietary very long chain fatty acids and phytanic acid, which in man is exclusively of dietary origin. Supplementation with oral docosahexaenoic acid has also proven ineffective.

Bibliography

Braverman N.E., Raymond G.V., Rizzo W.B., et al (2016). Peroxisome biogenesis disorders in the Zellweger spectrum: An overview of current diagnosis, clinical manifestations, and treatment guidelines. *Mol Genet Metab*. 117(3):313–21.

Cho S.Y., Chang Y.P., Park J.Y., et al (2011). Two novel PEX1 mutations in a patient with Zellweger syndrome: the first Korean case confirmed by biochemical, and molecular evidence. *Ann Clin Lab Sci*. 41(2):182–7.

Other Neonatal Peroxysomal Disorders

Clinical Features

The neonatal peroxysomal disorders are characterized by deficient peroxysomal biosynthesis. Zellweger disease is covered in Chapter 13, whereas infantile Refsum disease is described in a separate chapter. Here, neonatal adrenoleukodystrophy and rhizomelic chondrodysplasia punctata are included as the two most prominent peroxysomal biogenesis disorders after Zellweger disease.

Neonatal adrenoleukodystrophy has clinical features in common with Zellweger disease and adrenoleukodystrophy, but is less severe. Survival typically reaches the third year. Hepatopathy is common and liver peroxysomes are absent or reduced in number or appear enlarged. Mitochondrial abnormalities are also common.

In rhizomelic chondrodysplasia punctata, the proximal limbs are significantly shortened (rhizomelic). Facial dysmorphic features are also common, as are cataracts and ichthyosis. There is microcephaly and sensorineural deafness in the context of severely abnormal psychomotor development, which are apparent at birth. Endochondral bone formation is abnormal, bone epiphyses are stippled and vertebral bodies display coronal clefts. The disease follows a milder course than Zellweger disease. Most affected children die before their sixth birthday.

Pathology

In neonatal adrenoleukodystrophy, the white matter is severely abnormal, much more so than in Zellweger disease. Brain weight can be increased. Heterotopic Purkinje cells and neuronal loss can be present. Polymicrogyria and macrophages are characteristic features and resemble Zellweger disease. However, demyelination is severe and accompanied by a prominent perivascular lymphocytic infiltration. The adrenal glands are atrophic and contain striated adrenocortical cells.

In rhizomelic chondrodysplasia punctata, hepatic peroxysomes are absent or irregularly shaped. Milder forms of the disease are associated with chondrodysplasia without rhizomelia. The brain can be reduced in weight, but dysgenesis is absent. The white matter may be microscopically normal. Fragmentation of the inferior olives and cerebellar atrophy has been documented. Purkinje and cerebellar granule cells die from apoptosis.

Pathophysiology

Mutations in PEX7 account for all cases of rhizomelic chondrodysplasia punctata. PEX7 is the receptor for peroxisome targeting sequence 2. This target sequence is located in peroxysomal enzymes that synthesize the phospholipid plasmalogen and alpha-oxidize branched-chain fatty acids. Consequently, plasmalogen levels can be severely reduced and phytanic acid is not oxidized, leading to its accumulation in plasma. However, peroxysomal structure appears preserved in rhizomelic chondrodysplasia punctata.

Diagnosis

In rhizomelic chondrodysplasia punctata, red blood cell plasmalogen is very diminished, whereas very long chain fatty acids are normal. Pristanic acid is normal and phytanic acid is increased, leading to a reduced pristanic:phytanic acid ratio.

Treatment

None effective.

Bibliography

Klouwer F.C., Berendse K., Ferdinandusse S., et al (2015). Zellweger spectrum disorders: Clinical overview and management approach. *Orphanet J Rare Dis*. 10:151.

Pyruvate Dehydrogenase Deficiency

A girl was born at 37 weeks gestation with a nuchal cord and apnea after a pregnancy characterized by intrauterine growth retardation and cerebral ventriculomegaly with periventricular leukomalacia. Her Apgar scores had been 5 at 1 minute and 8 at 5 minutes. A first-born brother had died at several months of age. Metabolic acidosis was noted on the first day of life of the girl, with a lactate acid level of 9.3 mM (normal: 1.3–2.3). She did not latch when offered oral nutrition and had no gag reflex. Lethargy was prominent. Her tone was very diminished and she exhibited a paucity of spontaneous movements. Tendon reflexes were hypoactive. Further testing revealed blood pyruvate of 0.45 mM (normal: 0.03 – 0.11) and lactic aciduria. MR imaging confirmed earlier findings. Cerebrospinal fluid lactate was 10.7 mM (normal: 1.3 – 2.4). Pyruvate dehydrogenase activity in skin fibroblasts was 36% of normal. She harbored a deletion in the pyruvate dehydrogenase gene PDHA1. At 14 weeks of age, she experienced seizures that eventually included infantile spasms. A ketogenic diet was initiated at 5 months of age for prominent seizures refractory to anticonvulsants and thiamine. A gastrostomy was placed at 1 year of age for poor weight gain and dysphagia. At 2 years of age, seizures persisted, although they were less frequent (about 90% fewer seizures were noted after the ketogenic diet). Her development had been minimal: She seemed to recognize her parents visually and made vocal noises. She could only lift her head briefly. Eye fixation was poor and she could not track light. She smiled spontaneously.

Pyruvate Dehydrogenase Deficiency

Onset: At birth, with metabolic acidosis, decreased activity and hypotonia.
Additional manifestations: Agenesis of the corpus callosum, subtly dysmorphic features, seizures and ataxia. Leigh syndrome.

Disease mechanism: Cerebral cortical dysgenesis and deficit in conversion of pyruvate to acetyl coenzyme A, resulting in incomplete glucose metabolism and excess lactate production.
Testing: Elevated lactate and alanine in bodily fluids.
Treatment: Thiamine in responsive cases, ketogenic diet and dichloroacetate.
Research highlights: Reduction of pyruvate dehydrogenase activity in mice, with a variety of metabolic effects that can be restored by the downstream metabolite acetate.

Table 15.1 Principal characteristics of pyruvate dehydrogenase deficiency forms

Biochemical variants of pyruvate dehydrogenase deficiency	Inheritance	Principal manifestation
E1a	X-linked	Lactic acidosis
E1b	Autosomal recessive	Episodic ataxia
E2	Autosomal recessive	Cerebral dysgenesis
E3	Autosomal recessive	Infantile epilepsy
Pyruvate dehydrogenase phosphatase	Autosomal recessive	Leigh syndrome
Pyruvate dehydrogenase X or E3-binding protein	Autosomal recessive	Lactic acidosis
Lipoyltransferase	Autosomal recessive	Lactic acidosis
Short-chain enoyl-coenzyme A hydratase	Autosomal recessive	Leigh syndrome

Clinical Features

Defects in the pyruvate dehydrogenase complex, the largest enzyme in the organism, are a frequent cause of lactic acidosis, epilepsy, hypotonia, and death from metabolic acidosis in the neonatal period. The acidosis is due principally to lactic acidemia and leads to depressed activity and impaired alertness, often resulting in death if untreated. The facial features of

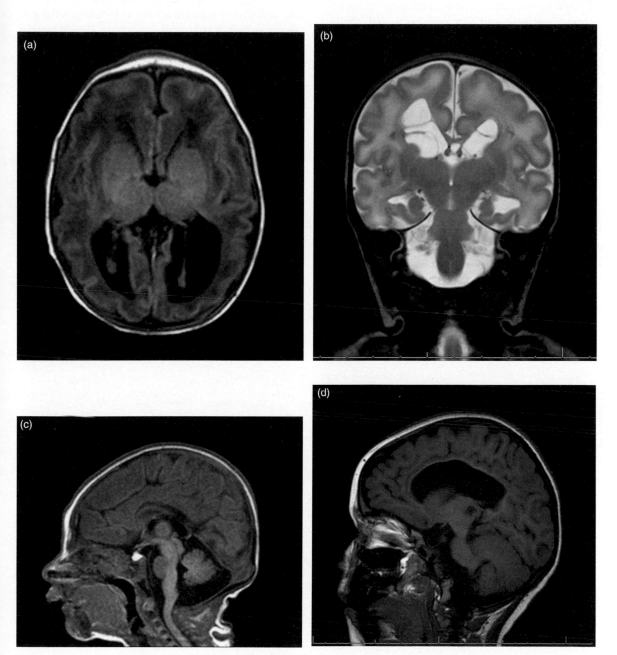

Figure 15.1 (a) to (c). Cranial MR imaging of a 6-day-old girl with pyruvate dehydrogenase deficiency due to mutation of the E1 alpha subunit. The corpus callosum is markedly thin. There is a paucity of myelination, especially in the posterior limbs of the internal capsule. Multiple large cysts communicate with the ventricles, which are also enlarged. (d). MR imaging of a 6-year-old girl with pyruvate dehydrogenase deficiency due to mutation of the gene LIPT1 – thalamic necrosis in the setting of a hypoplastic corpus callosum.

affected children resemble those of infants with fetal alcoholic syndrome, with thin upper lip, prominent philtrum, and depressed nasal bridge. Seizures are common. In some cases, the phenotype is that of Leigh syndrome.

Symptoms vary considerably in children with pyruvate dehydrogenase complex deficiency, and almost equal numbers of boys and girls have been affected, despite the location of the frequently mutated E1 alpha subunit gene in the X chromosome, a paradox perhaps explained by selective female X-inactivation. Thus, the phenotype of PDH deficiency is dictated by mutation severity (especially in males) and by the pattern of X-inactivation in females. Mutation of any one of several pyruvate dehydrogenase subunits, regulatory molecules, and metabolically-related enzymes can lead to an array of loosely related phenotypes.

Milder variants can present during infancy, childhood, or even adulthood with episodic cerebellar ataxia, which may occur spontaneously, be precipitated by carbohydrate intake, or occur in conjunction with mild infections. Dystonic attacks, alternating hemiplegia and progressive peripheral neuropathy may occur. Lactic acidosis is usually not found during testing of these children, but mild postprandial hyperlactatemia may occur.

Pathology

The brain is diminished in weight. There is agenesis or hypoplasia of the corpus callosum (Figure 15.1). Gross migration abnormalities include pachygyria, polymicrogyria and periventricular nodular heterotopias. Additional malformations include cerebellar and brainstem hypoplasia with hypoplastic dentate nuclei and pyramidal tracts. Associated clastic lesions included asymmetric leukomalacia, reactive gliosis, large pseudocysts of germinolysis, and basal ganglia calcifications. Subtle cerebral dysgenesis includes large pyramidal neurons trapped in superficial cortical layers. There can be prominent astrocytic hypertrophy.

Pathophysiology

Pyruvate dehydrogenase deficiency predominantly manifests as encephalopathy and lactic acidosis. The principal metabolic defect is deficient mitochondrial conversion of pyruvate into acetyl coenzyme A, which enters the tricarboxylic acid cycle (Figure 15.2). Pyruvate dehydrogenase is a mitochondrial matrix enzyme complex that catalyzes the oxidative decarboxylation of pyruvate to form acetyl-CoA, nicotinamide adenine dinucleotide

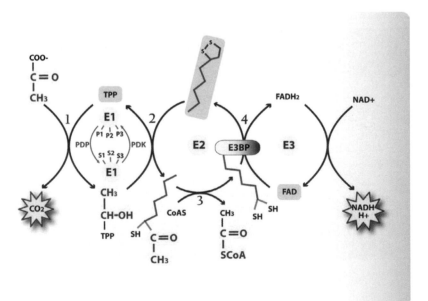

Figure 15.2 Schematic diagram illustrating metabolic steps catalyzed by the three subunits of pyruvate dehydrogenase E1, E2, and E3. Under aerobic conditions, pyruvate is transported into the mitochondrion where it is converted into acetyl coenzyme A (CoA) by the pyruvate dehydrogenase complex in irreversible fashion. When this flux is disrupted, pyruvate concentration rises together with lactate and alanine levels. ATP production and derived reactions are decreased. TPP: thiamine pyrophosphate; NAD+/NADH: nicotinamide adenine dinucleotide; FADH2: flavin adenine dinucleotide; PDP: Pyruvate dehydrogenase phosphatase; PDK: Pyruvate dehydrogenase kinase; E3BP: E3-subunit binding protein. Figure courtesy of I. Marin-Valencia.

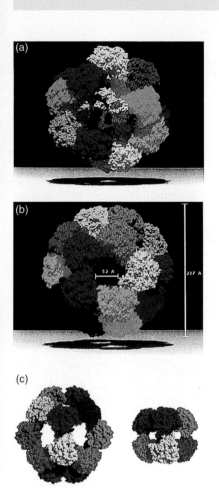

Figure 15.3 Space-filling representation (using programs MOLSCRIPT and RASTER3D) of the 60-subunit truncated dodecahedral E2p core of the *B. stearothermophilus* pyruvate dehydrogenase multienzyme complex. Each of the 20 trimers is colored differently. (a) View along the threefold axis with the central trimer depicted with different colors per protomer. (b) View along the fivefold axis showing the large opening ("windows") that allow CoA to enter and approach its binding pocket from the internal cavity of the oligomer. The outer diameter of the hollow particle is ~237 Å, and the solvent-accessible inner space has a diameter of ~118 Å. (c) View along the twofold axis showing the trimer–trimer subunit interaction and comparison with the cubic E2p core of *A. vinelandii*. The height of the cubic core is ~125 Å and the cross section of the windows is ~30 Å. Reproduced with permission from Izard T et al. Principles of quasi-equivalence and Euclidean geometry govern the assembly of cubic and dodecahedral cores of pyruvate dehydrogenase complexes. *Proc Natl Acad Sci U S A*. 1999; 96: 1240–5.

(NADH), and CO_2 (Figure 15.3). Pyruvate dehydrogenase is heavily regulated, with a specific kinase leading to its deactivation and a phosphatase to its activation. Alanine levels are elevated as the result of elevated pyruvate. Lactate is another downstream metabolite of pyruvate in an interconversion catalyzed by lactate dehydrogenase. Thus, there are two principal types of consequences: excess acidosis with consequent secondary disarray, and deficit of acetyl coenzyme A formation to fuel the tricarboxylic acid cycle. The latter mechanism is thought to impact glutamate and GABA synthesis, with consequent impact on neural excitability.

Diagnosis

The diagnosis requires measurements of lactate and pyruvate in plasma and cerebrospinal fluid (lactate: pyruvate ratio < 15), analysis of amino acids in plasma (hyperalaninemia) and of organic acids in urine (lactic and pyruvic acids) and neuroradiological investigations, including proton magnetic resonance spectroscopy to detect lactate. Enzymatic analysis of fibroblast or muscle PDH activity is often performed.

Treatment

A ketogenic diet together with thiamine supplementation can afford substantial benefit in responsive cases. The ketogenic diet is a source of acetyl coenzyme A independent of glycolysis. Dichloroacetate, a pyruvate dehydrogenase kinase inhibitor, is sometimes temporarily used to enhance lactate clearance.

Bibliography

Ganetzky R.D., Bloom K., Ahrens-Nicklas R., et al ECHS1 deficiency as a cause of severe neonatal lactic acidosis. *JIMD Rep.* [in press].

Pirot N., Crahes M., Adle-Biassette H., et al (2016). Phenotypic and neuropathological characterization of fetal pyruvate dehydrogenase deficiency. *J Neuropathol Exp Neurol.* 75(3):227–38.

Neonatal Pyruvate Carboxylase Deficiency

A female was born at term after a normal delivery. At 27 weeks gestation, brain ventriculomegaly was detected by routine ultrasonography and confirmed by fetal magnetic resonance imaging. She had a low birth-weight of 2115 g (−3.1SD), was 46 cm in length (−2.6SD) and had a normal head circumference of 34 cm. At 15 h of life, lethargy, hyperpnea, and truncal hypotonia appeared. Antibiotics were started, but no microorganism was detected. Bloodwork revealed severe metabolic acidosis (pH 6.94, pCO_2 12 mm Hg, pO_2 87 mm Hg, bicarbonate 2.4 mM and base excess −27.7 mM) with lactate 18 mM (normal: 1.3–2.3) and ammonia 179 μM (normal in the neonatal period: < 110), and glucose 40 mg/dl (normal: 45–88). Repeat testing revealed a pyruvate level of 0.56 mM (normal: 0.06–0.12), lactate level of 21.2 mM and an elevated lactate to pyruvate ratio of 38.0 (normal: 10.1–35.5). Neurological examination showed generalized hypokinesia, with almost absent spontaneous movements, poor blinking, and limb rigidity. Some dysmorphic features such as a thin upper lip, a wide philtrum and small palpebral fissures were observed. She also exhibited horizontal pendular nystagmus. Electroencephalography showed a burst suppression pattern. A cranial MR imaging study was obtained (Figure 16.1). She died of respiratory arrest on the 5th day of life.

Pyruvate Carboxylase Deficiency

Onset: Lactic acidosis within 72 hr of birth in the neonatal form (type B).
Additional manifestations: Neonatal form: Seizures, hypotonia, and depressed alertness; hepatomegaly and renal tubular acidosis. Infantile form (type A): Pyramidal tract dysfunction, ataxia, and episodic metabolic decompensation. Benign form (type C): Intellectual impairment and intermittent acidosis.
Disease mechanism: Failure of tricarboxylic acid cycle carbon replenishment via deficiency of oxaloacetate generation from pyruvate.
Testing: Characteristic blood and urinary biochemical profile depending on disease type (A, B, or C). Enzyme activity determination in fibroblasts or liver.
Treatment: Triheptanoin, biotin, or orthotopic liver transplantation.
Research highlights: Determination of the role of anaplerosis, or carbon replenishment, by glial cells in the broader context of neural function.

Clinical Features

Pyruvate carboxylase deficiency is an autosomal recessive disease due to mutation of the pyruvate carboxylase gene. The enzyme catalyzes the conversion of pyruvate to oxaloacetate when abundant acetyl coenzyme A is available, thus replenishing tricarboxylic acid cycle intermediates in the mitochondrial matrix. The enzyme is bound to biotin. Pyruvate carboxylase is involved in gluconeogenesis, lipogenesis, and neurotransmitter synthesis. Pyruvate carboxylase deficiency presents with three degrees of phenotypic severity.

An infantile form (A) with moderate lactic acidosis, mental and motor deficits, hypotonia, pyramidal tract dysfunction, ataxia, and seizures leading to death in infancy. Episodes of vomiting, acidosis, and tachypnea can be triggered by metabolic imbalance or infection.

A severe neonatal form (B), presenting as severe lactic acidosis, hypoglycemia, hepatomegaly, depressed consciousness, and severely abnormal development. Abnormal limb and ocular movements are common findings. Early death is also common.

A rare benign form (C) causes episodic acidosis and moderate mental impairment compatible with survival and near-normal neurological performance.

Table 16.1 Types and clinical severity of pyruvate carboxylase deficiency

Pyruvate carboxylase deficiency form	Severity
A: Infantile	Mild
B: Neonatal	Severe
C: Benign	Intermittent

Pathology

Brain structural abnormalities are frequently detected in type A and B individuals by magnetic resonance imaging (Figure 16.1). The neuroradiological findings reported in these individuals include ischemic-like lesions, ventricular dilatation, periventricular cysts (identified almost invariably in type B individuals), reduced myelination, and subcortical leukodystrophy among other abnormalities (Figure 16.2). These findings are usually detected in symptomatic neonates or infants, although ischemic-like lesions can be detected prenatally in type B deficiency.

Pathophysiology

A salient feature of pyruvate carboxylase deficiency is the conjunction of central nervous system maldevelopment (hypotrophy) and degeneration, which often dominate the phenotype. Neurological manifestations are prominent as the result of primary glial dysfunction. In astrocytes, the anaplerotic function of pyruvate carboxylase is required for gluconeogenesis and glycogen synthesis and to replenish α-ketoglutarate removed from the tricarboxylic acid cycle for the synthesis of glutamine, the main neuronal precursor of both glutamate and γ-aminobutyric acid. Pyruvate carboxylase is also involved in myelin lipid synthesis in oligodendrocytes, which may underlie the paucity of myelin and abundance of white matter lesions typical of the disease.

Pyruvate carboxylase is critical for gluconeogenesis in both liver and kidney. This phenomenon probably accounts for the hypoglycemia that can manifest during fasting, metabolic imbalance or, paradoxically, even in postprandial states. Furthermore, in the liver, the disease leads to decreased oxaloacetate availability, resulting in impaired acetyl coenzyme A oxidation which can then be diverted into ketone body and fatty

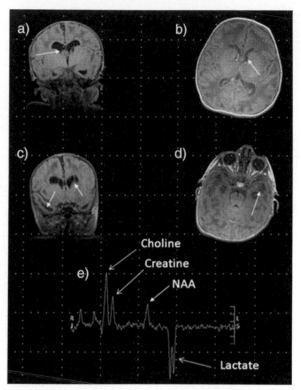

Figure 16.1 a to d. MR images of an infant with pyruvate carboxylase deficiency including T2-weighted images demonstrating periventricular white matter cysts and a global signal abnormality of the white matter signal. There is involvement of the temporal lobes and periventricular zones. e. Spectroscopy reveals a lactate peak manifested as an inverted doublet. The NAA (N-acetylaspartate) peak is diminished in amplitude (possibly revealing neuronal loss) and the choline peak is elevated (possibly due to white matter damage) compared to age-matched controls (not shown). Reproduced with permission from Ortez C et al. Infantile parkinsonism and GABAergic hypotransmission in a patient with pyruvate carboxylase deficiency. *Gene.* 2013; 532(2):302–6.

acid synthesis. This can explain the lipid droplet accumulation that is often found in hepatocytes (steatosis) and associated hepatomegaly.

Diagnosis

Assay of pyruvate carboxylase activity in fibroblasts, lymphocytes, and other tissues except muscle is definitive.

Type B pyruvate carboxylase deficiency is associated with the most characteristic analytical abnormalities. Brain MR imaging reveals cystic periventricular leukomalacia. Hyperammonemia with mild hypercitrullinemia, high lactate-to-pyruvate ratio, paradoxical

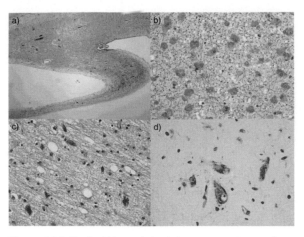

Figure 16.2 Cerebral histopathological examination in an infant affected by pyruvare carboxylase deficiency revealing periventricular cysts (a), numerous gemistocytic astrocytes (b) in the white matter with focal spongiosis (c) and neurons with central chromatolysis in the substantia nigra (d). Reproduced with permission from Ortez C et al. Infantile parkinsonism and GABAergic hypotransmission in a patient with pyruvate carboxylase deficiency. *Gene.* 2013; 532(2):302–6.

postprandial ketosis, and low glutamate comprise a suggestive metabolic profile, mostly due to depletion of intracellular aspartate and oxaloacetate. Renal tubular acidosis has also been reported. Moderate hyperammonemia (100–150 μM) is also observed in type B disease. An elevation of total cholesterol or its precursors (mevalonic acid) may occur in Type A and B forms.

Constant or intermittent metabolic acidosis caused by elevated lactate levels is typical of all forms of pyruvate carboxylase deficiency. Ketoacidosis is also present and contributes to the metabolic acidosis. Type A and B affected individuals usually manifest chronic metabolic acidosis with elevated lactate and ketosis, and Type C affected individuals tend to manifest these features only intermittently during metabolic stress.

Pyruvate carboxylase deficiency in general causes an increase in pyruvate levels, which is subsequently converted to lactate resulting in lactic acidemia, a reaction that can be enhanced by the administration of carbohydrates. The lactate:pyruvate ratio is a useful indicator of the underlying cause of lactic acidemia. However, only Type B affected individuals exhibit an elevated ratio (>25), reflecting a reduced redox state (high NADH/NAD ratio) in cytoplasm.

Treatment

The foremost goal of therapies for pyruvate carboxylase deficiency is the restoration of substrate flux into the tricarboxylic acid cycle with the objective of suppressing unmitigated catabolism and to activate synthetic pathways. Dietary treatment, however, has traditionally included limited options, since a high-fat diet increases ketoacidosis, and high-carbohydrate diets exacerbate lactic acidosis. The use of an exogenous source of substrate for enhancement of ATP production, such as the anaplerotic compound triheptanoin (a triglyceride containing three 7-carbon fatty acids (heptanoate)) may provide the necessary source of both oxaloacetate and acetyl coenzyme A to accomplish this goal. Triheptanoin is metabolized mainly in the liver converting one molecule of triheptanoin into one molecule of glycerol and three molecules of heptanoic acid. Heptanoate undergoes a partial cycle of β-oxidation in the liver to produce 5-carbon ketone bodies (β-ketopentanoate and β-hydroxypentanoate), which can then be exported to the blood.

Treatment with co-factors involved in pyruvate metabolism and supplements of the tricarboxylic acid cycle seem to ameliorate mostly biochemical disturbances without exerting significant impact on the neurological manifestations of the disease. A child with type A deficiency responded to oral biotin, manifesting improving lactic acidosis and cerebral myelination without impact on other neurological abnormalities. Treatment with high doses of citrate and aspartate has been used in type B children, resulting in an increase of oxaloacetate and metabolites of the tricarboxylic acid cycle and improvement of lactic acidosis. However, ketosis was not resolved and there was no significant amelioration of neurological abnormalities.

Orthotopic liver transplantation was performed in an infant with type B deficiency, resulting in decreased ketone body levels and an improvement in renal tubular function, but little effect on lactic acidemia or neurological performance.

Bibliography

Marin-Valencia I., Roe C.R., Pascual J.M. (2010). Pyruvate carboxylase deficiency: Mechanisms, mimics and anaplerosis. *Mol Genet Metab.* 101(1):9–17.

Ortez C., Jou C., Cortès-Saladelafont E., et al (2013). Infantile parkinsonism and GABAergic hypotransmission in a patient with pyruvate carboxylase deficiency. *Gene.* 532(2):302–6.

17 Tricarboxylic Acid Cycle Disorders

A girl was born uneventfully to first cousin parents. Her mother was given insulin for late onset diabetes mellitus at 5 months' gestation. Two siblings had died in the neonatal period under unexplained circumstances and a third one was severely ill. One brother and two sisters were healthy. Poor sucking, vomiting, and failure to thrive were noted in the first 2 weeks of life. Hypertonic episodes of the upper limbs were noted from the age of 6 months. At 14 months of age, she displayed moderate microcephaly (head circumference −2.5 SD), trunk hypotonia, hypertonic and dystonic posture of the limbs, and her development was abnormal. CT scan of the brain showed dilation of pericerebral spaces and ventricles and MR imaging revealed increased signal intensity in the white matter. She was neutropenic. Histopathological examination of the liver and the jejunum was normal, while changes in the skeletal muscle included abnormal variation in fiber diameter with predominance and hypertrophy of type II fibers. The Gomori trichrome stain was normal. Cerebrospinal fluid lactate and pyruvate were elevated about 2-fold over the normal maximum. Urinary organic acid analyses showed major excretion of fumaric acid and, to a lesser extent, of a-ketoglutaric acid. Other tricarboxylic acid cycle intermediates, including succinic acid, were present in normal amounts. Fumarase activity in lymphocytes was 0.5% of that of control. The child had inherited a homozygous mutation in the fumarase gene.

Tricarboxylic Acid Cycle Disorders

Onset: Hypotonia, lethargy, and seizures shortly after birth. Amniotic fluid volume dysregulation (oligo or polihydramnios) during gestation.
Additional manifestations: Leigh syndrome, microcephaly and cerebral dysgenesis. Epilepsy is common.

Disease mechanism: Failure of production of tricarboxylic acid cycle-related metabolites with widespread functional impact.
Testing: Urinary determination of cycle byproducts and enzymatic assay of several tissues.
Treatment: None effective.
Research highlights: Investigation of the role of tricarboxylic acid cycle intermediates as oncometabolites.

Clinical Features

Several tricarboxylic acid enzymes are susceptible to mutations that cause severe mitochondrial dysfunction. They are inherited in autosomal recessive fashion. Most present in the neonatal period, while some may manifest progressively in early infancy. Polyhydramnios, oligohydramnios, intrauterine growth retardation, and premature birth are reported in approximately one-third of cases.

Defects of aconitase, of the E3 component of the alpha-ketoglutarate dehydrogenase complex, of succinate dehydrogenase, of fumarase (also known as fumarate hydratase) and of succinyl-CoA synthetase are collectively associated with profound encephalopathy and with the excretion of specific metabolic precursors and byproducts. The manifestations of these disorders are pleomorphic.

Aconitase deficiency is characterized by onset between ages 2 and 6 months of cerebellar and retinal degeneration. Truncal hypotonia, athetosis, and seizures can be prominent. Affected children also manifest profound psychomotor retardation, with few achieving rolling, sitting, or recognition of family. They also develop progressive optic atrophy and retinal degeneration. Brain MR imaging illustrates progressive cerebral and cerebellar degeneration.

E3 (dihydrolipoamide dehydrogenase, which is also shared by the pyruvate dehydrogenase complex)

55

deficiency, a multifaceted disorder, causes accumulation of pyruvate and branched-chain amino acids in plasma and excretion of branched-chain alpha-keto acids in urine.

In the case of succinate dehydrogenase deficiency (which is also part of the mitochondrial respiratory chain and known as complex II), mutations of subunit A may cause Leigh syndrome (or optic atrophy in the elderly), while mutations in subunits B, C, and D are associated with paraganglioma, and mutations in subunits B and D are associated with pheochromocytoma and severely reduced tumor succinate dehydrogenase activity.

Fumarate hydratase mutations, which cause structural brain malformations such as microcephaly, dysmorphic facial features (frontal bossing, depressed nasal bridge, and hypertelorism), and neonatal polycythemia, are independently associated with uterine and cutaneous leiomyomas and with papillary renal cell cancer. However, succinate dehydrogenase- and fumarase-related tumors are inherited in an autosomal dominant fashion. Fumarate hydratase deficiency results in severe neonatal and early infantile encephalopathy that is characterized by poor feeding, failure to thrive, hypotonia, lethargy, and refractory seizures.

Succinyl-CoA synthetase complex (succinate-CoA ligase, encoded by the gene SUCLA2) defects present early in life as Leigh syndrome associated with mitochondrial DNA depletion. Affected neonates manifest accumulation of succinyl carnitine and mild methylmalonic aciduria.

Pathology

The most common finding is a small brain, which is indicative of cerebral underdevelopment. This may appear in radiological studies as cerebral atrophy or ventriculomegaly. When the prominent ventricles of normocephalic children are shunted, the cerebrospinal fluid spaces may collapse, allowing for the eventual manifestation of true microcephaly. This occurs without clinical improvement. Additional findings detected by MR imaging may include white matter abnormalities described as either delayed myelination or hypomyelination, deficient closure of the Sylvian opercula, and brainstem hypoplasia. The corpus callosum may be thin or absent. Diffuse bilateral polymicrogyria may also occur.

Pathophysiology

Surprisingly, severe reductions in the activity of tricarboxylic acid enzymes are compatible with life beyond several months or even years, allowing for a rich symptomatology. The basis for this seems to be the redundancy of many if not most energy metabolism reactions. However, all of these disorders are associated with severe neurological dysfunction. It is suspected that the mechanisms involved in tricarboxylic acid defects are multiple, as illustrated by their diverse clinical manifestations including from mitochondrial DNA depletion to Leigh syndrome to tumorigenesis. This notion defies the simplistic contention that the manifestations of these disorders arise simply from energy failure.

Diagnosis

Urinary organic acid analysis may be highly indicative of specific tricarboxylic acid defects. Enzyme assays conducted in skin fibroblasts or liver are available.

Treatment

None effective. Seizures, when present, are generally refractory to anticonvulsants.

Bibliography

Bourgeron T., Chretien D., Poggi-Bach J., et al (1994). Mutation of the fumarase gene in two siblings with progressive encephalopathy and fumarase deficiency. *J Clin Invest*. 93(6):2514–18.

Pithukpakorn M. (2005). Disorders of pyruvate metabolism and the tricarboxylic acid cycle. *Mol Genet Metab*. 85 (4):243–6.

Other Newborn Mitochondrial Disorders

A 2-week-old boy manifested profound generalized weakness, hypotonia, hyporeflexia, macroglossia, and severe lactic acidosis. The infant improved spontaneously: he held his head at 4 1/2 months, rolled over at 7 months, and walked by 16 months. At 33 months of age, he exhibited mild proximal weakness. Macroglossia disappeared by age 4 months. Blood lactic acid declined steadily and was normal by 14 months of age. Histochemical and ultrastructural studies of muscle biopsy specimens obtained at 1 and 7 months of age showed excessive mitochondria, lipid, and glycogen; a third biopsy at age 36 months showed only atrophy of scattered fibers. Cytochrome c oxidase stain was positive in fewer than 5% of fibers in the first biopsy, in approximately 60% of fibers in the second biopsy, and in all fibers in the third biopsy. Biochemical analysis showed an isolated defect of cytochrome c oxidase activity, which was only 8% of the lowest control level in the first biopsy; the activity increased to 47% in the second biopsy and was greater than normal in the third.

Other Newborn Mitochondrial Disorders

Onset: Variable, with reduced intrauterine growth or neonatal hypotonia and lethargy.

Additional manifestations: Multiorgan failure with predilection for kidney, liver, pancreas, or bone marrow.

Disease mechanism: Stimulation of aerobic metabolism coinciding with birth and early extrauterine life.

Testing: Blood metabolic profiling can reveal lactic acidosis. Sampling of accessible tissues for histological indicators of mitochondrial dysfunction.

Treatment: Supportive care in the case of reversible cytochrome c oxidase-deficient infantile myopathy and coenzyme Q10 in responsive forms of coenzyme Q10 deficiency.

Research highlights: High-throughput DNA sequencing coupled with functional prediction and experimental validation to discover mutated nuclear genes.

Clinical Features

The neonatal mitochondrial disorders comprise severe syndromes that manifest pre or postnatally and often affect multiple organ systems. Several salient syndromes are recognized.

Aminoglycoside-induced hearing loss is a relatively common occurrence among ill newborns due to the use of antibiotics such as gentamycin for suspected infection. It is associated with mutations in at least two mitochondrial-encoded genes, including MTRNR1 (encoding mitochondrial 12S ribosomal RNA) and MTCO1, which codifies for subunit I of cytochrome c oxidase. The mechanism of ototoxicity of aminoglycosides is thought to involve interference with the production of ATP in the mitochondria of hair cells in the cochlea. The aminoglycosides include kanamycin, gentamicin, tobramycin, neomycin, and streptomycin.

GRACILE syndrome comprises growth retardation, aminoaciduria, cholestasis, iron overload, lactic acidosis, and early death. It is associated with mutation of BCS1L, which encodes an ATPase necessary for the insertion of the Rieske protein into complex III. There is intrauterine growth retardation and affected infants are consequently small for gestational age. They develop Fanconi-type aminoaciduria, cholestasis with progressive liver dysfunction, and iron overload with hemosiderosis of the liver. About half of them die in the first few days and the others within weeks after birth. The disease is dominated by liver failure and there are no dysmorphic or neurological features.

Table 18.1 Mitochondrial disorders of the newborn

Neonatal mitochondrial disorder	Genes	Principal organs involved
Aminoglycoside-induced hearing loss	MTRNR1, MTCO1	Inner ear
GRACILE syndrome	BCS1L	Liver, kidney
Pearson syndrome	Mitochondrial DNA deletion	Bone marrow, pancreas
Cytochrome c oxidase deficiency	COX6B1	Brain
Reversible cytochrome c oxidase-deficiency	Mitochondrial tRNAGlu	Skeletal muscle
Complex I deficiency	NDUFA1, NFUFB11	Brain
Primary coenzyme Q10 deficiency	COQ1, COQ2	Brain, muscle
Thymidine kinase 2 deficiency	TK2	Muscle
Hepatocerebral syndromes	DGUOK, MPV17	Liver, brain
Arginyl-transfer RNA synthetase mutations	RARS1	Brain

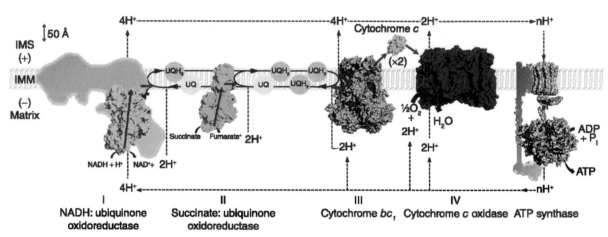

Figure 18.1 Overview of the respiratory chain and ATP synthase. Complexes are scaled to a 50 Å inner mitochondrial membrane. Red arrows represent the transfer of the two electrons produced by the oxidation of NADH or succinate by complex I or II respectively. These electrons are transferred to complex III via the pool of ubiquinone and then to complex IV via soluble cytochrome c. The number of protons, n, required to form ATP is dependent on the number of c subunits in the membrane segment of ATP synthase. Yeast mitochondria have ten c subunits. Hence, passage of ten protons will cause one complete rotation of the rotor and formation of three ATP, giving a value for n of 3.33. The protein complexes were drawn using PyMOL. Reproduced with permission from Rich PR et al. The mitochondrial respiratory chain. *Essays Biochem.* 2010. 47; 1–23.

Pearson syndrome is usually lethal and is caused by a single mitochondrial DNA deletion ranging in size from 1.1 to 10 kb. The syndrome includes refractory sideroblastic anemia, pancytopenia, and exocrine pancreas dysfunction. Pancreatic dysfunction is manifested by steatorrhea. Familial cases have been associated with clinical and neuropathological features of Leigh syndrome. The mitochondrial DNA deletion is usually more abundant in blood than in other tissues.

Cytochrome c oxidase deficiency leads to a severe neonatal syndrome associated with early or fetal death or to reversible infantile myopathy. The severe syndrome is due to homozygous mutation of the nuclear gene COX6B1, which impacts the respiratory chain (Figure 18.1). Children who survive the immediate neonatal period manifest low weight, poor suck, and abnormal breathing, which can evolve to ataxia, weakness, and visual and severe intellectual dysfunction.

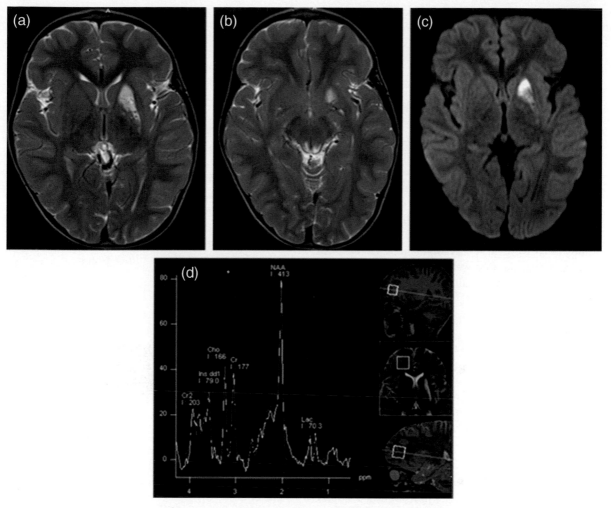

Figure 18.2 Complex I deficiency. **a** and **b.** Axial T2-weighted MR imaging demonstrates abnormal hyperintensity signal lesions in the basal ganglia, especially in the putamen. **c.** Diffusion-weighted MR imaging shows restricted diffusion at the same location. **d.** Magnetic resonance spectroscopy with illustrating a lactate peak in the cortex. Reproduced with permission from Longo MG et al. Brain Imaging and Genetic Risk in the Pediatric Population, Part 1. *Neuroimaging Clin N Amer.* 2015. 25(1), 31–51.

Reversible cytochrome c oxidase-deficient infantile myopathy is associated with congenital hypotonia, severe lactic acidosis and muscle cytochrome c oxidase deficiency detectable both histologically and enzymatically. With adequate support, the hypotonia improves spontaneously, lactic acidosis disappears and muscle tissue reverts to normal. In all cases, a homoplasmic m.T14674C or G mutation in the tRNAGlu of the mitochondrial DNA can be found.

Complex I deficiency is relatively common among the mitochondrial disorders of newborns. Two complex I subunits (NDUFA1 and NFUFB11) are encoded by genes located on the X chromosome.

Hemizygous mutations in NDFUA1 have been associated with disease, including Leigh syndrome (Figure 18.2).

Primary coenzyme Q10 deficiency causes four syndromes: encephalomyopathy, cerebellar ataxia, isolated myopathy, or infantile multisystemic disease. The latter is the only phenotype that manifests in the neonatal period. Defects of the gene COQ1, which regulates the first step in coenzyme Q10 biosynthesis (decaprenyl diphosphate synthase subunit 2, PDSS2), lead to neonatal hypotonia, refractory seizures, episodic vomiting, and nephrosis. MR imaging of the brain can reveal symmetrical abnormalities of the basal ganglia suggestive of Leigh syndrome. Mutations in the gene COQ2, which encodes the second biosynthetic enzyme, are associated with infantile encephalomyopathy and nephrosis followed by multiorgan failure. In some cases, coenzyme Q10 supplementation may be effective.

Thymidine kinase 2 mutations can lead to weakness and hypotonia at birth with a mean age at death of 3.5 years. Skeletal muscle is the main target tissue, but the anterior horn cells of the spinal cord may be severely affected such that the clinical presentation may resemble spinal muscular atrophy.

A fatal hepatocerebral syndrome due to mutations in the gene DGUOK (deoxyguanosine kinase) leads to neonatal liver failure, nystagmus, hypotonia, and abnormal neurological developmental. Onset is at birth or within the first weeks of life. A similar hepatocerebral syndrome is caused by MPV17 mutations, which code for an abnormal mitochondrial inner membrane protein.

Arginyl-transfer RNA synthetase (RARS1) mutations can lead to neonatal hypotonic and lethargy with cerebellar vermian hypoplasia and early death. In the infant, RARS1 mutations cause hypomyelinating leukodystrophy-9, associated with severe spasticity of the lower limbs, mild spasticity of the upper limbs, nystagmus, and mental retardation.

Pathology

Muscle biopsy of fresh frozen tissue provides a test bed in which to assay specific mitochondrial complex deficiencies both histochemically and enzymatically. MR imaging of the brain can reveal the lesions characteristic of Leigh syndrome, ventriculomegaly, cerebellar hypoplasia or an abnormal white matter composition. Some of these disorders also cause lactic acidemia. In Pearson syndrome, bone marrow examination reveals ringed sideroblasts, normoblasts with excessive deposits of iron in mitochondria detected by iron stains.

Pathophysiology

The disease mechanism of most mitochondrial diseases is unknown or remains poorly understood. Anaerobic glycolysis is the major source of cellular energy in the fetus. This may account for the relatively low prevalence of fetal loss in well-established mitochondrial diseases. In contrast, the rapidly increasing energy requirements of the neonate can explain the frequent neonatal presentation of these disorders. The all-or-none nature of Mendelian disorders, which contrasts with the heteroplasmic nature of mitochondrial DNA mutations may explain why severe mutations in nuclear genes cause early onset and often rapidly fatal diseases whereas mitochondrial DNA-related disorders tend to manifest later in life and follow a relatively milder course.

Diagnosis

Blood metabolic profiling can reveal lactic acidosis. Sampling of accessible tissues allows access to histological, biochemical, or enzymatic indicators of mitochondrial dysfunction.

Treatment

None effective except in some cases of coenzyme Q10 deficiency, which may respond to supplementation with this cofactor. Standard medical care can afford sufficient time (months or years) for reversible cytochrome c oxidase-deficient infantile myopathy to subside.

Bibliography

DiMauro S., Garone C. (2011). Metabolic disorders of fetal life: Glycogenoses and mitochondrial defects of the mitochondrial respiratory chain. *Semin Fetal Neonatal Med.* 16(4):181–89.

DiMauro S., Nicholson J.F., Hays A.P., et al (1983). Benign infantile mitochondrial myopathy due to reversible cytochrome c oxidase deficiency. *Ann Neurol.* 14(2):226–34.

Chapter 19

Organic Acidemias of the Newborn

*A girl was born at 40 weeks gestation via elective cesarean section because of a prenatal finding of hydrocephalus. At birth, she displayed small supra-orbital ridges with long eyelashes, a small jaw and neck and prominent lips. There were mild joint contractures and a murmur was audible. Cardiomyopathy was soon noted and treated. She was hypotonic in the neck and poorly reactive to her environment. However, she could perceive light and sound and exhibited erratic irregular eye movements. Her limbs were rigid and her tendon reflexes abnormally brisk. Her plantar responses were flexor. Her urine contained 2-D-hydroxyglutaric acid and hydroxymethyl-glutaric acid and her plasma an excess of the glutaric acid conjugate of acylcarnitine, indicating the diagnosis of 2-D-hydroxyglutaric acidemia. A cerebrospinal fluid reservoir was inserted and serially drained within hours of delivery. This was replaced with a ventriculoperitoneal shunt the second week of life without resolution of ventriculomegaly (**Figure 19.1**). She remained largely immobile and nonreactive and would smile only on certain days. At one month of life, she manifested flexor infantile spasms, which became as frequent as one every five minutes. She was treated with anticonvulsants, but her seizures evolved to daily myoclonic events. Her serum transaminases became elevated, but a hepatic biopsy was normal. At 10 years old, her neurological development had remained stagnant and daily seizures persisted.*

Organic Acidemias of the Newborn

Onset: Irritability, feeding difficulties, vomiting, and metabolic acidosis at birth.

Additional manifestations: Cardiomyopathy, nephropathy, epilepsy, and dysmorphic features. Unusual body odor in select disorders.

Disease mechanism: Accumulation of acidic protein catabolism byproducts following removal of the amino group of amino acids.

Testing: Relatively specific patterns of organic aciduria, aided by determination of urinary acylglycines and serum acylcarnitines.

Treatment: Hemodialysis, enzyme cofactor supplementation in select disorders, and repletion of excess carnitine consumption. Specific infant nutrition formulas.

Research highlights: Chemical and clinical phenotype correlations aided by an increased identification of affected neonates via newborn screening.

Clinical Features

The organic acidemias result from deficient amino acid catabolism. As a group, the organic acidemias affect 1 in 10,000 births and are usually heritable in autosomal recessive fashion. The manifestations of organic acidemia range from asymptomatic findings in urinary organic acid analysis to severe encephalopathy, cardiopathy, or nephropathy. The most severe disorders present in the newborn.

Following the first feedings, the neonate becomes irritable, feeds with difficulty, and vomits. Lethargy, hypotonia, and weakness ensue over time. The first diagnostic assays usually reveal metabolic acidosis, hyperammonemia, and ketonuria.

Additional manifestations are more variable and include seizures, cardiomyopathy, hepatopathy, and nephropathy with renal failure.

Some of the most significant organic acidemias are summarized here.

Table 19.1 Some organic acidemias that affect the newborn

Organic acidemia	Neonatal and infantile manifestations	Enzyme defect
2-D-hydroxyglutaric acidemia	Hypotonia Blindness Facial dysmorphic features Cardiomyopathy Epilepsy	D-2-hydroxyglutarate dehydrogenase or isocitrate dehydrogenase 2 (Figure 19.2 and 3)
2-L-hydroxyglutaric acidemia	Hypotonia Seizures Abnormal white matter (Figure 19.1) Cerebellar hypoplasia Basal ganglia injury	L-2-hydroxyglutarate dehydrogenase or solute carrier family 25 member 1 (SLC25A1) in combined 2-D- and 2-L-hydroxyglutaric acidemia
Glutaric acidemia type I	Frontotemporal (opercular) hipoplasia (Figure 19.4) Subdural hematoma Retinal hemorrhages Pallidal injury Encephalopathy crises after minor illnesses Generalized dystonia	Glutaryl-coenzyme A dehydrogenase (Figure 19.5)
Methylmalonic acidemia	Encephalopathy crises Epilepsy Dyskinetic movement disorders Basal ganglia injury (Figure 19.6) Renal failure Pancreatitis	Methylmalonyl-coenzyme A mutase (Figure 19.7)
Propionic acidemia	Hypotonia Lethargy and coma Seizures Neutropenia Metabolic stroke Cerebral edema Basal ganglia injury (Figure 19.8) Spastic quadriparesis Athetosis	Propionyl-coenzyme A carboxylase

Pathology

In children expiring during an acute metabolic crisis, cerebral hypoxic–ischemic changes can be prominent.

Alzheimer type II astroglial proliferation has been observed in select disorders associated with selective glial vulnerability such as propionic acidemia. White matter spongiosis or microscopic edema has also been observed.

Excitocity, typical of glutaric acidemia type 1, is associated with severe neuronal loss with postsynaptic vacuolation and with fibrillary gliosis in the striatum and cortex.

Pathophysiology

During the course of protein degradation, the amino group of amino acids is removed, yielding weak acids that can be toxic to cells when they accumulate in excess. Once produced in an amount that exceeds a critical level, these metabolites may accumulate beyond toxic levels due to limited efflux through the blood brain barrier.

Severe acidosis and hyperammonemia are additional independent pathogenic factors.

Excitotoxicity due to excess excitatory amino acids action via glutamatergic (NMDA (N-methyl-D-aspartate) and non-NMDA) receptors, impairment of

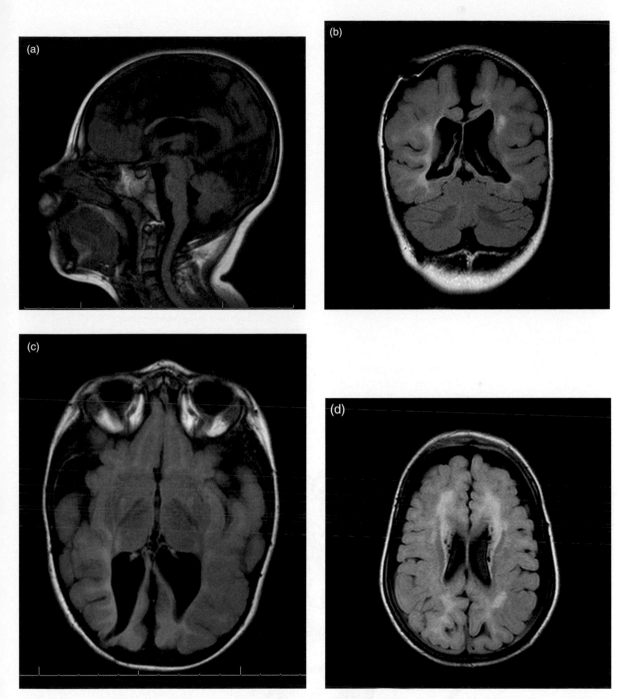

Figure 19.1 a to d: MR imaging of a 7-year-old child with 2-D-hydroxyglutaric aciduria. There is absence of normal white matter, whereas the remainder white matter is possibly dysmyelinated or gliotic. The gyral pattern is simplified, with underopercularization. There is also occipital lobe encephalomalacia, perhaps relating to additional ischemic injury. e: Chest X ray of the same child illustrating cardiomegaly caused associated with cardiomyopathy.

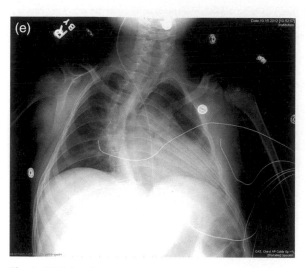

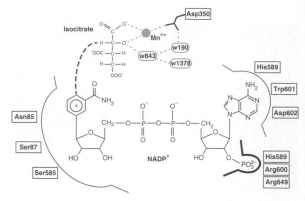

Figure 19.1 (*cont.*)

Figure 19.2 Mechanism of isocitrate dehydrogenase 2. Schematic diagram illustrating the interactions of the cofactor NADP+, isocitrate-Mn2+, and nearby amino acid residues in isocitrate dehydrogenase 2. The residues shown in the thick square (His589, Arg600, and Arg649) denote those essential for the cofactor recognition. In this diagram, isocitrate-Mn2+, Asp350, and three water molecules (w843, w190, and w1378) are also included. The thick dotted line represents the pathway of hydride transfer. Reproduced with permission from Yasutake Y et al. Crystal structure of the monomeric isocitrate dehydrogenase in the presence of NADP+: insight into the cofactor recognition, catalysis, and evolution. *J Biol Chem.* 2003; 278(38):36897–904.

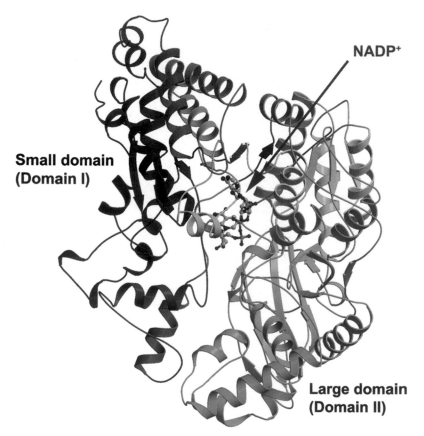

Figure 19.3 Ribbon diagram of the isocitrate dehydrogenase in complex with cofactor NADP+. The structure of the AvIDH consists of two domains, a small domain (Domain I) and a large domain (Domain II). The NADP+ was located at the interdomain cleft and interacted with domain I. The model is colored according to the sequence by a rainbow color ramp from blue at the N-terminal segment to red at the C-terminal segment. The bound NADP+ is represented as a ball-and-stick model. Reproduced with permission from Yasutake Y et al. Crystal structure of the monomeric isocitrate dehydrogenase in the presence of NADP+: insight into the cofactor recognition, catalysis, and evolution. *J Biol Chem.* 2003; 278(38):36897–904.

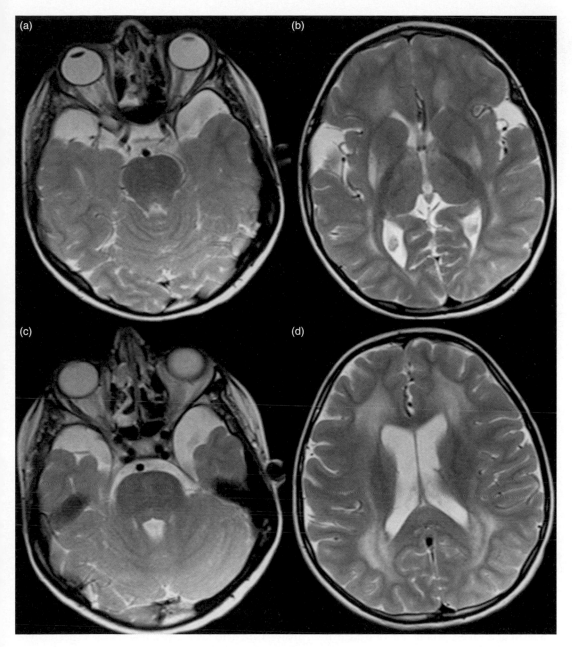

Figure 19.4 a to **d.** Glutaric aciduria I. Axial T2-weighted MR images illustrating widening cerebrospinal fluid spaces anterior to temporal lobes enlargement of the sylvian fissures and increased signal intensities in bilateral lentiform nuclei and periventricular deep white matter Reproduced with permission from Kurtcan et al. MRS features during encephalopathic crisis period in 11 years old case with GA-1. *Brain and Development.* 2015. 37(5), 546–551. **e.** Sequential MR imaging of a child between the ages of 19 days and 36 months (T2-weighted images, except for fluid attenuated inversion recovery images, right upper corner). MR images document normalization of frontotemporal hypoplasia (unilateral long arrows) and disappearance of subependymal pseudocysts (short arrows) and cavum vergae. The term newborn has an immature pattern of gyration and myelination normally observed at 34–35 weeks postconceptional age with too shallow and less branched sulci (arrowheads) and slightly, diffusely T2 hyperintense white matter. The adult gyral pattern is normally reached by 3 months, and on follow-up study, gyration is adequate for age. Myelination at 24 months is still insufficient in the subcortical temporal and frontal white matter, but at 36 months myelination is complete and the MR images are now normal. Reproduced with permission from Harting I et al. Dynamic changes of striatal and extrastriatal abnormalities in glutaric aciduria type I. *Brain.* 2009;132(Pt 7):1764–82.

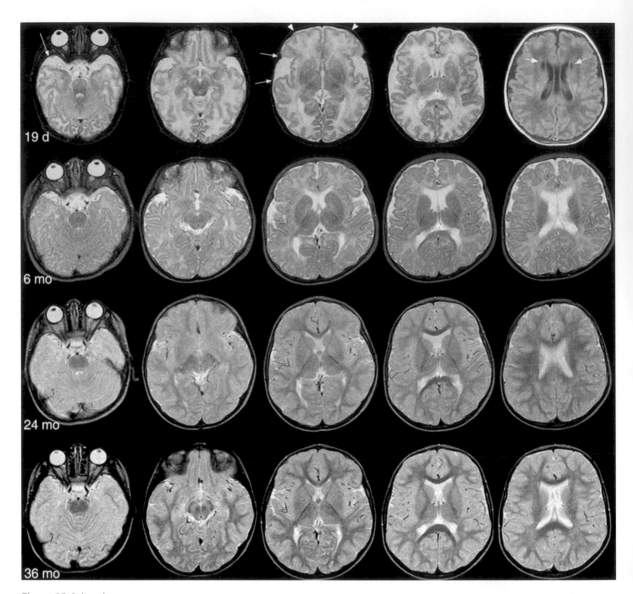

Figure 19.4 *(cont.)*

energy metabolism and excess production of oxidative substances have been postulated in specific disorders.

Organic acids that accumulate in excess can inhibit bioenergetics in brain and other high energy dependent tissues, leading to secondary mitochondrial impairment.

Diagnosis

Routine plasma assays document acidosis, elevated lactate and pyruvate, increased ammonia, and decreased bicarbonate in severe cases. Specific patterns of metabolites detectable via urinary organic acid

analysis are detectable depending on each specific type of organic acidemia. Analysis of urinary acylglycine conjugates can further help identify specific disorders. Plasma acylcarnitine analysis may also illustrate deficiency in select metabolic reactions.

Treatment

The first general intervention when organic acidemia is suspected is cessation of dietary protein administration while maintaining adequate caloric balance. This can be achieved via intravenous glucose administration.

(a)

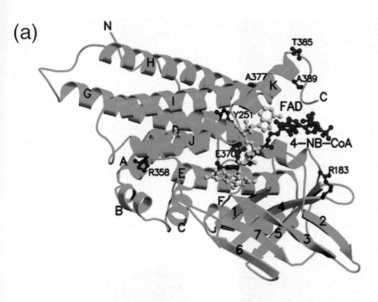

(b)

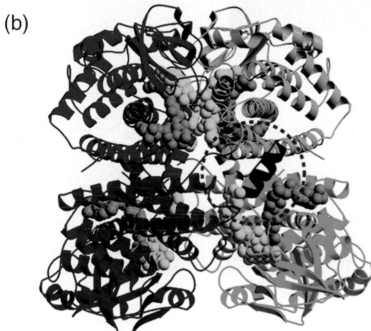

Figure 19.5 Overall polypeptide fold of glutaryl-CoA dehydrogenase. Ribbon diagram of a monomer (a) and a tetramer (b) of glutaryl-CoA dehydrogenase. Gold and purple subunits form one dimer, and green and blue subunits make the other dimer of the tetramer. Red dotted circle surrounding the dark green helix (helix K) of the green subunit depicts the subunit interface. Reproduced with permission from Fu Z, et al. Crystal structures of human glutaryl-CoA dehydrogenase with and without an alternate substrate: structural bases of dehydrogenation and decarboxylation reactions. *Biochemistry.* 2004; 43(30): 9674–84.

Hemodialysis has been used as a first-line, short term treatment to alleviate blood and tissue organic acid accumulation.

In some cases, cofactor supplementation aids catalysis by the defective enzyme and improves disease manifestations. These include cobalamine-responsive methylmalonic acidemia, riboflavin glutaryl coenzyme A dehydrogenase deficiency (glutaric acidemia type 1) and biotin-responsive holocarboxylase synthetase deficiency.

Special infant diet formulas are available depending on the enzymatic defect. These formulas contain only the minimum necessary quantities of the amino acid that cannot be normally metabolized while providing other proteins, fats, and carbohydrates.

Liver and renal transplantation have been performed in methylmalonic acidemia and maple syrup urine disease.

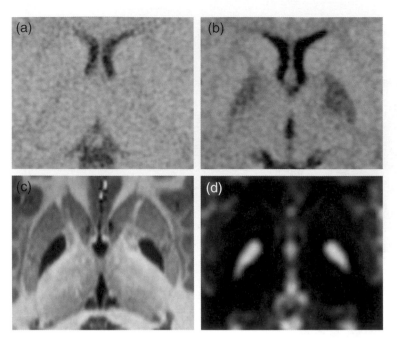

Figure 19.6 Progression of a globus pallidus infarct in methylmalonic aciduria. This 16-month-old child was known to have methylmalonic aciduria that had been diagnosed 6 months previously. Within 24 hours after onset of symptoms from gastroenteritis, she became lethargic and was taken to the emergency department. **a.** Computerized tomography at the time of admission to the hospital appears normal. **b.** Computerized tomography scan 35 hours later shows distinct hypoattenuating abnormalities involving the entirety of each globus pallidus. Diffusion weighted MR imaging performed 1 week later showed restricted diffusion in each globus pallidus (image not shown). **c.** High-resolution MR images and T2-weighted images (**d**) acquired 7.5 years later demonstrate bilateral complete globus pallidus infarcts. Reproduced with permission from Baker EH et al. MRI characteristics of globus pallidus infarcts in isolated methylmalonic acidemia. *AJNR Am J Neuroradiol.* 2015; 36(1): 194–201.

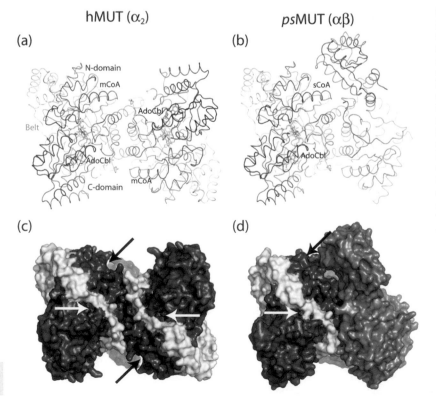

Figure 19.7 Dimeric assembly of human and bacterial methylmalonyl-coenzyme A mutase (MUT). Cartoon and surface representations of the human MUT homodimer (a, c) and *Propionibacterium shermanii* MUT heterodimer (b, d). Catalytic subunits (a) are colored according to domain architecture (N-domain, blue; C-domain, magenta; interdomain belt, yellow). The bacterial regulatory subunit (ß) is colored gray. In panels c and d, the cofactor binding pocket and substrate binding channel are indicated by white arrow and black arrow, respectively. mCoA: malonyl-coenzyme A; Cbl: cobalamin; sCoA: succinyl-coenzyme A. Reproduced with permission from Froese DS et al. Structures of the human GTPase MMAA and vitamin B12-dependent methylmalonyl-CoA mutase and insight into their complex formation. *J Biol Chem.* 2010; 285(49): 38204-13.

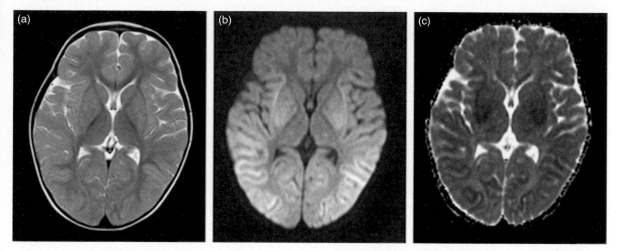

Figure 19.8 Neuroimaging findings in propionic acidemia. Male child, symptomatic from day 4 of life, diagnosed at the age of 4 months. An MR imaging study was obtained at the age of 5 years when he developed acute encephalopathy. Cerebral cortices especially of the temporal and occipital lobes and the basal ganglia (caudate and lentiform nuclei) are swollen and mildly hyperintense on axial T2 weighthed images (a). Hyperintensity on diffusion weigthed images (b) and low intensity on absolute diffusion coefficient maps (c) suggestive of restricted diffusion are seen in the affected regions. Reproduced with permission from Baumgartner MR et al. Proposed guidelines for the diagnosis and management of methylmalonic and propionic acidemia. *Orphanet J Rare Dis.* 2014; 9:130.

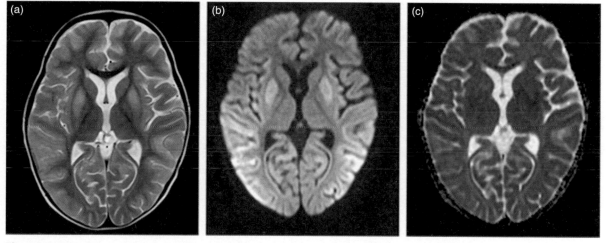

Figure 19.9 Propionic acidemia. Continuation of studies performed in the same child from Figure 19.8. A week later, a repeat MR study shows more intense T2 signal changes in the involved regions, more prominent in the putamina (a). Although a higher signal intensity is noted in the cortices and basal ganglia on diffusion weigthed images (b), with disappearance of low signal of the cortices and presence of higher signal intensity on absolute diffusion coefficient maps (c), there is pseudonormalization of diffusion restriction. Reproduced with permission from Baumgartner MR et al. Proposed guidelines for the diagnosis and management of methylmalonic and propionic acidemia. *Orphanet J Rare Dis.* 2014; 9:130.

Bibliography

Burlina A.B., Bonafé L., Zacchello F. (1999). Clinical and biochemical approach to the neonate with a suspected inborn error of amino acid and organic acid metabolism. *Semin Perinatol.* 23(2):162–73.

Seashore M.R., Seashore C.J. (2005). Newborn screening and the pediatric practitioner. *Semin Perinatol.* 29(3):182–8.

Molybdenum Cofactor Deficiency

*A term female baby was the first child of non-consanguineous parents. Her mother had reported sustained abdominal trembling similar to the vibration of a mobile telephone during the third trimester. Prenatal ultrasonography revealed an enlarged cisterna magna. She was delivered by cesarean section because of decelerating fetal heartbeat. Her initial activity level was appropriate following a one minute Apgar score of 7 and a five minute Apgar score of 9, but she soon became progressive tachypneic. When 14 hours old, clonic seizures with upward gaze were noted. Brain ultrasonography (**Figure 20.1**) revealed multicystic leukoencephalopathy of the parietal areas. Brain MR imaging confirmed and expanded this finding. Elevated urine sulfite was detected (80 mg/L) in the context of a normal serum uric acid (5.5 mg/dL). Isolated sulfite oxidase deficiency was confirmed by the demonstration of a maternally inherited nonsense mutation and a paternally inherited missense mutation in the SUOX gene.*

Treatment: Molybdenum may benefit children with gephryn mutations.
Research highlights: Administration of molybdenum cofactor precursors to infants early in the disease course.

Clinical Features

All molybdenum-containing enzymes require the same molybdenum cofactor, which is synthesized via a highly conserved set of biochemical reactions all organisms. Four molybdenum dependent-enzymes are known in man: aldehyde oxidase, mitochondrial amidoxime reducing component, xanthine oxidoreductase, and sulfite oxidase. Consequently, autosomal recessive mutations in genes that encode biosynthetic molybdenum cofactor enzymes impact the activities of all molybdenum-dependent enzymes and result in a combined form of molybdenum cofactor deficiency which is clinically indistinguishable from isolated sulfite oxidase deficiency. In contrast, sulfite oxidase defects are caused by autosomal recessive mutations in the gene for the corresponding enzyme. Isolated sulfite oxidase deficiency and the combined deficiency of all molybdenum cofactor-dependent enzymes, however, can be differentiated by biochemical assays demonstrating elevated xanthine and decreased uric acid as a result of the simultaneous loss of xanthine oxidoreductase deficiency in combined molybdenum cofactor deficiency.

Molybdenum cofactor and sulfite oxidase deficiency are predominantly neurological disorders and may not be immediately apparent at birth. On occasion, nonspecific facial dysmorphic features, of which a coarsened facies is the most common, are noted. Within hours or days of birth, however, feeding

Molybdenum Cofactor Deficiency

Onset: Facial dysmorphic features, intractable neonatal seizures, and feeding difficulties.
Additional manifestations: Opisthotonus and exaggerated startle reflex. Brain cyst formation and dislocated lens.
Disease mechanism: Elevated sulfite levels lead to progressive neurological damage.
Testing: Elevated urinary sulfites and decreased plasma uric acid. Elevated serum xanthine in the context of decreased uric acid differentiates molybdenum cofactor deficiency from sulfite oxidase deficiency.

difficulties are accompanied by seizures refractory to anticonvulsants. Opisthotonus and an exaggerated startle reaction may be prominent. Some children have been diagnosed with hypoxic–ischemic encephalopathy and neonatal hyperekplexia based on these findings alone. The appearance of progressive cerebral atrophy and ventricular dilatation, however, help eventually rule out these conditions (Figure 20.1). Children who survive the neonatal period in most cases manifest severe mental retardation as well as dislocated lenses and usually do not learn to sit or speak.

Pathology

Generalized cerebral atrophy, microgyria, and ventricular enlargement are common features of both molybdenum cofactor and sulfite oxidase deficiency. Additional features of these diseases are identifiable radiologically and may include multicystic white matter lesions, symmetrical lesions of the globi pallidi and subthalamic regions, pontocerebellar hypoplasia with retrocerebellar cyst, Dandy-Walker malformation and dysgenesis of corpus callosum (Figure 20.2). In a few cases, cerebral edema has been prominent.

Pathophysiology

Elevated sulfite levels lead to progressive neurological damage, while the contribution of other potentially detrimental metabolites such as taurine, S-sulfocysteine, and thiosulfate to the disease progression is not yet known.

In contrast to molybdenum itself, molybdenum cofactor or its precursors cannot be derived from nutritional sources. This phenomenon, together with an absence of endogenous recycling reactions, requires all of the molybdenum cofactor to be synthesized de novo (Figures 20.3 and 20.4). All proteins involved in molybdenum cofactor biosynthesis are

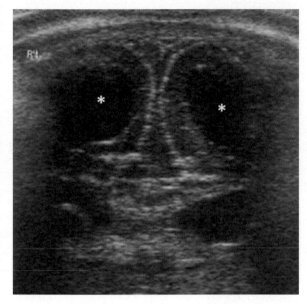

Figure 20.1 Sulfite oxidase deficiency in a newborn. Ultrasonography via the anterior fontanelle reveals cystic leukoencephalopathy (asterisks) in coronal view. Reproduced with permission from Chen LW et al, Prenatal multicystic encephalopathy in isolated sulfite oxidase deficiency with a novel mutation. *Pediatr Neurol.* 2014; 51(1): 181–82.

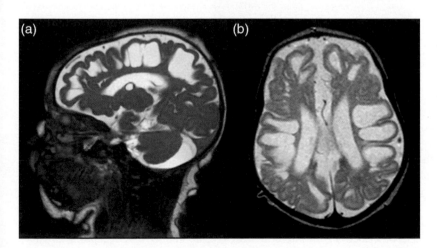

Figure 20.2 Sagittal magnetic resonance image with 3-mm slice thickness using fast imaging using steady-state acquisition sequence (FIESTA) (a) and axial T2-weighted magnetic resonance image (b) reveal extensive cystic encephalomalacia. Reproduced with permission from Chen LW et al, Prenatal multicystic encephalopathy in isolated sulfite oxidase deficiency with a novel mutation. *Pediatr Neurol.* 2014; 51(1): 181–82.

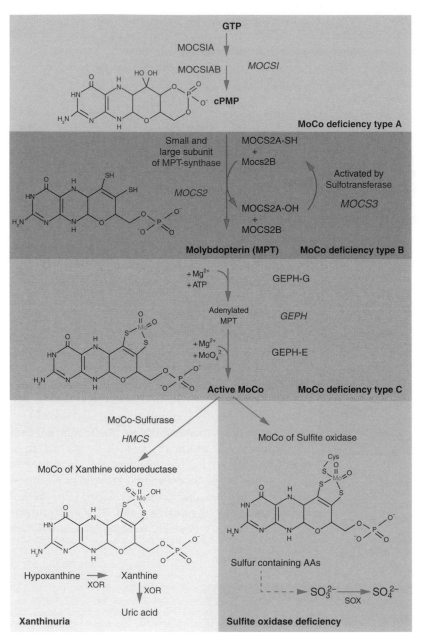

Figure 20.3 Biosynthesis of molybdemun cofactor via an ancient pathway common to all free-living species and types of diseases as a consequence of mutations in the different genes. MOCS1A belongs to the superfamily of S-adenosylmethionine-dependent radical enzymes, members of which catalyze the formation of radicals by a protein-bound [4Fe-4S] cluster. It is speculated that the B domain of the MOCS1AB fusion protein might function as a radical acceptor. The two MOCS2 proteins A and B are subunits of molybdopterin synthase incorporating sulfur groups delivered by the MOCS3 sulfurylase. Finally, molybdenum is attached to these sulfur groups in a two-step reaction catalyzed by the GPHN-encoded two-domain protein gephyrin. Reproduced with permission from Reiss J et al. Molybdenum cofactor deficiency: Mutations in GPHN, MOCS1, and MOCS2. *Hum Mutat.* 2011; 32(1): 10–18.

encoded by autosomal genes and heterozygous mutations are asymptomatic. Homozygosity for nonfunctional mutant forms of any of these proteins abolishes molybdenum cofactor biosynthesis completely, thereby impacting the activity of all the molybdenum cofactor-dependent enzymes, including sulfite oxidase (Figure 20.5).

The majority of mutations that cause molybdenum cofactor deficiency have been described in the genes of molybdenum cofactor synthesis step 1 and molybdenum cofactor synthesis step 2 with a few affected individuals harboring mutations in the gephrin gene GPHN.

Gephrin is a multifunctional protein involved in molybdemun cofactor biosynthesis and in molecular assembly, anchoring inhibitory neurotransmitter receptors to the postsynaptic cytoskeleton. Gephrin interacts with glycine and GABA receptors, possibly

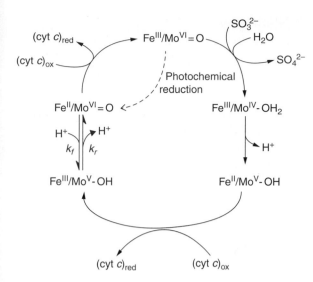

Figure 20.4 Proposed oxidation state changes occurring at the Mo and Fe centers of native animal sulfite oxidase during the catalytic oxidation of sulfite and the concomitant reduction of cytochrome (cyt c). Only the equatorial oxygen atom among the ligands of Mo is shown. Reproduced with permission from Feng C et al. Sulfite oxidizing enzymes. *Biochim Biophys Acta*. 2007; 1774(5):527–39.

influencing the molecular composition of inhibitory synapses. Some mutations in gephrin can also cause startle disease.

Diagnosis

Molybdenum cofactor deficiency and sulfite oxidase deficiency are often associated with decreased serum uric acid and elevated urine sulfites. Elevated serum xanthine in the context of decreased uric acid is characteristic of molybdenum cofactor deficiency, in contrast with sulfite oxidase deficiency, in which xanthine is normal.

Treatment

Using a mouse model of molybdenum cofactor deficiency, gene therapy with adeno-associated vectors has proven feasible. Although the phenotype may be reverted by injection of capsids carrying a molybdenum cofactor synthesis step 1 expression cassette, long term experiments reveal an increased risk for malignancies.

In man, administration of high levels of inorganic molybdenum has proven ineffective. However, this approach may be feasible in individuals with gephrin mutations on the basis of cell culture evidence. A diet

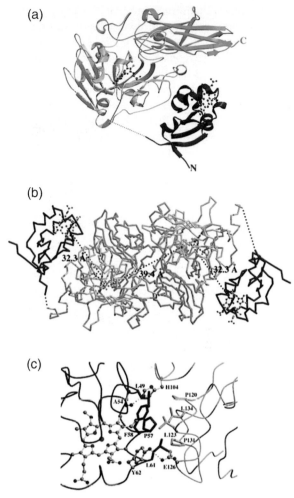

Figure 20.5 Structure of sulfite oxidase. **a.** The monomer with the N-terminal domain drawn in red, the Mo-cofacor domain in yellow, and the C-terminal domain in green. The N and the C terminals are labeled with N and C, respectively. The dotted line between domains I and II indicates the loop region. The Mo-cofactor and the heme are shown in ball-and-stick representation with the Fe atom in purple and the Mo atom in green. **b.** Ca trace of the sulfite oxidase dimer. The gray dotted lines connect the metal centers of the cofactors and indicate the distances between the Mo and Fe within the monomer and the Mo-Mo distance between the two monomers. **c.** Interface between the N-terminal and the Mo-cofactor domain. Aliphatic residues are shown in all-bonds representation whereas the heme and residues involved in hydrogen bonding are shown in ball-and-stick representation. Dotted lines indicate hydrogen bonds. Reproduced with permission from Kisker C et al. Molecular basis of sulfite oxidase deficiency from the structure of sulfite oxidase. *Cell*. 1997; 91(7):973–83.

low in sulfur amino acids has in some cases resulted in a significant reduction of abnormal sulfur metabolites, although no neurological improvement could be observed.

Intravenous administration of the molybdenum cofactor precursor cyclic pyranopterin monophosphate (also known as precursor Z or cPMP) was used in a child homozygous for a molybdenum cofactor synthesis step 1B (mutation Gly588Arg), which is associated with defective cPMP synthesis. Normalization of the previously elevated levels of S-sulfocysteine and thiosulfate was achieved and the child regained her level of alertness and remains seizure-free.

Bibliography

Chen L.W., Tsai Y.S., Huang C.C. (2014). Prenatal multicystic encephalopathy in isolated sulfite oxidase deficiency with a novel mutation. *Pediatr Neurol.* 51(1):181–2.

Reiss J., Hahnewald R. (2011). Molybdenum cofactor deficiency: Mutations in GPHN, MOCS1, and MOCS2. *Hum Mutat.* 32(1):10–18.

Urea Cycle Defects

A full-term, 3-day-old infant presented to the emergency department with poor feeding, increased work of breathing and encephalopathy one day after having been discharged from the hospital in good health. On the evening after discharge, his parents noted that he became sleepy and lost interest in feeding over the next 12 hours. The following morning, they noted that his breathing was rapid. His general examination at presentation revealed suprasternal retractions, a flat anterior fontanelle and an enlarged liver. Neurologic examination was notable for marked encephalopathy, as he did not open his eyes or react to stimulation. His suck was weak and poorly coordinated and his gag reflex was absent. He lay in a frog-legged position; however, tone was increased in all 4 extremities. There were no spontaneous movements or motor response to noxious stimulation. Tendon reflexes were symmetrically brisk without ankle clonus. Head CT in the emergency room revealed cerebral edema. Ammonia was elevated at 770 µM (reference <49 µM). Arterial blood gas showed a mild respiratory alkalosis. Serum glucose and anion gap were normal. Low blood citrulline in conjunction high orotic acid, high glutamine and alanine, and normal arginine indicated ornithine transcarbamylase deficiency.

Testing: Plasma ammonia and amino acids and urinary orotic acid are indicative of individual urea cycle defects. Enzyme assay identifies specific defects.
Treatment: Reduction of protein intake, prevention of hypercatabolism, and detoxification of excess ammonia via hemofiltration. Liver transplantation.
Research highlights: Correlation between symptom severity and flux through the cycle in carriers of ornithine transcarbamylase deficiency.

Urea Cycle Defects

Onset: Lethargy and feeding difficulties in the newborn. Intellectual disability in the older child in milder forms.
Additional manifestations: Coma and seizures in newborns. Dietary protein intolerance later in life with episodic hyperammonemia.
Disease mechanism: Osmolar excess due to hyperammonemia. Accumulation of glutamate with excitotoxicity and decreased nitric oxide synthesis.

Clinical Features

The urea cycle disorders result from defects in the metabolism of waste nitrogen arising from the breakdown of protein and other nitrogen-containing molecules. The incidence of urea cycle defects is 1 in 8,500 births. These disorders include ornithine transcarbamoylase deficiency, argininosuccinate lyase deficiency, carbamoyl phosphate synthetase deficiency, citrullinemia (or argininosuccinate deficiency) and argininemia (or arginase deficiency). In addition, they may also be considered to include deficiency of N-acetylglutamate synthase, which results in defective synthesis of the carbamoyl phosphate synthetase activator N-acetylglutamate, and deficiency of the mitochondrial ornithine transporter, which causes the hyperornithinemia-hyperammonemia-homocitrullinuria syndrome. Lastly, deficiency of the glutamate-aspartate antiporter citrin causes primarily hepatic disease. With the exception of ornithine transcarbamylase deficiency, which is an X-lined disorder, all are heritable in autosomal recessive fashion.

Newborns with a severe urea cycle disorder are initially normal but soon develop cerebral edema, lethargy, stupor or coma, feeding difficulties, hyper or hypoventilation, hypothermia, seizures (in about 50 percent of cases), and rigidity or posturing

Table 21.1 Urea cycle and related disorders

Enzyme defects	Gene	Transporter defects	Gene
Ornithine transcarbamylase	OTC	Ornithine /citrulline transporter ORNT1	SLC25A15
Argininosuccinate lyase	ASL	Glutamate/ aspartate antiporter citrin	SLC25A13
Carbamoyl phosphate synthetase	CPS1		
Citrullinemia	ASS1		
Arginase	ARG1		
N-acetylglutamate synthase	NAGS		

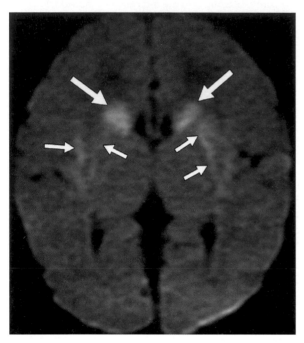

Figure 21.1 2-week-old boy with urea cycle disorder and encephalopathy who presented with recurrent vomiting and lethargy. Axial diffusion-weighted MR image shows areas of diffusion hyperintensity involving head of bilateral caudate nuclei (large arrows) with some putaminal involvement (small arrows). Reproduced with permission from Ibrahim M et al. Inborn errors of metabolism: combining clinical and radiologic clues to solve the mystery. *AJR Am J Roentgenol.* 2014; 203(3): W315–27.

(Figure 21.1). An encephalopathic, slow-wave EEG pattern may be observed during hyperammonemia, whereas cerebral atrophy may be seen on cranial MR imaging after an episode resolves. In milder deficiencies of these enzymes and in arginase deficiency, ammonia accumulation may be subtle or only precipitated by other illnesses, pregnancy, or other forms of metabolic stress at any time later in life. Such precipitants include surgery, prolonged fasting and the puerperium. Sleep disorders, delusions, hallucinations, and psychosis may occur during decompensation episodes.

Carbamoylphosphate synthetase deficiency is the most severe of the urea cycle defects (Figure 21.2). Individuals with complete deficiency develop hyperammonemia in the newborn period. Children who are successfully rescued from crises remain at significant risk for repeated episodes of hyperammonemia. Deficiency of N-acetylglutamate synthase defects resemble carbamoylphosphate synthetase deficiency, as the latter is rendered inactive in the absence of the former.

Ornithine transcarbamylase deficiency in males is as severe as carbamoylphosphate synthetase deficiency (Figure 21.3). Approximately 15 percent of carrier females also develop hyperammonemia during their lifetime and many require chronic treatment to avoid it. Carrier women who do not manifest symptoms of hyperammonemia may display intellectual deficits.

In citrullinemia type I, the hyperammonemia can also be severe. However, affected individuals are able to incorporate a fraction of nitrogen into urea cycle intermediates, rendering the treatment of citrullinemia type I more feasible.

Argininosuccinic aciduria can also present with acute hyperammonemia in the neonatal period. This enzyme defect is past the reaction in the metabolic cycle in which all the waste nitrogen has been incorporated into cycle intermediates. Some individuals develop hepatomegaly with elevation of serum transaminases. Liver biopsy shows enlarged hepatocytes, which may progress to fibrosis. Trichorrhexis nodosa with brittle hair is also an associated feature, which responds favorably to arginine supplementation. Significant intellectual impairment can be manifest even in the absence of episodes of hyperammonemic coma.

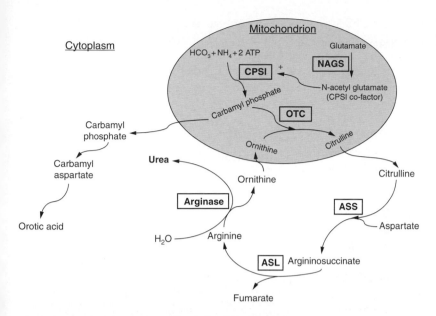

Figure 21.2 The urea cycle. ASL: argininosuccinic acid lyase; ASS: argininosuccinic acid synthetase; CPSI: carbamoyl phosphate synthetase I; NAGS: N-acetylglutamate synthetase; OTC: ornithine transcarbamylase. Reproduced with permission from Gelfand AA, Sznewajs A, Glass HC, Jelin AC, Sherr EH. Clinical Reasoning: An encephalopathic 3-day-old infant. *Neurology.* 2011; 77(1): e1–5.

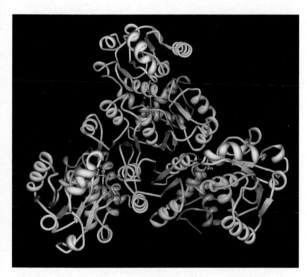

Figure 21.3 Ribbon representation of the ornithine transcarbamylase trimer. The three carbamoylphosphates are represented in ball and stick format. Reproduced with permission from Shi D et al. Human ornithine transcarbamylase: crystallographic insights into substrate recognition and conformational changes. *Biochem J.* 2001; 354(Pt 3): 501–9.

Arginase deficiency leads to hyperammonemia more rarely. Instead, affected individuals develop progressive spasticity resembling hereditary spastic paraplegia and can also manifest tremor, ataxia, and choreoathetosis. Somatic growth may also be impaired. Enzymatic assays help determine the specific defect.

The hyperornithinemia-hyperammonemia-homo-citrullinuria syndrome is due to ornithine translocase deficiency and presents acutely with episodes of vomiting, depressed consciousness, or coma and hepatitis. Alternatively, affected individuals may demonstrate aversion to protein-rich foods, intellectual disability, myoclonic seizures, ataxia and pyramidal tract dysfunction.

Citrin deficiency can manifest with neonatal intrahepatic cholestasis, in older children as failure to thrive and dyslipidemia and in adults as recurrent hyperammonemia with neuropsychiatric disturbances (as part of citrullinemia type II).

Pathology

Acute hyperammonenia is associated with cerebral edema, spongiosis of the white matter and basal ganglia and cortical neuronal loss. Alzheimer type II glial cells may be found, but not invariably. Females afflicted by severe ornithine transcarbamylase deficiency who survive the neonatal period can exhibit cystic destruction of the cerebral hemispheres with atrophy and ulegyria. The cerebellum and Ammon's horn are usually spared. Early hypomyelination and cerebellar heterotopias have also been described, indicating perhaps a prenatal onset of pathological mechanisms.

Pathophysiology

Ammonia, in its ionic form, is generated in all tissues and can diffuse freely across the blood–brain barrier and into the brain. Ammonia is normally maintained at relatively low concentrations (40–50 µM in the brain) via the action of glutaminase (or glutamine synthetase), which is localized inside the astrocyte. Glutamine synthetase is responsible for the synthesis of glutamine from ammonia and glutamate, leading to a glutamate–glutamine cycle: Glutamate synthesized and released by neurons in the course of synaptic transmission is taken up by astrocytes after it exerts its synaptic action. Astrocytic glutamate is then converted to glutamine by the action of glutamine synthetase. Glutamine is then exported back to the neuron, closing the cycle. Glutamine produced by this cycle is osmotically active and can cause Alzheimer type II astrocytosis and cytotoxic edema. An additional plausible mechanism is exerted via excess glutamate (NMDA-type) receptor activation, which results in excitotoxic injury.

Glutamine that is cleaved back to ammonia upon entering the mitochondria produces oxygen reactive species and induces the mitochondrial permeability transition, resulting in modified oxidative phosphorylation and cessation of ATP production, ultimately potentially leading to cerebral energetic deficit.

Nitric oxide is produced from arginine in a reaction catalyzed by nitric oxide synthase. This reaction is inhibited by arginine deficiency typical of the urea cycle defects, leading as a result to decreased nitric oxide production and potential consequent vasoconstriction or vasospasm.

Diagnosis

Plasma ammonia and amino acids and urinary orotic acid are useful for the diagnosis of individual urea cycle defects. Blood pH and CO_2 may vary depending on the degree of cerebral edema and hyper or hypoventilation, but initially reflects respiratory alkalosis. In neonates, the normal ammonia level is higher than in adults (which is typically less than 35 µM or less than 100 µM in neonates). An elevated plasma ammonia level greater than 150 µM in neonates and 100 µM in older children and adults in association with a normal anion gap and a normal blood glucose level is an indication of a urea cycle defect. Elevations or reductions of arginine, citrulline, and argininosuccinate help identify each defect in the context of the cycle.

Treatment

The treatment of urea cycle defects proceeds depending on the level of emergency imposed by the development of hyperammonemia and resulting cerebral edema. Urgent measures include stopping protein intake, intravenous glucose to halt protein catabolism and nitrogen scavengers such as sodium benzoate, sodium phenylbutyrate or sodium phenylacetate together with L-arginine or citrulline to increase ammonia excretion via the urea cycle. Hemofiltration is used in refractory hyperammonemia.

Maintenance therapy includes a reduced-protein diet. This mainstay of long-term management is based upon minimizing the nitrogen load on the urea cycle. The amount of natural protein tolerated by each individual is determined, aided by titration against ammonia.

Liver transplantation has been performed in all urea cycle defects except in N-acetylglutamate synthase deficiency and the hyperornithinemia-hyperammonemia-homocitrullinuria syndrome. This intervention is curative, allowing for the termination of the low-protein diet.

Bibliography

Gelfand A.A., Sznewajs A., Glass H.C., et al. (2011). Clinical Reasoning: An encephalopathic 3-day-old infant. *Neurology*. 77(1):e1–5.

Häberle J., Boddaert N., Burlina A., et al. (2012). Suggested guidelines for the diagnosis and management of urea cycle disorders. *Orphanet J Rare Dis*. 7:32.

Helman G., Pacheco-Colón I., Gropman A.L. (2014). The urea cycle disorders. *Semin Neurol*. 34(3):341–9.

Holocarboxylase Synthetase Deficiency and Biotinidase Deficiency

A girl was the second child of consanguineous parents. A 6-year-old brother was healthy. Birth was unremarkable but, when 1-hour-old, she experienced respiratory distress and septicemia was suspected (her C-reactive protein was elevated) and treated. She was discharged from the hospital at 7 days old. At 2 week old, her skin turned dry and squamous and 2 weeks later she began to lose her hair. At 6 weeks old she had become lethargic, did not make eye contact, was hypotonic and jittery, had a tense fontanelle and hypoactive infant reflexes, was hypothermic (body temperature 35.5°C), and exhibited ankle clonus and tonic clonic seizures. She had oral candidiasis, generalized seborrheic dermatitis and alopecia. Serum and cerebrospinal fluid lactate was elevated. Biotinidase deficiency was diagnosed and treated with oral biotin (10 mg daily). 10 days later, her cutaneous manifestations had normalized and her seizures disappeared. Lactate levels also normalized. At 18 months, she remained asymptomatic except for recurrent local fungal infections and had developed normally.

Holocarboxylase Synthetase and Biotinidase Deficiency

Onset: Severe neonatal acidosis and skin rash in holocarboxylase synthetase deficiency and, additionally, infantile seizures and hypotonia in biotinidase deficiency.
Additional manifestations: Lethargy and coma. Apnea or tachypnea. Necrotizing myelopathy with deafness and optic atrophy resembling demyelinating disease.
Disease mechanism: Lack of incorporation of biotin to apoenzymes, which is required for the activity of four carboxylases.

Testing: Characteristic pattern of organic aciduria, hyperammonemia, and direct enzymatic determination of carboxylase activity in holocarboxylase synthetase deficiency. Similar organic aciduria and biotinidase activity determination in plasma in biotinidase deficiency.
Treatment: Biotin, adjusted for enzyme affinity to the cofactor.
Research highlights: Regulation of transcription factors NF-κB and Sp1/3 by biotin, relevant to immunological and inflammatory processes.

Clinical Features

The cofactor biotin is attached to and removed from its target carboxylases enzymatically. Two forms of biotin metabolic defects result from deficient incorporation or from defective release of biotin from its apoenzymes: holocarboxylase synthetase deficiency and biotinidase deficiency, respectively.

Holocarboxylase deficiency is inherited as an autosomal recessive disorder. Newborns with the disorder manifest hypotonia, lethargy and coma, feeding and respiratory difficulties, seizures, and severe acidosis. Skin rash and alopecia are common. The respiratory abnormalities include apnea or tachypnea. Hyperammonemia and organic aciduria are common. When untreated, the disease leads to intractable epilepsy and death. Milder and late-onset forms of the disease have been recognized, with a more favorable outcome.

Biotinidase deficiency is also inherited in autosomal recessive fashion, affecting 1 in 61,000 individuals. Children may manifest the disease in the neonatal period, but infantile presentations with onset at 3–6 months of age are more common. Seizures are often the first sign of the disease, followed by hypotonia. Seizure types include partial seizures, infantile spasms, and myoclonic and generalized tonic-clonic

Table 22.1 Biotin-dependent enzymes

Enzyme	Principal role
Pyruvate carboxylase	Gluconeogenesis
Propionyl-coenzyme A carboxylase	Branch-chain amino acid and odd-chain fatty acid catabolism
Beta-methylcrotonyl-coenzyme A carboxylase	Leucine catabolism
Acetyl-coenzyme A carboxylase	Fatty acid biosynthesis

events. Hyperventilation, stridor, and apnea may also occur. Skin rash, alopecia, and skin fungal infections due to cellular immune dysfunction are common. Optic atrophy and deafness ensue after a prolonged period of time. Juvenile and adolescent onset of the disease is also possible, with spastic paraparesis and optic neuropathy.

Pathology

The brains of children with holocarboxylase synthetase deficiency have been studied by MR imaging. When abnormalities are present, they involve loss of the white-grey matter demarcation and decreased density of the white matter in a scattered fashion. Often, however, there are no detectable abnormalities.

In biotinidase deficiency, Purkinje cells degenerate in the context of Bergmann glial proliferation. Vascular proliferation and macrophagic infiltration can occur in the spinal cord, indicating subacute necrotizing myelopathy. Other abnormalities detectable by imaging have ranged from atrophy to decreased white matter attenuation, cysts, ventriculomegaly, and subdural effusions.

Pathophysiology

Biotin is a B-vitamin that serves as a cofactor to four carboxylases: pyruvate carboxylase, propionyl-coenzyme A carboxylase, beta-methylcrotonyl-coenzyme A carboxylase and acetyl coenzyme A carboxylase.

The carbonyl group of biotin is covalently attached to the epsilon-amino group of the carboxylases via an amide bond. This attachment is mediated by holocarboxylase synthetase. Biotin leaves the carboxylases via cleavage of the amide bond by biotinidase once the carboxylases have been proteolytically degraded.

In holocarboxylase synthetase deficiency, the four carboxylases remain underbiotinylated. This leads to accumulation of organic acid substrates that produce acidosis and block the urea cycle, inducing hyperammonemia. Some disease-causing holocarboxylase synthetase mutations tend to raise the Michaelis constant (Km) of the enzyme for biotin. There is a negative correlation between Km and the age of onset of holocarboxylase synthetase deficiency. Another set of mutations affect enzyme maximum velocity (Vmax). Generally speaking, mutations within the biotin-binding region of the enzyme increase Km, whereas mutations located elsewhere in the protein raise the Km. The implication of this is that biotin supplementation is usually effective in treating Km-associated mutations.

Serum biotinidase is primarily synthesized in the liver. The brain possesses very low biotinidase activity, thus relying on biotin transported from the blood. A major function of the enzyme is the recycling of biotin from carboxylases, but additional roles may also be clinically relevant. One such role is to serve as a biotin-binding protein in serum. Another is to biotinylate other proteins such as histones.

Diagnosis

Holocarboxylase deficiency leads to a characteristic accumulation of urinary beta-hydroxyisovalerate, beta-methylcrotonylglycine, beta-hydroxypropionate, methylcitrate, and lactate arising from deficiency of multiple carboxylases. Leukocyte, amniocyte, or fibroblast enzyme activity assays are available for some of the biotin-dependent carboxylases. These assays normalize in the presence of biotin. Direct measurement of holocarboxylase synthetase is also feasible.

In biotinidase deficiency, neurological and biochemical cerebrospinal fluid abnormalities such as increased lactate and organic acids precede serum biochemical abnormalities. The pattern of organic aciduria is similar to that typical of holocarboxylase synthetase deficiency. Direct serum assay of biotinidase activity can be performed. Additional sources for enzymatic determination include leukocytes and skin fibroblasts. Serum biotinidase activity is unaltered in biotin deficiency. Biotinidase deficiency is commonly part of newborn screening programs.

Treatment

Most individuals with holocarboxylase synthetase and biotinidase deficiency experience marked improvement upon supplementation with biotin. Individuals harboring holocarboxylase synthetase mutants with higher Km require greater doses of biotin and may not be fully responsive.

Bibliography

Haagerup A., Andersen J.B., Blichfeldt S., et al. (1997). Biotinidase deficiency: Two cases of very early presentation. *Dev Med Child Neurol.* 39(12):832–5.

Wolf B. (2012). Biotinidase deficiency: "if you have to have an inherited metabolic disease, this is the one to have". *Genet Med.* 14(6):565–75.

Disorders of Pyridoxine Metabolism

A girl was born via spontaneous vaginal delivery at 38 weeks' gestation. Examination revealed mild hypotonia and excessive jitteriness. On the fifth day of life, she exhibited events concerning for seizures, characterized by nonsuppressible rhythmic movements of her extremities with associated eye deviation and oxygen desaturation. Video EEG monitoring confirmed that these events were myoclonic-tonic and brief tonic seizures. The EEG background showed excessive multifocal sharp-wave discharges and discontinuity for her postconceptual age. She received intravenous pyridoxine (200 mg) with no appreciable change in the EEG background. She was continued on phenobarbital and oral pyridoxine as other diagnostic testing was performed. Cerebrospinal fluid analysis for monoamine metabolites showed a profile suggestive of pyridoxine-dependent seizures. ALDH7A1 DNA sequencing demonstrated two inherited heterozygous mutations. Pyridoxine dose was increased to 150 mg daily and she was successfully weaned off phenobarbital. At 28 months of age, her development, exam, and EEG remained normal

Disorders of Pyridoxine Metabolism

Onset: Pharmacoresistant neonatal epilepsy.
Additional manifestations: Evolving seizures including status epilepticus and early death. Depressed consciousness and cerebral dysgenesis including corpus callosum hypoplasia. Emesis and abdominal distension.
Disease mechanism: Pyridoxine-dependent epilepsy is caused by antiquitin (ALDH7A1) mutations; pyridoxal-5′-phosphate-responsive epileptic encephalopathy is caused by mutation of pyridoxamine 5′-phosphate oxidase (PNPO); and tissue nonspecific isoenzyme of alkaline

phosphatase can lead to hypophosphatasemia and is coded by the gene ALPL.
Testing: Accumulation of α-aminoadipic semialdehyde, piperideine-6-carboxylate and pipecolic acid in urine, plasma or cerebrospinal fluid.
Treatment: Intravenous pyridoxine followed by oral pyridoxine or pyridoxal-5′-phosphate.
Research highlights: Dietary lysine restriction for the treatment of antiquitin deficiency.

Clinical Features

The disorders of pyridoxine metabolism include three entities: pyridoxine-dependent epilepsy, usually caused by antiquitin (ALDH7A1) mutations; pyridoxal-5′-phosphate-responsive epileptic encephalopathy (caused by mutation of pyridoxamine 5′-phosphate oxidase or PNPO); and tissue nonspecific isoenzyme of alkaline phosphatase (coded by the ALPL gene) deficiency.

Pyridoxine dependent epilepsy due to antiquitin mutations affects about 1 in 500,000 newborns, although many more children manifest epilepsy responsive to pyridoxine. Newborns with pyridoxine dependent epilepsy are not deficient in pyridoxine. They manifest depressed alertness and seizures that remain intractable with antiepileptic drugs and that can only be ameliorated when pharmacologic doses of pyridoxine are administered and followed by maintenance pyridoxine therapy (Figure 23.1). Seizures include partial motor seizures, generalized tonic seizures, or myoclonus, and can evolve to infantile spasms or recurrent status epilepticus. In some instances, mothers report rhythmic fetal movements suggestive of intrauterine seizures. If untreated, death from status epilepticus may ensue. Among several incorrect diagnoses, the manifestations of pyridoxine dependent epilepsy have been attributed to coexisting

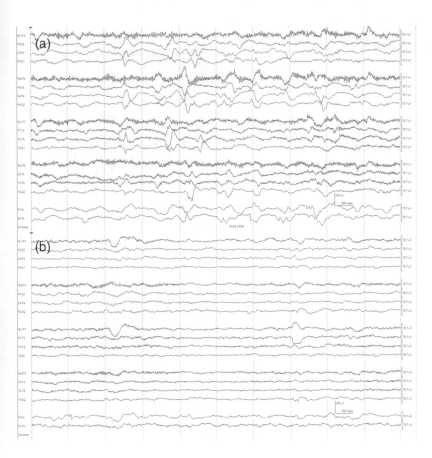

Figure 23.1 EEG response in an infant without pyridoxine-dependent epilepsy. EEG from patient without pyridoxine dependency showing response to intravenous pyridoxine. a. Wake epoch before treatment shows an abnormal and invariant background with almost continuous epileptiform discharges. b. Wake epoch after treatment with intravenous pyridoxine showing normal background for age. Reproduced with permission from Cirillo M, Venkatesan C, Millichap JJ, Stack CV, Nordli DR Jr. Case report: Intravenous and oral pyridoxine trial for diagnosis of pyridoxine-dependent epilepsy. *Pediatrics*. 2015; 136(1):e257–61.

hypoxic-ischemic encephalopathy, neonatal lactic acidosis, hypoglycemia, electrolyte disturbances, hypothyroidism, and diabetes insipidus. In most but not all cases, parenteral or oral pyridoxine rapidly results in seizure control, with improvement in the encephalopathy, allowing for the discontinuation of all antiepileptic medications that were previously instituted. Pyridoxine, however, needs to be maintained throughout life to prevent seizure recurrence. Presentations after the third month of life are atypical. Associated manifestations include emesis, abdominal distention, lethargy or excessive alertness, irritability, paroxysmal facial grimacing, and abnormal eye movements. In older children, a reduction in the cognitive or verbal IQ, particularly in measures of expressive language, along with a low normal motor or performance IQ has been noted. Adolescents may manifest severe social interaction disability and obsessive compulsive disorder.

Pyridoxal-5′-phosphate-responsive epileptic encephalopathy is caused by mutation of pyridoxamine 5′-phosphate oxidase (PNPO) and presents in a similar fashion to pyridoxine dependent epilepsy. This includes pharmacoresistant neonatal seizures and encephalopathy. Most children do not respond to pyridoxine but due to continuous supplementation of elevated doses of pyridoxal-5′-phosphate.

Deficiency of tissue nonspecific isoenzyme of alkaline phosphatase leads to impaired absorption and metabolism of vitamin B6. The disorder is associated with neonatal seizures responsive to pyridoxine and with deficient bone mineralization.

Pathology

Cranial imaging may demonstrate gray and white matter atrophy, hydrocephalus, corpus callosum hypoplasia, mega cisterna magna, and cortical dysplasia. About one-third of children with pyridoxine dependent epilepsy suffer from birth asphyxia.

The cellular composition of the brain may display abnormal radial neuronal organization as in type Ia focal cortical dysplasia. Heterotopic neurons may be present in subcortical white matter. Cortical astrogliosis, hippocampal sclerosis, and status marmoratus of the basal ganglia are also common.

Pathophysiology

Vitamin B6 is an essential nutrient. However, pyridoxine deficiency is rare because the six vitamers of vitamin B6 (the alcohol pyridoxine, the aldehyde pyridoxal, the amine pyridoxamine, and their respective 5′-phosphorylated esters) are ubiquitous in human food. After absorption, pyridoxine, pyridoxamine and pyridoxal may be phosphorylated and systemically distributed with the remainder three vitamers (Figure 23.2). Pyridoxal-5′-phosphate is the only biologically active vitamer and it participates in over 140 reactions as a cofactor, including transamination of amino acids, decarboxylation reactions, modulation of the activity of steroid hormones and regulation of gene expression. It also participates in the actions of dopamine, serotonin, glutamate, and GABA. Specifically, glutamic acid decarboxylase, the enzyme that converts the excitatory neurotransmitter glutamic acid into the inhibitory neurotransmitter GABA, is dependent on pyridoxal-5′-phosphate.

Antiquitin, an aldehyde dehydrogenase part of the lysine degradation pathway, is encoded by the ALDH7A1 gene (Figure 23.3). Lysine catabolism in particularly important in brain and liver. Antiquitin deficiency results in the accumulation of

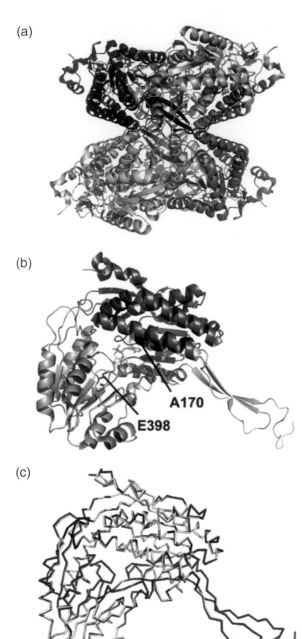

Figure 23.3 Structure of antiquitin. a. Tetrameric antiquitin forms a dimer-of-dimer in the crystal structure. The pale and dark green subunits form a dimer that interacts with the red and pink dimer to form an overall tetrameric structure of antiquitin. b. Each monomer of antiquitin contains a NAD+-binding domain (blue), a catalytic domain (pink), and an oligomerization domain (green). The bound NAD+ molecule is colored in yellow. Residues (Ala170 and Glu398) implicated in pyridoxine-dependent epilepsy are indicated in red. c. Superimposition of Ca trace of seabream (red) and human (yellow) antiquitin. Reproduced with permission from Tang WK et al. The crystal structure of seabream antiquitin reveals the structural basis of its substrate specificity. *FEBS Lett.* 2008; 582(20):3090–6.

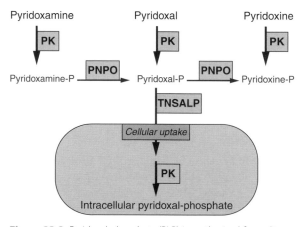

Figure 23.2 Pyridoxal phosphate (PLP) is synthesized from dietary pyridoxal, pyridoxamine, or pyridoxine by pyridoxal kinase (PK) and pyridox(am)ine 5′-phosphate oxidase (PNPO). Cellular uptake involves membrane-bound tissue nonspecific alkaline phosphatase (TNSALP).

α-aminoadipic semialdehyde, piperideine-6-carboxylate, and pipecolic acid, which may exert deleterious effects. Missense mutations in ALDH7A1 can be divided into three categories: affecting NAD$^+$ cofactor binding or catalysis, altering the substrate binding pocket, and potentially disrupting dimer or tetramer antiquitin assembly.

The enzyme encoded by the PNPO gene catalyzes the terminal, rate-limiting step in the synthesis of pyridoxal-5′-phosphate from dietary pyridoxine and pyridoxamine. PNPO mutations result in deficiency of pyridoxal-5′-phosphate. Additional determinants of brain pyridoxal phosphate level may include dietary lysine intake, catabolic state, pyridoxine intake, prenatal pyridoxine intake, and infection.

Diagnosis

The diagnosis can sometimes be made after the administration of pyridoxine aided by continuous electroencephalographic recording. Care must be taken to treat any resulting apnea requiring intubation after a first administration of pyridoxine.

Antiquitin deficiency results in the accumulation of α-aminoadipic semialdehyde, piperideine-6-carboxylate and pipecolic acid, which serve as diagnostic markers in urine, plasma, and cerebrospinal fluid. Accumulation of α-aminoadipic semialdehyde results in an intracellular reduction in pyridoxal-5′-phosphate.

Treatment

The treatment of antiquitin deficiency includes lifelong supplementation of pyridoxine in pharmacologic doses. In the seizing infant, an initial or more doses of pyridoxine can be given intravenously followed by oral supplementation. Some individuals with medically intractable epilepsy and unresponsiveness to pyridoxine respond to the administration of pyridoxal-5′-phosphate. Pyridoxal-5′-phosphate can substitute pyridoxine in antiquitin deficiency.

Some children with antiquitin deficiency who had an unclear response to pyridoxine may exhibit a favorable response to folinic acid.

Dietary lysine restriction leads to significant decrease of potentially neurotoxic compounds in body fluids and has shown some potential benefit in terms of seizure control and neurodevelopmental outcome.

Bibliography

Cirillo M., Venkatesan C., Millichap J.J., et al. (2015). Case report: Intravenous and oral pyridoxine trial for diagnosis of pyridoxine-dependent epilepsy. *Pediatrics.* 136(1):e257–61.

Clayton P.T. (2006). B6-responsive disorders: A model of vitamin dependency. *J Inherit Metab Dis.* 29(2–3):317–26.

Jansen L.A., Hevner R.F., Roden W.H., et al. (2014). Glial localization of antiquitin: Implications for pyridoxine-dependent epilepsy. *Ann Neurol.* 75(1):22–32.

Chapter 24

Maple Syrup Urine Disease

A boy manifested fluctuating consciousness, hyper- tonia, and myoclonic jerks during the first week of life. He was the product of a consanguineous union. A diagnosis of maple syrup urine disease was made in the second week. A double volume exchange transfusion and assisted ventilation were instituted. After one further week, he improved while receiving the appropriate therapeutic diet. However, his infancy was punctuated by frequent metabolic decompensa- tions despite dietary compliance, which were triggered by mild intercurrent illnesses. He also exhibited mild spastic paraparesis, myoclonic jerks, gastroesophageal reflux, and a hyperactive airway. His psychomotor development was also abnormal: At 28 months, his developmental level corresponded to 20 months (Bayley Scales of Infant and Toddler Development). He received a liver transplant at the age of 3 years and 4 months and a repeat transplant after another 6 months, with good metabolic control of his disorder. Five years post-transplant, he was attending a regular school at grade level.

Treatment: Exchange transfusion, peritoneal dialysis, and continuous hemofiltration have been used acutely. Dietary reduction of branched amino acids. Liver and hepatocyte transplantation. Differentiation of human amnion epithelial cells into hepatocytes for liver transplantation.
Research highlights: Structure-based design of inhibitors of the enzyme kinase that result in decreased phosphorylation of the complex, increasing its activity.

Clinical Features

Maple syrup urine disease is an autosomal dominant disorder of branched amino acid (leucine, isoleucine, and valine) degradation caused by deficiency of the branched-chain α-ketoacid dehydrogenase complex with a frequency of 1 in 185,000 newborns. Although the neonatal form of the disorder is fairly uniform, the branched-chain α-ketoacid dehydrogenase complex is encoded by several genetic loci (a heterotetrameric E1 decarboxylase component including two identical E1α and two identical E1β subunits, an E2 transacylase component with 24 identical subunits and a homodi- meric dihydrolipoamide dehydrogenase E3 compon- ent), accounting for significant clinical heterogeneity.

In the common form of the disease, children appear normal at birth, but develop encephalopathy within 4–7 days. This presentation occurs in three- fourths of individuals with the disease. Feeding diffi- culties and vomiting are followed by alternating rigid- ity and hypotonia. Dystonic extension of the arms resembling decerebrate rigidity is often observed. A maple syrup or burnt sugar odor is present in the diapers. Seizures and coma may ensue, leading to early death in some cases. This may be associated with cerebral edema (Figure 24.1). Children who sur- vive are prone to metabolic crises and neurological deterioration, which may be precipitated by infections. Long-term neurological sequelae include mental

Maple Syrup Urine Disease

Onset: In the common form, feeding difficulties and progressive encephalopathy within 4–7 days of birth.
Additional manifestations: Spongiform degeneration of the white matter. Intermediate severity and intermittent forms with episodic ketoacidosis may occur. A thiamine-responsive form associated with E2 mutations is treatable. An E3-associated form causes Leigh syndrome.
Disease mechanism: Competition of leucine with other amino acids for brain transport. Inhibition of several enzymes by leucine and branched chain keto acids.
Testing: Accumulation of branched chain amino acids and branched chain keto acids in biological fluids.

Table 24.1 Types and features of maple syrup urine disease

Forms of maple syrup urine disease	Characteristics
Common	Severe white matter damage
Intermediate	Mental retardation without ketoacidosis
Intermittent	Episodic ketoacidosis and normal development
Thiamine-responsive E2 deficient	Treatable mental retardation
Dihydrolipoamide dehydrogenase (E3)-deficient	Infantile lactic acidosis and Leigh syndrome

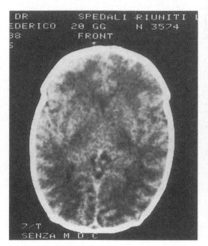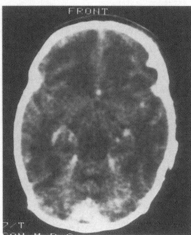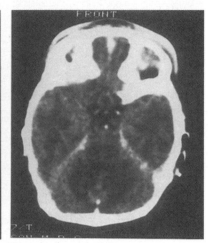

Figure 24.1 Non-contrast computerized tomography in maple syrup urine disease. Low density is present in the white matter of cerebral hemispheres, but also involving the pallida and thalami, the brainstem and cerebellar white matter. Small ventricles are also noticeable. Reproduced with permission from Taccone A et al. Computed tomography in maple syrup urine disease. *Eur J Radiol.* 1992; 14(3):207–12.

retardation, spasticity, hypotonia, cortical blindness, dystonia, ptosis, ophthalmoplegia, and facial nerve paralysis.

The thiamine responsive form of maple syrup urine disease is characterized by mental retardation and excess branch chain amino acid and keto acid accumulation. Treatment with thiamine reverses these abnormalities after weeks or months. Mutations in E2 subunit cause this form of the disease.

Dihydrolipoamide dehydrogenase (E3) deficiency is characterized by lactic acidosis with modest elevations in branched chain amino acids and keto acids. Because E3 is shared by pyruvate, α-ketoglutarate, and branched chain α-ketoacid dehydrogenases its deficiency causes impairment of all three enzymes. Infants develop lactic acidosis between 8 weeks and 6 months of age in association with progressive deterioration that includes movement disorders, hypotonia and seizures. Death usually ensues within the first year of life. The neuropathology is typical of Leigh syndrome.

Pathology

The principal site of pathology is the white matter. There is decreased myelination with no demyelination or neuronal degeneration (Figure 24.2). Spongy degeneration of the white matter is associated with a decreased number of oligodendroglial cells. The pyramidal tracts of the spinal cord, the myelin around the dentate nuclei, the corpus callosum and the cerebral hemispheres are most affected. Moderate astrocytic hypertrophy is present in these structures. In the cerebellum, necrosis of the granular cell layer can be prominent.

Pathophysiology

The E1 and E2 components of the enzyme are specific for the dehydrogenase complex, whereas the E3 component is common among the three α-ketoacid dehydrogenases. In addition, the complex contains a kinase and a phosphatase that regulate its activity

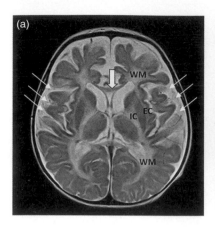
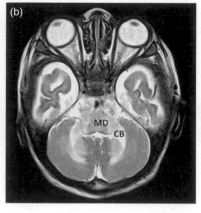

Figure 24.2 MR imaging in maple syrup urine disease. T2 weighted MR images showing hyperintense signal in the cerebral white matter (WM), internal capsule (IC), external capsule (EC), cerebellum (CB), medulla (MD), thinned corpus callosum (wide arrows), and widening of the frontoparietal sulci (small arrows). Reproduced with permission from Srinivasan KG. Typical neuroradiological diagnosis of maple syrup urine disease as a precursor to clinical diagnosis. A case report. *Neuroradiol J.* 2009; 22(5):564–7.

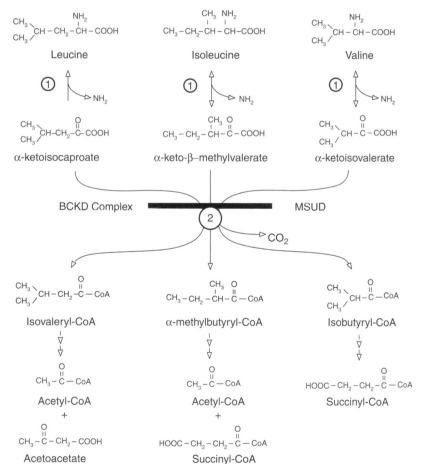

Figure 24.3 Oxidative degradation of the branched chain amino acids leucine, isoleucine, and valine. The transamination of these amino acids is catalyzed by a single branched-chain aminotransferase (reaction 1) that exists as both the cytosolic and mitochondrial isoforms. The oxidative decarboxylation of branched chain keto acids is catalyzed by the single mitochondrial branched-chain a-ketoacid dehydrogenase complex (reaction 2). The metabolic block at the second reaction results in maple syrup urine disease. Reproduced with permission from Chuang DT et al. Lessons from genetic disorders of branched-chain amino acid metabolism. *J Nutr.* 2006; 136(1 Suppl):243S–9S.

via phosphorylation. This regulation has been exploited with therapeutic purposes.

The oxidative degradation of branched-chain amino acids begins with reversible transamination in mitochondria by coupling with α-ketoglutarate to give rise to the corresponding branched chain α-ketoacids (Figures 24.3). The oxidation of these ketoacids occurs primarily in the liver, followed by extrahepatic tissues including kidney, muscle, heart, brain and adipose tissues and involves

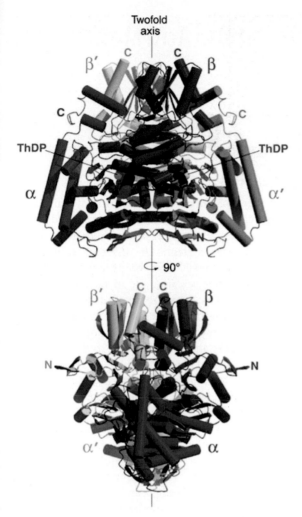

Figure 24.4 Overall structure of the branched-chain α-ketoacid dehydrogenase complex heterotetramer in two orthogonal orientations rotated about the vertical axis. The secondary structure elements are depicted as cylinders for helices and arrows for strands. The chain termini in the different subunits are labeled N and C, and the four subunits (α, purple; ß, red; α', blue; ß', yellow) are in color. In essentially all instances, disease severity correlates well with the predicted effect of the mutation on the structure, stability, and cofactor or K$^+$ binding by the enzyme. In severe cases, cofactor binding is essentially prohibited, or proper assembly made impossible. Reproduced with permission from AEvarsson A et al. Crystal structure of human branched-chain alpha-ketoacid dehydrogenase and the molecular basis of multienzyme complex deficiency in maple syrup urine disease. *Structure*. 2000; 8(3):277–91.

decarboxylation by the branched-chain α-ketoacid dehydrogenase complex that is deficient in maple syrup urine disease (Figure 24.4).

Leucine competes with other large neutral amino acids that utilize a specific transporter for transport across the blood–brain barrier. Because some of these amino acids, such as phenylalanine and tyrosine, are precursors of neurotransmitters, this competition for transport may interfere with neurotransmitter synthesis.

Leucine and branched chain keto acids also inhibit pyruvate dehydrogenase, α-ketoglutarate dehydrogenase and mitochondrial respiration. Additionally, they may also contribute to neurotoxicity via increased lipid peroxidation and excess oxidant production.

Diagnosis

The diagnosis can be established by the demonstration of excessive accumulation of branched chain amino acids and branched chain keto acids in biological fluids.

Treatment

Exchange transfusion, peritoneal dialysis, and continuous hemofiltration are used at presentation for the common disease form. The mainstay of chronic therapy is dietary reduction of branched chain amino acids.

Hepatic and hepatocyte transplantation is effective in diet-refractory cases, as may be transplantation of human amnion epithelial cells after differentiation into hepatocytes.

Inhibitors of the complex kinase such as α-chloroisocaproate, phenylpyruvate, clofibric acid, and phenylbutyrate increase the amount of active (dephosphorylated) branched alpha-keto acid dehydrogenase.

Bibliography

Burrage L.C., Nagamani S.C., Campeau P.M., et al. (2014). Branched-chain amino acid metabolism: From rare Mendelian diseases to more common disorders. *Hum Mol Genet.* 23(R1):R1–8.

Chin H.L., Aw M.M., Quak S.H., et al. (2015). Two consecutive partial liver transplants in a patient with classic maple syrup urine disease. *Mol Genet Metab Rep.* 4:49–52.

Other Inborn Errors of Amino Acid Metabolism

A 2-day-old girl presented with poor feeding, hiccups, and shallow breathing. Antenatally, her mother noticed increased fetal movements from 20 weeks of gestation. After discharge from the hospital, the mother noticed frequent hiccups. Examination revealed hypotonia with shallow breathing and frequent apneic episodes, which required ventilatory support. Soon she developed frequent myoclonic jerks. Her plasma glycine level was 1751 μM (normal range: 200–600 μM) and her cerebrospinal fluid glycine level 416 μM (normal range: 0–10 μM). Computed tomography of the head did not show any abnormalities but EEG revealed a burst suppression pattern. She expired on her sixth day of life.

Other Inborn Errors of Amino Acid Metabolism

Manifestations: Several disorders of amino acid metabolism present in the newborn or young infant with severe encephalopathy. Among these, glycine encephalopathy manifests with seizures, whereas lysinuric protein intolerance presents with hyperammonemia similar to urea cycle defects. In contrast, hepatorenal tyrosinemia is associated with crises of painful neuropathy.

Additional manifestations: Incomplete, intermittent, or late forms of these disorders exist and can remain undiagnosed.

Testing: Amino acid determination in plasma, urine, and cerebrospinal fluid.

Treatment: A general approach includes restricting or supplementing the involved amino acid to correct the biochemical defect, in addition to supplying additional depleted metabolites.

Clinical Features

Glycine encephalopathy, also known as non-ketotic hyperglycinemia, is an autosomal recessive disorder of glycine degradation caused by mutations in the glycine cleavage system. The disorder exhibits an incidence of 1 in 60,000. Newborns manifest lethargy, hypotonia, apneic seizures, and myoclonic jerks. On occasion, mothers report rhythmic fetal movements reminiscent of seizures. MR imaging can demonstrate lesions in the myelin of the posterior limb of the internal capsule and of long tracts in the brainstem (Figures 25.1 and 25.2). EEG may reveal burst-suppression that evolves into hypsarrhythmia or multifocal spikes (Figure 25.3). The presenting episode can often be overcome in three weeks. Sequelae of the presenting episode include intractable seizures and mental retardation. Mild and episodic disease forms are associated with epilepsy, mental retardation or movement disorders. A transient form of neonatal hyperglycinemia is benign and resolves spontaneously. Four subunits comprise the glycine cleavage system, including glycine dehydrogenase or P, encoded by GLDC; aminomethyltransferase or T, encoded by AMT; lipoamide dehydrogenase or L; and the lipoic acid-containing cleavage system or H, encoded by GCSH (Figures 25.4 and 25.5). Glycine encephalopathy leads to disproportionately elevated of glycine in the cerebrospinal fluid in addition to more modest elevations in blood and urine. Enzymatic confirmation of the diagnosis is based upon measurement of glycine cleavage system activity in liver tissue. Treatment with sodium benzoate to reduce plasma concentration of glycine and N-methyl D-aspartate receptor antagonists such as dextromethorphan, ketamine, and felbamate is feasible.

Lysinuric protein intolerance is an autosomal recessive disorder of lysine degradation that manifests

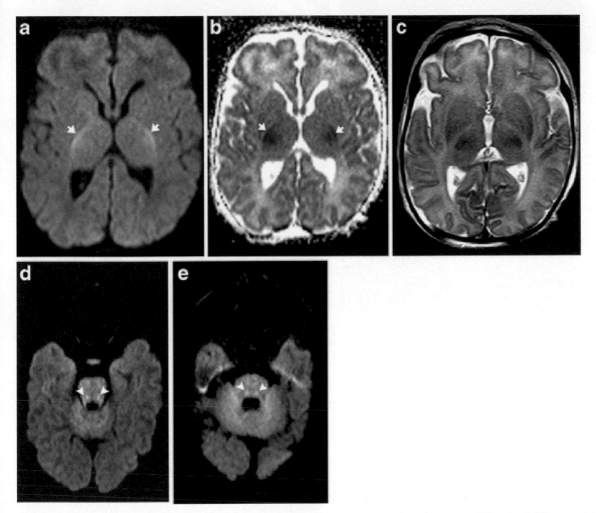

Figure 25.1 Glycine encephalopathy. A 4-day-old neonate presented with encephalopathy and respiratory failure. Axial diffusion-weighted MR images (a) and apparent diffusion coefficient map (b) show restricted diffusion in the posterior limbs of the internal capsules (arrows). Axial T2 weighted image (c) at the same level shows no signal abnormality. Axial diffusion-weighted MR images (d, e) at the level of pons show restricted diffusion in the dorsal midbrain and pons. Reproduced with permission from Kanekar S et al. Characteristic MRI findings in neonatal nonketotic hyperglycinemia due to sequence changes in GLDC gene encoding the enzyme glycine decarboxylase. *Metab Brain Dis*. 2013; 28(4):717–20.

when nutrition with elevated protein content such as infant formula is initiated. The disease is caused by mutation of the dibasic amino acid transporter y$^+$LAT-1, encoded by SLC7A7. Transport of the dibasic amino acids lysine, arginine, and ornithine is defective in the basolateral membranes of epithelial cells of renal tubules and small intestine. These amino acids are excreted in large quantities in the urine, particularly in the case of lysine, in the context of decreased intestinal absorption. Deficiency in urea cycle intermediates such as ornithine and arginine can lead to hyperammonemia, which is prominent after protein ingestion. Newborns or infants display difficulties with feeding soon after formula is administered. Lethargy and coma are associated with hyperammonemia. Obligatory nasogastric

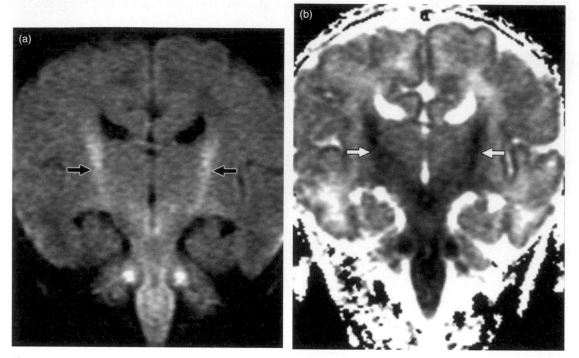

Figure 25.2 Five-day-old boy with nonketotic hyperglycinemia. Diffusion-weighted imaging (a) and apparent diffusion coefficient (b) maps show diffusion restriction due to myelin vacuolation within pyramidal tracks (arrows), middle cerebellar peduncles and dentate nuclei. Reproduced with permission from Thomas B et al. MRI of childhood epilepsy due to inborn errors of metabolism. *AJR Am J Roentgenol.* 2010; 194(5):W367–74.

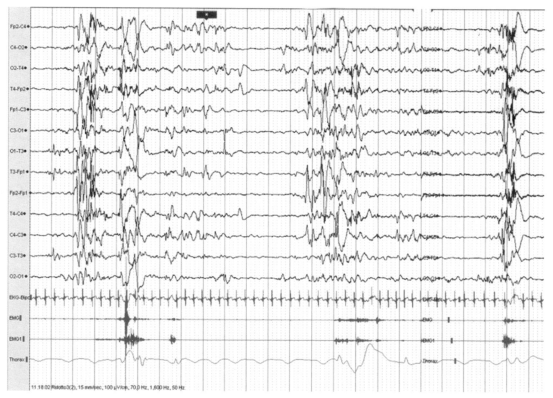

Figure 25.3 Glycine encephalopathy. The EEG recording shows a suppression-burst pattern characterized by a succession of bursts of paroxysmal activity separated by episodes of flat or low-amplitude tracing. Reproduced with permission from Belcastro V et al. A novel AMT gene mutation in a newborn with nonketotic hyperglycinemia and early myoclonic encephalopathy. *Eur J Paediatr Neurol.* 2016; 20(1):192–5.

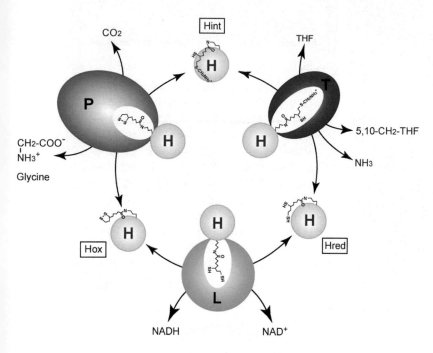

Figure 25.4 Outline of the reversible reaction of the glycine cleavage system (GCS). P, T, L, and H are the protein components of GCS. Hox, Hint, and Hred represent H-proteins bearing covalently attached lipoate (oxidized form), aminomethyllipoate, and dihydrolipoate, respectively. Reproduced with permission from Okamura-Ikeda K et al. Crystal structure of aminomethyltransferase in complex with dihydrolipoyl-H-protein of the glycine cleavage system: implications for recognition of lipoyl protein substrate, disease-related mutations, and reaction mechanism. *J Biol Chem.* 2010; 285 (24):18684–92.

nutrition, which is often instituted in this situation, can be fatal. Hepato and splenomegaly eventually develop, together with pulmonary alveolar proteinosis. In mild cases, there is hypotonia and failure to thrive with autoimmune disorders and immune deficiency. Older children are prone to fractures and bone maturity is delayed. Marked hepatomegaly is typically found in later age children, in the context of obesity, and pancytopenia. Intellectual attainment may be a function of the frequency and severity of previous hyperammonemic episodes. Treatment includes citrulline supplementation to replete the urea cycle via the replenishment of arginine and ornithine, together with lysine supplementation. Because of protein aversion and consequent low consumption of meat protein in the older child, secondary carnitine deficiency can be treated with levocarnitine supplementation. Hyperammonemia is treated as in urea cycle defects.

Hepatorenal tyrosinemia or tyrosinemia type 1 is caused by autosomal recessive deficiency of fumarylacetoacetate hydrolase. In its most severe form, it presents in early infancy with hepatic failure and coagulopathy. In milder cases, nephropathy manifests insidiously, with hypophosphatemic rickets and renal Fanconi syndrome. Terminal liver disease results in cirrhosis and hepatocellular carcinoma. Crises of painful paresthesia are associated with neuropathy, which can lead to phrenic nerve dysfunction and death before the second decade of life. In tyrosinemia, the neurotoxin delta amino-levulinic acid accumulates. Additionally, alpha-fetoprotein and succinylacetate are elevated. The disease is the result of insufficient catalysis of tyrosine by fumarylacetoacetate hydrolase, with associated accumulation of tyrosine, which is converted into fumarylacetoacetone. The latter gives rise to excess succinylacetoacetate and succinylacetone. These toxic metabolites elicit an endoplasmic reticulum stress response and induce chromosomal instability, cell cycle arrest, and apoptosis. The treatment of tyrosinemia includes a diet restricted in phenylalanine and tyrosine until liver transplantation can be accomplished. Alternatively, nitisinone, a herbicide inhibitor of 4-hydroxyphenyopyruvic acid dioxygenase, reduces succinylacetone levels via block of the formation of maleylacetoacetic acid and fumarylacetoacetic acid.

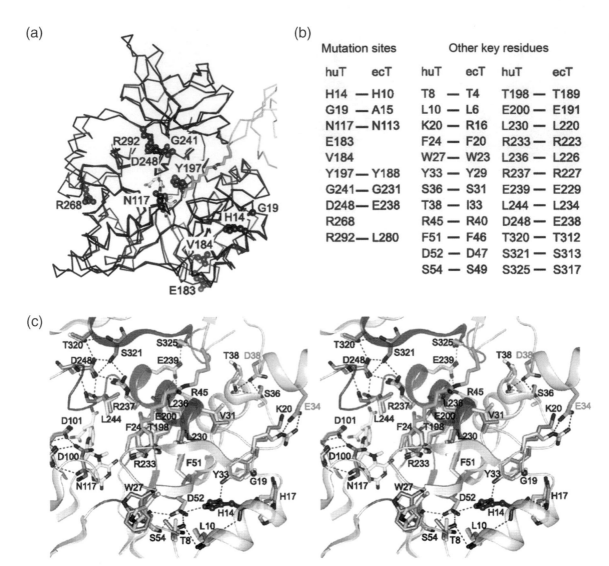

Figure 25.5 Structural comparison of human T-protein (huT) with *Escherichia coli* T-protein (ecT). a. non ketotic hyperglycinemia-related mutation sites mapped on the overall topology of superimposed huT and ecT. The structure of huT (red) is overlaid on that of ecT (blue) of the ecT·ecHred complex and represented in ribbon. Mutation residues of huT and the corresponding residues of ecT are shown in CPK and stick, respectively, with numbers for huT. ecHred is shown in ribbon colored in green with dihydrolipoyllysine in stick. 5-CH3-THF is shown in stick colored in yellow. b. alignment of key residues of huT and ecT. c. close-up view of the hydrogen bond networks assembling four highly conserved regions in T-protein. Key residues of huT (light blue) and ecT (pink) contributing to the assembly are represented in stick with numbers for huT. Mutant residues are depicted in ball-and-stick representation with atoms colored in red (carbon and oxygen) and blue (nitrogen) with red labels. Four highly conserved regions in the main chain of huT represented schematically (residues 51–56, 196–204, 229–248, and 229–328) are colored in red. The structure of ecHred of the complex and its residues are shown in schematically and stick, respectively, colored in green. Hydrogen bonds are drawn in broken lines. Reproduced with permission from Okamura-Ikeda K et al. Crystal structure of aminomethyltransferase in complex with dihydrolipoyl-H-protein of the glycine cleavage system: implications for recognition of lipoyl protein substrate, disease-related mutations, and reaction mechanism. *J Biol Chem.* 2010; 285(24):18684–92.

Bibliography

Iqbal M., Prasad M., Mordekar S.R. (2015). Nonketotic hyperglycinemia case series. *J Pediatr Neurosci.* 10(4):355–8.

Noble-Jamieson G., Jamieson N., Clayton P., et al. (1994). Neurological crisis in hereditary tyrosinaemia and complete reversal after liver transplantation. *Arch Dis Child.* 70(6):544–5.

Ogier de Baulny H., Schiff M., Dionisi-Vici C. (2012). Lysinuric protein intolerance (LPI): A multi organ disease by far more complex than a classic urea cycle disorder. *Mol Genet Metab.* 106(1):12–17.

Newborn Congenital Glycosylation Disorders

A well-formed girl became ill on her first day of life. The pregnancy, achieved via in vitro fertilization, had been complicated by oligohydramnios. The child was born at the 29th week of gestation by urgent cesarean section. Generalized edema and mild hypotonia were observed at birth. Her Apgar scores were 8 and 9 at 5 and 10 min, respectively. Within hours, she developed multifocal myoclonic seizures and clinical signs of anemia and bleeding episodes with coagulopathy and pancytopenia. In her third week, she exhibited diarrhea, nasogastric feeding intolerance, abdominal distension, ascites, and pericardial effusion. After a further week, frequent bleeding was associated with inferior vena cava thrombosis. Heart failure led to liver congestion, portal hypertension, and hepatosplenomegaly. Her edema progressed. Generalized tonic clonic seizures appeared in the 6th week of life. She died at 2 months of age from multiple organ failure. Autopsy revealed steatofibrosis with cholestasis, cerebral cortical and cerebellar atrophy or degeneration and optic atrophy. She harbored two heterozygous mutations in the ALG8 gene, causative of alpha-1,3-glucosyltransferase deficiency.

Testing: In general, plasma transferrin isoform analysis.
Treatment: Mannose for phosphomannose isomerase deficiency. No effective therapy for the others
Research highlights: Continued identification of an expanding array of phenotypes and causative enzymes.

Clinical Features

The congenital glycosylation disorders constitute a family of mostly autosomal recessive anabolic defects with multiorgan manifestations. Several dozen defects are recognized. The most frequent congenital glycosylation defect is phosphomannose isomerase type 2, which is covered in a separate chapter since the majority of disease manifestations become prominent in the infant. Here are described the congenital glycosylation disorders with a severe neonatal presentation. They all share a common general mechanism: the defective incorporation of oligosaccharide chains to proteins or other macromolecules. These disorders include defects in *N*-glycosylation, *O*-glycosylation and glypiation or synthesis of glycosylphosphatidylinositol. Additionally, the glycosylation defects include the galactosemias, in which there is abnormal *N*-glycan formation, and mucolipidoses II and III, which are associated with impaired attachment of mannose-6-phosphate to proteins. The disorders of *O*-glycosylation include limb-girdle muscular dystrophies, type 2 lyssencephaly and congenital muscular dystrophies.

The diagnostic test for most types of *N*-linked congenital glycosylation defects is plasma transferrin isoform analysis to determine the number and composition of sialylated *N*-linked oligosaccharide residues bound to transferrin. Only the most salient features of each neonatal disorder are summarized here. Each disorder is abbreviated with a responsible

Newborn Congenital Glycosylation Disorders

Onset: Pre or perinatal multiorgan dysfunction with primary or secondary (i.e., due to hypoglycemia or other metabolic imbalance) neurological manifestations.
Additional manifestations: Dysmorphic cranial and other somatic features. Progressive visceral, hematological, and immunological failure often leading to early death. Epilepsy, hydrocephalus, and microcephaly are common.
Disease mechanism: Generally autosomal recessive, with exceptions. Multiple mechanisms dependent upon the biological function of the mutant glycoprotein.

enzyme symbol followed by –CDG (denoting congenital disorder of glycosyation)

- PMM2-CDG (CDG-Ia), the result of phosphomannomutase 2 mutations, is discussed separately.
- MPI-CDG (CDG-Ib) is caused by mutations in phosphomannose isomerase. There is predominantly extraneurological involvement, but the disease may present with hypoglycemic seizures. Cyclic vomiting, failure to thrive, hepatic fibrosis, and protein-losing enteropathy are characteristic. This disorder is treatable with mannose.
- ALG6-CDG (CDG-Ic) is the result of mutations in alpha-1,3-glucosyltransferase and may lead to hypotonia, poor head tone, abnormal development, ataxia, strabismus, and epilepsy.
- ALG3-CDG (CDG-Id) is due to a defect in endoplasmic reticulum mannosyltransferase VI and is accompanied by microcephaly, epilepsy, and severe visual impairment.
- DPM1-CDG (CDG-Ie) is caused by deficiency of dolichol-phosphate mannosyltransferase subunit 1. It is associated with microcephaly, epilepsy, hypertelorism, small hands with dysplastic nails, and knee contractures.
- MPDU1-CDG (CDG-If), due to mutations in mannose-P-dolichol synthase leads to severe psychomotor retardation, seizures, failure to thrive, dry skin, and scaling with erythroderma, and impaired vision.
- ALG12-CDG (CDG-Ig) is caused by deficiency of dolichyl-P-mannose: Man-7-GlcNAc-2-PP-dolichyl-alpha-6-mannosyltransferase and is associated with dysmorphic features, hypotonia, feeding difficulties, severely abnormal intellectual development, progressive microcephaly and impaired immunity.
- ALG8-CDG (CDG-Ih) is due to mutations in dolichyl-P-glucose: Glc-1-Man-9-GlcNAc-2-PP-dolichyl-alpha-3-glucosyltransferase. When it affects the nervous system, the disorder leads to hepatointestinal dysfunction, hypotonia, epilepsy, and abnormal development.
- ALG2-CDG (CDG-Ii) or alpha-1,3-mannosyltransferase deficiency is associated with cataracts, colobomas, infantile spasms, and severely abnormal development.

- DPAGT1-CDG (CDG-Ij) or dolichol phosphate n-acetylglucosamine-1-phosphotransferase, is associated with hypotonia, intractable epilepsy, abnormal development, and microcephaly.
- ALG1-CDG (CDG-Ik), a relatively frequent defect, is due to deficiency of mannosyltransferase 1. The disorder leads to severely abnormal development, hypotonia, and early-onset intractable epilepsy.
- ALG9-CDG (CDG-IL) arises from mutations in mannosyltransferase 7–9 deficiency and leads to microcephaly, hypotonia, abnormal development, epilepsy, and hepatomegaly.
- DOLK-CDG (CDG-Im), or dolichol kinase deficiency, leads to dilated cardiomyopathy, epilepsy, hypotonia, ichthyosis, and abnormal cognitive development.
- RFT1-CDG (CDG-In), due to mutations in requiring fifty three 1 homolog, is associated with severe mental retardation with limited development, hypotonia, epilepsy, myoclonus, decreased visual function, and sensorineural deafness.
- ALG11-CDG (CDG-Ip) or alpha-1, 2-mannosyltransferase deficiency, is associated with dysmorphic features, microcephaly, hypotonia, failure to thrive, and intractable epilepsy.
- SRD5A3-CDG (CDG-Iq), the result of mutations in steroid 5-alpha-reductase 2-like 1, is associated with ocular coloboma, optic nerve hypoplasia, hypotonia, and intellectual disability.
- DDOST-CDG (CDG-Ir) or dolichyl-diphosphooligosaccharide-protein glycosyltransferase deficiency leads to failure to thrive, abnormal development, hypotonia, strabismus, and hepatic dysfunction.
- MOGS-CDG (CDG-IIb) or glucosidase I deficiency leads to hypotonia, craniofacial dysmorphism, hypoplastic genitalia, epilepsy, feeding difficulties, hypoventilation, and generalized edema.
- SLC35C1-CDG (CDG-IIc) arises from mutation of the GDP-fucose transmembrane transporter FucT1 (or SLC35C1) and results in microcephaly, hypotonia, abnormal craniofacial features, and immune deficiency.
- B4GALT1-CDG (CDG-IId) or beta-1,4-galactosyltransferase deficiency is associated with Dandy-Walker malformation, hydrocephalus,

coagulation abnormalities, and elevated plasma creatine kinase.

- SLC35A2-CDG is an X-linked disorder caused by mutation of the UDP-galactose transporter SLC35A2. The principal manifestation is early-onset epileptic encephalopathy with developmental regression.
- COG6-CDG (CDG-IIL) or component of oligomeric Golgi complex 6 deficiency leads to intractable epilepsy, vitamin K deficiency, and intracranial bleeding.

Bibliography

Freeze H.H., Eklund E.A., Ng B.G., et al. (2015). Neurological aspects of human glycosylation disorders. *Annu Rev Neurosci.* 38:105–25.

Vesela K., Honzik T., Hansikova H., et al. (2009). A new case of ALG8 deficiency (CDG Ih). *J Inherit Metab Dis.* 32 Suppl 1.

Wolfe L.A., Krasnewich D. (2013). Congenital disorders of glycosylation and intellectual disability. *Dev Disabil Res Rev.* 17(3):211–25.

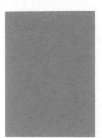

Disorders of Infancy

Phenylketonuria

An 8-year-old girl was evaluated for mental retardation. She was the second child of a consanguineous couple (first cousins). Gestation and delivery were uneventful. Neonatal screening was not performed. Infant development was globally abnormal and she never acquired verbal language. At the age of 15 months, she exhibited myoclonic seizures with spontaneous resolution. She starting attending a school for autistic children from the second year of life. At evaluation, she was of normal weight and stature, with a head circumference of 49 cm (3rd centile). She also displayed light brown hair, which was different from the dark-haired family pattern. She was hyperactive and exhibited ataxic gait, limb dysmetria, intention tremors of the upper extremities and flapping. She did not interact with other children and followed rigid routines, with abnormal interest for rotatory objects such as wheels or blenders. She fulfilled DSM-IV criteria for typical autistic disorder.

Phenylketonuria

Onset: Infantile mental retardation.
Additional manifestations: Epilepsy, spastic paraparesis, and microcephaly. Treated phenylketonuria can also be associated with intellectual dysfunction. Adults may manifest a progressive motor disorder.
Disease mechanism: Autosomal recessive dysfunction of phenylalanine hydroxylase. This leads to the accumulation of phenylacetic acid, phenylpyruvic acid and phenylacetylglutamine and to deficiency of tyrosine. Abnormal protein synthesis, myelin synthesis and biogenic amine production.
Testing: Screening of blood on filter paper followed by determination of phenylalanine and tyrosine.

Treatment: Phenylalanine-restricted, tyrosine-supplemented diet. Diets containing neutral amino acids that compete with phenylalanine transport.
Research highlights: Enzyme substitution therapy using direct administration of phenylalanine ammonia-lyase. This enzyme has also been provided by genetically modified intestinal flora.

Clinical Features

Phenylketonuria, caused by autosomal recessive loss of function of the hepatic enzyme phenylalanine mono oxygenase, which is also known as phenylalanine hydroxylase, occurs in 1 in 10,000 newborns. Its principal manifestations include mental retardation with an IQ usually lower than 30, microcephaly, spastic paraparesis, and epilepsy. Children often exhibit fair skin, blond hair, and blue eyes. Later, in the third or fourth decade the disease evolves into a progressive motor disorder.

Treated phenylketonuria is also associated with reduced intelligence, white matter abnormalities, and cognitive decline in adulthood, especially when the therapeutic diet is not completely adhered to.

Maternal phenylketonuria leads to a distinct syndrome of neonatal microcephaly with cardiac abnormalities that is discussed separately. The white matter is preserved in this disorder.

Pathology

The most common feature of untreated phenylketonuria is microcephaly, with a brain weight of about 80 percent of the normal weight. White matter abnormalities are also common and range from spongiosis and poor myelination in younger children to focal myelin degradation with neutral fat accumulation in adults (Figure 27.1). Glial proliferation accompanies

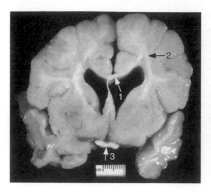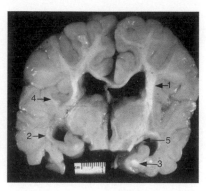

Figure 27.1 Neuropathology of phenylketonuria. Left: Coronal section at temporal tip illustrating large lateral ventricles with rounded corners. Corpus callosum is narrow and slightly myelinated (arrow 1). Anterior corona radiata is partly myelinated (arrow 2) as is anterior limb of internal capsule. There is no myelin in external and extreme capsules. Subcortical U-fibers are not yet myelinated. White matter of temporal pole is not myelinated. Optic chiasm is well myelinated and of normal bulk (arrow 3). Gray matter bulk of cortex, caudate, and putamen is normal for age. Right: Coronal section through posterior thalamus again shows large lateral ventricles including temporal horns. Corpus callosum is very thin. Posterior limb of internal capsule is somewhat thin, but well myelinated (arrow 1). Proximal optic radiation is very thin (arrow 2). Cingulum is myelinated in parahippocampal gyrus (arrow 3) but not in gyrus cinguli. Auditory radiation is myelinated in transverse gyrus of Heschl (arrow 4) and optic tract lateral to crus pedunculi is myelinated and of normal bulk (arrow 5). Gray matter bulk of cortex and thalamus is normal for age. Reproduced with permission from Koch R, Verma S, Gilles FH. Neuropathology of a 4-month-old infant born to a woman with phenylketonuria. *Dev Med Child Neurol.* 2008; 50(3):230–3.

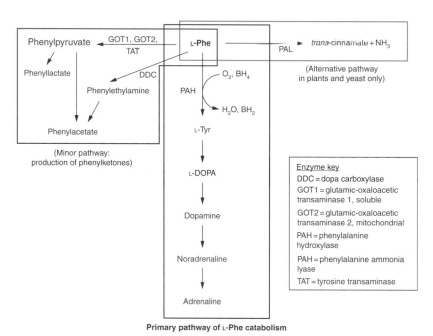

Primary pathway of L-Phe catabolism

Figure 27.2 Metabolic pathway of L-Phe. The primary pathway (blue box) is the catalytic conversion of l-phe to l-Tyr by phenylalanine hydroxylase (PAH). In phenylketonuria (PKU), the deficiency of PAH enzyme leads to the production of phenylketones by an alternative pathway (red box). A third pathway (green box) can be found in plants and yeast involving the enzyme phenylalanine ammonia lyase (PAL). Reproduced with permission from Ho G et al. Phenylketonuria: translating research into novel therapies. *Transl Pediatr.* 2014; 3(2):49–62.

these abnormalities, which predominantly involve the centrum semiovale, optic nerves, and long tracts of the brainstem. Neuronal maturation abnormalities are less frequent, including increased density of cortical neurons, reduced neuronal size and Nissl contents, and simplified dendrites and spines.

Pathophysiology

The relevant metabolic reactions are represented in Figure 27.2 and the enzyme structure in Figure 27.3. The brain does not contain phenylalanine mono oxygenase. Thus, the main consequences of phenylketonuria derive from the accumulation of phenylalanine and its metabolites (phenylacetic acid, phenylpyruvic acid, and phenylacetylglutamine) and from deficiency of tyrosine, which becomes an essential amino acid. Phenylalanine may compete with other neutral amino acids for transport into the brain, which could become deficient in neural tissue. As a result, protein synthesis, myelin synthesis, and biogenic amine production are impacted. Further, high concentrations of phenylalanine can lead to crystallization into neurotoxic amyloid-like fibrils that form pathological aggregates.

Diagnosis

Screening for phenylketonuria can be conducted on a drop of blood collected on filter paper. Confirmatory testing involves quantitative determination of phenylalanine and tyrosine in blood. In common phenylketonuria, phenylalanine is elevated while tyrosine is decreased. The presence of phenylpyruvate in the urine yields a positive green-colored reaction upon exposure to $FeCl_3$ (ferric chloride).

Treatment

The clinical manifestations of phenylketonuria can be prevented by neonatal screening detection followed by lifelong restriction of dietary phenylalanine. Normally, about 90 percent of the dietary phenylalanine intake is converted into tyrosine; therefore the treatment includes tyrosine supplementation. Diets containing mixtures of neutral amino acids are intended to compete with transport of phenylalanine in the intestine and into the brain.

A subset of children with phenylketonuria is responsive to tetrahydrobiopterin (BH_4). This form of phenylketonuria is caused by mutations that cause deficient BH_4 synthesis or recycling. These children also require neurotransmitter precursors (L-dopa with carbidopa and 5-hydroxytryptophan) as part of their treatment.

Several types of viral vectors, including adeno-associated viral vectors, have been examined for their potential to correct phenylketonuria in mutant mice or hepatocytes derived from these mice. Direct injection of naked plasmid-DNA has been achieved, leading also to transient transgene expression. Fusion proteins have also been generated to specifically target the enzyme to the liver as a form of enzyme replacement therapy. Enzyme

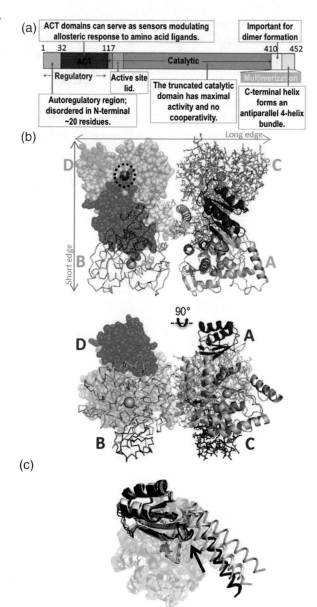

Figure 27.3 The structure of phenylalanine hydroxylase (PAH). a. The annotated domain structure of mammalian PAH. b. The 2.9 Å PAH crystal structure in orthogonal views, colored as in part A, subunit A is shown in ribbons; subunit B is as a Ca trace; subunit C is in sticks; and subunit D is in transparent spheres. In cyan, the subunits are labeled near the catalytic domain (top); in red, they are labeled near the regulatory domain (bottom). The dotted black circle illustrates the autoregulatory domain partially occluding the enzyme active site (iron, in orange sphere). c. Comparison of the subunit structures of full-length PAH and those of the composite homology model; the subunit overlay aligns residues 144–410. The four subunits of the full-length PAH structure (the diagonal pairs of subunits are illustrated using either black or white) are aligned with the two subunits of 2PAH (cyan) and the one subunit of 1PHZ (orange). The catalytic domain is in spheres, the regulatory domain is in ribbons, and the multimerization domain is as a Ca trace. The arrow denotes where the ACT domain and one helix of 2PAH conflict. Reproduced with permission from Arturo EC et al. First structure of full-length mammalian phenylalanine hydroxylase reveals the architecture of an autoinhibited tetramer. *Proc Natl Acad Sci U S A.* 2016; 113(9):2394–9.

substitution therapy using phenylalanine ammonia-lyase, an enzyme that catalyzes the conversion of phenylalanine into transcinnamic acid and insignificant amounts of ammonia, has also been attempted via intravenous infusion. However, a progressive immune reaction limits the viability of this replacement enzyme. Genetically modified probiotics including *Escherichia coli* may be useful as an alternative therapy. These organisms express elevated activities of phenylalanine ammonia-lyase in the intestine.

Bibliography

Al Hafid N., Christodoulou J. (2015). Phenylketonuria: a review of current and future treatments. *Transl Pediatr.* 4(4):304–17.

Koch R., Verma S., Gilles F.H. (2008). Neuropathology of a 4-month-old infant born to a woman with phenylketonuria. *Dev Med Child Neurol.* 50(3):230–3.

Steiner C.E., Acosta A.X., Guerreiro M.M., et al. (2007). Genotype and natural history in unrelated individuals with phenylketonuria and autistic behavior. *Arq Neuropsiquiatr.* 65(2A):202–5.

Infantile Organic Acidemias

A 15-year-old boy was evaluated for longstanding epilepsy. Family, pregnancy, and labor were unremarkable. A slightly abnormal psychomotor development had been evident in the first few months of life, although he had been able to stand and walk with aid. He also developed some communicative abilities. He then experienced a generalized seizure at the age of 18 months. At 18 to 24 months, his gait had worsened, with limb clumsiness. There was also language regression in the context of progressive overall intellectual deterioration. His seizures were treatable with just one medication and did not recur after the age of 8 years. By 15 years of age, he was wheelchair bound and completely dependent on others, even for feeding. He exhibited severe mental retardation, absent communicative abilities, pseudobulbar signs, bilateral optic atrophy, strabismus, hypoacusis, spastic tetraparesis, and choreodystonia in the upper limbs. His right plantar response was flexor and the left, extensor.

Infantile Organic Acidemias

Onset: Insidious, subtle, or frank mental retardation.
Additional manifestations: Encephalopathy crises, ketoacidosis, episodic gastrointestinal symptoms. Hypotonia. Protein intolerance.
Disease mechanism: Accumulation of excess endogenous acids as the result of impaired protein catabolism.

Testing: Specific patterns of organic aciduria, urinary acylglycines, and serum acylcarnitines, which are particularly informative during decompensations.
Treatment: Hemodialysis during life-threatening crises. Enzyme cofactor supplementation in select disorders and repletion of carnitine depleted via conjugation with organic acid derivatives. Specific dietary formulas and dietary protein restriction.
Research highlights: Detection in presymptomatic or early symptomatic state via newborn screening.

Clinical Features

Late-onset and milder variant forms of organic acidemias may present with an acute decompensation precipitated by a mild intercurrent illness, or with failure to thrive, hypotonia, slowly progressive mental retardation and a history of vomiting, protein intolerance, acidosis, or hypoglycemia. While these children exhibit milder chronic disease features, the neurological manifestations may be just as severe as those presenting earlier. Newborn screening can be beneficial to these infants as the initial crisis may be prevented. The general pathophysiology, pathology, diagnosis, and treatment have been separately described in Newborn Organic Acidemias. This chapter summarizes the most common organic acidemias that lead to slowly progressive manifestations or to episodic decompensation.

Table 28.1 Some organic acidemias that can manifest in infancy

Organic acidemia	Enzyme defect	Infantile and childhood manifestations
2-L-hydroxyglutaric aciduria	L-2-hydroxyglutarate dehydrogenase	Tumor formation (Figure 28.1) Failure to thrive Abnormal mental development White matter abnormalities (Figures 28.2 and 28.3)
Isovaleric acidemia	Isovaleryl-coenzyme A dehydrogenase	Peculiar odor Failure to thrive Encephalopathic crises
3-Methylglutaconic acidemia	3-Methylglutaconyl-coenzyme A hydratase	Abnormal mental development and dementia Dystonia Spasticity Quadriparesis Optic atrophy Leukoencephalopathy
Beta ketothiolase deficiency	Acetyl-coenzyme A acetyltransferase 1	Epilepsy Ketoacidosis, including: • Vomiting • Dyspnea • Lethargy and coma • Dehydration
Succinic semialdehyde dehydrogenase deficiency	Aldehyde dehydrogenase 5 family member A1	Hypotonia Abnormal intellectual development Epilepsy Ataxia Sleep disturbance Hyperactivity Hallucinations Obsessive-compulsive disorder
Glutaric acidemia type II	Electron transfer flavoprotein alpha subunit, electron transfer flavoprotein beta subunit or electron transfer flavoprotein dehydrogenase	Hypoglycemic crises Hepatomegaly Cardiomyopathy Brain malformation Peculiar odor
2-Methylbutyryl-CoA dehydrogenase deficiency	2-Methylbutyryl-CoA dehydrogenase	Failure to thrive Visual impairment Abnormal motor development Epilepsy

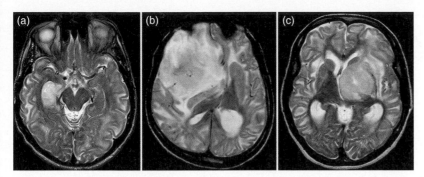

Figure 28.1 Axial T2-weighted MR images in 2-L-hydroxyglutaric aciduria. Subject (**a**) had an anaplastic astrocytoma in the right hippocampal area; subject 2 (**b**) was diagnosed with oligodendroglioma; and subject 3 (**c**) had a low-grade glioma in the left thalamus. Besides the obvious intra-axial mass lesions in all 3 cases, extensive, leukodystrophy-like changes, showing a centripetal gradient are conspicuous, which, in conjunction with additional abnormalities found in basal ganglia and dentate nuclei (not shown), are very suggestive of 2-L-hydroxyglutaric aciduria. Reproduced with permission from Patay Z et al. Cerebral neoplasms in L-2 hydroxyglutaric aciduria: 3 new cases and meta-analysis of literature data. *AJNR Am J Neuroradiol.* 2012; 33(5):940–3.

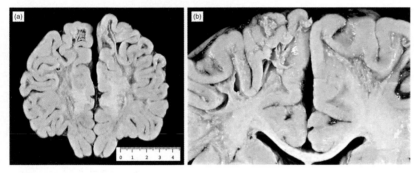

Figure 28.2 Sections of brain tissue in 2-L-hydroxyglutaric aciduria. **a.** Frontal coronal section showing massive demyelination, with a bland aspect of the white matter and cystic formation in peripheral subcortical areas. The scale is in centimeters. **b.** Detail of the demyelinated areas in a parietal section. Note the slightly atrophic, otherwise relatively preserved, aspect of the corpus callosum. Reproduced with permission from Seijo-Martínez M, Navarro C, Castro del Río M, Vila O, Puig M, Ribes A, Butron M. I-2-hydroxyglutaric aciduria: clinical, neuroimaging, and neuropathological findings. *Arch Neurol. 2005;* 62(4):666–70.

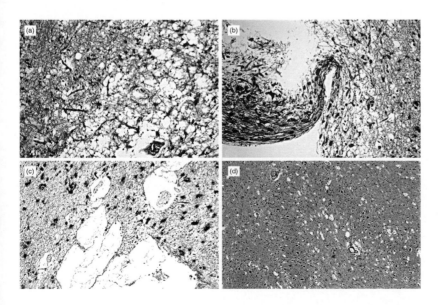

Figure 28.3 Histopathology in 2-L-hydroxyglutaric aciduria. Microscopic views of brain tissue. **a.** Cortex and white matter, showing severe spongiosis of the latter with mild involvement of the cortex (hematoxylin-eosin, original magnification ×10). **b.** Cystic areas surrounded by numerous hyperplastic astrocytes (hematoxylin-eosin, original magnification ×10). **c.** Immunodetection with glial fibrillary acidic protein. An elevated number of positive hyperplastic astrocytes surround the microcysts in the white matter (glial fibrillary acidic protein, original magnification ×20). **d.** Low-power image of the dentate nucleus. There is minimal neuronal loss, but spongiosis and vacuolation are present in the periphery of the nucleus (hematoxylin-eosin, original magnification ×5).

Bibliography

El-Hattab AW. (2015). Inborn errors of metabolism. *Clin Perinatol.* 42(2):413–39.

Seijo-Martínez M., Navarro C., Castro del Río M., et al. (2005). L-2-hydroxyglutaric aciduria: Clinical, neuroimaging, and neuropathological findings. *Arch Neurol.* 62(4):666–70.

Niemann–Pick Type A Disease

A boy was born at term after a normal pregnancy. He smiled at 6 weeks but head control was never attained. He manifested postprandial vomiting since the age of 1 month, although he gained weight continuously. He had had several bouts of upper respiratory infections. At the age of 6 months he was admitted to the hospital with bronchopneumonia. On admission, height and weight corresponded to the 75th percentile, the head circumference to the 50th. The skin had a dark yellowish-brown tan which was darker than that of his parents. Chest examination revealed pneumonia of the right middle and lower lobe. The prominent abdomen was almost completely filled by the enlarged liver and spleen. A minimal general opacity of the cornea was observed. At fundoscopy, the maculae appeared as brownish-red spots contrasting to the greyish-yellow color of the perimacular retina. No signs of visual impairment or signs of auditory loss or of unusual startle reactions to sounds could be demonstrated. Head control was poor; spontaneous movements were rare. There was generalized hypotonia and weak tendon reflexes. The sign of Babinski was absent. Motor development corresponded to 3 months. At 9 months, examination showed persistence of hypotonia and of weak tendon reflexes. Babinski's sign was now detected. No visual or hearing impairment could be substantiated. The size of the liver was slightly reduced, whereas the size of the spleen remained unchanged. Persistent vomiting remained and the boy ceased to thrive as well as before. Sudden death occurred at the age of 10 months.

Niemann–Pick Type A Disease

Onset: Hepatosplenomegaly within the first three months of life.
Additional manifestations: Progressive psychomotor regression, flaccidity, and hypotonia.

Cherry-red retinal spots or macular halos. Hepatic failure. Pulmonary compromise. Seizures are rare.
Disease mechanism: Accumulation of sphingomyelin and other lipids with reduced phosphocholine and ceramide. Reorganization of lipid rafts in the plasma membrane, which may impact signaling. In knockout mice this leads to abnormal synapse formation and function. Neuroinflammation.
Testing: Elevated serum triglycerides and low-density lipoprotein cholesterol with decreased high-density lipoprotein cholesterol.
Determination of acid sphingomyelinase activity in leukocytes or cultured skin fibroblasts.
Treatment: None effective.
Research highlights: Enzyme replacement therapy using human recombinant acid sphingomyelinase in knockout mutant mice with the visceral form of the disease (type B).

Clinical Features

Niemann–Pick type A and type B disease are caused by autosomal recessive loss of function of the lysosomal hydrolase acid sphingomyelinase. Type A disease is a neurovisceral storage disorder with relatively stereotypic features, whereas type B is primarily visceral and manifests a wider spectrum of severity. Type A children rarely survive beyond their second birthday, whereas type B individuals live into their fourth decade. Nevertheless, significantly overlapping forms may occur.

Children with Niemann–Pick type A disease are typically born normal. They develop hepatosplenomegaly over the first three months of life. About one-half of them manifest cherry red retinal spots or a red-brown halo around the macula. However, in contrast with Tay–Sachs disease, there is no hyperacusis or excess startle reflex nor macrocephaly. Seizures are also rare. Psychomotor deterioration ensues rapidly and normal milestones are rarely attained. Children become hypotonic and flaccid. Pulmonary infiltration is often apparent radiologically. Bone involvement is not clinically apparent.

Pathology

The liver and spleen are grossly enlarged. There are abundant mononuclear or, more rarely, multinuclear foamy macrophages in many organs (Figure 29.1).

These cells contain cholesterol and fill the pulp of the spleen, hepatic sinusoids, pulmonary alveoli, thymus, and lymph nodes. There is also vacuolation of lymphocytes. These inclusions and stored materials are composed of electrolucent granules and electrodense vacuoles and concentric lamellar structures (Figure 29.2).

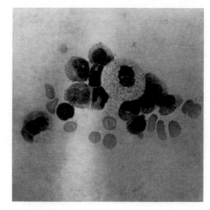

Figure 29.1 Bone marrow smear in Niemann-Pick A disease. Hematoxylin-eosin. Original magnification 900 ×, oil immersion. Vacuolated plasma cell. Reproduced with permission from da Silva V, Vassella F, Bischoff A, Spycher M, Wiesmann UN, Herschkowitz N. Niemann-Pick's disease. Clinical, biochemical and ultrastructural findings in a case of the infantile form. *J Neurol*. 1975; 211(1):61–8.

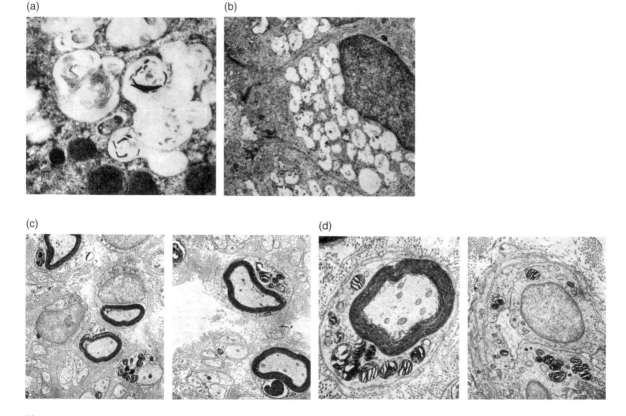

Figure 29.2 Pathology in Niemann–Pick A disease. Electron microscopic picture of hepatocytes. **a**. Magnification 27700x; OsO4 fixation. Lysosomes filled with membrane-like structures and with dense osmiophilic material. **b**. Magnification 14100x; OsO 4 fixation. Lysosomal vacuols in hepatocytes. **c** and **d**. Electron micrographs of transverse sections through the sural nerve in infantile Niemann–Pick's A disease. **c**. Within the Schwann cell cytoplasm of 2 myelinated and 4 unmyelinated nerve fibres inclusion bodies containing a dark substance are present. The inclusion bodies show in part a circular multimembraneous content, in part a more stratified appearance. **d**. Membrane bound bodies of apparent lysosomal origin similar to "zebra bodies" occupy a great part of the cytoplasma of the Schwann cell around a myelinated nerve fiber. Inclusion bodies of the same appearance are also present within endoneurial capillary endothelial cells. Reproduced with permission from da Silva V, Vassella F, Bischoff A, Spycher M, Wiesmann UN, Herschkowitz N. Niemann-Pick's disease. Clinical, biochemical and ultrastructural findings in a case of the infantile form. *J Neurol*. 1975; 211(1):61–8.

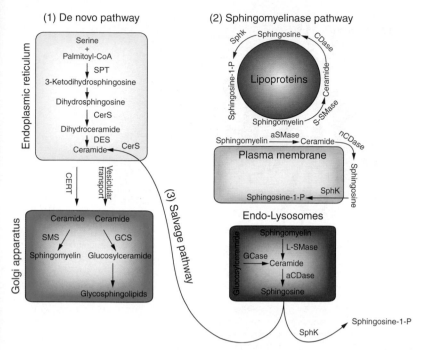

Figure 29.3 Sphingolipid metabolism. [1]De novo ceramide synthesis. Within the endoplasmic reticulum, serine and palmitoyl-coenzyme A are condensed by serine palmitoyltransferase (SPT) to form in the first step of the de novo sphingolipid synthesis. Subsequently, 3-ketosphinganine is metabolized to dihydrosphingosine. Dihydrosphingosine is acylated by (dihydro)ceramide synthase (CerS) producing dihydroceramide, which is then converted to ceramide by dihydroceramide desaturase (DES). Ceramide is then trafficked to the Golgi apparatus via vesicular transport or via the ceramide transfer protein (CERT) where it is the substrate for the synthesis of more complex sphingolipids, such as sphingomyelin and glycosphingolipids. [2] Sphingomyelinase pathway. The breakdown of sphingomyelin by aSMase within the endo-lysosomal system, at the outer leaflet of the plasma membrane, and in association with lipoproteins. Ceramide generated from the breakdown of SM can be deacylated by acid or neutral ceramidases (aCDase, nCDase) to yield free sphingosine. Sphingosine can be the substrate for either CerS, via the [3] ceramide salvage pathway or sphingosine kinases (SphK) to form ceramide and S1P, respectively. For simplicity, neutral and alkaline sphingomyelinases are not depicted in this diagram. Abbreviations: SPT – serine palmitoyltransferase; CerS – (dihydro)ceramide synthase; DES – dihydroceramide desaturase; CERT – ceramide transfer protein; SMS – sphingomyelin synthase; GCS – glucosylceramide synthase; aSMase – acid sphingomyelinase; S-SMase – secretory sphingomyelinase; L-SMase – lysosomal sphingomyelinase; GCase – glucosylceramidase; aCDase – acid ceramidase; nCDase – neutral ceramidase; SphK – sphingosine kinase. Reproduced with permission from Jenkins RW et al. Roles and regulation of secretory and lysosomal acid sphingomyelinase. *Cell Signal.* 2009; 21(6): 836–46.

MR imaging demonstrates atrophy of the cerebral cortex and the cerebellum. Irregular white matter hyperintensities may also be present upon T2-weighted examination. Macroscopically, the brain is diffusely atrophic. Microscopically, the changes are similar to infantile GM1 and GM2 gangliosidoses. Neurons with enlarged cell bodies are prominent throughout the brain, autonomic ganglia, dorsal root ganglia, and myenteric plexus. These neurons contain sphingomyelin, GM2, and GM2 gangliosides. Lipid storage is also prominent in macrophages and microglia, as is in retinal ganglion cells, amacrine and Müller cells, and conjunctiva and corneal epithelium.

Pathophysiology

Sphingomyelin is an important constituent of plasma membranes and of myelin (Figure 29.3).

In both Niemann–Pick type A and B diseases, mutations in the acid sphingomyelinase gene SMPD1 (or ASM) lead to enzymatic loss of function in association with a 50-fold increase in visceral sphingomyelin (Figure 29.4).

As the name indicates, the enzyme operates optimally at the reduced pH characteristic of the lysosomal interior, catalyzing the conversion of sphingomyelin into phosphocholine and ceramide (*N*-fatty-sphingosine). However, when cells are subject to stresses such as irradiation or heat shock, the enzyme translocates to the outer leaflet of the plasma membrane, where it degrades sphingomyelin into ceramide, perhaps in acidic microdomains. This leads to reorganization of lipid rafts in the plasma membrane, which may impact signaling. In knockout mice this leads to abnormal synapse formation and function. In addition to sphingomyelin, other lipids

109

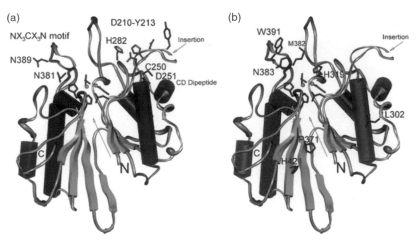

Figure 29.4 Secondary structure rendering of the model of the human acid sphingomyelinase phosphodiesterase domain. Secondary structures are indicated with red barrels (a-helices) and green arrows (ß-sheets). The amino and carboxyl termini of the domain are labeled with "N" and "C," respectively. The dimetal center, indicated with a red arrow, is located within the pseudo twofold symmetry axis of this domain. The highest confidence region, consisting of the side chains of five predicted conserved metal-coordinating residues (Asp206, Asp278, Asn318, His425, and His457) are shown in red. The metal ions are indicated with pink spheres. The 30-residue insertion is indicated with a black arrow. (a) The side chains of the conserved residues with respect to the dimetal center are shown in purple: Asn381 and Asn389 from the NX3CX3N motif; Asp210–Tyr213 and His282 from the cluster of hydrophilic/aromatic residues; and Cys250 and Asp251 from the CysAsp dipeptide. (b) The side chains of the Niemann-Pick mutation residues are indicated in blue in context to the dimetal center: Met382, Asn383, and Trp391 in or near the NX3CX3N motif; His319 in MM3; and Leu302, Pro371 and His421, predicted to lie outside of the dimetal center. Reproduced with permission from Seto M et al. A model of the acid sphingomyelinase phosphoesterase domain based on its remote structural homolog purple acid phosphatase. *Protein Sci.* 2004; 13(12): 3172–86.

such as bis(monoacylglycero)phosphate, cholesterol, glucocerebroside, and gangliosides GM2 and GM3 accumulate. In the brain of type A disease, sphingomyelin increases by 5- to 10-fold in the gray matter, whereas it remains normal in type B disease.

Cells deficient in sphingomyelinase are resistant to apoptosis. Irradiation or ischemia is less effective in knockout mice. This is probably related to deficient production of ceramide and consequent loss of reorganization of rafts into platforms.

The gene SMPD1 is paternally imprinted such that the maternal gene is preferentially expressed and this influences the phenotype. In some cases, abnormal clinical and laboratory findings have been noted in heterozygous individuals who carry only one SMPD1 mutation. Three common mutations (Arg469Leu, Leu302Pro, and frameshift Pro330) are prevalent in Ashkenazi Jews with type A disease, with a carrier frequency of 1 in 100, whereas 677delT is common in Israeli Arabs. Gln292Lys is associated with later onset disease and milder neurological involvement.

Diagnosis

The serum lipid profile is suggestive, with elevated serum triglycerides and low-density lipoprotein cholesterol in the context of decreased high-density lipoprotein cholesterol. Determination of acid sphingomyelinase activity in leukocytes or cultured skin fibroblasts is definitive.

Treatment

Bone marrow transplantation in knockout mice is moderately effective, as the neurological manifestations of the disease may prove refractory despite visceral disease amelioration. Direct intracranial injection of bone marrow cells is also inefficient in preventing neurological decline. Intravenously-administered replacement enzyme is effective in preventing visceral manifestations in mice, including inflammatory abnormalities, but not cerebral manifestations. Other treatment modalities attempted in mice include autologous hematopoietic stem cell gene therapy using retroviral vectors, liver gene therapy with adeno-associated virus constructs, and directly-injected of gene therapy vectors or recombinant enzyme in the brain.

Bibliography

da Silva V., Vassella F., Bischoff A., et al. (1975). Clinical, biochemical and ultrastructural findings in a case of the infantile form. *J Neurol.* 211(1):61–8. Niemann-Pick's disease.

Schuchman E.H., Wasserstein M.P. (2015). Types A and B Niemann-Pick disease *Best Pract Res Clin Endocrinol Metab.* 29(2):237–47.

Sialidosis

A baby was the first child of first cousins. The mother and father were healthy, but two of the mother's sisters had died at approximately one year of unknown causes. At birth, the infant had a peculiar appearance to her face, ascites, and periorbital edema. The edema cleared at the end of the first week. Two weeks later she returned to her family physician with diarrhea and was found to have hepatosplenomegaly. On examination at 6 weeks, she was thin, weighing 4.18 kg, (10th percentile). Her length was 57 cm (75th percentile), and her head circumference was 38.5 cm (50th percentile). Her face had the dish-shaped configuration common in type 1 GM gangliosidosis and her head was brachycephalic in shape. The bridge of her nose was flattened, and she had mild hypertelorism. The diarrhea responded to regular therapy. Two months later she returned to the hospital with watery diarrhea and tachypnea. She was sickly and emaciated, weighing 4.6 kg and responded only to painful stimuli. In addition to earlier findings, she now had a heart rate of 140. There was indrawing of her chest on breathing. Rales were heard over the right chest. She had moderate peripheral edema and the liver was now 5 cm below the right costal margin. She was treated with ampicillin and furosemide and placed in oxygen. Over a six-day period her chest and edema cleared. At 6 months she again returned to the hospital with a two-day history of fever and cough. She had a temperature of 40.5°C, grunting respirations, and rales. Her chest X-ray showed not only bilateral infiltrations but cardiomegaly. She did not respond to therapy and died two days after admission.

Sialidosis

Onset: Dysmorphic facial and skeletal features may be noticeable at birth.

Additional manifestations: Progressive psychomotor dysfunction, macular cherry-red spots and organomegaly. Hydrops fetalis has sometimes been an additional congenital manifestation.
Disease mechanism: Accumulation of sialylated glycoproteins, glycopeptides, and oligosaccharides in lysosomes. Extralysosomal dysfunction stemming from neuraminidase deficiency
Testing: Urinary determination of sialyloligosaccharides.
Treatment: None effective.
Research highlights: The Neu1 mouse model of neuraminidase deficiency recapitulates the human disorder.

Clinical Features

The glycoprotein storage disorders include several diseases that arise from lysosomal dysfunction. There is defective removal of the carbohydrate chains of glycoproteins due to mutation of lysosomal hydrolase genes. Although several disorders are well recognized as glycoprotein storage diseases, additional entities such as beta-galactosidase deficiency or mucopolysaccharidosis IVA may be classified among these disorders. The principal glycoprotein lysosomal storage disorders are summarized here.

In the mucolipidoses, there is combined tissue storage of lipids and mucopolysaccharides. Sialidosis follows two relatively well-defined clinical courses. In sialidosis type 1, there may be cherry-red retinal spots and progressive visual loss and myoclonus, whereas sialidosis type 2 is more severe (Figures 30.1 and 30.2). Some children with sialidosis type 1 do not manifest overt symptoms until late childhood. These children can also exhibit ataxia and epilepsy. Many affected individuals have been Italian. In contrast, mucolipidosis type I, also known as sialidosis type 2,

Table 30.1 Glycoprotein lysosomal storage disorders

Disorder	Defective enzyme	Accumulating compounds
Sialidosis	Sialidase (neuramidase)	Sialyloligosaccahrides
Galactosialidosis	Carboxypeptidase protective protein	Sialyloligosaccahrides
Alpha-mannosidosis	Alpha-mannosidase	Oligosaccharides
Beta-mannosidosis	Beta-mannosidase	Beta-mannosyl derivatives
Alpha-fucosidosis	Alpha-fucosidase	Oligosaccharides and glycolipids
Aspartylglucosaminuria	Glycosylasparaginase	Aspartylglucosamine and glycoasparagines
Schindler disease	Alpha-*N*-acetyl-galactosaminidase	Alpha-*N*-acetyl-galactosamine

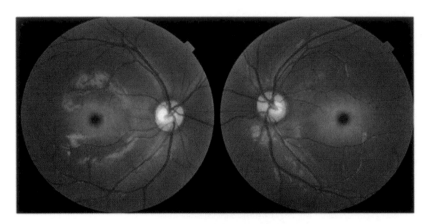

Figure 30.1 Fundus photographs, showing a cherry-red spot in both maculae in sialidosis. Reproduced with permission from Zou W et al. Fundus autofluorescence and optical coherence tomography of a macular cherry-red spot in a case report of sialidosis. *BMC Ophthalmol.* 2016; 16:30.

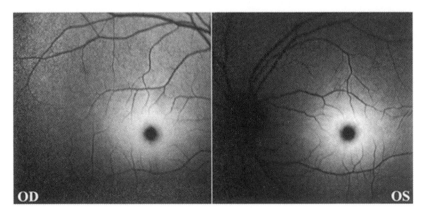

Figure 30.2 Fundus autofluorescence (FAF) imaging, showing bilateral hyperreflective areas surrounding the fovea in sialidosis. Reproduced with permission from Zou W et al. Fundus autofluorescence and optical coherence tomography of a macular cherry-red spot in a case report of sialidosis. *BMC Ophthalmol.* 2016; 16:30.

is caused by autosomal recessive neuramidase deficiency and is the best known sialidosis. Neuramidase is also named sialidase. Type 2 sialidosis is characterized by dysmorphic features, disostosis multiplex, cherry-red spots, organomegaly including cardiomegaly, and progressive psychomotor regression.

Pathology

There are vacuolated cells in the bone marrow, which is helpful for diagnostic reasons. In addition, the most characteristic disease feature is the vacuolation of neurons, oligodendrocytes, endothelial cells, and hepatocytes, among other visceral cells. Kupffer cells and histiocytes in the splenic pulp are particularly affected. These pathological changes are similar in type 1 and type 2 sialidosis. The vacuoles are limited by a membrane and contain floccular material. Spinal neurons, Schwann cells, and myenteric plexus neurons may contain concentric myelin layers. Intracytoplasmic storage of lipofuscin may also be conspicuous throughout the brain and in Kupffer cells. Neuronal loss is prominent in the thalamic lateral geniculate nucleus, substantia nigra, and gracile and cuneate nuclei. Loss of cerebellar Purkinje cells coexists with Bergmann glial proliferation.

Pathophysiology

The biochemical hallmark of sialidosis is the progressive accumulation of sialylated glycoproteins, glycopeptides, and oligosaccharides in the lysosomes of many cell types, as well as the excretion of sialyloligosaccharides in body fluids. There are four neuraminidases or sialidases. Neuraminidase 1 is localized inside the lysosome. Deficiency of sialidase 1 is more pronounced in sialidosis type 2 than in sialidosis type 1. In addition to their role in lysosomal catabolism, sialidases possess extralysosomal functions, which may be relevant for pathogenesis.

Diagnosis

Abnormal somatosensory evoked potentials with giant cortical waves can be detected in sialidosis type 1. An additional feature is that a prolonged P100 peak latency of the visual evoked potentials can also be found in most children even in early stage before the onset of visual symptoms. Urine samples can be analyzed by dimethylmethylene blue dye-binding assay or by multiplex assay based on enzymatic digestion of heparan sulfate, dermatan sulfate, and keratan sulfate followed by quantification by liquid chromatography and tandem mass spectrometry.

Treatment

There is no effective treatment.

Bibliography

Bonten E.J., Annunziata I., d'Azzo A. (2014). Lysosomal multienzyme complex: pros and cons of working together. *Cell Mol Life Sci.* 71(11):2017–32.

Gravel R.A., Lowden J.A., Callahan J.W., et al. (1979). Infantile sialidosis: a phenocopy of type 1 GM1 gangliosidosis distinguished by genetic complementation and urinary oligosaccharides. *Am J Hum Genet.* 31(6):669–79.

Heroman J.W., Rychwalski P., Barr C.C. (2008). Cherry red spot in sialidosis (mucolipidosis type I). *Arch Ophthalmol.* 126(2):270–1.

Galactosialidosis

A boy was the first child to consanguineous parents. Early psychomotor development was normal. He walked unsupported at 14 months of age, but walking and running were always clumsy. At 1½ years of age he developed attacks of pain in his feet and hands associated with hyperesthesia. The attacks were provoked by changes in temperature, exertion, or infections, and the pain was relieved by rest. They appeared up to four times a day and lasted several minutes. Nerve conduction studies were normal at 3 years of age, but at 5 years of age they revealed absent response of sensory nerve action potentials in the left sural nerve. Progressive visual loss was noted since 4 years of age, with intermittent divergent concomitant strabismus, which eventually became constant. At ten years of age, he was visually impaired, with reduced color vision and nystagmus. A thin retinal nerve fiber layer and a macular cherry-red spot were noted. He also exhibited bilateral exophthalmos, frontal bossing, maxillary hypoplasia and increased lumbar lordosis. Sensory examination was normal. The liver and spleen were of normal size and there were no angiokeratomas of the skin. There was mild weakness of all muscles, with difficulties standing on both heels. Tendon reflexes were increased, with bilateral ankle clonus and Babinski signs. Psychometric tests revealed a mild learning disability. X-ray of the skeleton showed dysostosis multiplex. Cardiological investigations and MR imaging of the brain and spine were normal.

early infantile form. Organomegaly, disostosis multiplex, teleangiectasia, and corneal opacification. Vascular occlusion may follow endothelial dysfunction.

Disease mechanism: Autosomal recessive combined loss of function of beta-galactosidase and sialidase due to mutation of protective protein/cathepsin A, mediated via the intralysosomal proteolytic degradation of the two unprotected enzymes.

Testing: Demonstration of excess urinary oligosaccharide excretion.

Treatment: None effective.

Research highlights: Sheep and murine models of the disease, which resemble the human disorder.

Clinical Features

Galactosialidosis is an autosomal recessive glycoprotein storage disorder due to combined deficiency of beta-galactosidase and neuraminidase 1 stemming from a defect of lysosomal protective protein/cathepsin A (PPCA). Three forms of galactosialidosis are recognized.

Most individuals with galactosialidosis manifest dysmorphic features, psychomotor regression, macular cherry-red spots, myoclonus, foam cells in the bone marrow and vacuolated lymphocytes. Type I galactosialidosis is clinically similar to sialidosis type 2.

Galactosialidosis

Onset: Variable in early or late infancy or in juvenile or adult life. Progressive psychomotor disability is common.

Additional manifestations: Three forms are recognized, of which the late infantile and the juvenile are milder in comparison with the severe

Table 31.1 Clinical phenotypes of galactosialidosis

Galactosialidosis type	Clinical severity
I: Early infantile	Severe
II: Late infantile	Mild
III: Juvenile and adult	Variable

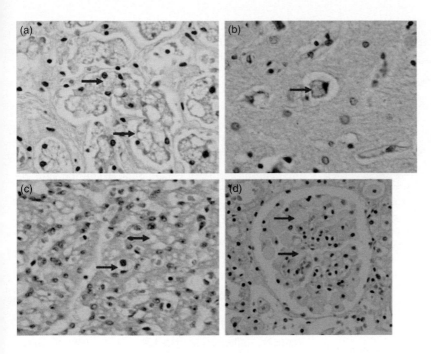

Figure 31.1 Galactosialidosis. Histopathologic findings with hematoxylin–eosin stain in (a) liver (300×); (b) brain (300×); (c) cardiac fiber (300×); and (d) kidney (250×). All arrows designate vacuoles at each cell. Reproduced with permission from Matsumoto N et al. A case of galactosialidosis with a homozygous Q49R point mutation. *Brain Dev.* 2008; 30(9):595–8.

In this form of the disease, coarse facies, hepatosplenomegaly, disostosis multiplex, and teleangiectasia are common. Infants rarely survive beyond the first year. As in sialidosis type 2, hydrops fetalis may occur. In type II galactosialidosis, the disease adopts a milder form characterized by late infantile coarsening of the face, hepatosplenomegaly, disostosis multiplex, and corneal opacification, resembling a mucopolysaccharidosis. Neurological abnormalities appear late in the disease course, in the context of intellectual disability. Seizures are rare. The juvenile or adult type occurs often in Japanese individuals. The face is mildly coarse and there are minor bone abnormalities. Macular cherry-red spots and angiokeratoma formation are common, but hepatosplenomegaly is rare. The main neurological abnormalities include myoclonus, ataxia, seizures and slowly progressive intellectual impairment.

Pathology

There are widespread changes in the nervous system. The optic nerve, thalamus, globus pallidus, and lateral geniculate body can be atrophic. Neuronal loss and fibrillary astrogliosis accompanies this atrophy. Neuronal storage, however, is found only in select structures such as Betz cells of the motor cortex, cells of the basal forebrain, neurons of the cranial nerve nuclei, anterior horn cells and cells of the trigeminal and spinal ganglia. In some cases, multiple cortical and subcortical infarcts have been associated with narrow blood vessels caused by storage material within the endothelium. Nerves can exhibit decreased nerve fiber density and vacuolated Schwann cells.

There is cytoplasmic vacuolation of many cell types, which is due to excess storage of oligosaccharides. In the severe infantile form, clear cytoplasmic vacuoles are conspicuous in hepatocytes, Kupffer cells, Schwann cells, fibroblasts, endothelium, lymphocytes and plasma cells (Figure 31.1). In the kidney, glomerular cells and tubular epithelial cells are finely vacuolated.

Pathophysiology

In galactosialidosis, the genetic defect resides in the gene CTSA, which encodes a dimeric protein with cathepsin A-like activity known as protective protein/cathepsin A (PPCA) (Figure 31.2). PPCA exists in a stabilized complex with beta-galactosidase and sialidase (alpha-neuraminidase).

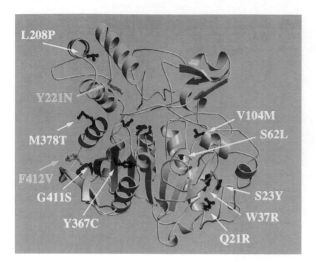

Figure 31.2 Schematic diagram of the PPCA (protective protein/cathepsin A) monomer, which is present as a dimer in the crystal structure. The core domain contains the catalytic triad (shown in blue). The cap domain consists of a three-helical bundle and a small mixed β-sheet involved in enzyme inactivation. The PPCA mutations found in galactosialidosis patients are shown in red (group 1) or green (group 2). Reproduced with permission from Rudenko G et al. The atomic model of the human protective protein/cathepsin A suggests a structural basis for galactosialidosis. *Proc Natl Acad Sci U S A.* 1998; 95(2):621–5.

Deficiency of PPCA thus leads to combined loss of function of beta-galactosidase and sialidase. This is mediated via the intralysosomal proteolytic degradation of the two unprotected enzymes, which is followed by accumulation of syalyloligosaccharides in lysosomes and fluids.

Diagnosis

The diagnosis of galactosialidosis is facilitated by the demonstration of excess oligosaccharide with *N*-acetylneuraminic acid at the nonreducing end. These compounds can be detected by thin-layer chromatography or high-performance liquid chromatography.

Treatment

There is no specific treatment.

Bibliography

Darin N., Kyllerman M., Hård A.L., et al. (2009). Juvenile galactosialidosis with attacks of neuropathic pain and absence of sialyloligosacchariduria. *Eur J Paediatr Neurol.* 13(6):553–5.

Infantile Ceroid Lipofuscinosis (Haltia-Santavuori Disease)

A 19-month-old girl was referred for assessment of severely abnormal development. Her initial development was normal: she gained head control, rolled over and sat at the age of 3, 5, and 9 months, respectively. Then, development slowed down: she crawled at 11 months and pulled to stand at 13 months. After that, psychomotor deterioration started: she lost learned gestures (clapping hands and waving bye–bye) at 14 months and then lost the capacity to smile, make eye contact and reach for objects at 18 months. At 19 months, she did not track objects with her eyes, did not crawl and sat unstably due to truncal ataxia. She displayed persistent hand mannerisms resembling those typical of Rett syndrome. Her weight was reduced (8,270 g) as was her height (72.8 cm). Head circumference was 46.1 cm (−0.4 SD). A cranial MR imaging study was performed (Figure 32.1). EEG showed bilateral central and parietal spikes with high voltage and slow background activities. At 23-months, she could not sit, fix her gaze and was experiencing sleep disturbances and myoclonic jerks of the extremities. Her head circumference had decreased to 41.3 cm (−3.9 SD). At 3 years of age, her EEG was isoelectric.

Testing: Demonstration of excessive storage for age in neurons of the intestinal myenteric or submucosal plexus and other accessible tissues.
Treatment: None effective.
Research highlights: Cysteamine bitartrate combined with N-acetylcysteine may lead to delay of isoelectric EEG and depletion of leukocyte granular osmiophilic deposits.

Clinical Features

The neuronal ceroid lipofuscinoses are common neurodegenerative disorders of children and adults generally characterized by progressive psychomotor and visual deterioration in association with excess deposition of autofluorescent lipofuscin pigment in the lysosomes of neural and other cells. Fifteen types of autosomal neuronal ceroid lipofuscinoses are recognized depending upon underlying genetic mechanism and age of onset. The term Batten disease is commonly used to refer to the neuronal ceroid lipofuscinosis although it properly refers to the juvenile form associated with locus CLN3.

Although all 15 loci are often classified together, the ceroid lipofuscinosis have relatively little in common such that, were it not for traditional reasons, they could be classified independently of one another. The major clinical types are the infantile, late infantile, juvenile, and adult forms, each represented by loci CLN1 to CLN4. However, this simplistic classification has expanded and it will probably continue to expand.

In general the ceroid lipofuscinosis are characterized by progressive neuronal loss which is more severe in the early-onset forms and is accompanied by glial proliferation. Preferential areas of cell loss include cortical GABAergic interneurons, thalamic relay cells, and Purkinje cells. Apoptosis or autophagy seems to mediate this neuronal cell loss.

Infantile neuronal ceroid lipofuscinosis CLN1 or Haltia-Santavuori disease occurs most often in

Infantile Ceroid Lipofuscinosis

Onset: Psychomotor delay and then regression by 15–18 months of age. Minimally abnormal development precedes frank regression.
Additional manifestations: Blindness. Progressive mental disturbance with aggression and hallucinations. Intractable seizures. Progressive flattening of the EEG to isoelectricity.
Disease mechanism: Autosomal recessive loss of function of palmitoyl-protein thioesterase 1, which is associated with accumulation of lipofuscin and widespread neuronal loss replaced by gliosis. Neuroinflammation.

Table 32.1 The neuronal ceroid lipofuscinoses

Form	Locus number	Inheritance	Gene name
Congenital	CLN10	Autosomal recessive	CTSD, Cathepsin D
Infantile (Haltia-Santavuori)	CLN1	Autosomal recessive	PPT1, Palmitoyl-protein thioesterase 1
Infantile (progressive myoclonic epilepsy)	CLN14	Autosomal recessive	KCTD7, potassium channel tetramerization domain 7
Late infantile (Jansky-Bielschowsly)	CLN2	Autosomal recessive	TPP1, tripeptidyl peptidase
Late infantile variant	CLN5	Autosomal recessive	Protein of unknown function
Late infantile variant (Lake-Cavanagh)	CLN6	Autosomal recessive	Protein of unknown function
Late infantile variant	CLN7	Autosomal recessive	MFSD8, major facilitator superfamily domain-containing protein 8
Late infantile variant (Northern epilepsy)	CLN8	Autosomal recessive	Protein containing TLC domain
Early juvenile variant	CLN9	Autosomal recessive	Unknown
Juvenile (Spielmeyer-Sjögren; Batten)	CLN3	Autosomal recessive	Battenin
Juvenile variant	CLN12	Autosomal recessive	ATP13A12, P-type ATPase 13A2
Adult (Kufs type A)	CLN4	Autosomal recessive	Unknown
Adult variant	CLN11	Autosomal recessive	GRN, progranulin
Adult variant (Kufs type B)	CLN13	Autosomal recessive	CTSF, cathepsin F
Adult variant (Parry)	CLN4B	Autosomal dominant	DNAJC5, cysteine string protein alpha

Finland. There is psychomotor retardation and later regression starting at 10–18 months of age. Hypotonia, clumsiness and slow head growth may be noted earlier. Visual dysfunction is prominent before 2 years of age and is due to progressive optic atrophy with retinal hypopigmentation and poorly reactive pupils. Myoclonic and seizures follow and sleep is abnormal. In advanced stages, aggression and hallucinations may occur. The EEG demonstrates slowing and eventually becomes flat due to neuronal loss.

Pathology

The head circumference is reduced and the skull is excessively thick. The brain is atrophic, with narrow gyri and wide sulci (Figures 32.1 and 32.2). The cerebellum and brainstem are also atrophic, in contrast with a grossly normal appearing spinal cord. Three pathological stages have been described. In the first stage, which spans up to 2.5 years of age, there are colorless or yellow neuronal storage granules with marked astrocytic hyperplasia. In the next stage (2.5–4 years of age), there is extensive cortical

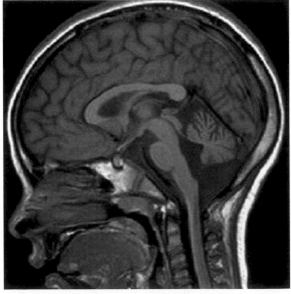

Figure 32.1 5-year-old girl with neuronal ceroid lipofuscinosis. Sagittal T1 MR imaging shows diffuse cerebellar atrophy. Reproduced with permission from Thomas B et al. MRI of childhood epilepsy due to inborn errors of metabolism. *AJR Am J Roentgenol.* 2010; 194(5):W367–74.

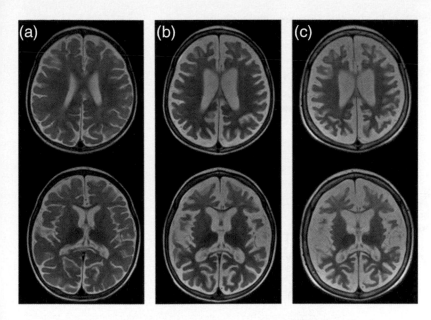

Figure 32.2 T2-weighted axial brain MR imaging in neuronal ceroid lipofuscinosis at the age of 19 months (a), 23 months (b), and 3 years (c) Thalamic hypointensity to the white matter and to the basal ganglia and thin periventricular intermittent high signal rims are seen from the early stage. Brain atrophy is severe and progressive. Reproduced with permission from Niida Y et al. A girl with infantile neuronal ceroid lipofuscinosis caused by novel PPT1 mutation and paternal uniparental isodisomy of chromosome 1. *Brain Dev.* 2016; 38(7):674–7.

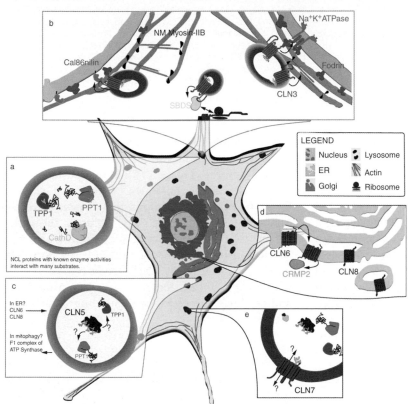

Figure 32.3 The interactions and locations of neuronal ceroid lipofuscinosis proteins. **a.** Soluble NCL proteins with known enzymatic activity: PPT1, TPP1, and cathepsin D (CathD), are localized to the lysosome and interact with their substrates in the lysosome lumen. **b.** CLN3 has been reported to localize to several subcellular locations and, as described in the text for the purposes of this review, is depicted in the lysosomal membrane, and interacts with several proteins including proteins at the cell periphery. CLN3 interacts with SBDS, calsenilin, and myosin-IIB through the C-terminus, and the fodrin-Na⁺–K⁺–ATPase complex through a cytosolic loop. CLN3 most likely does not interact with all of these proteins at the same time, but rather these interactions are probably dynamic. **c.** CLN5 is a highly glycosylated protein is localized to the lysosome. It has potential interactions with NCL proteins and has been shown to interact with CLN6 and CLN8, potentially in the ER. Interactions of CLN5 and PPT1 have been described with the F1-complex of the ATP-Synthase, which may occur during mitochondrial degradation. **d.** CLN6 and CLN8 are both transmembrane proteins that reside in the ER, and CLN6 interacts with CRMP-2. **e.** CLN7, a putative transporter (MFSD8) resides in the lysosomal membrane, but the interactions or function of CLN7/MFSD8 has not been elucidated. A representative lysosome (red) is highlighted for each NCL protein, though these lysosomal proteins probably exist together in many lysosomes. Reproduced with permission from Getty AL et al. Interactions of the proteins of neuronal ceroid lipofuscinosis: clues to function. *Cell Mol Life Sci.* 2011; 68(3):453–74.

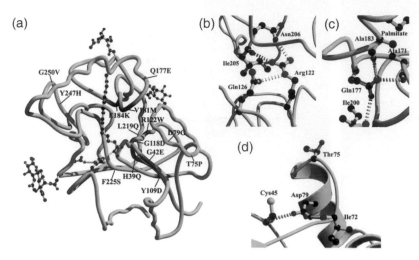

Figure 32.4 Palmitoyl Protein Thioesterase-1 (PPT1). Neuronal ceroid lipofuscinosis (NCL) mutations in PPT1. **a.** Sites of clinical NCL mutations in PPT1 are mapped onto the peptide backbone. Infantile NCL mutations are displayed in red, a mutation causing late infantile NCL symptoms is in blue, and juvenile NCL mutations are in green. **b.** The most common infantile NCL mutation (Arg122Trp) leads to the loss of three hydrogen bonds and a steric and polarity mismatch with the surrounding residues, resulting in misfolded protein. **c.** The Gln177Glu mutation is predicted to cause the loss of hydrogen bonds to Ala171 and Ala183, two residues that contact palmitate. This mutation results in a less severe phenotype that is clinically indistinguishable from late infantile NCL. **d.** Two mutations on α1 lead to juvenile NCL. Trp75Pro may alter the beginning of α1 due to the conformational restraints on Pro, and Asp79Glu loses hydrogen bonds to Cys45 and Ile72. Reproduced with permission from Bellizzi JJ 3rd et al. The crystal structure of palmitoyl protein thioesterase 1 and the molecular basis of infantile neuronal ceroid lipofuscinosis. *Proc Natl Acad Sci* U S A. 2000; 97(9):4573–8.

neuronal loss with astrocytic hyperplasia and macrophagic infiltration. In the last stage (after 4 years) cortical neurons are almost completely absent and there is secondary white matter degeneration. Nevertheless, the pyramidal cells of Betz in the precentral gyrus, the pyramidal neurons of the hippocampal CA1 and CA4 regions, and the spinal anterior horn cells are relatively preserved. In the retina, there is loss of photoreceptor, bipolar, and ganglion cells and replacement by glia. Accumulation of pigment is notable, in addition to neurons, in sweat glands, skeletal and smooth muscles, endothelial cells, and macrophages. Neurons in the myenteric and submucosal plexuses are affected and are thus sometimes used for diagnostic purposes. The stored material is autofluorescent under ultraviolet light. It contains sphingolipid activator proteins Sap A and D but not subunit C of the mitochondrial ATP synthase. In contrast with the late infantile and juvenile forms of ceroid lipofuscinosis, there are no vacuolated lymphocytes.

Pathophysiology

Disease severity is correlated with residual enzyme activity. The PPT1 enzyme, palmitoyl-protein thioesterase 1, can remove long chain fatty acids from cysteine residues in proteins that are targeted to the lysosome (Figure 32.3). However, its natural substrate remains unknown. Later-onset disease forms occur with mutations that preserve greater catalytic activity (Figure 32.4). Among the earliest disease events is synaptic pathology, which can be demonstrated before significant cell loss has taken place. Curiously, cell loss is not correlated with the amount of storage material. Neuroinflammation is a suspected compounding pathogenic mechanism.

Diagnosis

Determination of PPT1 enzyme activity or tissue diagnosis via the identification of lipofuscin granular inclusions in neurons and other tissues. Visual evoked potentials and EEG serve to document severe dysfunction in advanced disease stages.

Treatment

None effective, as epilepsy is generally refractory to therapy. In general, however, valproate and lamotrigine are relatively more effective. Other anti-convulsants may exacerbate myoclonus. Experimental treatments have focused on enzyme replacement, stem cell transplantation or viral vector introduction. Oral cysteamine bitartrate and N-acetylcysteine is associated with delay of isoelectric EEG, depletion of leukocyte granular osmiophilic deposits, and subjective benefits.

Bibliography

Niida Y., Yokoi A., Kuroda M., et al. (2016). A girl with infantile neuronal ceroid lipofuscinosis caused by novel PPT1 mutation and paternal uniparental isodisomy of chromosome 1. *Brain Dev*. pii:S0387–7604.

Anderson G.W., Goebel H.H., Simonati A. (2013). Human pathology in NCL. *Biochim Biophys Acta*. 1832(11):1807–26.

Farber Disease

A two-and-a-half-year old child presented with progressive regression of psychomotor capacities and joint nodules. He was born to cousin parents. The child was normal until 5 months of age, when he lost the ability to hold his neck or sit with support. At about that time, he developed multiple small swollen lesions on his scalp and joints. His voice became hoarse and he experienced repeated chest infections. He later developed dysphagia and lost weight markedly. Examination revealed multiple soft, irregular subcentimeter-size nodules over scalp, dorsal aspects of joints and spine. Joint movements were painful. The child's weight and head circumference were abnormally small. He could not hold his head erect. There was no cherry-red spot in the retina nor hepatosplenomegaly. MR imaging of the brain revealed marked cerebral hypoplasia.

Farber Lipogranulomatosis

Onset: First few months of life, with painful joints, subcutaneous nodules and hoarseness.
Additional manifestations: Pulmonary infiltration and hepatosplenomegaly. Abnormal psychomotor development and regression, progressive myoclonic epilepsy or motor neuron disease. Death often ensues in the second year of life.
Disease mechanism: Autosomal recessive deficiency of acid ceramidase, encoded by the lysosomal enzyme ASAH1. Ceramidase is a ubiquitous byproduct of cell membrane catabolism with toxic and inflammatory properties.
Testing: Assay of ceramidase enzymatic activity in plasma, white blood cells or fibroblasts.
Treatment: Hematopoietic stem cell transplantation in children without neurological involvement.
Research highlights: Heterozygous ASAH1 mice or missense mutant mice expressing affected individual-identified mutations in ASAH1 develop the disease, with high levels of ceramide accumulation.

Clinical Features

Farber lipogranulomatosis is a lysosomal storage disease characterized by autosomal recessive loss of function of acid ceramidase, an enzyme that hydrolyzes ceramide and which is encoded by the gene ASAH1. Several phenotypes are recognized and there have been attempts at classifying them into distinct disease categories. However, Farber disease variants display a syndromic continuum rather than discrete forms.

In the most common of Farber disease, onset is between 2 weeks and 4 months of age, with psychomotor deterioration. Arthropathy, subcutaneous nodules and laryngeal dysfunction are the most common associated features and may dominate the phenotype or even predate neurological manifestations (Figure 33.1). The subcutaneous nodules are most prominent over the joints and can be accompanied by pain upon mobilization. Visceral dysfunction associated with hepatosplenomegaly and other forms of multiorgan involvement can be fatal. A poor cry that progresses to aphonia is also characteristic. In those who survive visceral failure or pulmonary infections constitute the usual cause of death. The mechanism underlying the neurological manifestations involves anterior horn cell loss and neuropathy. Progressive muscular atrophy, hypotonia, and diminished tendon reflexes are common. One-third of affected individuals exhibit a mild cherry-red spot in the retina, which is usually asymptomatic.

A genetically related but clinically distinct syndrome includes spinal muscular atrophy with progressive myoclonic epilepsy, which is caused by less severe loss of acid ceramidase enzymatic function. Children afflicted by this form of the disease develop normally until about 5 years of age, when progressive walking difficulties, frequent falls, and hand tremor first become apparent. Myoclonic seizures appear years later. Facial weakness and denervation signs can be prominent in the context of a normal brain

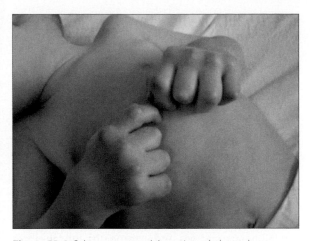

Figure 33.1 Subcutaneous nodules at interphalangeal articulations in Farber disease. Reproduced with permission from Ekici B et al. Farber disease: A clinical diagnosis. *J Pediatr Neurosci.* 2012; 7(2):154–5.

configuration detected by MR imaging. Respiratory infections may be prominent.

Hypomorphic mutations in ASAH1 may also result in an osteoarticular phenotype with a juvenile phase resembling rheumatoid arthritis and evolving to osteolysis. This phenotype lacks neurological manifestations.

Pathology

The typical subcutaneous nodules of Farber disease are granulomatous lesions that contain lipid cytoplasmic inclusions named Farber bodies. The inclusions display a curvilinear tubular structure (Figure 33.2). Additional granulomatous infiltration is present in subcutaneous tissues and joints. Lesions rich in foam macrophages can be symptomatic and are prominent in the larynx, lungs, and heart valves.

(a) (b) (c)

(d)

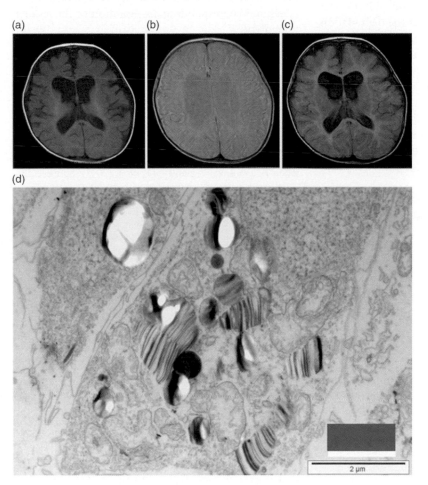

Figure 33.2. MR imaging and electron microscopy images in Farber disease. The T1 weighted and T2 weighted, and FLAIR magnetic resonance images of the brain (a, b, and c, respectively) illustrate diffuse loss of white matter volume predominantly along the occipital horns of the lateral ventricle with associated dilatation of the supratentorial and infratentorial ventricular system. d. Electron microscopy of a skin biopsy from a male child with Farber disease. Reproduced with permission from Chedrawi AK et al. Novel V97G ASAH1 mutation found in Farber disease patients: unique appearance of the disease with an intermediate severity, and marked early involvement of central and peripheral nervous system. *Brain Dev.* 2012; 34(5):400-4.

In the nervous system, abundant storage material is present in the cytoplasm of neurons. Lipid accumulation is conspicuous in anterior horn cells, brainstem nuclei, basal ganglia, and cerebellum, with more limited cortical involvement. Autonomic ganglia cells and Schwann cells are also affected.

Pathophysiology

Farber disease is associated with negligible or significantly reduced activity of N-acylsphingosine amidohydrolase (acid ceramidase). Ceramide levels can exceed 60-fold over normal and ceramide accumulation in liver, kidney, and brain correlates with disease severity. Acid ceramidase not only hydrolyzes ceramide into sphingosine within acidic cellular compartments, but can also synthesize ceramide from sphingosine at neutral pH when located in another compartment. Acid ceramidase exists in a complex with other lipid hydrolases and requires a polypeptide cofactor (saposin C and D) for full hydrolytic activity. It is thought that the degradation of membrane-bound ceramide takes place inside lysosomes that contain the enzyme, cofactors, and negatively charged lipids. Large quantities of ceramide originate from the degradation of complex membrane sphingolipids.

In skin, ceramide metabolism is particularly important because ceramides with alkyl chains up to 36 carbon atoms in length are abundant, conferring water impermeability. Ceramide accumulation probably leads to granuloma formation.

Additional functions for ceramide are possible. In particular, apoptosis, cellular stress response, and cytokine expression are thought to be mediated by ceramides.

Absence of acid ceramidase is embryonic lethal in mice, which may be related to cell death triggered by ceramide accumulation.

Diagnosis

Enzymatic assay of acid ceramidase using *N*-lauroyl-sphingosine as substrate in leukocytes, plasma, fibroblasts, or amniocytes.

Treatment

Bone marrow transplantation leads to regression of subcutaneous nodules and arthropathy but does not impact neurological decline. Successful hematopoietic stem cell transplantation has been conducted in children without neurologic manifestations.

Lentivectors including human ceramidase have been infused in neonates, with decrease in ceramidase levels and corresponding amelioration of the lesional phenotype.

Bibliography

Ahmad A., Mazhar A.U., Anwar M. (2009). Farber disease: A rare neurodegenerative disorder. *J Coll Physicians Surg Pak.* Jan;19(1):67–8.

Sands M.S. (2013). Farber disease: understanding a fatal childhood disorder and dissecting ceramide biology. *EMBO Mol Med.* Jun;5(6):799–801.

Zhou J., Tawk M., Tiziano F.D., et al. (2012). Spinal muscular atrophy associated with progressive myoclonic epilepsy is caused by mutations in ASAH1. *Am J Hum Genet.* Jul 13;91(1):5–14.

Chapter 34

Infantile Sialic Acid Storage Disease

A four-year-old girl was evaluated because of impaired speech and ambulatory abilities. She was the second child of consanguineous parents. She had experienced abnormal development, with head control at 4.5 months, unsupported sitting at 14 months, and walking at 2.5 years with prominent athetosis. Her weight and head circumference were normal but her height was below the third percentile for age. She exhibited a slightly coarse appearance with a broad face, flat nasal bridge, and high palate. Her neurological evaluation revealed mild mental retardation and ataxia. There was no visceromegaly or ocular abnormalities. MR imaging demonstrated only an overly thin corpus callosum. She had learnt to use a single word at the age of 2.5 years and at the age of 8 years she uttered only three words. Her receptive language development was better than her speech production.

Infantile Sialic Acid Storage Disease

Onset: Regression of motor and intellectual accomplishments in infancy. Hydrops fetalis or coarse facies may be apparent earlier.
Additional manifestations: Hepatosplenomegaly, disostosis, cardiomegaly, and nephrotic syndrome. Death is common in the first year of life. Salla disease is a milder form of the disorder without organomegaly or skeletal manifestations.
Disease mechanism: Autosomal recessive deficiency the lysosomal sialic acid transporter sialin, encoded by SLC17A5. Sialin also transports aspartate and glutamate into synaptic vesicles.
Testing: Assay of urine sialic acid or demonstration of excess cellular or intralysosomal sialic acid.
Treatment: None effective.
Research highlights: Direct transport measurements in whole cells by redirecting recombinant lysosomal transporters to the cell surface.

Clinical Features

Autosomal recessive infantile sialic acid storage disease and adult free sialic acid storage disorder or Salla disease result from the accumulation of sialic acid in lysosomes. The prevalence of free sialic acid storage disorder is highest in the Salla region of Finland, from which the name derives. Infantile sialic acid storage disease occurs in all populations.

In infantile sialic acid storage disease, affected individuals may manifest intrauterine abnormalities such as hydrops fetalis or exhibit coarse dysmorphic features at birth. Many newborns, however, are normal and only manifest the disease later. These infants experience regression of motor and intellectual accomplishments. Hepatosplenomegaly, cardiomegaly, nephrotic syndrome, and ascites are also common in infancy. Skeletal abnormalities include irregular metaphyses, osteopenia, club feet, short femurs, fractures, hip dysplasia, anterior beaking of the dorsal vertebrae or hypoplasia of the distal phalanges. Death usually ensues in the first year of life.

The first signs of Salla disease are hypotonia and nystagmus at 3–6 months of age in the context of a coarse facies. Later in infancy and childhood, ataxia, dysarthria and other forms of gait impairment become gradually noticeable. These motor abnormalities persist and remain more pronounced than cognitive impairment throughout the second decade of life. Ataxia, however, can subside between the ages of 10 and 15 years. In addition to dysmyelination of the cerebrum, which is detectable by MR imaging, nerve dysmyelination may occur, leading to polyneuropathy. Motor development continues into the third decade in the context of progressive athetosis and spasticity. Intellectual development also continues into the fourth decade. Eventually, motor disability remains severe, whereas cognitive capacities related to verbal comprehension and interactive abilities remain stable throughout adulthood. Survival, however, is often limited to the fifth decade, with some individuals manifesting late-onset epilepsy. There is no organomegaly or skeletal disostosis.

Pathology

MR imaging demonstrates cortical, basal, and cerebellar atrophy. There is progressive dysmyelination across the cerebrum. The corpus callosum is hypoplastic. MR spectroscopy illustrates increase of *N*-acetylaspartate and reduction of choline.

Microscopically, there is excess storage material inside many cell types (Figure 34.1). This material is enclosed in membrane-bound vacuoles, which represent lysosomes. Vacuolated lymphocytes, renal

tubular epithelium, hepatocytes and Kupffer cells, macrophages, Schwann cells, and endothelial cells are prominent. In the brain, neurons and glia demonstrate similar storage. There is loss of axons and extensive gliosis. Axonal spheroids and microcalcifications may be present.

Pathophysiology

Salla disease and infantile sialic acid storage disease are caused by defective transport of sialic acid across the lysosomal membrane to the cytosol, resulting in accumulation of intralysosomal sialic acid. Both are due to mutations in the SLC17A5 gene, which encodes the transporter sialin (Figure 34.2). Sialic acid (N-acetylneuraminic acid) is a negatively charged

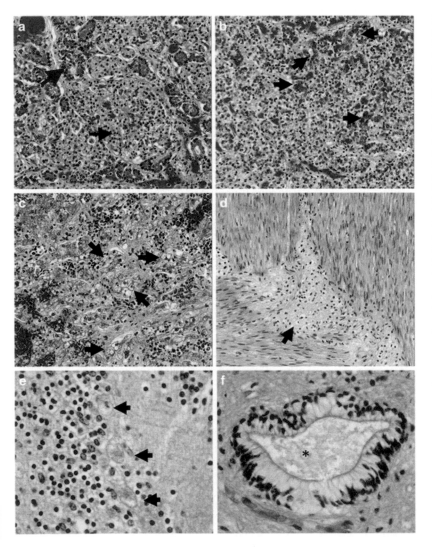

Figure 34.1. Pathologic findings in sialic acid storage disease. a. Section through pancreas showing enlarged, vacuolated islet cells (black arrow), with relatively normal-appearing acinar cells (blue arrow) at periphery. b. Pituitary gland contains a majority of pale, vacuolated cells with a foamy appearance; some acidophilic cells with a superimposed foamy quality (arrows) are seen. c. Sections of liver show granular, swollen, pale, foamy cells throughout (some clusters indicated by arrows). The stored material does not stain by Oil Red-O or periodic acid-Schiff histochemical stains (not shown). d. Ganglion cells of the myenteric plexus (arrow) have enlarged, pale cytoplasm with a foamy quality. e. Cerebellar cortex: three Purkinje cells are swollen, with cytoplasmic accumulation of foamy storage material and loss of Nissl substance (arrows). f. Ependymal canal, spinal cord: ependymal cells have a clear cytoplasm due to presence of storage material (asterisk indicates center of canal). Reproduced with permission from Lines MA et al. Infantile sialic acid storage disease: Two unrelated Inuit cases homozygous for a common novel SLC17A5 mutation. *JIMD Rep.* 2014; 12:79–84.

(a)

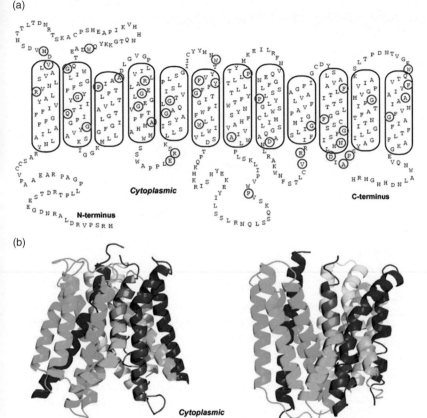

Figure 34.2 Conserved residues in the SLC17 family of proteins. a. PredictProtein-derived topology model for human sialin sequence with manual adjustments. The circled residues are conserved among all nine SLC17 proteins across vertebrate species in which the proteins have been identified. b. Inward (cytoplasmic)-facing and outward (lumenal/extracellular)-facing models of sialin based on structures of the bacterial multiple facilitator superfamily transporters GlpT and FucP, respectively. Structures are sequentially color coded from blue at the N-terminus to red at the C-terminus. Reproduced with permission from Reimer RJ. SLC17: A functionally diverse family of organic anion transporters. *Mol Aspects Med.* 2013; 34(2–3):350–9.

(b)

sugar generated during the degradation of cell membrane and other constituents. Lysosomal sialidases remove sialic acid residues from its conjugates, which are then exported to the cytosol for reutilization or further degradation.

Sialin is also responsible for membrane potential-driven aspartate and glutamate transport into synaptic vesicles.

The majority of sialin mutations are associated with loss of transporter activity or with retention of the protein inside the endoplasmic reticulum, while mutations associated with milder forms of the disease lead to reduced transporter function.

Diagnosis

Urinary excretion of sialic acid exceeds 100-fold of normal. Additional diagnostic methods include the demonstration of elevated fibroblast concentrations of free sialic acid and of excess sialic acid inside lysosomes.

Treatment

There is no effective form of therapy.

Bibliography

Coker M., Kalkan-Uçar S., Kitiş O., et al. (2009). Salla disease in Turkish children: Severe and conventional type. *Turk J Pediatr.* 51(6):605–9.

Paavola L.E., Remes A.M., Harila M.J., et al. (2015). A 13-year follow-up of Finnish patients with Salla disease. *J Neurodev Disord.* 7(1):20.

Sagné C., Gasnier B. (2008). Molecular physiology and pathophysiology of lysosomal membrane transporters. *J Inherit Metab Dis.* 31(2):258–66.

Childhood Congenital Disorders of Glycosylation

A 14-month-old female displayed poor ability to fix and follow, nystagmus, intermittent esotropia and foveal hypoplasia. She was born at 39 weeks via an uncomplicated spontaneous vaginal delivery and her weight was normal. However, in the newborn period she failed to thrive and eventually received gastrostomy tube placement for feeding. In the first few months of life, she was diagnosed with neurosensory hearing loss and poor truncal muscle tone. Magnetic resonance imaging showed severe vermian cerebellar hypoplasia. At 6 months of age, she was diagnosed with phosphomannomutase type 2 deficiency after her transferrin isoform assay showed severe hypoglycosylation. Three months later, she developed ventricular hypertrophy and pericardial effusions. She also had hypothyroidism and chronic normocytic anemia.

Childhood Congenital Disorders of Glycosylation

Onset: First few months of life with hypotonia, dysmorphism, and strabismus.
Additional manifestations: In phosphomannomutase 2 deficiency, visceral manifestations affect every organ except the lung and can lead to multiorgan failure and death in the multisystem form. Cerebellar degeneration, eye movement disorders, stroke-like events, and neuropathy.
Disease mechanism: Autosomal recessive deficiency of enzymes involved in the transfer of glycan residues to most proteins, leading to decrease protein biological activity and premature degradation. Phosphomannomutase 2 deficiency is the most common defect.
Testing : Assay of hypoglycosylated forms of serum transferrin. Additional glycoproteins such as thyroglobulin and antithrombin III are used to complement transferrin testing.

Treatment: None effective for phosphomannomutase 2 deficiency.
Research highlights: Rectification of protein glycosylation *in vitro* via administration of mannose combined with inhibition of phosphomannose isomerase.

Clinical Features

The glycosylation of protein and lipids is a ubiquitous biological process. The congenital disorders of glycosylation, also known as carbohydrate deficient glycoprotein syndromes, are multisystem disorders characterized by defective glycoprotein biosynthesis or regulation. They comprise disorders of *N*-linked glycosylation (the attachment of oligosaccharide or glycan to the nitrogen atom of asparagine in a protein), of *O*-linked glycosylation (the attachment of a sugar molecule to an oxygen atom in an amino acid residue in a protein) and of lysosomal glycoprotein degradation.

Of these, the first are the most common and are often simply termed congenital glycosylation disorders. The disorders of *O*-linked glycosylation include congenital muscular dystrophies, type 2 lyssencephaly and limb-girdle dystrophies. The glycoprotein degradation disorders or glycoproteinoses result from specific deficiencies in lysosomal hydrolases that break down glycoproteins.

Over 100 disease-causing genes are primarily involved in *N*-linked glycosylation and other aspects of glycan regulation. They also include disorders that were identified earlier: the galactosemias and mucolipidoses types II and III, in which there is abnormal *N*-glycation or lack of addition of mannose-6-phosphate to lysosomal enzymes, respectively.

Phosphomannomutase 2 – Congenital Disorder of Glycosylation (PMM2-CDG, also known as CDG-Ia) is the most common congenital *N*-linked glycosylation defect, with a prevalence of 1 in 20,000 and is heritable in autosomal recessive fashion. The first signs of phosphomannomutase 2 deficiency usually become apparent during the first months of life. However, the phenotypic diversity is broad such that four general phases or types of phosphomannomutase 2 deficiency are recognized. They include, in decreasing order of severity: hydrops fetalis (which is often fatal), infantile multisystem, late-infantile with childhood ataxia and intellectual disability, and adult phase with stable disability.

The infantile multisystem form or phase of phosphomannomutase 2 deficiency is progressive. Dysmorphic features, including inverted nipples and abnormal fat pads, are often present but may disappear with age. Digestive system manifestations (vomiting, diarrhea, hepatic failure) can dominate the phenotype in about half of the affected individuals, but are always associated with truncal hypotonia and strabismus. Eye movement abnormalities can be prominent. All organs (with the exception of the lungs) are often involved, but often in transient or reversible fashion. Hepatic fibrosis and renal dysfunction of varying severity are always present. Lymphedema has been associated with a maldeveloped lymphatics system. Hypertrophic cardiomyopathy with transient myocardial ischemia has been noted. In contrast, some infants manifest potentially lethal signs of organ involvement such as prominent hepatopathy, pericardial effusion, nephrotic syndrome, renal cysts, or multiorgan failure. Unexplained coma may also occur. 20 percent of affected infants die within their first year from refractory hypoalbuminemia or respiratory dysfunction associated with aspiration pneumonia. The other half of affected individuals (those without systemic manifestations) display hypotonia, cerebellar atrophy or hypoplasia, strabismus, and intellectual impairment.

During the late-infantile form of phosphomannomutase 2 deficiency, children manifest facial hypotonia and esophoria. Seizures, when present, are usually treatable. Stroke-like events are often preceded by intercurrent infection and may include ictal or postictal paralysis, focal cerebral edema or necrosis or frank ischemic infarction. IQ usually ranges from 40 to 70. Progressive peripheral neuropathy may begin in this phase as may retinitis pigmentosa due to progressive photoreceptor degeneration (Figure 35.1).

The last or adult phase is characterized by intellectual disability, hypogonadism, skeletal deformities and osteoporosis and progressive cerebellar ataxia. Coagulopathy, when present, is associated with decreased concentrations of factors IV, IX, and XI, antithrombin III, protein C, and protein S.

Pathology

An enlarged cisterna magna and superior cerebellar cistern related to olivopontocerebellar degeneration is observed in late infancy to early childhood in phosphomannomutase 2 deficiency. The anterior part of the cerebellum is preferentially atrophied. Dandy-Walker malformations and small white matter cysts have also been reported. Slowly progressive cerebral and cerebellar atrophy is common during the first decade of life, followed by stabilization of the encephalic mass.

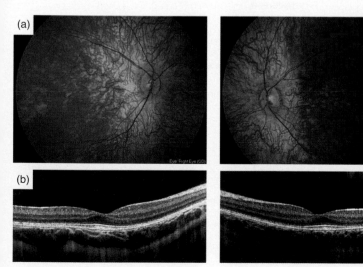

Figure 35.1 a. Fundoscopic images in a congenital glycosylation defect (phosphomannomutase deficiency) showing diffuse hypopigmentation of fundus with attenuation of the retinal vessels. b. Optical coherence tomography revealing loss of the outer retina throughout the macula. Reproduced with permission from Messenger WB et al. Ophthalmic findings in an infant with phosphomannomutase deficiency. *Doc Ophthalmol.* 2014; 128(2):149–53.

Neuronal loss and gliosis is widespread in the central nervous system. In the cerebellum, loss of Purkinje cells and axonal torpedo formation are conspicuous. Demyelination and Schwann cell inclusions are present in the peripheral nervous system.

The liver may be enlarged. Liver biopsy may demonstrate lamellar inclusions in macrophages and in hepatocyte lysosomes but not in Kupffer cell lysosomes. The heart can display hypertrophic cardiomyopathy and the skeletal muscle mild myopathic abnormalities with focal myofibrillary disorganization on electron microscopic examination.

Pathophysiology

N-glycosylation takes place inside the endoplasmic reticulum and Golgi apparatus of all cells (Figure 35.2). Glycosylation of a protein can vary widely depending on the cell type where the glycoprotein is produced. Also, for all proteins, a family of slightly different glycoforms is generated. In the early phase of glycosylation, a limited number of glycoproteins is produced in the endoplasmic reticulum. Then, in the Golgi apparatus, wider structural diversity is conferred through the rest of the glycosylation

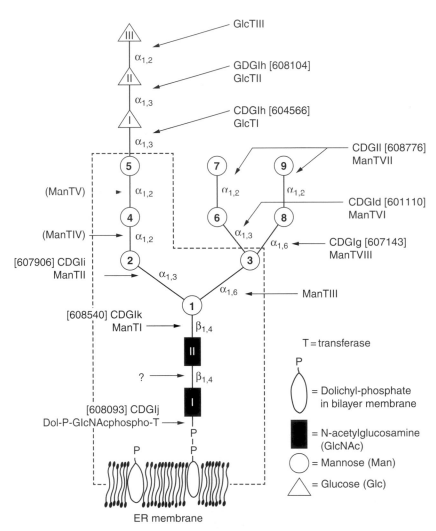

Figure 35.2 *N*-glycosylation reactions. Dolichyl-pyrophosphate bound high-mannose, end-product of assembly stage in *N*-glycosylation: Gly3Man9GlcNAc2-PP-Dol. Covalent glycosidic linkages shown and sequence of addition of building blocks indicated by Roman (GlcNAc and Glc) or Arabic (Man) numerals inside trivial monosaccharide symbols. Metabolic blocks causing corresponding CDG-I phenotypes represented by arrow at appropriate assembly step. *N*-glycan part assembled at cytoplasmic side of ER membrane enclosed inside dashed line. (?): assembly enzyme unknown. Reproduced with permission from Leroy JG. Congenital disorders of N-glycosylation including diseases associated with O- as well as N-glycosylation defects. *Pediatr Res.* 2006; 60(6):643–56.

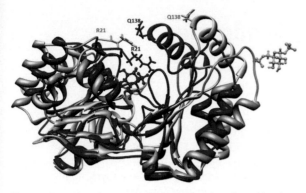

Figure 35.3 Phosphomannomutase closure along ligand binding. The initial model in open conformation is shown in pale blue, and the model in closed conformation is shown in dark blue. Side chains of two residues that come close upon domain closure, Arg21 and Gln138, are shown as sticks. The initial and final positions of the ligand are shown in pink and red, respectively, with a ball and stick representation. Reproduced with permission from Andreotti G et al. Conformational response to ligand binding in phosphomannomutase 2: insights into inborn glycosylation disorder. *J Biol Chem.* 2014; 289(50):34900–10.

process. Hypoglycosylated proteins are generally biologically hypoactive, are structurally unstable and can activate the unfolded protein response.

Phosphomannomutase is encoded by the PMM2 gene and catalyzes the transformation of mannose-6-phosphate into mannose-1-phosphate, which is a substrate for the formation of dolichol-pyrophosphate-oligosaccharides (Figure 35.3). These oligosaccharides form secondary branches on proteins inside the endoplasmic reticulum. Cells transport exogenous mannose and convert it to mannose-6-phosphate using hexokinase. Alternatively, mannose-6-phosphate can be formed from fructose-6-phosphate via phosphomannose isomerase. Both exogenous glucose and glycogen-derived glucose can contribute to this process. The majority of mannose in *N*-glycans is derived from glucose in most cells.

Diagnosis

Assay of plasma transferrin glycoforms is commonly used to screen for congenital glycosylation disorders, as the abundance of the different transferrin species

report on the status of glycosylation reactions. Testing can also be performed in cerebrospinal fluid, newborn screening blood cards, or urine. False positives occur in alcoholism, galactosemia, and hereditary fructose intolerance. False negatives have been reported in preterm infants and in cases of phosphomannomutase 2 deficiency early in the disease course.

Additional assays complement transferrin analysis by probing the abundance or activity of unrelated glycoproteins in plasma such as thyroid binding globulin concentration or protein C, protein S, antithrombin III, and factor IX activities.

Treatment

Serum mannose concentrations are decreased in phosphomannomutase 2 deficiency and mannose supplementation of cultured fibroblasts corrects hypoglycosylation. Nevertheless, increased serum mannose achieved via dietary supplementation does not improve clinical or biochemical abnormalities in children with phosphomannomutase 2 deficiency because most mannose-6-phosphate is catabolized by phosphomannose isomerase. However, hydrophobic, membrane-permeant forms of mannose generated by acylation of mannose-1-phosphate can normalize glycosylation in fibroblasts. Nevertheless, these compounds are toxic. Additionally, inhibition of phosphomannose isomerase in fibroblasts and other cells by MLS0315771, a benzoisothiazolone, leads to diversion of mannose-6-phosphate into a favorable *N*-glycosylation pattern.

Bibliography

Freeze H.H. (2009). Towards a therapy for phosphomannomutase 2 deficiency, the defect in CDG-Ia patients. *Biochim Biophys Acta.* Sep;1792(9):835–40.

Grünewald S. (2009). The clinical spectrum of phosphomannomutase 2 deficiency (CDG-Ia). *Biochim Biophys Acta.* Sep;1792(9):827–34.

Messenger W.B, Yang P., Pennesi M.E. (2014). Ophthalmic findings in an infant with phosphomannomutase deficiency. *Doc Ophthalmol.* Apr;128(2):149–53.

Chapter 36

Creatine Deficiency Syndromes

A boy was born to consanguineous parents by cesarean section due to failure of labor progression. He started walking at the age of 13 months, but his speech was absent then. At the age of 2 years and 6 months, he was still communicating using single words and knew only about 20 words. He then started having drop attacks consisting of generalized tonic stiffening lasting a few seconds. This was associated with eye deviation to the left and, at times, with right-arm jerks. Generalized tonic-clonic seizures appeared later but remained infrequent. EEG showed a slow background in wakefulness, excessive delta activity in sleep, and frequent generalized bursts of 1 to 2-Hz spike and polyspike slow wave discharges. He was diagnosed with Lennox-Gastaut syndrome. Valproate controlled his seizures for the next five years. At 4 years, he was able to combine two words and at the age of 6 years, he was still using two-word sentences and was able to give his full name. At 7 years, he again started to have drop attacks. Over the following year, he had three generalized myoclonic seizures per week, despite valproate treatment. Follow-up, at the age of 8 years and 6 months, showed no progress in his development. At 10 years of age he was diagnosed with familial guanidinoacetate methyltransferase deficiency. Creatine supplementation resulted in cessation of seizures and improvement in all areas of his development. EEG at the age of 12 years was normal.

myopathy and progressive extrapyramidal symptoms may appear in infancy.

Disease mechanism: Deficiency of enzymes involved in the neural synthesis of creatine (arginine-glycine amidinotransferase and guanidinoacetate methyltransferase) or in creatine transport via SLC6A8 into the central nervous system.

Testing: Low guanidinoacetate in urine or plasma for arginine-glycine amidinotransferase deficiency; elevated guanidinoacetate in guanidinoacetate methyltransferase deficiency. Elevated ratio of urinary creatine/creatinine in creatine transporter deficiency.

Treatment: Oral high-dose creatine-monohydrate and other disorder-specific dietary interventions.

Research highlights: Oxidative damage and apoptosis in cultured cells from affected individuals.

Clinical Features

The creatine deficiency syndromes include two autosomal recessive disorders of creatine synthesis: arginine-glycine amidinotransferase and guanidinoacetate methyltransferase deficiencies and the X-linked deficiency of the creatine transporter. The estimated incidence of guanidinoacetate methyltransferase deficiency, the most common of the three disorders, is close to 1 in 1,000,000 newborns. The creatine deficiency syndromes generally lead to intellectual impairment with prominent speech underdevelopment and, often, epilepsy. They are also commonly associated with febrile convulsions. However, there are manifestations specific to each syndrome: in guanidinoacetate methyltransferase deficiency, additional progressive extrapyramidal symptoms are superimposed onto intractable epilepsy, whereas myopathy is a distinctive feature of arginine-glycine amidinotransferase deficiency, which is the least common of the creatine

Creatine Deficiency Syndromes

Onset: Three months to three years with developmental arrest and febrile seizures.
Additional manifestations: Three types of syndromes are recognized. Absent or poor expressive language may be associated with dysmorphic features. In some syndromes,

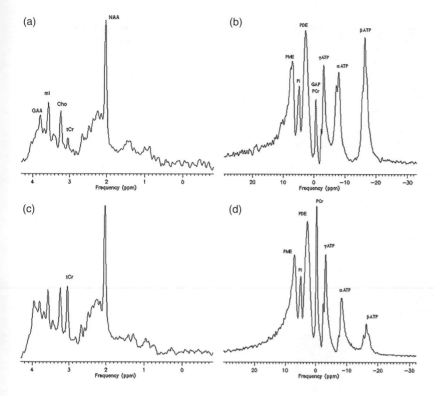

Figure 36.1 Single-voxel proton spectroscopy (left panels) and whole-brain phosphorous spectroscopy (right panels) of a child with cerebral creatine deficiency, before (**a** and **b**) and after (**c** and **d**) 6 months of therapy with creatine and guanidinoacetate (GAA)-lowering diet restrictions. The baseline studies demonstrate, besides a strong reduction of tCr and PCr peaks, an abnormal peak of guanidinoacetate (GAA) at 3.8 ppm on proton spectrum (**a**), of GAA-phosphate (GAA-P) at -0.5 ppm on phosphorous spectrum (**b**), and a high level of brain ATP. In contrast, in the on-therapy spectra, the GAA and GAA-P peak are not resolved, ATP turns to normal but there is an incomplete recovery of the tCr and PCr signal intensity. Reproduced with permission from Bianchi MC et al. Treatment monitoring of brain creatine deficiency syndromes: a [1]H- and ^{31}P-MR spectroscopy study. *AJNR Am J Neuroradiol.* 2007; 28(3):548–54.

deficiency syndromes. In all three syndromes, dysmorphic abnormalities can be present, including microcephaly, broad forehead, midface hypoplasia, high-arched palate, ear malformations, deeply set eyes and fifth finger clinodactyly. Additional distinct clinical features help differentiate among the three disorders.

In guanidinoacetate methyltransferase deficiency, a severe, early onset (noticeable between 10 months and 3 years of age) refractory epileptic encephalopathy is associated with general development arrest or neurologic deterioration, movement disorders including chorea, athetosis, dystonia, or ataxia, and severe mental disability. Epilepsy and its associated electroencephalographic abnormalities are refractory to anticonvulsants, but respond to treatment with creatine monohydrate. Seizures can take multiple forms, but atonic drop attacks and generalized seizures are the most frequent. Lennox-Gastaut syndrome and late-onset West syndrome have been reported. Multifocal spikes and generalized <3-Hz-spike and slow waves are commonly detected in the electroencephalogram. Additional manifestations include hyperactivity, abnormal social interactions, and aggressive and self-injurious behavior.

Arginine-glycine amidinotransferase deficiency, the least frequent of the three syndromes, is characterized by intellectual impairment and severe language dysfunction without epilepsy other than febrile seizures. Myopathy leads to hypotonia and weakness. Movement disorders have not been observed.

In males with deficiency of the creatine transporter SLC6A8, epilepsy is generally less severe. Seizures can be generalized tonic-clonic or simple or complex partial. Hypotonia is common. Speech acquisition is delayed, with first words expressed at about 3 years of age, which may not progress beyond single-word utterances. Ataxia, dystonia, or athetosis can also be present. Hyperactivity and attention disorder are associated with abnormal social interactions.

Pathology

There is little anatomical information available for the creatine deficiency syndromes. MR imaging has documented signal changes in the globus pallidus in all three syndromes. Brain MR spectroscopy can be diagnostic, as it illustrates a diminished creatine abundance (Figure 36.1).

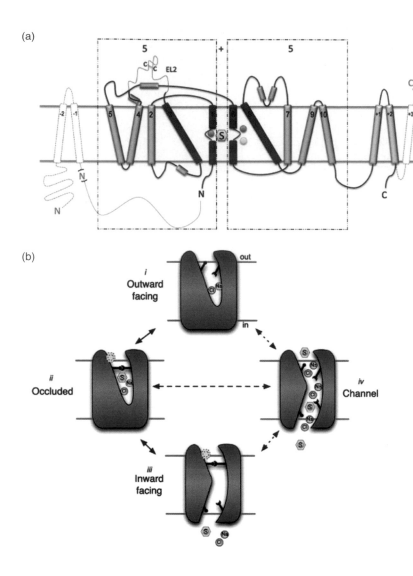

Figure 36.2 Structural aspects of the SLC6 family. (a) Helical architecture of the LeuT fold transporters. The 5 + 5 (LeuT fold) motif is represented as 2D where transmembrane domains (TMs) 1, 3, 6 and 8 form the substrate binding helices (red cylinders) and combine with TMs 2, 4 and 5 and 7, 9 and10 (blue), respectively, to form the antiparallel pentahelical domains (demarcated by the dashed boxes). TMs 11 and 12 (dark gray cylinders, labeled +1 and +2, respectively) are located peripheral to the 5 + 5 motif. The black lines represent densities resolved in the LeuT crystal structures. Gray solid lines represent additional regions found in eukaryotic SLC6 proteins. Other LeuT fold proteins, such as vSGLT, possess the 5 + 5 core but also have additional N and C terminal helices (dashed gray lines and light gray cylinders). Substrate (S), Na^+ (purple spheres) and Cl^- (green sphere) are also represented. (b) Illustration of alternating access and channel modes of transport. Substrate and ions access the binding site of the outward facing transporter (i) via the open outer gate (black sticks), outer gate closes yielding the occluded state (ii) which then transitions to the inward facing state (iii) releasing substrate and ions to cytosol (though controversial, this transition is proposed to be driven by a second substrate molecule (dashed line hexagon) binding to the S2 site). The transporter then rectifies to the outward facing structure (i). The transporter may undergo a lower probability transition (dashed lines) to a channel state (iv) where both gates are open simultaneously. Reproduced with permission from Pramod AB et al. SLC6 transporters: Structure, function, regulation, disease association and therapeutics. *Mol Aspects Med.* 2013; 34(2–3):197–219.

Pathophysiology

Creatine and its derivative phosphocreatine constitute an energy donor system through the creatine-phosphocreatine-creatine kinase reaction, allowing the regeneration of ATP. Creatine is also endowed with potential neuromodulator properties. It used to be held that most, if not all, of brain creatine was of extracerebral origin. However, creatine does cross the blood-brain barrier only poorly, such that the central nervous system supplies at least part of its creatine needs by neural synthesis. Arginine-glycine amidinotransferase and guanidinoacetate methyltransferase, the two enzymes of the creatine synthesis pathway, are abundant throughout the central nervous system, indicating autonomous brain creatine synthesis. This, however, is paradoxical when considering the syndrome of the creatine transporter deficiency, which causes creatine deficiency despite preserved neural expression of the two synthetic enzymes. A solution to the paradox is provided by the fact that brain cells take up guanidinoacetate and convert it to creatine. Guanidinoacetate uptake is competed by creatine. This suggests that in most brain regions, guanidinoacetate is transported from arginine-glycine amidinotransferase- and guanidinoacetate methyltransferase-expressing cells through the transporter SLC6A8 to allow creatine synthesis, thereby explaining creatine deficiency in the SLC6A8-deficient brain (Figure 36.2).

In cultured neural cells, an 85 percent decrease in guanidinoacetate methyltransferase protein is insufficient to cause creatine deficiency, but leads to guanidinoacetate accumulation. This is associated with excess axonal sprouting and decreased natural apoptosis, and is followed by induction of non-apoptotic cell death.

In fibroblast cultures, oxidative damage probably contributes toward the disease mechanism in the more severe forms of the syndromes. This is based on the detection of elevated intracellular reactive oxygen species content and apoptotic cells. An altered cell cycle is also characteristic of some fibroblast cell lines generated from individuals with creatine deficiency syndromes.

Diagnosis

Guanidinoacetate is the immediate product in the creatine biosynthetic process. Low guanidinoacetate concentrations in urine, plasma, and cerebrospinal fluid are characteristic diagnostic markers for arginine-glycine amidinotransferase deficiency, while elevated guanidinoacetate concentrations are characteristic of guanidinoacetate methyltransferase deficiency. An elevated ratio of urinary creatine/creatinine excretion is diagnostic in males with creatine transporter deficiency with 100 percent specificity. However, this test has a high false-positive rate due to dietary factors or dilute urine samples and lacks sensitivity in females. Plasma guanidinoacetate has 100 percent specificity for both arginine-glycine amidinotransferase and guanidinoacetate methyltransferase deficiencies, but arginine-glycine amidinotransferase deficiency exhibits decreased sensitivity in this assay.

All creatine disorders can be investigated through measurement of creatine metabolites in other body fluids or via brain proton magnetic resonance spectroscopy. Absence creatine in the presence of a normal choline and N-acetyl aspartate levels in MR spectroscopic spectra is unique to the cerebral creatine deficiency syndromes.

Infants with guanidinoacetate methyltransferase deficiency can also be identified from elevated guanidinoacetate in newborn blood spots.

Treatment

A common treatment is oral supplementation of high-dose creatine-monohydrate for all three disorders. Guanidinoacetate-reducing interventions such as high-dose L-ornithine, or arginine-restricted diet can be additionally employed in guanidinoacetate methyltransferase deficiency. Other interventions for guanidinoacetate methyltransferase deficiency have included various combinations of L-ornithine, sodium benzoate (to decrease glycine), and protein restricted diets.

Supplementation of substrates for intracerebral creatine synthesis (arginine or glycine) has been additionally used to treat deficiency of the creatine transporter SLC6A8. However, in males with creatine transporter deficiency, creatine supplementation alone does not improve clinical outcome and does not result in replenished cerebral creatine levels.

The SLC6A8 null mice have been treated with the creatine analog cyclocreatine. Brain cyclocreatine and cyclocreatine phosphate were detected after several weeks of cyclocreatine treatment. Treated mice exhibited improvement in several abilities such as enhanced novel object recognition, spatial orientation, and recall performance.

Bibliography

Braissant O., Henry H., Béard E., et al. (2011). Creatine deficiency syndromes and the importance of creatine synthesis in the brain. *Amino Acids*; 40(5):1315–24.

Clark J.F., Cecil K.M. (2015). Diagnostic methods and recommendations for the cerebral creatine deficiency syndromes. *Pediatr Res.* 77(3):398–405.

Chapter 37

Pompe Disease

A newborn received an X-ray of the chest that demonstrated cardiomegaly. His stay in the nursery was prolonged 2 weeks for this reason, but no treatment was instituted. He remained otherwise healthy until 4 months of age, when a set immunizations triggered fever, loss of appetite, and tachypnea. Myocardial function deteriorated and his cardiomyopathy evolved to dilated, necessitating treatment at that time. At five months of age, he appeared intellectually normal but displayed a paucity of spontaneous limb movements. He could maintain a sitting position and could reach for objects, however. Cry was weak and his tongue was normal. He had large bilateral testicular hernias. There was soft hepatomegaly of three fingers across. Muscles were prominent and firm to palpation. Reflexes were normal.

Pompe Disease

Onset: Neonatal or infantile cardiomyopathy, or progressive weakness and flaccidity.
Additional manifestations: Macroglossia with fasciculations, asymptomatic hepatomegaly, hypotonia, and respiratory failure.
Disease mechanism: Dysfunction of aerobic glycolysis in skeletal muscle, which is dependent upon a steady supply and breakdown of glycogen. Secondary nutrient sensor dysregulation.
Testing: Enzymatic assay in white blood cells or muscle biopsy illustrating cytoplasmic and lysosomal glycogen accumulation.
Treatment: High-protein diet with aerobic exercise or enzyme replacement therapy using recombinant human alpha-glucosidase infusions. Affected individuals with no detectable enzyme develop immune intolerance to the recombinant enzyme.
Research highlights: Autophagy in the null acid maltase mouse model.

Clinical Features

There are 15 forms of glycogen storage disease associated with specific defects of glycogen synthesis, glycogen breakdown, or glycolysis. Pompe disease is caused by autosomal recessive deficiency of acid maltase, also known as alpha-glucosidase and glycogen storage disease type II, an enzyme that degrades glycogen inside lysosomes. Two forms of Pompe disease are recognized: An infantile and a later-onset, milder form.

The mild form of Pompe disease manifests in childhood or even in adulthood and may follow a slow clinical course over many years. Limb girdle and respiratory muscles are predominantly affected. The latter can be serially assessed by measuring the forced vital capacity. Tongue fasciculations indicative of brainstem motor neuron dysfunction can be prominent. Dilation of small and large cerebral arteries is common and may be associated with cerebral infarction. Cardiac involvement may be absent. Urinary and bowel incontinence may occur. Neuropathy

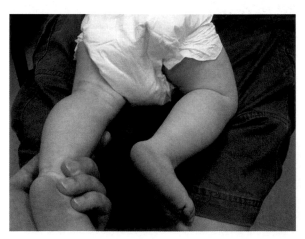

Figure 37.1 Calf muscle hypertrophy in an infant with Pompe disease.

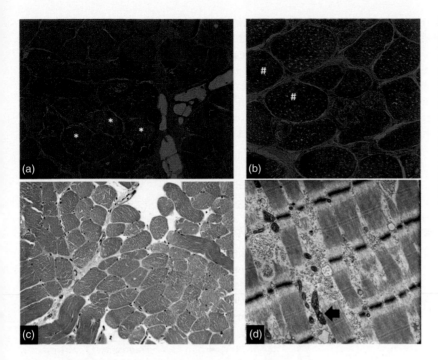

Figure 37.2 Histological examination of muscle biopsies of two subjects (**a** and **b**, and **c** and **d**, respectively) with Pompe disease. Muscle biopsy (**a**) from one child shows extensive vacuolar changes (asterisk) and positive acid phosphatase aggregates (#) in panel **b**. The muscle biopsy (**c**) from the other child is essentially unremarkable while the muscle electron micrograph (**d**) shows membrane bound glycogen deposits and mildly distorted mitochondrial morphology. Reproduced with permission from Dasouki M et al. Pompe disease: literature review and case series. *Neurol Clin.* 2014; 32(3):751–76.

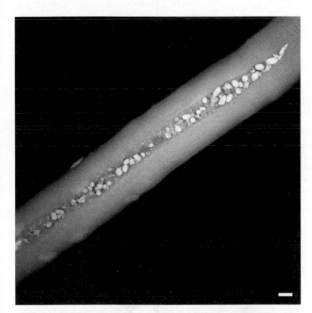

Figure 37.3 Autofluorescent lipofuscin inclusions in a muscle biopsy from an individual with a childhood form of Pompe disease. The child was diagnosed during a family study and began therapy at 7 years of age. The biopsy was taken prior to the initiation of enzyme replacement therapy. Bar: 10 μm. Reproduced with permission from Lim JA et al. Pompe disease: from pathophysiology to therapy and back again. *Front Aging Neurosci.* 2014; 6:177.

may also become symptomatic. Eventually, most affected individuals require ambulatory and respiratory support and life expectancy is decreased compared to the general population. Enzyme activity is not related to disease severity in older individuals.

The infantile form is more severe and is associated with nearly absent residual enzyme activity (Figure 37.1). Cardiomyopathy dominates the phenotype. Cardiac involvement may be asymptomatic in the neonatal period but eventually becomes the leading manifestation. Within the first few months of life, macroglossia, hepatomegaly, weakness, and hypotonia appear and progress rapidly. There is a high incidence of hypoventilation and obstructive sleep apnea. Paradoxically, despite morphological liver involvement, there is no functional hepatopathy. Death typically ensues before one year of age.

Pathology

The entire heart is enlarged, with thickened ventricular walls. The contractile apparatus of skeletal muscle is deformed due to massive free and intralysosomal glycogen deposition (Figure 37.2). There is also extensive glycogen accumulation in the heart, liver and central and peripheral nervous systems. The pattern of accumulation includes neurons and glial cells of the white matter, brainstem, and cerebellum, with relative sparing of cerebellar Purkinje cells. Glycogen deposition is also extensive in spinal ganglionic neurons, myenteric plexus, and Schwann cells. However, accumulation is more marked in brainstem and spinal cord neurons. Vacuolar degeneration of the cerebral arteries with aneurysm formation has been reported.

Glycogen accumulation is predominantly intralysosomal, in the form of beta-particles, but there is also excess cytoplasmic glycogen (Figure 37.3). The transit of cytosolic to intralysosomal glycogen involves autophagy, such that an animal model deficient in autophagy only in skeletal muscle exhibited lower lysosomal glycogen deposition (Figure 37.4).

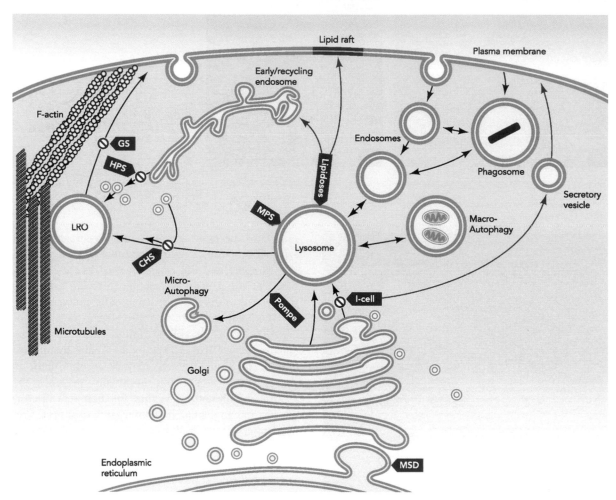

Figure 37.4 Stylized cell showing the functions that can be disrupted in lysosomal storage disorders. Pompe disease involves a lysosomal hydrolase defect that results in the inability to degrade autophagocytozed vesicular glycogen. The mucopolysaccharidoses (MPS) involve different defects in either a processing enzyme, glycosidase, or sulphatase and impact on glycosaminoglycan degradation within the lysosome. The sphingolipidoses (lipidoses) involve different hydrolase defects that alter the lysosomal catabolism of lipids. I-cell disease involves a Golgi processing enzyme defect, altering the traffic of soluble lysosomal hydrolsases to the lysosome and causing the secretion of these enzymes. Multiple sulphatase deficiency (MSD) prevents the active site processing of sulphatases in the endoplasmic reticulum, generating catalytically inactive sulphatase proteins. The hereditary albinism syndromes Chediak-Higashi (CHS), Hermansky-Pudlak (HPS), and Griscelli (GS) each impact on different aspects of vesicular traffic, altering the biogenesis of lysosomal-related organelles (LRO). Because of the dynamic interrelationship of the endosome lysosome system, these primary defects can have a secondary impact on other lysosomal function. Reproduced with permission from Parkinson-Lawrence EJ et al. Lysosomal storage disease: Revealing lysosomal function and physiology. *Physiology* (Bethesda). 2010; 25(2):102–15.

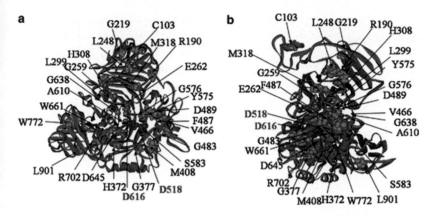

Figure 37.5 Locations of the amino acid residues that cause processing/transport defects in human acid alpha-glucosidase when substituted. The backbones are displayed as a ribbon model. The positions of both the catalytic residues (red) and the residues subject to substitution (orange) are displayed as space filling models. Front view (a) and side view (b). Reproduced with permission from Sugawara K et al. Structural modeling of mutant alpha-glucosidases resulting in a processing/transport defect in Pompe disease. *J Hum Genet*. 2009; 54(6):324–30.

Pathophysiology

In Pompe disease, muscle glycogen is increased by as much as ten-fold as the result of mutations in acid maltase (Figure 37.5). The concentration of glycogen in normal skeletal muscle is 1g per 100g of tissue, whereas liver contains up to 6g per 100g of tissue. Yet, muscle and neural manifestations predominate in Pompe disease, usually without any functional liver involvement.

Muscle relies on four energy sources: a) oxidative phosphorylation, which is linked to aerobic glycolysis, b) anaerobic glycolysis, c) creatine kinase, and d) adenylate kinase. Of these, aerobic glycolysis is predominantly impaired in Pompe disease.

Systemic metabolic abnormalities are common. There is evidence for disturbed energy metabolism contributing to a chronic catabolic state and for diminished plasma methylation capacity and elevated levels of insulin-like growth factor type 1 and its carrier protein insulin-like growth factor binding protein 3. This suggest nutrient sensor disturbance as an additional pathogenic mechanism.

Diagnosis

The clinical features of infantile acid maltase deficiency may be associated to other helpful findings in non-invasive testing, although muscle biopsy or enzymatic analysis of white blood cells is often necessary to establish the diagnosis. An elevation in creatine kinase can be noted in Pompe disease, whereas myotonia is detectable by electromyography (Figure 37.6).

The urinary glucose tetrasaccharide, $Glc\alpha1$-$6Glc\alpha1$-$4Glc\alpha1$-$4Glc$ (Glc4), is a biomarker of glycogen accumulation and tissue damage and is elevated

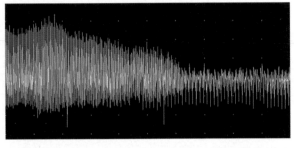

Figure 37.6 Myotonic discharge from lumbar paraspinal muscle in Pompe disease Gain: 1 s/div, 50 µV/div. Reproduced with permission from Beltran Papsdorf TB et al. Pearls & Oy-sters: clues to the diagnosis of adult-onset acid maltase deficiency. *Neurology*. 2014; 82(9):e73–5.

in individuals with Pompe disease. Baseline urinary Glc4 is elevated in neonates with infantile-onset Pompe disease identified through newborn screening.

Treatment

A combination of high-protein diet and aerobic exercise proves useful in older individuals with acid maltase deficiency.

Periodic enzyme replacement therapy with recombinant human alpha-glucosidase has proven helpful. However, cross-reactive immunologic material-negative individuals, who lack detectable endogenous enzyme, develop an immune response to the recombinant enzyme that can render the therapy ineffective. Long term enzyme replacement therapy is beneficial. Cognitive development at school age ranges between normal and mildly abnormal in long-term survivors with Pompe disease treated with this therapeutic modality.

Bibliography

Angelini C. (2015). Spectrum of metabolic myopathies. *Biochim Biophys Acta*. 1852(4):615–21.

Boustany R.M. (2013). Lysosomal storage diseases–the horizon expands. *Nat Rev Neurol*.; 9(10):583–98.

Pascual J.M, Roe C.R. (2013). Systemic metabolic abnormalities in adult-onset acid maltase deficiency: Beyond muscle glycogen accumulation. *JAMA Neurol*. 70(6):756–63.

Chapter 38

Alpers–Huttenlocher Disease

An abnormally developed speech and motor perform-ance were noted in a girl at the age of two years. At three years of age, she developed epilepsy and six months later experienced migrainous attacks associ-ated with vomiting, vertigo, and transient left-sided weakness. At the age of four years she suffered a 10-day episode of headache and vomiting culminating in seizures and coma. At the age of five years she developed status epilepticus. MR imaging of the brain suggested chronic ischemia of the grey matter. A month later she was noted to have nystagmus, hypotonia of the lower limbs and absent knee jerks. Liver function derangement was also noted. Her epi-lepsy continued to worsen and she died at the age of five years and six months.

Clinical Features

Progressive hepatocerebral degeneration with onset in infancy is a feature of several mitochondrial diseases characterized by mitochondrial DNA depletion as the result of deficient mitochondrial genome maintenance.

In Alpers–Huttenlocher disease, epilepsy is usually the presenting manifestation, which can occur in a previously abnormally developed infant. Early sei-zures involve the occipital lobe and are associated with vomiting, headache, and myoclonus. These sei-zures are usually treatable early in the disease course. However, epilepsy becomes increasingly refractory and generalized. Most affected individuals then experi-ence epilepsia partialis continua or convulsive status

Alpers–Huttenlocher Disease

Onset: Epilepsy of the occipital lobe.
Additional manifestations: Stepwise decline in overall neural performance. Hepatic failure and toxic sensitivity to valproate are common. Myoclonus, blindness, and overall regression are also the norm. Seizures become intractable, with epilepsia partialis continua or status epilepticus. Death ensues in about 4 years.
Disease mechanism: Mitochondrial DNA depletion or multiple deletions caused by deficient mitochondrial genome maintenance due to mutations in the nuclear gene codifying gamma polymerase 1 (POLG1).
Testing: MR imaging demonstrates poliodystrophy and cerebrospinal fluid contains elevated protein and lactate. Hepatic biopsy illustrates characteristic changes.
Treatment: None effective.
Research highlights: Site-directed mutagenesis of the human, *Drosophila* and yeast protein allow for structural and functional enzyme predictions.

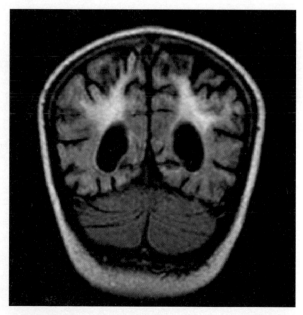

Figure 38.1 Magnetic resonance image of the brain of a child with Alpers disease at 4 years of age. Coronal FLAIR of the occipital region showing atrophy of both occipital lobes and high signal intensity in the white matter. Reproduced with permission from Kollberg G et al. POLG1 mutations associated with progressive encephalopathy in childhood. *J Neuropathol Exp Neurol.* 2006; 65(8):758–68.

epilepticus late into their disease course. Valproic acid can trigger liver failure, but hepatopathy is an invariant feature of the disorder even in the absence of hepatotoxicity. Hepatic dysfunction leading to hypoglycemia can precede or follow the encephalopathy. Disease progression follows a stepwise course, which can be accelerated by intercurrent illnesses. Late stages of the disease include migraine, cerebral cortical blindness, myoclonus, and intractable epilepsy. Early death in about four years is common.

In the hepatocerebral form of mitochondrial DNA depletion, infants can be severely growth-retarded and manifest hypoglycemia. Progressive hepatic failure and icterus may dominate the phenotype. Seizures are not common.

Pathology

The Alpers–Huttenlocher phenotype is a poliodystrophy or gray matter degenerative disease. The cerebral cortex is variably affected, but it reveals a constant involvement of the calcarine visual cortex with microscopic changes including spongiosis, neuronal loss, and astrocytosis (Figure 38.1).

The characteristic hepatic microscopic features of Alpers–Huttenlocher disease include microvesicular steatosis, bile duct proliferation, hepatocyte loss, bridging fibrosis or cirrhosis, collapse of liver cell plates, parenchymal disarray or disorganization of normal lobular architecture, regenerative nodules, and oncocytic change (mitochondrial proliferation associated with intensely eosinophilic cytoplasm) in scattered hepatocytes not affected by steatosis (Figure 38.2).

Deficiencies of electron transport chain enzymatic activities in muscle and liver not specific for Alpers–Huttenlocher disease are common and variable, ranging from normal to single and multiple respiratory chain complex deficiencies.

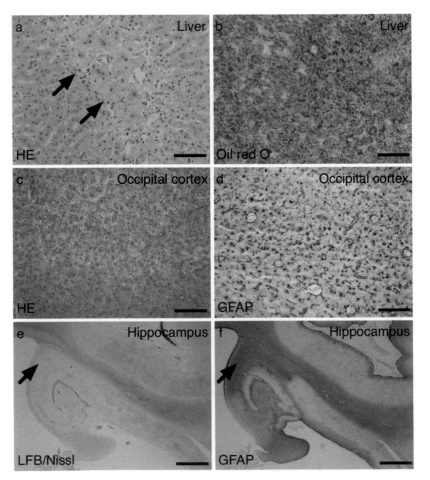

Figure 38.2 Liver and brain pathology in Alpers disease. Post-mortem liver samples from a child (a and c) showed perivenular foci of enlarged hepatocytes with fine vacuolation (arrows). On lipid staining with oil red O (b) of frozen sections there was diffuse lipid deposition. Sample of the cerebral cortex from the occipital lobe showed full thickness neuronal loss with vacuolation and astrocytosis (c and d). Samples of the hippocampi (e and f) showed segmental neuronal loss, most marked from CA1 (arrow) and gliosis in a similar pattern (f-GFAP). Scale bars, a and b = 100 μm; c and d = 200 μm; e and f = 2 mm. Reproduced with permission from Rajakulendran S et al. A clinical, and genetic study of homozygous A467T POLG-related mitochondrial disease. *PLoS One.* 2016; 11(1):e0145500.

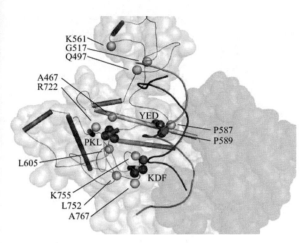

Figure 38.3 Alpers disease mutations in DNA polymerase γ. Alpers Cluster 2 mutations that affect the upstream DNA-binding channel of Polγ. Amino acid residues affected by Alpers Cluster 2 mutations in POLG1 are shown as yellow spheres. Other Polγ residues are shown in brown. DNA is indicated by orange (template) and brown (primer) strands. The spacer domain is also shown as a transparent surface representation in pale gray and the exo domain is shown in purple. Reproduced with permission from Euro L et al. Clustering of Alpers disease mutations and catalytic defects in biochemical variants reveal new features of molecular mechanism of the human mitochondrial replicase, Pol γ. *Nucleic Acids Res.* 2011; 39(21):9072–84.

Pathophysiology

Alpers–Huttenlocher disease is caused by mutations in the nuclear gene POLG1, which encodes the catalytic subunit of DNA polymerase gamma (POLG) (Figure 38.3). POLG is the only enzyme responsible for the replication and repair of the DNA in mitochondria. The most common homozygous POLG1 mutation causative of Alpers–Huttenlocher disease, Ala467Thr, is also associated with multiple mitochondrial DNA deletions in the clinical settings of mitochondrial encephalomyopathy, lactic acidosis and stroke-like episodes (MELAS), myoclonic epilepsy, myopathy and sensory ataxia (MEMSA), or of sensory ataxic neuropathy, dysarthria and ophthalmoplegia (SANDO). The mitochondrial DNA background plays an important role in modifying the disease phenotype but nuclear modifiers, epigenetic and environmental factors may also influence the severity of disease.

Although the ~200 reported Alpers–Huttenlocher mutations scatter across the entire POLG1 gene, they cluster in separate functional regions of the enzyme tridimensional structure (Figure 38.4). Cluster 1 mutations are located in the active site region, causing reduced polymerase activity, which is potentially compounded by reduced DNA binding. Cluster 2 mutations map to the upstream DNA-binding channel, resulting in reduced DNA-binding affinity, but are too distant from the catalytic site to significantly affect directly polymerase activity. Cluster 2 mutations are recessively inherited, whereas cluster 1 mutations may be either dominant or recessive, depending on the severity of the biochemical defect. Cluster 3 mutations are located in the partitioning loop or its neighboring areas such as the orienter module. They may alter the balance of polymerase and exonuclease activities of the enzyme. Cluster 4 mutations are located on the surface of the exonuclease domain along the interface of the distal accessory subunit. These mutations probably reduce the stimulation induced by the distal accessory subunit, which enhances polymerase rate and reduces exonuclease activity. Cluster 3 and 4 mutations may probably cause increased mutagenesis in the mitochondrial DNA in vivo, a phenotype that associated in yeast models with amino acid alterations within these clusters. Cluster 5 mutations are located on the distal surface of the intrinsic processivity subdomain. Their distant location and lack of biochemical consequence suggest that this region is involved in replisome contacts.

The most common mutation, Ala467Thr, affects a highly conserved amino acid located in the spacer or linker domain of the polymerase (cluster 2). Mutagenesis of this conserved region in the corresponding protein of the fruit fly *Drosophila* alters the activity, processivity and DNA-binding affinity of the enzyme. The molecular mechanism likely involves the disruption of interactions between the catalytic subunit of the enzyme and a homodimeric accessory subunit (encoded by POLG2).

Diagnosis

Several clinical findings facilitate the diagnosis. The combination of reduced muscle electron transport chain function (isolated complex IV or a combination I, III, and IV electron transport complex defects), dicarboxylic aciduria, fulminant or severe hepatic failure, refractory epilepsy, lactic acidosis, mitochondrial DNA content reduction to about 30 percent and elevated cerebral spinal fluid protein (> 100 mg/dL) is highly suggestive of Alpers–Huttenlocher disease.

MR imaging illustrates cerebral volume loss at the expense of the cerebral cortex with ventriculomegaly.

143

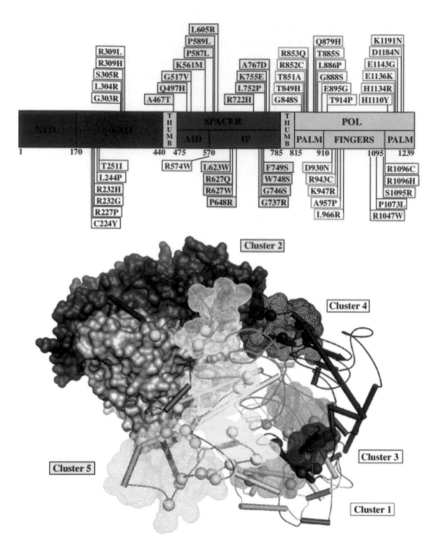

Figure 38.4 Alpers disease mutations clustering within functional modules in the catalytic subunit of Pol γ. Upper panel: schematic diagram of the POLG1 gene showing the distribution of recessive Alpers disease mutations. AID and IP in the spacer domain refer to the accessory (subunit) interacting and intrinsic processivity subdomains, respectively, that are discussed in the text; NTD refers to the N-terminal domain. Lower panel: tertiary structural representation of the apoenzyme form of Pol γ with modeled DNA, identifying the positions of five functional modules (shown in mesh) that are defined by clusters of amino acid residues (shown as spheres) affected by Alpers disease mutations as follows: Cluster 1, green; Cluster 2, yellow; Cluster 3, red; Cluster 4, blue; Cluster 5, cyan. The domains of Pol γ A are shown as surface representations, and in part as secondary structural elements (SSEs) that are colored as depicted in A. The proximal and distal accessory subunits are shown as surface representations in light and dark gray, respectively. Primer–template DNA was docked and is displayed as orange ribbons. Reproduced with permission from Euro L et al. Clustering of Alpers disease mutations and catalytic defects in biochemical variants reveal new features of molecular mechanism of the human mitochondrial replicase, Pol γ. *Nucleic Acids Res.* 2011; 39(21):9072–84.

Electroencephalogram in the advanced disease state may show multifocal paroxysmal activity with high-amplitude delta slowing (200–1000 microvolts) and spikes and polyspikes (10–100 microvolts, 12–25 Hz). Visual evoked potentials are abnormal in the context of a normal electroretinogram.

Polymerase gamma mutations do not always induce mitochondrial DNA depletion in blood cells. Rather, mitochondrial DNA depletion (with a mean 35 percent residual mitochondrial DNA content) is detectable in skeletal muscle or liver. However, muscle and liver mitochondrial DNA depletion may lag behind disease symptoms.

Deficiency in polymerase gamma enzymatic activity ($\leq$ 10 percent of normal activity) is also detectable in skeletal muscle or liver.

Treatment

Liver transplantation has been performed, but the outcome has been poor.

The therapeutic potential of antioxidants is illustrated by the attenuation of cardiomyopathy in mice with mutations that inactivate POLG exonuclease function by overexpression of catalase, an enzyme that reduces oxidative damage. Yeast harboring the homologous disease-associated mutations in the mitochondrial polymerase display a reduction in mitochondrial dysfunction after exposure to antioxidants such as dihydrolipoic acid.

Similarly, the suppression of disease-associated mutations by ribonucleotide reductase overexpression is effective in the case of other nucleotide-binding defective mutants. Thus, adequate nucleotide levels may be required for proper mitochondrial DNA replication, offering a potential therapeutic opportunity.

POLG1 mutant mice that undergo exercise training are phenotypically indistinguishable from normal mice and also exhibit a similar frequency of mutant mitochondrial DNA and cytochrome c oxidase. Perhaps exercise promotes mitochondrial biogenesis via PGC-1α (peroxisome proliferator-activated receptor gamma coactivator 1-alpha), facilitating either the dilution of mutant mitochondrial DNA or targeting dysfunctional mitochondrial DNA for destruction.

Bibliography

Saneto R.P., Cohen B.H., Copeland W.C., et al. (2013). Alpers-Huttenlocher syndrome. *Pediatr Neurol.* 48(3):167–78.

Chapter 39

Leigh Syndrome

A boy, aged 7 months 3 weeks, was normal until six weeks before admission to the hospital when he stopped crying, lay very still, and slept for long periods, only waking when disturbed. He did not suck and had to be fed by spoon. Sweating was increased during this period. At the onset of the baby's illness his sister was at home with a cold, sneezing and coughing a good deal. The boy's pupils were small with no reaction to light, or appreciation of light; ophthalmoscopy showed a bilateral optic atrophy. The infant appeared to be deaf. Both upper and lower limbs were markedly spastic. Reflexes were not obtained. There were bilateral extensor responses. The child rapidly worsened and became comatose after 3 days following admission, dying in terminal hyperpyrexia later the same day.

Leigh Syndrome

Onset: Sudden or rapidly evolving loss of postural tone and prostration at 7 months of age in the setting of a child with previously abnormal intellectual and motor development. A minor unrelated illness is usually the immediate prodrome to the syndrome.
Additional manifestations: Hypotonia and subsequent rigidity. Respiratory dysfunction, optic atrophy, and ataxia. Seizures, when present, tend to be manageable. The disease follows a static, fully incapacitating course with lack of volitional development and motor incapacity or a stepwise declining course.
Disease mechanism: Mitochondrial dysfunction caused by mutations in the nuclear or the mitochondrial DNA with high heteroplasmy.
Testing: MR imaging illustrating necrosis of the brainstem and striatum or thalamus often accompanied by leukoencephalopathy. Enzymatic

assay of muscle or fibroblast mitochondrial function and genotyping.
Treatment: None effective.
Research highlights: Complex I deficient mice by knockout of the NDUFS4 gene illustrate progressive glial activation and neuronal necrosis.

Clinical Features

Leigh syndrome is characterized by subacute, near-simultaneous necrosis of specific non-adjacent regions of the central nervous system in association with dysfunctional mitochondria that result from any one of numerous genetic mutations in either the nuclear or the mitochondrial genome. The incidence is 1 in 40,000 newborn children. Onset can be any time during infancy, with a median age of 7 months. During an extended prodromic period, infants usually exhibit abnormal intellectual and motor development. Then, a minor illness such as a urinary tract infection, gastroenteritis, or respiratory infection is abruptly followed by prostration out of proportion to the precipitant illness, with development of severe neurological signs and symptoms. The specific manifestations of Leigh syndrome vary to some extent, but they usually appear subacutely (over the course of days or weeks) and can be generally grouped in abnormalities of respiration, nutrition, tone, and movement coordination. Seizures, when present, are usually treatable. The most common chronic manifestations include hypotonia that evolves to rigidity, optic atrophy, spasticity, generalized dystonia, and optic atrophy. Feeding difficulties almost invariably necessitate gastrostomy. Despite the genetic heterogeneity of the syndrome, two general clinical courses can be recognized: a static course characterized by arrested development and little change after the initial episode and a relapsing, stepwise course associated with lesion extension which is often detectable by MR imaging. A worse outcome is associated with younger age of disease onset, genetically identified disease, seizures, brainstem lesions detected by MR imaging, failure to gain weight, and frequent stepwise deterioration necessitating admission to hospital. The median age at death is 2.5 years.

Pathology

There is bilateral spongy necrosis of the brainstem, diencephalon and basal ganglia in a symmetric fashion, which is detectable by MR imaging (Figures 39.1–39.8). Regions affected include the caudate nucleus, putamen, periaqueductal area, and tegmentum. Lesions are also often found in the centrum semiovale, cerebellar white matter and nuclei and the gray and white matter in the spinal cord. Histologically, there is spongy rarefaction and excessive vascularity. Mononuclear cell infiltrates may cuff small vessels.

Muscle abnormalities are common. In the case of SURF1 (surfeit locus protein 1) mutations, there is uniformly decreased cytochrome c oxidase staining. Ragged red fibers are unusual but lipid accumulation and fiber size variability are common.

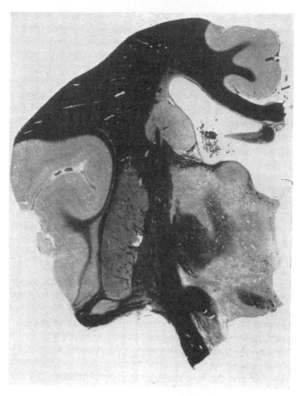

Figure 39.2 Periaqueductal grey matter of the mid-brain, showing microglial proliferation, compound granular cells, and a proliferation of capillaries and precapillaries. Nissl × 350. Reproduced with permission from Leigh D. Subacute necrotizing encephalomyelopathy in an infant. *J Neurol Neurosurg Psychiatry.* 1951; 14(3):216–21.

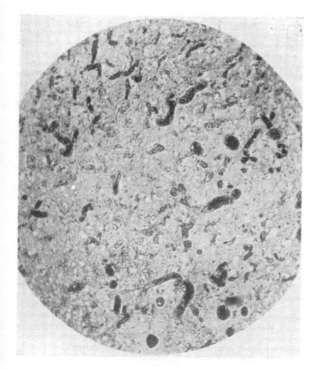

Figure 39.1 Leigh syndrome. Vascular proliferation in the anterior nucleus of the thalamus. Perdrau's silver stain × 90. Reproduced with permission from Leigh D. Subacute necrotizing encephalomyelopathy in an infant. *J Neurol Neurosurg Psychiatry.* 1951; 14(3):216–21.

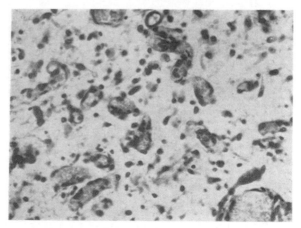

Figure 39.3 Thalamus at mid-dorsal level, showing destruction particularly of the anterior nucleus, nucleus magnocellularis, and the midline nuclei. Note sparing of subthalamic nucleus (corpus Luysii). Heidenhain's myelin stain × 2. Reproduced with permission from Leigh D. Subacute necrotizing encephalomyelopathy in an infant. *J Neurol Neurosurg Psychiatry.* 1951; 14(3):216–21.

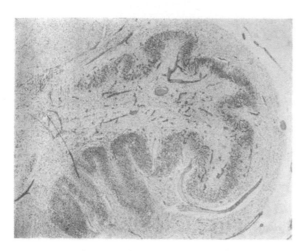

Figure 39.4 Inferior olive showing preservation of the dorso-medial portion of the nucleus. An intense glio-mesodermal reaction, with destruction of olivary nerve cells, can be seen in the dorsolateral and ventral portion of the olive. Nissl × 20. Reproduced with permission from Leigh D. Subacute necrotizing encephalomyelopathy in an infant. *J Neurol Neurosurg Psychiatry*. 1951; 14(3):216–21.

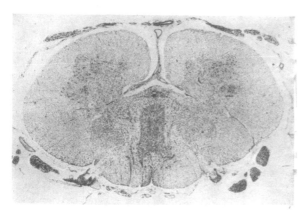

Figure 39.5 Spinal cord, fifth cervical segment. Vascular and glial proliferation in the columns of Goll. Nissl × 11.5. Reproduced with permission from Leigh D. Subacute necrotizing encephalomyelopathy in an infant. *J Neurol Neurosurg Psychiatry*. 1951; 14(3):216–21.

Pathophysiology

Leigh syndrome can be caused by mutations in more than 35 genes of both nuclear and mitochondrial origin, which lead to dysfunction of any of the five complexes of the respiratory chain or of pyruvate dehydrogenase. Nuclear DNA mutations are transmissible in a Mendelian fashion, including autosomal recessive and X-linked modes of inheritance. In what follows, the most common molecular causes of Leigh syndrome are discussed.

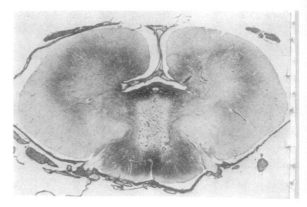

Figure 39.6 The same cord segment showing gliosis of the dorsal portions of the posterior columns and around the central canal. Holzer × 11.5. Reproduced with permission from Leigh D. Subacute necrotizing encephalomyelopathy in an infant. *J Neurol Neurosurg Psychiatry*. 1951; 14(3):216–21.

Complex I Deficiency. Complex I (NADH: ubiquinone oxidoreductase) is the first enzymatic constituent of the mitochondrial respiratory chain. It transfers electrons from NADH to ubiquinone, catalyzing the redox-driven proton translocation that maintains the electrochemical gradient across the inner mitochondrial membrane. Complex I is the largest multisubunit ensemble of the chain, containing 45 subunits. Seven subunits are encoded by mitochondrial DNA and 38 subunits are encoded by nuclear DNA. In addition, there are multiple assembly proteins involved in maintaining the integrity of the complex. Of these, at least ten assembly proteins of nuclear DNA origin have been associated with mitochondrial diseases. However, there are many candidate genes involved in complex I assembly, suggesting that more nuclear-encoded genes will be discovered. Deficiency of complex I is the most commonly identified cause of childhood-onset mitochondrial disease, accounting for approximately a third of all cases of oxidative phosphorylation disorders. Leigh syndrome due to complex I deficiency can result from mitochondrial or nuclear DNA-encoded mutations, but the majority of cases are due to nuclear DNA mutations.

NDUFS4 (NADH dehydrogenase iron-sulfur protein 4) knockout mice have served to model Leigh syndrome due to complex I deficiency. In these mice, activation of caspase 8 implies the initiation of the extrinsic apoptotic pathway. However, the predominant cell loss mechanism is necrotic, suggesting a switch from apoptosis to necrosis in affected neurons.

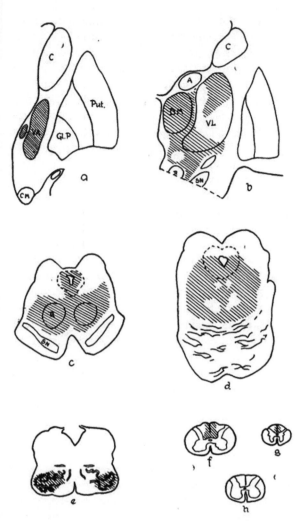

Figure 39.7 Hatched areas indicate the situations of the lesions at various coronal levels of the thalamus, brain stem, and spinal cord. Reproduced with permission from Leigh D. Subacute necrotizing encephalomyelopathy in an infant. *J Neurol Neurosurg Psychiatry.* 1951; 14(3):216–21.

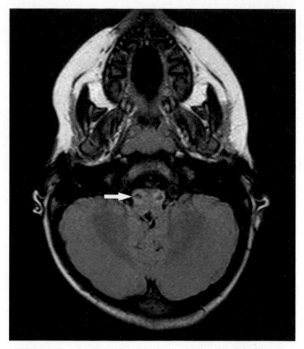

Figure 39.8 MR imaging in a 3-year-old child with Leigh syndrome illustrating transsynaptic olivary hypertrophy, a degenerative phenomenon.

Table 39.1 Frequent causes of Leigh syndrome

Defect	Mode of inheritance	Relative frequency
Complex I	Autosomal recessive; mitochondrial	++++
Complex II	Autosomal recessive	+
Complex IV	Autosomal recessive	+++
Complex V	Autosomal recessive; mitochondrial	++
tRNA$^{Leu(UUR)}$	Mitochondrial	+
tRNA^{Lys}	Mitochondrial	+
Coenzyme Q10	Autosomal recessive	+
Pyruvate dehydrogenase complex	X-linked recessive; autosomal recessive	+++

Complex II Deficiency. Complex II is the smallest complex of the respiratory chain and all of its four subunits are nuclear DNA-encoded. Complex II is located on the inner mitochondrial membrane, where it oxidizes FADH$_2$, transferring electrons to ubiquinone as part of the electron transport chain. Only two (A and B) of its four subunits are responsible for this electron transfer activity. Mutations in complex II are relatively rare, as is complex II deficiency in Leigh syndrome. Mutations in subunit A are associated with autosomal recessive mitochondrial disorders, including Leigh syndrome.

Complex IV Deficiency. Cytochrome c oxidase (COX or complex IV) is comprised of 13 subunits, three of which are encoded by mitochondrial DNA, with the rest being nuclear-encoded. Complex IV is involved in the last step of electron transfer in the respiratory chain. The most common cause of nuclear-encoded mutation in Leigh syndrome is deficiency of complex IV. This may be brought about by mutation of any of the cytochrome c oxidase subunits or by deficiency of genes that control complex IV assembly. In particular, mutations in the nuclear DNA-encoded assembly gene SURF1 are a relatively frequent cause of Leigh syndrome. Truncating mutations in the SURF1 gene are particularly common and result in rapid degradation of SURF1, which leads to the absence of functional SURF1 protein. The loss of SURF1 reduces the formation of normal complex IV, impacting the mitochondrial respiratory chain. Brainstem lesions are particularly common in children with Leigh syndrome due to SURF1 mutations. However, these children tend to follow a relatively milder course.

Complex V Deficiency. The ATP synthase or complex V is a multisubunit assembly embedded in the inner mitochondrial membrane. It contains a membrane-inserted hydrophobic domain and a hydrophilic ATPase domain that faces the mitochondrial lumen. Complex V deficiency may be the result of mutations in either the nuclear or the mitochondrial genome, as 14 of its subunits are nuclear DNA-encoded, whereas the remainder two subunits are mitochondrial DNA-encoded. The mitochondrial ATPase 6 gene encodes an important subunit of complex V. Mutations in this gene result in the most common maternally inherited form of Leigh syndrome (MILS), constituting the most frequent mitochondrial DNA mutation found in Leigh syndrome. The ATPase 6 subunit is part of the proton channel of complex V, resulting, when mutated, in loss of ATP-synthetic activity. A specific nucleotide change (T to G and T to C) at the mitochondrial DNA position 8993 is usually responsible for this phenotype. Because of its mitochondrial DNA origin, over 90 percent of mutant mitochondrial DNA heteroplasmy is required for the development of maternally inherited Leigh syndrome. This form of Leigh syndrome is characterized by a rapidly progressive course involving the basal ganglia and the brainstem. Lower abundance (50 percent) heteroplasmic mutation of the same nucleotide in ATPase 6 causes the different phenotype of neuropathy, ataxia, and retinitis pigmentosa (NARP).

tRNALeu(UUR) Mutations. The A3243G point mutation in the mitochondrial DNA is one of the most frequent causes of mitochondrial disease. The mutation leads to loss of function of the tRNA$^{Leu(UUR)}$ gene. This single substitution accounts for disorders as diverse as mitochondrial encephalomyopathy with lactic acidosis and stroke-like episodes (MELAS), hypertrophic cardiomyopathy, diabetes, myoclonic epilepsy with ragged-red fibers (MERRF) syndrome, isolated neuropathy, progressive external ophthalmoplegia, Kearns-Sayre syndrome, or Leigh syndrome. For unknown reasons, the degree of heteroplasmy of the A3243G mutation is not correlated with disease severity or with phenotype. In cases of Leigh syndrome, the phenotype is characterized by apneic episodes, ataxia, and bilateral striatal lesions detected by MR imaging. Ragged-red fibers, typical of MELAS muscle, may be absent in A3243G-associated Leigh syndrome.

tRNALys Mutations. G8363A is an infrequent mitochondrial DNA tRNA^{Lys} gene mutation that has been associated with MERRF syndrome, psychiatric abnormalities, cardiomyopathy and deafness, multiple lipomas, or Leigh syndrome. The effects of this mutation on the respiratory chain are diverse, with cytochrome c oxidase deficiency and ragged-red fibers sometimes found in muscle. Enzymatic analysis of the mitochondrial respiratory chain may show defective complex I and IV activity. The sibling of a G8363A Leigh syndrome child who harbored G8363A at 60 percent heteroplasmy developed a syndrome resembling autism in his second year of life, with loss of previously acquired language, hyperactivity with toe-walking, abnormal social interactions, stereotyped mannerisms, restricted interests, self-injurious behavior, and seizures. Because autistic traits are not uncommon and because this child lacked any evidence of mitochondrial injury by MR imaging, causation is not established.

Coenzyme Q10 Deficiency. Coenzyme Q10 is a lipophilic molecule that functions as an electron carrier and is involved in the transfer of electrons from complex I and complex II to complex III. Because of its electron binding capacity, coenzyme Q10 is an antioxidant. Mutations in the synthetic pathway of coenzyme Q10 involving decaprenyl diphosphate synthase subunit 2 are associated with a multisystem disorder that includes Leigh syndrome. These individuals also suffer from nephrotic syndrome and focal seizures.

Pyruvate Dehydrogenase Deficiency. Pyruvate dehydrogenase is one of the largest and most complex multisubunit enzyme complexes of the organism.

It catalyzes the intramitochondrial conversion of pyruvate into acetyl coenzyme A, thus constituting the entryway into the tricarboxylic acid cycle. Children with pyruvate dehydrogenase deficiency have an earlier onset, often at birth or between 3 and 6 months, and tend to follow a more severe course. Most deaths occur within the first 3 years of life. After that period, the disease is associated with prolonged survival. Leigh syndrome can be caused by mutations in any of the genes that encode the three major subunits of the complex or its regulatory phosphatase. It is hypothesized that a common effect of these Leigh-associated mutations is a reduction of flux through the tricarboxylic acid cycle. Deficiency of the X-linked E1 alpha subunit of pyruvate dehydrogenase is the most common etiology of Leigh syndrome. Because of this linkage to the X-chromosome, males usually manifest more severe disease. Females, however, can also manifest a severe phenotype perhaps because of skewed unfavorable X-inactivation. Leigh syndrome has also been associated with the E3 subunit of pyruvate dehydrogenase, which is transmissible in autosomal recessive fashion.

Diagnosis

Because Leigh syndrome is a heterogeneous disease, diagnostic criteria have been put forth. The purpose of such classifications is not only to always ensure that children are properly categorized for diagnostic and prognostic reasons and counseling, but also that gene discovery efforts utilize subject populations as homogeneous as possible. These schemes usually include progressive neurological disease with motor and intellectual abnormalities, signs, and symptoms of brainstem or basal ganglia disease, elevated lactate levels in blood or cerebrospinal fluid and relatively characteristic symmetric necrotic lesions in the basal ganglia and brainstem. However, there are unsatisfactory aspects to such a system, such that there is no universally agreed guideline. But if these criteria seem necessarily vague, even more uncertainty arises from the variable manifestations of individual mitochondrial DNA mutations.

Enzymatic analysis of the respiratory chain and pyruvate dehydrogenase is commonly accomplished in fresh-frozen muscle biopsy samples or cultured fibroblasts. Other diagnostic methods such as blue native gel electrophoresis and ultrastructural analysis of muscle can also aid with the diagnosis, as can muscle histochemical staining for cytochrome c oxidase, succinate dehydrogenase, and the Gomori trichrome method to assess the presence of ragged-red fibers. Ultrastructural changes in mitochondria can often be seen.

Because of the variability in these diagnostic methods, genotyping constitutes the best standard in the case of nuclear DNA mutations and of high-abundance mitochondrial DNA mutations.

Treatment

There is no treatment for Leigh syndrome, just as a widely beneficial therapy for mitochondrial disorders in general remains unavailable. One or more dietary antioxidants are commonly employed, but their actual mechanism of action and clinical benefits are largely unknown or absent. EPI-743, a coenzyme Q10 analog, has been suggested to improve clinical outcomes in cases of genetically confirmed Leigh syndrome as part of preliminary research, as has been in individuals with Leber's hereditary optic neuropathy.

Bibliography

Gerards M., Sallevelt S.C., Smeets H.J. (2016). Leigh syndrome: Resolving the clinical and genetic heterogeneity paves the way for treatment options. *Mol Genet Metab.* 117(3):300–12.

Leigh D. (1951). Subacute necrotizing encephalomyelopathy in an infant. *J Neurol Neurosurg Psychiatry.* 14(3):216–21.

Infantile Dopamine Transporter Deficiency

Following a normal pregnancy and birth, a neonate exhibited excessive irritability and feeding difficulties. Parkinsonism-dystonia was manifest by 6 months of age and was followed by the development of pyramidal tract dysfunction. The child was initially misdiagnosed with cerebral palsy. By 12 months, there was parkinsonism, dystonia, and pyramidal tract signs in the setting of globally abnormal development. MR imaging brain scans were unremarkable. The clinical response to multiple therapeutic agents thought to modulate neurotransmission was poor. Insertion of a deep-brain stimulator device in the child resulted in mild improvement of dystonia and rigidity. The disease progressed, with worsening symptoms of parkinsonism, dystonia, and hypertonicity in the context of relatively preserved comprehension. There was no psychiatric or conduct disorder.

Dopamine Transporter Deficiency

Onset: Parkinsonism and dystonia at about 6 months of age with prior irritability and feeding difficulties.

Additional manifestations: Progressive hypotonia is followed by spasticity. Hyperkinetic symptoms such as dystonia, chorea or dyskinesia or hypokinetic and other parkinsonian features, or mixed hyperkinetic and hypokinetic phenomena. Hyperkinetic movements diminish during childhood. Oculomotor abnormalities can include ocular flutter and oculogyric crises. A mild juvenile form causing dystonia-parkinsonism has also been described.

Disease mechanism: Autosomal recessive loss of function of the dopamine transporter, which leads to depleted intracellular and excessive extracellular dopamine.

Testing: The cerebrospinal fluid ratio of homovanillic acid to 5-hydroxyindoleacetic acid is elevated, as is the excretion of urine homovanillic acid. Serum prolactin and creatine kinase may also be increased. Genotyping is available.

Treatment: None effective. Dopaminergic agents or deep brain stimulation has been associated with limited clinical benefit

Research highlights: Null dopamine transporter mice are only hyperactive but have served to test several cellular mechanisms stemming from reduced dopamine reuptake.

Clinical Features

Dopamine transporter (DAT) deficiency is an autosomal recessive disorder of neurotransmission associated with loss of function of the neuronal dopamine transporter, encoded by SLC6A3. Clinically, dopamine transporter mutations are a cause of infantile parkinsonism-dystonia but also of a milder, later onset juvenile parkinsonism-dystonia phenotype.

Affected individuals with infantile dopamine transporter deficiency manifest at about 6 months of age with a variable movement disorder in the context of axial hypotonia, irritability, and feeding difficulties, although the hypotonia may become apparent later. Abnormal movements include hyperkinetic symptoms such as dystonia, chorea, or dyskinesia (including orolingual dyskinesia), hypokinetic and other parkinsonian features, or mixed hyperkinetic and hypokinetic phenomena. Hyperkinetic movements tend to diminish during childhood. Dystonia includes oromandibular manifestations, dystonic upper extremity posturing or severe generalized dystonic crises. Parkinsonian manifestations include early or later bradykinesia, cogwheel rigidity, hypomimia, and resting tremor. Pyramidal tract dysfunction may supervene in early childhood. Oculomotor abnormalities are variable and include ocular flutter, saccade initiation failure, slow saccadic eye movements, eyelid myoclonus, and oculogyric crises.

Motor and cognitive development is abnormal, although cognitive performance exceeds motor abilities. Speech remains generally undeveloped. Although life-span can be significantly decreased, prolonged survival is associated with severe bradykinesia or akinesia.

Pathology

There are no pathological reports available. Brain MR imaging scans are generally unremarkable and proton MR spectroscopy is normal.

Pathophysiology

The dopamine transporter is a Na^+/Cl^--dependent neurotransmitter sodium symporter. The transporter contains 12 transmembrane domains lining a gated channel with two predominant conformations: open to the extracellular or intracellular fluid (Figure 40.1). Upon dopamine binding to its primary binding site in addition to Na^+ and Cl^-, the transporter undergoes a conformational change from outward-facing to inward-facing, thus translocating dopamine. In the majority of infantile cases, the mutant human transporters retain 0–5 percent residual transport activity whereas the human mutants found in juvenile cases retain higher residual activity in association with some residual or even normal levels of expression of mature transporter at the cell surface. In contrast, surface expression of mature transporters in the infantile disease form is severely reduced or absent.

Dopaminergic neurons expressing the dopamine transporter are located predominantly in the substantia nigra pars compacta, with projections to the striatum via the nigrostriatal pathway, and in the ventral tegmental area of the midbrain, with mesocorticolimbic projections to the nucleus accumbens, hippocampus, and other corticolimbic structures.

The dopamine transporter regulates the amplitude and duration of dopaminergic action at presynaptic and postsynaptic receptors such that its loss of function may lead to downregulation or desensitization of postsynaptic dopamine receptors. Insufficient uptake of dopamine into presynaptic neurons probably also causes accumulation of extracellular dopamine, resulting in dopamine degradation and increased homovanillic acid in the cerebrospinal fluid. However, dopamine transporter defects do not affect serotonin synthesis, such that the concentration of 5-hydroxyindoleacetic acid in the cerebrospinal fluid is normal, accounting for an increased ratio of homovanillic acid to 5-hydroxyindoleacetic acid. Deficient dopamine reuptake may also lead to depletion of presynaptic dopamine stores and insufficient releasable synaptic vesicular contents. Excess extraneuronal dopamine could also overstimulate presynaptic D2 autoreceptors (D3 receptors), resulting in inhibition of tyrosine hydroxylase thereby decreasing dopamine production.

Mechanisms underlying the loss of DAT transport function include reduced expression of DAT, loss of dopamine recognition by DAT due to reduced binding affinity, and lack of glycosylation to form mature DAT, which is known to negatively affect trafficking to the cell surface and transport function of DAT.

SLC6A3 knockout mice are hyperactive and have served to corroborate several of the potential consequences of decreased dopamine reuptake.

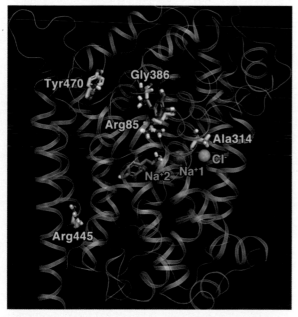

Figure 40.1 Structural homology modeling of the dopamine transporter based on LeuT. Transmembrane domains and loops are in grey; mutated amino acids affected by missense mutations in yellow and bound ions in purple (Na+) and green (Cl-). Reproduced with permission from Ng J, Zhen J, Meyer E, Erreger K, Li Y, Kakar N, Ahmad J, Thiele H, Kubisch C, Rider NL, Morton DH, Strauss KA, Puffenberger EG, D'Agnano D, Anikster Y, Carducci C, Hyland K, Rotstein M, Leuzzi V, Borck G, Reith ME, Kurian MA. Dopamine transporter deficiency syndrome: phenotypic spectrum from infancy to adulthood. *Brain*. 2014; 137(Pt 4):1107–19.

Diagnosis

All affected individuals harbor homozygous or compound heterozygous mutations in SLC6A3.

153

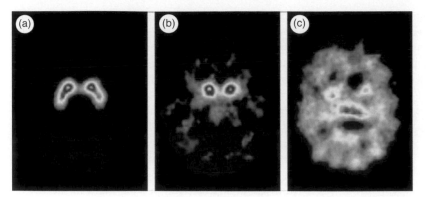

Figure 40.2. Nuclear brain imaging with single photon emission ioflupane ^{123}I scan in a normal subject (a), an individual with juvenile parkinsonism of unknown etiology (b), and a child with dopamine transporter deficiency (c). Reproduced with permission from Kurian MA et al. Clinical and molecular characterisation of hereditary dopamine transporter deficiency syndrome: an observational cohort and experimental study. *Lancet Neurol.* 2011; 10(1):54–62.

The cerebrospinal fluid ratio of homovanillic acid to 5-hydroxyindoleacetic acid is elevated, as is the excretion of urine homovanillic acid. Serum prolactin and creatine kinase may also be increased. Nuclear medicine imaging using ioflupane ^{123}I shows loss of dopamine transporter activity in the basal ganglia in the context of high background activity (Figure 40.2). The high background is also characteristic of adult affected individuals with poor uptake in the basal nuclei and could be attributed to unbound ioflupane I[123] circulating in blood, although this remains unproven.

Treatment

A variety of agents including drugs generally considered muscle relaxants, dopaminergic, anticholinergic, antiglutamatergic, and γ-aminobutyric acid [GABA]-ergic agents) and deep brain stimulation are either ineffective or largely insufficient, as is levodopa combined with carbidopa or the dopamine agonists ropinirole and pramipexole. Dietary tyrosine restriction has also proven ineffective.

Bibliography

Kurian M.A., Zhen J., Cheng S.Y., et al. (2009). Homozygous loss-of-function mutations in the gene encoding the dopamine transporter are associated with infantile parkinsonism-dystonia. *J Clin Invest.* 119(6):1595–603.

Ng J., Zhen J., Meyer E., et al. (2014). Dopamine transporter deficiency syndrome: Phenotypic spectrum from infancy to adulthood. *Brain.* 137(Pt 4):1107–19.

Canavan Disease

A 50-day-old boy with progressive irritability had been born to an unrelated healthy couple. The pregnancy was unremarkable except for increased fetal movement. He was born at term by spontaneous vaginal delivery. The Apgar scores were 10 and 10 in the first and fifth minute, respectively. However, hypertonia in the lower limbs was noted by the obstetrician. Birth weight was 3.9 kg (90th centile), length was 50 cm (50th centile), and head circumference was 34 cm (50th centile). Two of the child's sisters had severe psychomotor disabilities. They never achieved the ability to smile response, roll, crawl, sit independently, or babble. Both girls gradually developed spasticity in upper and lower limbs and became unresponsive to auditory and visual stimuli. The older sister died at 22 months, and the younger died at 11 months. A third pregnancy was intentionally aborted. At 50-days of age, the boy's head circumference was 38 cm (50th centile). He failed to fix or follow a visual target and he did not smile. He also manifested axial hypotonia and lower limb symmetric hypertonia accompanied by brisk deep tendon reflexes.

Canavan Disease

Onset: Hypotonia, including head lag, at 3 months of age.

Additional manifestations: Feeding difficulties, macrocephaly and optic atrophy. Progressive spasticity and rigidity can replace hypotonia. Seizures are usually mild. Neonatal and mild juvenile forms are also recognized.

Disease mechanism: Autosomal recessive loss of function of the aspartoacylase enzyme, which is important for myelin production. Aspartoacylase cleaves N-acetylaspartate into acetate and aspartate. Spongiform degeneration of the white matter may be due to increased osmotic pressure.

Testing: Increased levels of N-acetylaspartate in the brain and other tissues. This can be detected by routine proton MR spectroscopy. Genotyping for two common Ashkenazi and other common mutation, or for de novo variants is widely available.

Treatment: Systemic or intrathecal administration of adeno-associated virus constructs containing aspartoacylase or stem cells has been followed by biochemical benefit circumscribed to areas of penetration of the therapeutic agent.

Research highlights: Null mice and spontaneously mutant tremor rats have served as a testbed for adeno-associated, stem cell, and enzyme replacement therapies.

Clinical Features

Known as spongy leukodystrophy or aspartoacylase deficiency, Canavan disease is an autosomal recessive disorder prevalent among Ashkenazi Jews. Although the predominant form affects infants, a neonatal and a milder juvenile form have been described. Onset in the more common infantile form is at 3 months of life with hypotonia leading to head lag. Poor visual fixation, irritability, and impaired sucking become apparent later. Developmental regression, nystagmus with optic atrophy and macrocephaly develop during the first year, which are followed by spasticity. Mild epilepsy ensues in the second year of life. Death often occurs in the first decade.

Pathology

Brain weight is 50 percent greater than normal during the first 2 years of life but then decreases to normal as cerebral atrophy progresses. There is little myelin, including at the U-fibers, which blurs the cortical gray-white matter junction (Figure 41.1). The cortex can appear normal, but the white matter is gray,

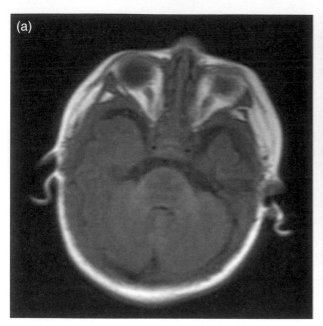
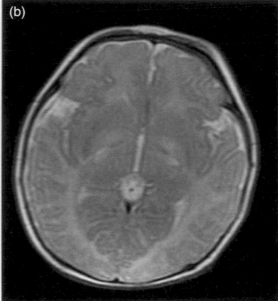

Figure 41.1 Brain magnetic resonance image in Canavan disease. a. T1-weighted image reveals hypomyelination of pontine tegmentum. b. Indicates hypomyelination of posterior limb of internal capsule and posterior part of sub-cortical deep white matter in a T2-weighted image. Reproduced with permission from Zhang H et al. Two novel missense mutations in the aspartoacylase gene in a Chinese patient with congenital Canavan disease. *Brain Dev.* 2010; 32(10):879–82.

gelatinous, and sunken in, with cyst formation (Figure 41.2). There are numerous vacuoles in the white matter which are devoid of solid material. These vacuoles may be lined by myelin basic protein and span 200 μm in diameter. They are more prominent at the gray-white matter junction. Astrocytosis is present, including Alzheimer type I and type II glia (Figure 41.3). Oligodendrocytes are lost late in the disease course. Axons are preserved, with occasional spheroid formation. The white matter can be replaced by astrocytes, capillaries, and macrophages. Astrocytes are swollen and contain elongated mitochondria with central crystalline cores surrounded by abnormal cristae.

Pathophysiology

Two mutations in the aspartoacylase gene account for 98 percent of Ashkenazi affected individuals and another mutation for 60 percent of non-Ashkenazi affected individuals. Aspartoacylase hydrolyzes N-acetylaspartate to acetate and aspartate in oligodendroglial cell bodies (Figure 41.4). Consequently, N-acetyl aspartate accumulates in the brain and also in body fluids, reaching high millimolar concentrations. The biological function of N-acetylaspartate remains unclear and it was even considered inert,

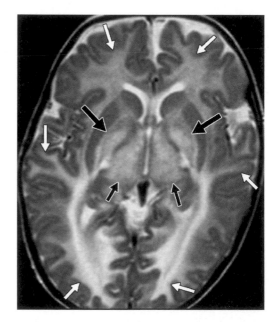

Figure 41.2 Two-year-old girl with Canavan disease who presented with macrocephaly, seizures, and hypotonia. Axial T2-weighted MR imaging at level of lentiform nuclei shows diffuse hyperintensity within cerebral hemispheric white matter (white arrows), thalami (small black arrows), and globus pallidi (large black arrows). Reproduced with permission from Ibrahim M et al. Inborn errors of metabolism: combining clinical and radiologic clues to solve the mystery. *AJR Am J Roentgenol.* 2014; 203(3): W315–27.

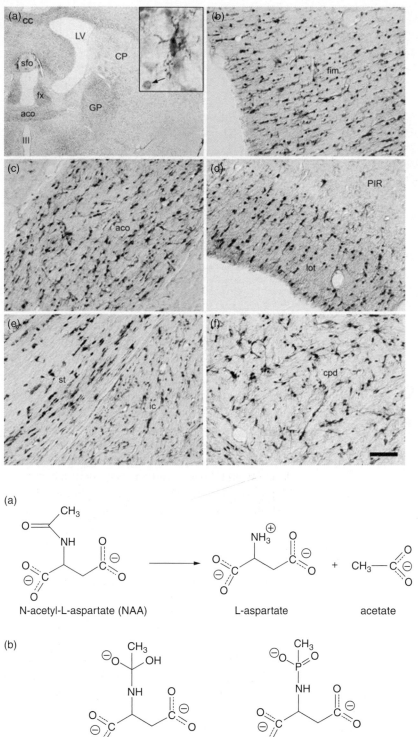

Figure 41.3 Expression of aspartoacylase (ASPA) in the rat brain. In the corpus callosum most if not all oligodendrocytes are immunoreactive for ASPA to some degree, ranging from very lightly to intensely stained (cc). The great majority of immunoreactive oligodendrocytes in the corpus callosum and external capsule are Type I/II morphologically, with more than one cellular process. ASPA is expressed in oligodendrocyte cell bodies, nuclei, proximal processes, and in some finer more distal processes, but it is not expressed throughout entire oligodendrocyte arborizations. In addition to the corpus callosum, all telencephalic fiber pathways contain numerous oligodendrocytes that expressed ASPA protein, including the fornix (a), fimbria (b), anterior commissure (c), lateral olfactory tract (d), internal capsule and stria terminalis (e) and cerebral peduncles (f). Many of the oligodendrocytes in these forebrain pathways exhibit Type I/II morphology, and are often arranged in rows or clusters with oligodendrocyte cell bodies in direct contact with one another. Reproduced with permission from Moffett JR et al. Extensive aspartoacylase expression in the rat central nervous system. *Glia.* 2011; 59(10):1414–34.

Figure 41.4 a. Deacetylation reaction catalyzed by aspartoacylase. b. Structure of the putative reaction intermediate (i) that would be formed in a carboxypeptidase-like mechanism for the deacetylation of N-acetyl-l-aspartate and structure of the phosphonamidate analogue of this intermediate (ii) that was cocrystallized with human aspartoacylase. Reproduced with permission from Le Coq J et al. Examination of the mechanism of human brain aspartoacylase through the binding of an intermediate analogue. *Biochemistry.* 2008; 47(11):3484–92.

(a)

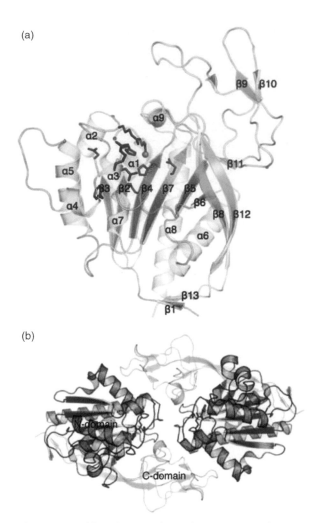

(b)

Figure 41.5 Ribbon diagrams of recombinant aspartoacylase (rASPA) monomer and dimer. a. N-domain of rASPA is color-coded in cyan and red. C-domain is color-coded in yellow and green. Residues His-21, Gly-22, Glu-24, Asn-54, Arg-63, Asn-70, Arg-71, Phe-73, Asp-114, His-116, and Glu-178 (blue sticks) are highly conserved in the AstE-AspA family and delineate the active site. Zn^{2+} is shown as a pink sphere. b. The rASPA dimer observed in the asymmetric unit of the rASPA crystals is shown in ribbon representation. Both the N-domain (red) and C-domain (green) of the rASPA monomers are involved in formation of the dimer interface. Residues His-21, Glu-24, and His-116 (blue sticks) coordinate Zn^{2+} (pink sphere). Reproduced with permission from Bitto E et al. Structure of aspartoacylase, the brain enzyme impaired in Canavan disease. *Proc Natl Acad Sci U S A.* 2007; 104(2):456–61.

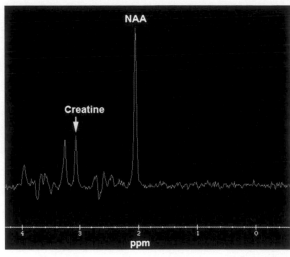

Figure 41.6 MR spectroscopy in an infant with Canavan disease. The proton spectrum of the left posterior lobe reveals the characteristic high NAA peak of Canavan disease, which should not be present for a normal infant under 4 months old. Reproduced with permission from Zhang H et al. Two novel missense mutations in the aspartoacylase gene in a Chinese patient with congenital Canavan disease. *Brain Dev.* 2010; 32(10):879–82.

giving the brain a characteristic spongiform appearance. The structural effect of the common mutations on aspartoacylase is known: For example, the loss of hydrogen bonding interactions with the carboxylate side chain of the commonly mutated Glu285 disturbs the active site architecture, leading to altered substrate binding and lower catalytic activity (Figure 41.5). Aspartoacylase is also expressed by Schwann cells, but nerve function is usually spared in Canavan disease.

Diagnosis

Genotyping is widely available. The common Ashkenazi mutations in the aspartoacylase gene are Glu285Ala and Tyr321X lead to loss of function, as does the non-Ashkenazi frequent mutation Ala306-Glu. Other mutations also occur at relative high frequencies and confer mild disease severity. They are usually combined with one of the most common severe mutations. Proton MR spectroscopy reveals increased concentration of N-acetylaspartate, as does analysis of urine (Figure 41.6).

Treatment

Acetazolamide can be used to decrease cerebrospinal fluid pressure. Several interventions lead to

but it may be important in the synthesis of myelin, as acetate derived from N-acetylaspartate is used for conversion of lignoceric acid to the myelin constituent cerebronic acid. Thus, a deficit of brain acetate was initially postulated as a disease mechanism. N-acetylaspartate is most concentrated in the cerebral cortex and it may attract water, which accumulates, amelioration of the biochemical phenotype of mutant mice or of the tremor rat, a spontaneous disease model. Among these, lithium citrate, given with the intent of reducing osmotic pressure, leads to no clinical improvement. Similarly, glycerol triacetate has been used to supply acetate to the brain but is also devoid of beneficial clinical efficacy. Gene therapy using adeno-associated virus 2 (AAV2) injected into affected individuals' brains was associated with no clinical improvement, but this may be due to a very restricted penetration of the enzyme. Enzyme replacement has focused on polyethylene glycol adducts of aspartoacylase injected intraperitoneally. This enzyme penetrates the brain and is accompanied by decreased N-acetylaspartate. Similar insufficient results have been obtained with hyaluronidase and aspartoacylase mixtures injected intraperitoneally in the mutant mouse. Stem cell administration leads to oligodendrocyte formation, but in insufficient numbers to myelinate the brain. AAV8 containing the recombinant gene injected intravenously significantly prolongs mutant mouse survival. Additional reduction of N-acetylaspartate synthetase or N-acetyltransferase-8 like protein in mice with aspartoacylase deficiency leads to normal myelin content, myelin sphingolipid composition, and little or no spongy myelin degeneration, indicating that N-acetylaspartate is an important mediator of the myelin dysfunction typical of the disease.

Bibliography

Matalon R., Michals-Matalon K., Surendran S., et al. (2006). Canavan disease: studies on the knockout mouse. *Adv Exp Med Biol.* 576:77–93.

Zhang H., Liu X., Gu X. (2010). Two novel missense mutations in the aspartoacylase gene in a Chinese patient with congenital Canavan disease. *Brain Dev.* 32(10):879–82.

Chapter 42

Cockayne Syndrome

A girl was evaluated at 14 months of age for microcephaly, abnormal global development and brain atrophy on CT scan (Figure 42.1). She was born at 39 weeks of gestation to non-consanguinous parents. The pregnancy was complicated by gestational hypertension requiring treatment. Fetal movements were normal. Intrauterine growth retardation was first noted at 32 weeks of gestation. Delivery occurred via cesarean section and birth weight was 1800 grams (50th percentile for 32 weeks gestational age). She rolled at 5–6 months of age but had not acquired independent sitting or walking at 3.5 years of age. She spoke her first word at one year of age but at 3.5 years she only had 2–3 words. She was able to transfer objects past midline and finger feed. Growth parameters at 14 months of age revealed a height of 63 cm (50th percentile for a 5 month old), weight of 5.67 kg (50th percentile for a 4 month old) and head circumference of 36.2 cm (50th percentile for a one month old female). Examination at 3.5 years of age revealed a height of 66.5 cm (50th percentile for a 7 month old), weight 6.3 kg (50th percentile for a 4 month old) and a head circumference of 37 cm (50th percentile for a 1 month old). She exhibited brachycephaly, coarse and sparse hair, deep set eyes, bulbous nasal tip, long philtrum and delayed dentition. Contractures were present at the knees and ankles. There was marked hypotonia with limb hypertonia. She had posterior polar cataracts, retinal dystrophy including optic atrophy, diffuse retinal atrophy, retinal blood vessel attenuation, macular blunting, and marked enophthalmos. From the time of initial assessment, she had recurrent vomiting and received a gastrostomy. Hypertension was present but the etiology was not known. She died at 4.5 years of age of respiratory distress.

Cockayne Syndrome

Onset: In the common form, failure to thrive, microcephaly and abnormal neurological and physical development noticeable between 1 and 2 years of age. The severe form is congenital and the milder form occurs in childhood.

Additional manifestations: Appearance of cachectic dwarfism. Progressive impairment of vision, hearing, and behavioral and intellectual performance. Photosensitivity. Leukodystrophy and cerebral calcification. Neuropathy. Seizures.

Disease mechanism: Autosomal recessive failure of DNA repair due to mutation of ERCC6 or ERCC8.

Testing: DNA repair assay on fibroblasts. Electromyography, nerve conduction testing or nerve biopsy illustrate neuropathy.

Treatment: None effective.

Research highlights: Mechanisms of DNA repair after radiation injury.

Clinical Features

Cockayne syndrome is an autosomal recessive disorder with an incidence of 2 in 1,000,000 newborns characterized by short stature and an appearance of premature aging. Additional features include a failure to gain weight and grow at the expected rate, microcephaly and impaired development of the nervous system with progressive neurological deterioration. Affected individuals exhibit extreme photosensitivity such that even a brief sun exposure can cause a sunburn. Other manifestations include hearing loss, eye abnormalities, severe tooth decay, bone abnormalities and changes in brain configuration such as leukodystrophy detectable by neuroimaging. Three forms of the disease are recognized.

Table 42.1 Clinical features of Cockayne syndrome

Cockayne syndrome type	Usual age at diagnosis	Principal manifestations
I, moderate or common form	Infancy	Growth failure Progressive neurologic dysfunction
II, severe form	Birth	Growth failure Absent neurologic development Structural ocular defects
III, mild form	Childhood	Milder similar abnormalities

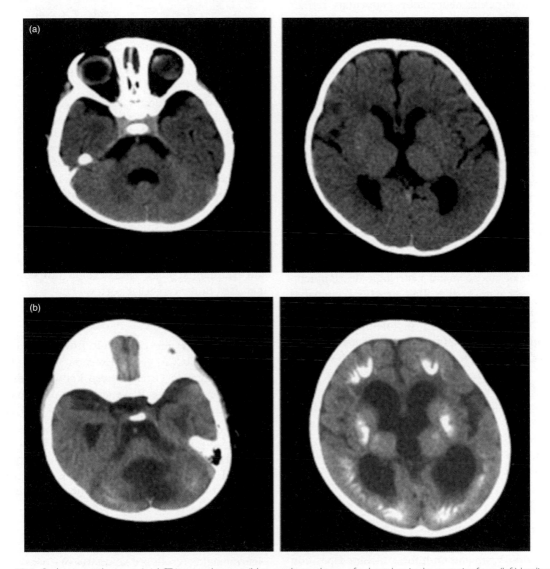

Figure 42.1 Cockayne syndrome. a. Axial CT images show a mild to moderate degree of volume loss in the posterior fossa (left) leading to a prominent fourth ventricle. Prominent sulci, lateral and third ventricles are also seen due to supratentorial volume loss (right). Note faint calcification in the right basal ganglia. b. Axial CT images show marked progression of brain atrophy involving the cerebellum, brain stem, basal ganglia, thalami and the cerebral hemispheres. Note calcifications in the cerebellar hemispheres (left), calcifications in the basal ganglia and thalami; and extensive subcortical white matter calcifications in the cerebral hemispheres (right). Reproduced with permission from Ghai SJ et al. Cockayne syndrome caused by paternally inherited 5 Mb deletion of 10q11.2 and a frameshift mutation of ERCC6. *Eur J Med Genet*. 2011; 54(3):272–6.

Type I Cockayne syndrome (common or moderate form) is characterized by normal prenatal growth followed by growth and developmental abnormalities that usually become apparent between the first and second year. Height, weight, and head circumference fall below the fifth percentile. Progressive impairment of vision, and hearing, behavioral and intellectual deterioration lead to severe disability. Additional, more variable features include cutaneous photosensitivity with or without thin or dry skin or hair, demyelinating neuropathy, pigmentary retinopathy and cataracts, sensorineural hearing loss, dental anomalies including dental caries, enamel hypoplasia and abnormal tooth number, size and shape, a characteristic physical appearance of cachectic dwarfism with thinning of the skin and hair, deeply set eyes, and a stooped standing posture. Undescended testes and delayed or absent sexual maturation may occur. No affected individuals have been able to reproduce. Radiographic findings include thickening of the calvarium, sclerotic epiphyses and vertebral and pelvic abnormalities. Neuroimaging studies reveal leukodystrophy and intracranial calcifications (Figure 42.1). Death typically occurs in the first or second decade.

Type II Cockayne syndrome (severe form) is associated with growth failure noticeable at birth with little or no postnatal neurologic development. Congenital cataracts and other structural anomalies of the eye (microphthalmos, microcornea, iris hypoplasia) may be prominent in one-third of cases. Affected children display early postnatal contractures of the spine leading to kyphosis or scoliosis and of the joints. Death usually occurs by seven years of age. This form of the disease overlaps with cerebrooculofacioskeletal syndrome and with Pena-Shokeir type II syndrome

Cockayne syndrome type III is more loosely defined, as it includes milder or incomplete forms with onset in childhood.

Pathology

Neuroimaging demonstrates a characteristic tigroid pattern of demyelination in the subcortical white matter of the brain and multifocal calcium deposition (Figure 42.2). There is relative preservation of neurons, except for the cerebellar cortex, and absence of senile plaques, amyloid, ubiquitin, or tau deposition. Apoptotic cell death might be involved in

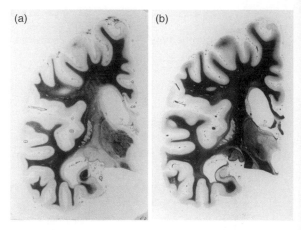

Figure 42.2 Neuropathology of Cockayne syndrome. The cerebral white matter at the plane of the lateral geniculate body. Severe fibrillary gliosis was observed on staining by the Holzer method (a), while myelinated fibers were found to be preserved in a section stained by the KB method (b). Reproduced with permission from Itoh M et al. Neurodegeneration in hereditary nucleotide repair disorders. *Brain Dev.* 1999; 21(5):326–33.

the cerebellar neurodegeneration. There is also a reduction of volume and patchy demyelination in the cerebral and cerebellar white matter and multifocal calcium deposition in the basal ganglia and cerebral white matter, respectively. Grumose or foamy spheroid bodies occur in the globus pallidus and substantia nigra and axonal torpedoes are increased in the cerebellar cortex.

Pathophysiology

Cockayne syndrome can result from mutations in either the ERCC6 gene (Excision Repair Cross-Complementation Group 6, also known as the CSB (Cockayne syndrome B) gene, which is responsible for two-thirds of cases) or the ERCC8 gene (Excision Repair Cross-Complementation Group 8, also known as the CSA (Cockayne syndrome A) gene, which accounts for about a third of cases). These genes are involved in repairing damaged DNA. DNA can be damaged by ultraviolet rays from the sun and by toxic chemicals, radiation, or free radicals.

Diagnosis

Neuroimaging results are suggestive of Cockayne syndrome. Electromyography, nerve conduction testing, and nerve biopsy can document neuropathy. A specific DNA repair assay on fibroblasts can confirm the diagnosis. The assay may demonstrate marked sensitivity to UV radiation, deficient recovery of RNA synthesis following UV damage and impaired repair of actively transcribed genes or transcription-coupled repair.

Treatment

There is no effective treatment.

Bibliography

Ghai S.J., Shago M., Shroff M., et al. (2011). Cockayne syndrome caused by paternally inherited 5 Mb deletion of 10q11.2 and a frameshift mutation of ERCC6. *Eur J Med Genet.* 54(3):272–6.

Itoh M., Hayashi M., Shioda K., et al. (1999). Neurodegeneration in hereditary nucleotide repair disorders. *Brain Dev.* 21(5):326–33.

Menkes Disease

A 3-month-old boy was evaluated for lethargy that developed over the course of 2 days. His pre and perinatal course were remarkable for intrauterine distress leading to urgent successful surgical delivery and for difficulty gaining weight, which was noted at 3 weeks. However, supplemental nutrition administered since then had had little effect. At presentation, he had to be awoken for feeds and did "fall right back to sleep." Weight was below the 3rd percentile for age. He was obtunded and hypotonic, with a significant head lag. Bloodwork revealed metabolic acidosis with a lactic acid level of 7.4 mM after hydration therapy. The following day, he had several 15–30 second seizures including left eye deviation followed by left neck deviation and left arm extension. Cranial MR imaging revealed meningeal contrast enhancement indicating meningitis (Figure 43.1), which was confirmed via cerebrospinal fluid analysis. He received phenobarbital and antibiotics for 21 days. After antibiotics were completed, his seizures recurred and became difficult to treat. His EEG was severely abnormal. Lethargy reappeared. More profound hypotonia was noted and he lost the ability to track visually. He also lost most of his hair. Repeat MR imaging illustrated encephalic lesions and resolution of meningitis (Figure 43.1). Repeat cerebrospinal fluid analysis revealed a lactate value of 6.3 mM. He developed severe neutropenia. A gastrostomy and a muscle biopsy (normal) were performed.

occipital horn syndrome, is non progressive and is associated with disostosis.

Disease mechanism: X-linked loss of function of the copper transporter MNK, encoded by ATP7A, leading to reduced copper incorporation into enzymes such as cytochrome c oxidase, lysyl oxidase, superoxide dismutase, peptidylglycine α-amidating mono-oxygenase, tyrosinase, dopamine-β-hydroxylase and ascorbic acid oxidase. An additional feature is altered immune function.

Testing: Reduced levels of serum ceruloplasmin and copper levels.

Treatment: Intramuscular or subcutaneous administration of copper-histidine.

Research highlights: *Mottled/brindled* spontaneously mutant mice receiving complementary therapies via lateral ventricle injections of adenovirus harboring a human ATP7A DNA construct and copper chloride exhibit prolonged survival and preservation of neural structure.

Clinical Features

Three phenotypes resulting from ATP7A defects are recognized: Menkes disease, occipital horn syndrome, and ATP7A-related distal motor neuropathy. Also known as kinky hair disease, Menkes disease is associated with copper deficiency, in contrast with Wilson's disease, which is characterized by copper accumulation. Menkes disease is an X-linked disorder with a frequency of 1 per 100,000 live male births. However, several girls have also been affected. Despite most children manifesting in infancy, a neonatal form has been described. The infants are pale and exhibit kinky (or, later, no) hair, accounting for the disease name. A variety of minimally symptomatic phenotypes, including ataxia or mental retardation have been recognized.

Menkes Disease

Onset: Kinky and rapidly thinning hair with pallor and growth retardation. Severe infection or subdural hematoma can be the first manifestation.

Additional manifestations: Propensity to bleeding and to fractures. Progressive combination of seizures and dementia. A milder disease form,

Most of the clinical manifestations can be explained by the deficient activities of various copper-containing enzymes. These include cytochrome c oxidase, lysyl oxidase, superoxide dismutase, peptidylglycine α-amidating mono-oxygenase, tyrosinase, dopamine-β-hydroxylase, and ascorbic acid oxidase. The disease is associated with progressive cerebral injury (Figure 43.1). The clinical manifestations of Menkes disease, however, are quite variable. In part, the variability can be explained by a large number of mutations. These include mutations that lead to splicing abnormalities, small duplications, nonsense mutations, and missense mutations and to aberrant protein fragments that may retain functional activity. All mutations detected have been unique for each given family, and almost all have been associated with a decreased level of mRNA for the copper-transporting ATPase.

In the neonatal form, symptoms include hypothermia, hypoglycemia, poor feeding, and impaired weight gain. Less often there is a fatal hemorrhagic diathesis and multiple congenital fractures (Figure 43.2). Cephalohematomas can be prominent in infants born vaginally. The appearance of hair is often unremarkable at birth; newborns can have little or no hair, or normally pigmented hair. Other affected individuals present with seizures, delayed development, or failure to thrive. The most striking finding is the abnormal hair. It is colorless and friable. On examination under the microscope, a variety of abnormalities are evident, most commonly pili torti (a hair shaft which is flattened and twisted 180 degrees on its axis) (Figure 43.3). Monilethrix (an elliptical swelling of the hair shafts with intervening tapered constrictions) and trichorrhexis nodosa (small beaded swelling of the hair shaft with fractures at regular intervals) are also seen. The optic discs are pale, and there are microcysts of the pigmentary epithelium and iris. Hydronephrosis, hydroureter, and diverticula or rupture of the bladder have been reported. Radiographs of long bones show a variety of abnormalities, including osteoporosis, metaphyseal spurring, a diaphyseal periosteal reaction and scalloping of the posterior aspects of the vertebral bodies. Skull radiographs may reveal the presence of wormian bones in the lambdoidal and posterior sagittal sutures. Neuroimaging studies frequently disclose cerebral atrophy, areas of low density within the cortex, impaired myelination and tortuous and enlarged intracranial vessels. The frequent presence of subdural hematomas has in many instances raised suspicion of intentional trauma.

The disease course is inexorably progressive, but the rate of neurologic deterioration varies significantly. There are recurrent infections of the respiratory and urinary tracts. Sepsis and meningitis are common and there is evidence for dysfunction of the cellular immune responses.

Pathology

In the skin, elastin fibers are reduced in number and consist of thin strands of amorphous elastin associated with numerous microfibrils. Cerebral and systemic arteries are tortuous, with irregular lumens and frayed and split intimal linings. These abnormalities reflect the failure in elastin and collagen cross-linking caused by a decrease in functional activity of copper-dependent lysyl oxidase.

Gross examination of the brain discloses diffuse atrophy and often unilateral or bilateral subdural hematomas. There is extensive focal degeneration of gray matter with neuronal loss and gliosis and an associated axonal degeneration in white matter. Cellular loss is prominent in the cerebellum. Purkinje cells are most affected. Many are lost and others show abnormal dendritic arborization (resembling a weeping willow) and perisomatic processes. Focal axonal swellings, typically described as torpedoes, are also observed. On electron microscopy, there are abundant mitochondrial abnormalities.

Anatomical changes within the brain are believed to result from reduced activity of the various copper-containing enzymes; in particular, from mitochondrial dysfunction, from vascular lesions, or from a combination of the two. In addition, copper is specifically protective toward N-methyl-D-aspartate (NMDA)-mediated excitotoxic cell death, whereas ATP7A is required to maintain a pool of copper in neurons.

Pathophysiology

The Menkes disease protein, ATP7A, allows cellular copper to cross intracellular membranes and to be also translocated from the trans-Golgi network to the plasma membrane in the presence of extracellular copper (Figure 43.4). The fundamental abnormality in this disease is thus the maldistribution of copper, which is unavailable as a cofactor of several enzymes including mitochondrial

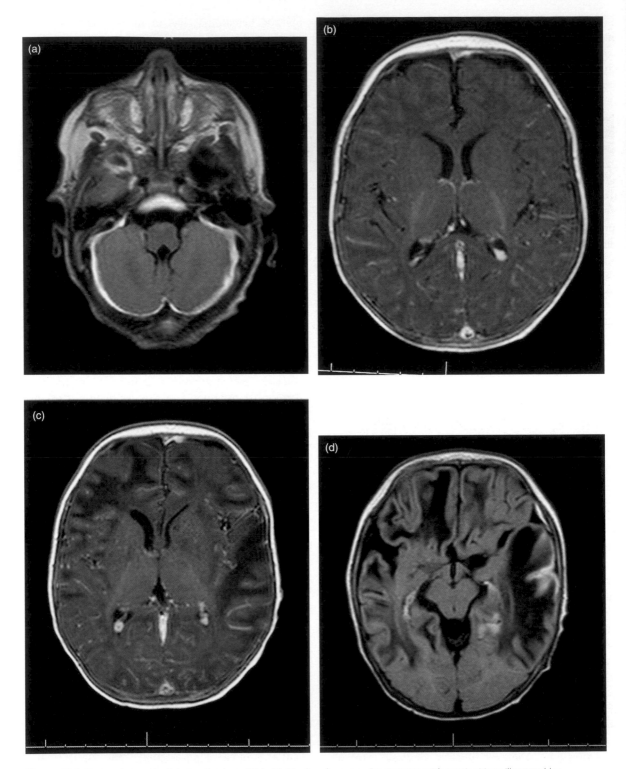

Figure 43.1 Progressive cerebral destruction in a child with Menkes disease. a. Presentation with meningitis as illustrated by contrast-enhanced FLAIR images. b. Study obtained at 5 months of age. c. Study at 6 months of age. d. Disease progression one month later. e. MR study obtained simultaneously with D. vascular tortuosity is appreciable. f. Cerebellar atrophy is apparent at 7 months of age.

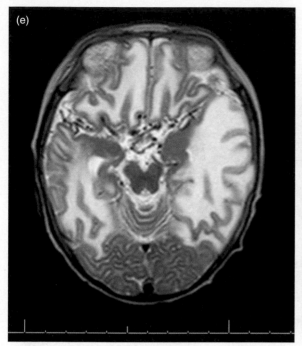

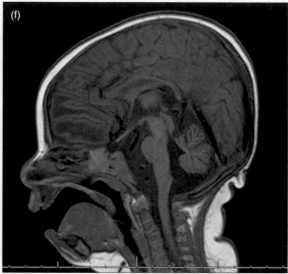

Figure 43.1 (*cont.*)

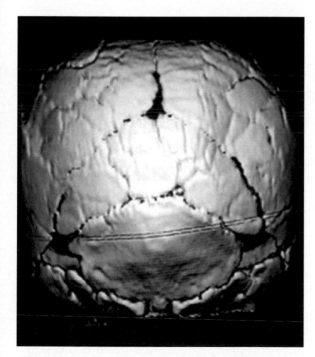

Figure 43.2 Eleven-week-old boy with Menkes disease. Three-dimensional shaded surface display of skull shows multiple wormian bones. Reproduced with permission from Thomas B et al. MRI of childhood epilepsy due to inborn errors of metabolism. *AJR Am J Roentgenol.* 2010; 194(5):W367–74.

cytochrome c oxidase, lysyl oxidase, superoxide dismutase, dopamine beta-hydroxylase, and tyrosinase. Thus, the main features of the disease include mitochondrial respiratory chain dysfunction (complex IV deficiency), deficiency of collagen cross-links resulting in hair and vascular abnormalities (elongated cerebral vessels and subdural effusions), neuronal degeneration (markedly affecting Purkinje cells), and deficient melanin production, all of which dominate disease manifestations.

ATP7A is located on Xq13. It encodes MNK, an energy-dependent, copper-transporting P-type membrane ATPase. The structural homology between ATP7A and ATP7B is high in the 3' two-thirds of the genes, but there is considerable divergence between them in the 5' one third. ATP7A is expressed in all tissues with the exception of liver. It consists of six metal-binding domains, eight transmembrane domains, and domains for phosphatase, phosphorylation and ATP binding. At basal copper levels, the protein is located in the trans-Golgi network, the sorting station for proteins exiting from the Golgi apparatus, where it is involved in copper uptake into its lumen. At increased intra- and extracellular copper concentrations, the MNK protein shifts toward the

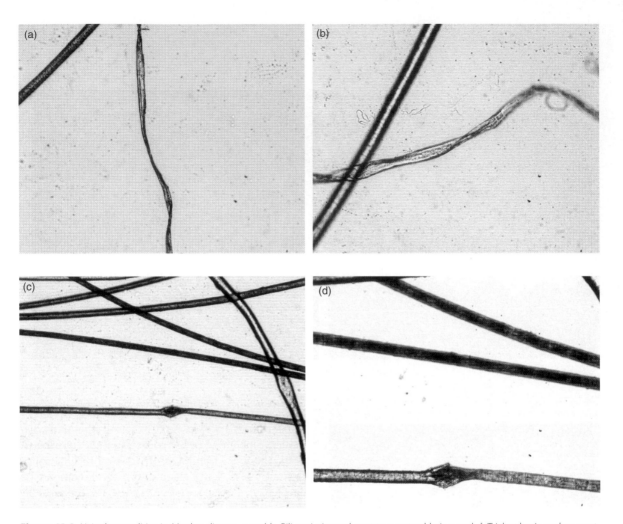

Figure 43.3 Hair abnormalities in Menkes disease. **a** and **b**. Pili torti pictured next to a normal hair. **c** and **d**. Trichorrhexis nodosa next to normal hair.

plasma membrane, presumably to enhance removal of excess copper from the cell.

The characteristic abnormality in copper metabolism as expressed in the human infant is a maldistribution of body copper, a result of defective copper transport across the placenta, the gastrointestinal tract and the blood–brain barrier. The consequence is a failure of copper incorporation into the essential enzymes cited above. Affected individuals absorb little or no orally administered copper; when the metal is given intravenously, they experience a prompt rise in serum copper and ceruloplasmin. As a result of impaired copper efflux, the copper content of cultured fibroblasts, myotubes, and lymphocytes derived from affected individuals is several times greater than normal.

Diagnosis

Reduced levels of serum ceruloplasmin and copper are diagnostic of Menkes disease. Urinary copper is variable: normal, reduced and even elevated levels have been reported. The ratio of urinary homovanillic acid/vanillylmandelic acid ratio is elevated.

Heterozygotes are mostly asymptomatic and do not manifest any biochemical abnormalities. However, areas of pili torti constitute between 30 and 50 percent of their hair. Prenatal diagnosis has been based on the increased copper content of cultured amniocytes and chorionic villus samples. The determination of abnormal catecholamine metabolites in plasma (for example, dopamine: norepinephrine ratio) and in cerebrospinal

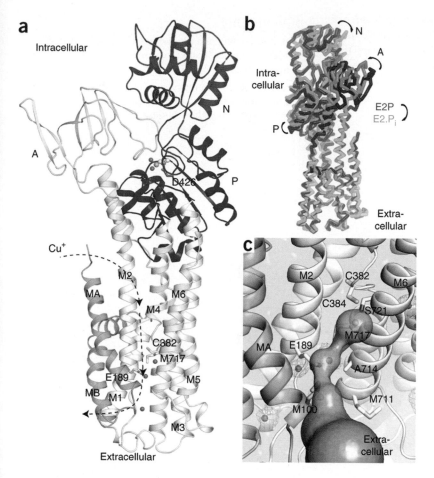

Figure 43.4 The Menkes protein is a copper-transporting P-type ATPase. **a.** Black arrows mark the direction of Cu+ transport. Crystal waters located in close vicinity to Cys382, Met717, and Glu189 are shown as red spheres. **b.** Superimpositions of the transmembrane domains of the E2P (purple) and E2.Pi (green) states. Intracellular domains change their configuration from the E2P to the E2.Pi state (black arrows) while the transmembrane domains remain rigid. **c.** Close-up view of the extrusion pathway with residual Fo – Fc electron density (green mesh at 2.5 s, before modeling) of BeF3–bound LpCopA, with key residues labeled. The opening from the high-affinity Cu+-coordinating residues Cys382, Cys384 and Met717 in the E2P conformation is displayed as a red surface and overlays with crystallographic water molecules as red spheres. Reproduced with permission from Andersson M et al. Copper-transporting P-type ATPases use a unique ion-release pathway. *Nat Struct Mol Biol.* 2014; 21(1):43–8.

fluid resulting from deficiency of dopamine-β-hydroxylase is sensitive and specific and may allow for earlier detection.

Treatment

Mottled/brindled mouse spontaneous mutants have served as a testbed for Menkes disease after they were confirmed to harbor mutations in ATP7A. These mice live less than 14 days and exhibit severe intestinal copper malabsorption associated with tremors and spasms that can be prevented by subcutaneous injection of copper.

In children, intramuscular or subcutaneous administration of copper-histidine affords protection against intellectual deterioration but is less effective in preventing other somatic complications. Because disease manifestations are the consequence of impaired activity of the various copper-containing enzymes, copper supplementation would seem to be a rational means of treating the disorder. However, neither oral nor parenteral administration of copper has been effective, even though the latter induces a rapid rise of both ceruloplasmin and copper. Copper replacement therapy employing subcutaneous injections of copper histidinate has been suggested, but due to the considerable clinical heterogeneity, the effectiveness of this therapy has been difficult to evaluate. Studies of affected individuals who share the same copper-responsive mutation treated at different ages suggest that early copper injection treatment may be associated with satisfactory outcomes, as also observed in a broader affected individual group treated neonatally. However, fetal copper injections from the 31st week of uterine life can prove ineffective.

In *mottled/ brindled* mutant mice, stimulation of noradrenergic function via intraperitoneal injection of L-threo-dihydroxyphenylserine, which is converted into norepinephrine by aromatic-L-amino acid decarboxylase, leads to increases in brain norepinephrine and related metabolites but does not prevent neocortical or hippocampal neuronal degeneration. However, neonatal mutant mice receiving complementary therapies via lateral ventricle injections of adenovirus harboring a human ATP7A DNA construct and copper chloride exhibit prolonged survival and preservation of neural structure.

Bibliography

Smpokou P., Samanta M., Berry G.T., et al. (2015). Menkes disease in affected females: The clinical disease spectrum. *Am J Med Genet A*. 167A(2):417–20.

Tümer Z. (2013). An overview and update of ATP7A mutations leading to Menkes disease and occipital horn syndrome. *Hum Mutat*. 34(3):417–29.

Infantile Refsum Disease

An 11-year-old boy was evaluated for severe mental retardation, deafness, and blindness. He was born via cesarean section because his mother had uterus bicornis. He remained healthy until one month of age, when he manifested transient cholestatic icterus, hepatomegaly, and hypoalphaproteinemia. He was irritable and had simian creases and a mild facial dysmorphic appearance. At 1 year of age, he had developed normally but exhibited mild generalized hypertonicity with normal reflexes and flexor plantar responses. By 2 years of age, he manifested nystagmus, pigment clumping throughout the retina, metaphyseal osteoporosis, hypocholesterolemia, and decreased vitamin E levels. By 4 years of age, his development was abnormal and he displayed sensorineural deafness. At 11 years, he was disproportionately underweight. He had a pectus excavatum and a high arched palate. Funduscopic exam revealed retinitis pigmentosa, macular degeneration, optic atrophy, and narrowed vessels. His mental abilities resembled those of a 3-year old child, without language development.

Infantile Refsum Disease

Onset: Retinitis pigmentosa. Abnormally slow infantile intellectual and motor development.
Additional manifestations: Progressive visual impairment and blindness, deafness, and neuropathy. Failure to thrive. Severe mental retardation. Hipocholesterolemia. Leukoencephalopathy.
Disease mechanism: Autosomal recessive defect in peroxysomal biogenesis due to mild decrease in the function of targeting proteins peroxins or their receptors with systemic metabolic consequences.
Testing: Very long chain fatty acids and phytanic are elevated in serum, especially late in the disease course.

Treatment: Dietary intake reduction of phytanic acid and orthotopic hepatic or hepatocyte transplantation.
Research highlights: Pex1-G844D homozygous mice that recapitulate growth retardation and fatty liver with cholestasis.

Clinical Features

Infantile Refsum disease or phytanic acid storage disease is part of the group of disorders known as Zellweger spectrum diseases, which also include Zellweger syndrome and neonatal adrenoleukodystrophy. Infants with Refsum disease exhibit minor dysmorphic features and hypocholesterolemia, onto which retinitis pigmentosa, sensorineural deafness, mental retardation, and failure to thrive supervene. The disease is the mildest of all peroxysomal diseases, with survival into the early teens. Progressive leukoencephalopathy can be prominent. Some affected individuals only manifest a central cerebellar leukodystrophy characterized by rapid regression. Progressive polyneuropathy may be a late but prominent disease feature.

Pathology

Involvement of the peritrigonal white matter, centrum semiovale, thalami, corpus callosum, and corticospinal tracts is detectable by MR imaging and suggests a peroxisomal disorder. The white matter contains a reduced number of myelinated axons in periventricular regions, corpus callosum, pyramidal tracts, and optic nerves. Perivascular spaces may exhibit abundant periodic acid–Schiff (PAS)-negative macrophages. Astrocytes may display lamellar inclusions. In the cerebellum, ectopic Purkinje cells may be found in the molecular layer.

Hepatomegaly with micronodular cirrhosis may be present. Hepatic macrophages are PAS-positive and contain angulate lysosomes. Hepatocytes are filled with spicular structures and may also contain abnormal mitochondria. In one infant, the auditory sensory epithelium and stria vascularis were severely underdeveloped.

Pathophysiology

The mechanism of infantile Refsum disease is discussed in Neonatal Peroxysomal Disorders.

Diagnosis

Very long chain fatty acids and phytanic are elevated in serum, in the context of reduced docosahexaenoic acid, although phytanic acid levels may be normal in early infancy.

Treatment

Dietary intake reduction of phytanic acid, which cannot be synthesized by man and is abundant in dairy products, has occasionally been associated with stabilization or improvement of neuropathy and with the acquisition of new developmental gains. Docosahexaenoic acid supplementation has no effect on growth or visual capacity.

Orthotopic liver and hepatocyte transplantation have led to amelioration of disease manifestations and rectification of serum biochemical parameters. Hypercatabolic states are thought to be associated with excess phytanic acid release from fat stores and this may lead to fulminant tetraparesis or cardiopathy. In such cases, plasmapheresis has been successfully instituted.

Bibliography

Hiebler S., Masuda T., Hacia J.G., et al. (2014). The Pex1-G844D mouse: A model for mild human Zellweger spectrum disorder *Mol Genet Metab.* 111(4): 522–32.

Poll-The B.T., Saudubray J.M., Ogier H.A., et al. (1987). Infantile Refsum disease: An inherited peroxisomal disorder. Comparison with Zellweger syndrome and neonatal adrenoleukodystrophy. *Eur J Pediatr.* 146(5):477–83.

Krabbe Disease

A well-monitored pregnancy culminated with the uneventful birth of a first son at term. At 3 months of age, his grandmother first noticed in him "a certain stiffness, like a tendency to arch his back when he was picked up." By the next month, inconsolable crying was occurring randomly many times during the day and often also at night. When he was 6 months old, the crying became almost permanent, especially when he was minimally disturbed, and the stiffness was now noticeable by just observing him unsuccessfully attempting to move in the crib (if he ever moved). He was never able to sit independently and lost all neck muscle control at about 7 months.

Krabbe Disease

Onset: Truncal rigidity between 3–5 months of age and irritability with loss of the ankle jerk. Optic nerve enlargement by MR imaging.
Additional manifestations: Progressive spasticity and lower motor neuron signs due to neuropathy; rigidity, blindness, and dementia in the infantile form. Treatable seizures. Elevated cerebrospinal fluid protein concentration. Death often ensues before the second birthday.
Disease mechanism: Autosomal recessive loss of function of GALC, encoding galactosylceramidase, with reduced myelin formation and maintenance. Additional features are the accumulation of toxic psychosine (galactosylsphingosine) in the nervous system and autoimmune response.
Testing: White blood cell enzymatic assay and genotyping via DNA sequencing and gene deletion assay. A pathogenic deletion (502T/del) comprising 30 kb of the coding region of GALC) is not uncommon. Mass spectrometric analysis in dried blood cards can be used for newborn screening.

Treatment: Hematopoietic stem cell transplantation in the presymptomatic infant (usually a sibling) or in the older, minimally symptomatic affected individual.
Research highlights: Development of gene, enzyme replacement, neural stem cell transplantation, substrate reduction, and chemical chaperone therapies and mechanisms of myelin breakdown using the *twitcher* mouse model.

Clinical Features

Krabbe disease (globoid cell leukodystrophy, which due to galactosylceramidase deficiency or, more rarely, to prosaposin deficiency) is often diagnosed in persons of Northern European (Swedish) ancestry at an incidence of 1 in 250,000 persons. Eighty-five percent of cases manifest the infantile form of the disease. Infants with Krabbe disease usually first present near the fifth month of life. This infantile form is rather stereotypic, in contrast with other variable presentations that occur at any stage of the lifespan and which also follow a heterogeneous (sometimes nonfatal) course. The manifestations of infantile Krabbe disease gradually evolve from subtle to very severe neurological dysfunction to, ultimately, a widespread lack of neural function by the end of the second year of life. Krabbe disease affects all myelinated structures (brain, spinal cord and nerve, including the optic nerve) and, as is common for some myelin disorders, an inflammatory reaction supervenes onto the primary dysmyelinating process. There are no extraneural manifestations. The disease usually evolves in four stages: a first stage including poor feeding, shoulder girdle hypotonia, gastroesophageal reflux and intermittent clasping of the thumbs; a second stage in which irritability, limb spasticity, extensor spasms, severe feeding difficulties and truncal weakness are prominent; a third phase with areflexia, treatable epilepsy, oculomotor dysfunction, and poor pupillary responses; and a fourth phase with dysautonomic features, unresponsiveness to stimuli and flaccidity. In contrast, late-onset Krabbe disease can include visual impairment, neuropathy with paresthesia or dysesthesia, intention tremor, spastic hemiparesis and cerebellar ataxia.

Pathology

Krabbe disease is predominantly a myelin (involving white matter and nerve) disease. The first sign of disease can be neuropathy, which becomes manifest as a loss of tendon reflexes. More commonly, however, abnormalities of infant arousal and posture indicating encephalopathy are first noted. The cerebral cortex is preserved or moderately atrophic (Figure 45.1). In contrast, the white matter of cerebrum, cerebellum, and anterior columns of the spinal cord is thin, grey-white, and of rubbery consistency. An early feature can be optic nerve enlargement. Foci of white matter necrosis and calcification may also be seen. Occasionally, the myelin of the cerebral hemispheres degenerates in a tigroid radial or linear pattern extending from the ventricular cavities to the cortex. U-fibers of the white matter tend to be preserved. Nerves are white, enlarged and stiff early in the disease course.

Microscopically, oligodendrocyte loss occurs early and prominently in the disease, leading to fibrillary astrocytosis. This phenomenon has implications for therapies that require oligodendrocyte integrity, such as intravenous enzyme infusions, a likely cause of treatment ineffectiveness. Globoid cells are visible in the white matter of the brain and spinal cord and appear in the fetus as early as 20 weeks' gestation. These phagocytic multinucleated cells are epithelioid in nature and tend to infiltrate areas of active demyelination, often clustering around blood vessels. Globoid cells contain galactoceramidase accumulation in polygonal or tubular intracellular structures. There is also abundant macrophagic infiltration in demyelination areas, which disappears in chronic forms of the disease.

Pathophysiology

Galactosylceramide, a byproduct of lysosomal sulfatide degradation, is normally degraded by galactosylceramidase (Figures 45.2 and 45.3). Galactosylceramidase is a glycoprotein generated by intralysosomal protease cleavage of a precursor molecule into two subunits. About 50 percent of cases harbor a large 30-kb gene deletion that eliminates one subunit and truncates the other. The pathophysiology of Krabbe disease includes

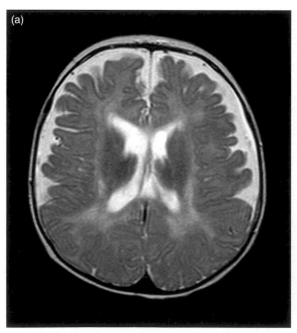
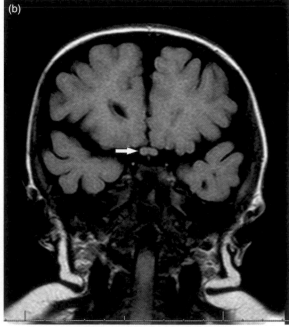

Figure 45.1 a and b: Magnetic resonance images of Krabbe disease in a 6-month-old boy. a. There is confluent, striated increased signal in the white matter, especially over the parietal and occipital lobes. b. The prechiasmatic optic nerves are enlarged.

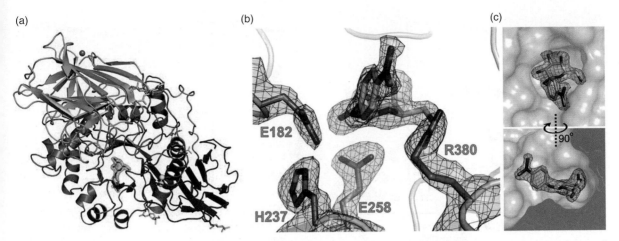

(a)   (b)   (c)

Figure 45.2 Structure of the wild-type galactosylceramidase GALC enzyme in complex with substrate. a. Ribbon diagram showing the overall structure of GALC with the substrate 4NßDG bound in the active site. The electron density (blue) is shown for uncleaved substrate bound in the active site pocket of GALC. Surface glycans (pink sticks) are shown. b. Detail of the GALC active site with bound, uncleaved substrate showing active site residues (sticks) and electron density (as above). c. Surface representation of the GALC active site (gray) with the substrate and electron density shown (as above). Reproduced with permission from Hill CH et al. Structural snapshots illustrate the catalytic cycle of β-galactocerebrosidase, the defective enzyme in Krabbe disease. *Proc Natl Acad Sci U S A.* 2013; 110(51):20479–84.

two paradoxes. First, there is no uniform correlation between clinical severity (i.e., infantile or late onset forms of the disease) and the residual level of enzymatic activity measured *in vitro*. Second, despite a loss of function of galactosylceramidase, there is no excessive accumulation of galactosylceramide, its natural substrate, in the brain. This is due to very early loss of oligodendrocytes, which are the galactosylceramidase containing cells. Because of this selective oligodendrocyte death, myelination in the infantile form of the disease does not progress beyond early stages. Globoid cells, however, contain galactosylceramidase. In contrast, galactosylsphingosine (psychosine), a metabolite produced during normal myelination, accumulates significantly and is responsible for an array of secondary neurochemical abnormalities. In normal circumstances, psychosine is barely detectable. In fact, psychosine can induce the transformation of microglia into the characteristic Krabbe multinucleated globoid cells. Cytokinesis (the separation of cytoplasm following mitosis) is not completed in these cells, whereas nuclear division proceeds. The signals inhibiting cytokinesis in these cells are transmitted through the orphan G-protein coupled receptor TDAG8 (T-cell associated gene 8), acting through an increase of cAMP. Psychosine and some structurally related lysosphingolipids such as glucosylsphingosine or sphingosylphosphorylcholine are ligands for this receptor. The affinity constant (Km) of psychosine for the

TDAG8 receptor is around 3 μM, a concentration not reached under physiologic conditions. In Krabbe disease, however, psychosine accumulates to high micromolar concentration allowing activation of the TDAG8 receptor Psychosine can also inhibit protein kinase C translocation to the plasma membrane, and cytochrome c oxidase and induce the apoptosis of oligodendrocytes and nerve Schwann cells. Insulin like growth factor I (IGF-1) inhibits oligodendrocyte precursor apoptosis and promotes oligodendrocyte development. In oligodendrocytes IGF-1 acts through the activation of the antiapoptotic PI3K (phosphatidylinositide 3-kinase)-Akt (Protein kinase B)/PKB or the MAPK (mitogen-activated protein kinase)/Erk (extracellular signal-regulated protein kinase) 1–2 signal transduction pathways. In murine oligodendrocyte precursor cells psychosine causes a decrease in both Akt und ERK1–2 phosphorylation accompanied by an activation of caspase 3, resulting in apoptosis. Another target of psychosine is phospholipase A2, which cleaves the membrane lipid phosphatidylcholine into lysophosphatidylcholine and arachidonic acid, which causes generation of reactive oxygen species and free radicals. AMP activated protein kinase (AMPK) regulates of glucose and lipid metabolism. Psychosine downregulates AMPK activity which leads to a preponderance of biosynthetic pathways. Oligodendrocytes treated with psychosine display enhanced synthesis of fatty acids and cholesterol, while catabolic

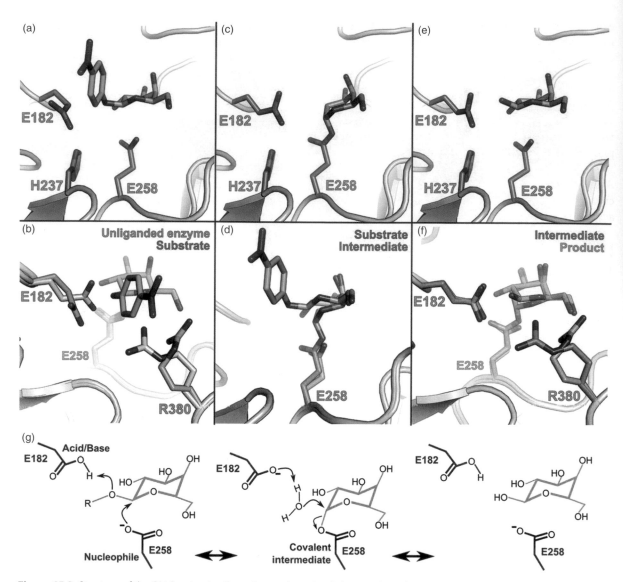

Figure 45.3 Structures of the GALC active site illustrating conformational changes along the reaction coordinate. **a.** Wild-type enzyme in complex with substrate 4NßDG (green). **b.** Overlay of the GALC active site residues in the absence (gray) and presence (green) of substrate. **c.** Covalent intermediate structure illustrating D-galactal (orange) covalently attached to the catalytic nucleophile. **d.** Movement of E258 and the pyranose ring between substrate binding (green) and covalent linkage with the inhibitor D-galactal (orange). **e.** Enzyme–product complex formed following extended incubation with substrate illustrating catalytic activity of GALC *in crystallo*. **f.** The two different conformations of the R380 side chain in the covalent intermediate (orange) and product (pink) complexes. **g.** Schematic representation of the proposed retaining two-step glycosidic bond hydrolysis reaction. Reproduced with permission from Hill CH et al. Structural snapshots illustrate the catalytic cycle of β-galactocerebrosidase, the defective enzyme in Krabbe disease. *Proc Natl Acad Sci U S A.* 2013; 110(51):20479–84.

β-oxidation is inhibited. Thus, the inhibition of AMPK by psychosine favors energy consuming over energy generating pathways. The resulting lower energy could also contribute to oligodendrocyte loss. In addition to direct toxicity, psychosine can stimulate the production of toxic nitric oxide induced by cytokines.

Krabbe disease is not exclusively a myelin disease, however, as neuronal cell bodies, axons, and the neuromuscular junction can be affected. Neurons and microglia often contain inclusions rich in ubiquitin and α-synuclein, as in Parkinson's disease.

An early feature of Krabbe disease is axonopathy before significant demyelination takes place. Axons exhibit impairment of fast transport and are lost early in the disease course. Psychosine induces lipid raft clustering and consequent defective recruitment of signaling molecules, leading to the impairment of axonal transport. Contributing to this phenomenon, psychosine activates axonal PP1 (protein phosphatase 1) and GSK3β (glycogen synthase kinase 3 beta), which accumulates in the axon together with phosphorylated kinesin light chains.

In the neuromuscular junction, inactivation of the Akt pathway and activation of the proteasome coincide with synaptic transmission failure. There is also accumulation of psychosine in muscle.

Diagnosis

The cerebrospinal fluid protein concentration is elevated. Brain MR imaging can illustrate leukodystrophy and myelopathy (of the anterior columns) early in the disease course, sometimes with optic nerve enlargement. Enzyme activity in leukocytes, amniotic fluid or chorionic villus cells is often below 5 percent of normal. Newborn screening using tandem mass spectroscopy of Guthrie blood cards is available. Genetic testing of the gene encoding galactosylcerebrosidase GALC is often performed. Except for c.G857A (encoding Gly270Asp), which is associated with late-onset Krabbe disease, most point mutations are family-specific. Alternatively, a minority of affected individuals are thought to harbor a prosaposin (PSAP) mutation.

Treatment

Among several natural animal forms of galactosylceramidase deficiency, the *twitcher* mouse model, a therapeutic testbed for late infantile Krabbe disease, has allowed some insights into the disorder. Additional animals with galactosylceramidase suitable for therapeutic development are dogs and monkeys. However, despite significant efforts, treatment for Krabbe disease remains unsatisfactory. This may be compounded by the fact that the cellular pathology of Krabbe disease is multifocal. Hematopoietic stem cell transplantation aims to supply normal macrophages expressing the deficient enzyme that can penetrate the central nervous system, supplying galactosylcerebrosidase to the myelinating tissue. Other therapies have included substrate reduction, chaperone drug administration (aimed to stabilize residual galactosylceramidase), and cytokines. However, the impact of these treatments has been modest in terms of interrupting neurological deterioration in animals. Gene therapy using viral vector injection into blood or brain has also met with limited success. In some cases, the disease appears to progress suddenly and rapidly in the treated *twitcher* mouse after a prolonged period of neurological recovery due to unknown factors. Enzyme replacement therapy has also been investigated, despite concerns that oligodendrocyte and Schwann cell loss is an early feature of the disease.

Bibliography

Graziano A.C., Cardile V. (2015). History, genetic, and recent advances on Krabbe disease. *Gene.* 555(1):2–13.

Li Y., Sands M.S. (2014). Experimental therapies in the murine model of globoid cell leukodystrophy. *Pediatr Neurol.* 51(5):600–6.

Infantile Ascending Hereditary Spastic Paraplegia

Chapter

46

A girl, the product of a consanguineous union, was evaluated for severe motor disability. A brother was normal. Abnormal motor development was observed during the girl's first year of life. She sat up at the age of 12 months, was able to stand up at 18 months and walked with support at 3 years. At 7 years old, she could walk short distances with a walker, but spasticity in lower limbs was present. Subsequently, an ascending progression of motor difficulties was observed: she was wheelchair bound at 12 years, when upper limb weakness started and needed computer assistance to write at 16 years old, when her voice became weaker. Now 22 years old, she needs a talker for oral communication and has no swallowing difficulties. In contrast, cognitive functions are preserved and she works with computer aids in a sheltered workshop.

Motor development impairment and disease progression were even more severe in her younger affected sister: she walked with support at 6 years, was wheelchair bound with hand use difficulties at 10 years and needed a talker at 12 years. Now 20 years old, swallowing difficulties are present. She also works with computer aids in a sheltered workshop.

Infantile Ascending Hereditary Spastic Paraplegia

Onset: Insidiously progressive weakness and spasticity in the lower limbs at 12–24 months of age.
Additional manifestations: The disorder is allelic with juvenile primary lateral sclerosis and juvenile amyotrophic lateral sclerosis. Progression of spasticity and paresis reaching the bulbar musculature and gaze palsy.
Disease mechanism: Perturbation of endosomal dynamics. Alsin, the defective protein, binds to small GTPase RAB5 and functions as a guanine nucleotide exchange factor for RAB5.

Testing: None specific other than genotyping.
Treatment: None effective.
Research highlights: Alsin-depleted murine spinal motor neurons can be rescued from defective survival and axon growth by co-cultured astrocytes via an unidentified soluble protective factor.

Clinical Features

Infantile ascending hereditary spastic paraplegia is characterized by childhood-onset pure spastic paraparesis followed by rapid ascent of paresis to the upper limb and oropharyngeal muscles. It is associated with autosomal recessive loss of function mutations in ALS2, a gene that encodes alsin, a member of the guanine nucleotide exchange factors for the small GTPase RAB5. Infantile ascending hereditary spastic paraplegia is allelic with juvenile primary and amyotrophic lateral sclerosis.

The disease manifests in infancy and progresses within the first decade of life, ultimately leading to severe tetraparesis and bulbar syndrome in the second decade, in the context of preserved mental function. Affected individuals are usually confined to a wheelchair by the age of 17 years. In contrast, in ALS2-related juvenile primary lateral sclerosis, all the affected individuals manifest impaired ocular motility ranging from slow voluntary eye movements to gaze paresis, which is thought to be associated with involvement of the upper motor neurons in the frontal cortex (area 8) that control ocular motility. The principal clinical differences between juvenile primary lateral sclerosis and infantile ascending hereditary spastic paraplegia are earlier motor impairment and a more rapid course with possible scoliosis in infantile ascending hereditary spastic paraplegia, and the presence of oculomotor dysfunction in juvenile primary lateral sclerosis.

178

Pathology

MR imaging demonstrates hyperintensities in posterior periventricular areas. Additional imaging features include brain cortical atrophy predominant in the motor areas, mild cerebellar atrophy, and bilateral hyperintense signal in the posterior arm of the internal capsule and brainstem.

Pathophysiology

Alsin binds to small GTPase RAB5 and functions as a guanine nucleotide exchange factor for RAB5. The C terminus of alsin carries a domain that mediates the activation of RAB5 via a guanine-nucleotide exchanging reaction and the endosomal localization of ALS2. The N-terminal region containing another specialized domain that acts suppressive in its membrane localization. The middle alsin domain enhances C-terminal domain-mediated endosome fusion. Thus, a perturbation of endosomal dynamics caused by loss of the alsin functional domain that confers RAB5 guanine exchange factor activity might underlie neuronal dysfunction and degeneration.

A long isoform of ALS2 binds to mutant superoxide dismutase 1 (SOD1) and protects motor neurons from toxicity induced by mutant SOD1. In contrast, a short isoform of alsin and truncating pathogenic ALS2 mutations do not protect neurons from mutant SOD1 toxicity.

Diagnosis

There is no specific diagnostic method other than genetic analysis.

Treatment

There is no effective therapy.

Bibliography

Eymard-Pierre E., Yamanaka K., Haeussler M., et al. (2006). Novel missense mutation in ALS2 gene results in infantile ascending hereditary spastic paralysis. *Ann Neurol.* 59(6):976–80.

Racis L., Tessa A., Pugliatti M., et al. (2014). Infantile-onset ascending hereditary spastic paralysis: A case report and brief literature review. *Eur J Paediatr Neurol.* 18(2):235–9.

Metachromatic Leukodystrophy and Multiple Sulfatase Deficiency

A 2-year-old girl presented with walking difficulties. Developmental milestones were attained normally until the age of 9 months. At 10 months, however, she could not rise without help. At 11 months, she could stand up and take a few steps with help. Independent walking was acquired at 17 months. Speech emerged normally and social skill development was age-appropriate. From the age of 20 months, the parents noticed regression of previously acquired skills, as she developed spastic gait, dysarthria, and became progressively irritable. Exam at 31 months of age revealed dysarthria, slow swallow reflex, mild spasticity predominating distally in the lower extremities, normal muscle power, hyporeflexia, and extensor plantar responses. Gait analysis showed truncal hypotonia with excessive lateral trunk-swing and ataxia with an enlarged base. By 4 years of age she developed slowly progressive visual loss leading to blindness, feeding difficulties, and language regression. Spasticity increased further. Arylsulfatase A leukocyte activity was normal on two occasions. However, the study of glycolipids in the urine sediment revealed massive excretion of sulfatides, dihexosylceramide sulfates, and globotriaosylceramides. This suggested metachromatic leukodystrophy due to deficiency of cerebroside sulfatase activator (saposin-B deficiency). The diagnosis was confirmed by identification of two mutations in the PSAP gene, Asn215Lys, of paternal origin, and Met1Val, of maternal origin.

neuropathy and dementia in the common late infantile form. Treatable seizures. Death often ensues before the second decade. Multiple sulfatase deficiency, a related disorder, is also associated with features of mucopolysaccaridosis.

Disease mechanism: Autosomal recessive loss of function of ARSA, encoding arylsulfatase A, which results in widespread metachromatic sulfatide deposition with demyelination. Autophagosomes are increased and exhibit defective fusion with lysosomes. Multiple sulfatase deficiency is due to mutation of SUMF1, which impairs the modification of a critical active site cysteine present in all sulfatases.

Testing: White blood cell enzymatic assay and genotyping by DNA sequencing. A null exon 2 splice site mutation in ARSA is common. The late infantile form exhibits no enzymatic activity, whereas other disease forms are associated with minimal residual arylsulfatase A activity.

Treatment: Hematopoietic stem cell transplantation in the minimally symptomatic child to preserve intellectual capacity.

Research highlights: Gene, enzyme replacement and neural stem cell transplantation and mechanisms of demyelination by lysosulfatide using mice.

Clinical Features

Metachromatic leukodystrophy is a lysosomal sulfatide storage disorder of central and peripheral myelin that affects 1 in 40,000 to 1 in 160,000 individuals depending on ethnicity, with an overrepresentation among consanguineous populations. In metachromatic leukodystrophy, autosomal recessive mutations in the gene ARSA, encoding arylsulfatase A, lead to accumulation of sulfatide in multiple (but not all) tissues and to its urinary excretion. Notably, 1 to 2% of all persons are deficient in arylsulfatase A activity

Metachromatic Leukodystrophy

Onset: Motor dysfunction with spasticity in the second year of life. White matter signal abnormality in MR imaging.

Additional manifestations: Combination of spasticity and lower motor neuron signs due to and excrete small amounts of sulfatide without clinical consequence, a condition termed pseudodeficiency. Three major subtypes of the disease have been described: Late infantile (50% of cases), juvenile (30 percent), and adult (20 percent). The late infantile form presents between 1 and 2 years of age with gait abnormalities due to spasticity progressing to a widespread motor and intellectual disorder. More rarely, a seizure can be the first significant indication of the disease. Dysarthria, dementia, rigidity, visual and auditory impairment, and epilepsy may ensue. Many late infantile affected individuals do not learn to speak in complete sentences. Loss of expressive language is typical before 3 years of age. In juvenile affected individuals, language regression is more insidious and impaired concentration and behavior are followed by impairment of reading, writing, and calculating about four years after disease onset. The end stage of the disease comprises tonic spasms, decerebrate posture and unresponsiveness. Death often occurs before the age of 5 years. Juvenile metachromatic leukodystrophy occurs between 4 and 12 years and is more insidious. Dysarthria and intellectual and behavioral dysfunction can precede or become more prominent than motor manifestations, while seizures are uncommon. Incontinence may be present. The end stage of the disease is ultimately similar to the late infantile form. Adult metachromatic leukodystrophy occurs at any mature age, with a predilection for the fourth and fifth decades. Neuropathy or behavioral dysfunction can be the initial complaints. Progression is more variable and leads to a similar end stage as the other two forms.

Multiple sulfatide deficiency is far rarer and is due to impaired sulfatide metabolism as a result of SUMF1 (sulfatide modifying factor 1) mutation, which catalyzes the posttranslational modification of several sulfatases. The disease combines features of late infantile metachromatic leukodystrophy with mild features of mucopolisaccharidosis. The latter can appear late in the course of the disease and include ichthyosis, coarse facial features, joint stiffness, and skeletal abnormalities. Hepatosplenomegaly can be an associated manifestation.

Pathology

In addition to the brain, sulfatides accumulate in metachromatic leukodystrophy in quantities detectable by pathological staining in kidney, macrophages, sweat gland epithelial cells, hepatic Kupffer cells and bile duct epithelium, adrenal medullar and pancreatic Langerhans islets. Gallbladder polyps have been reported. The brain is the most affected organ, exhibiting metachromatic granule accumulation. These granules contain sulfatides (galactolipids), cholesterol, and phosphatides. This leads to demyelination with reactive astrocytosis, conferring the white matter a firm and grey appearance. Oligodendrocytes are early targets of the disease and are severely affected. However, volume loss of the grey matter is also an early disease feature. Nerves are also segmentally demyelinated and exhibit axonal loss. Schwann cells and endoneurial macrophages contain metachromatic granules.

In multiple sulfatase deficiency, metachromatic material accumulates together with mucopolysaccharides, leading to leukodystrophy with hydrocephalus and meningeal fibrosis (Figure 47.1). Periventricular dilatation and hydrocephalus, commonly found in mucopolysaccharidosis, may ensue.

Pathophysiology

Lysosomal sulfatide accumulation constitutes the central biochemical defect of all forms of metachromatic leukodystrophy. Despite widespread sulfatide deposition in many tissues, the white matter bears most of the disease impact, reacting with degenerative changes. In addition, accumulation of sulfogalactosylsphingosine (lysosulfatide) is toxic to myelin cells. There is no correlation between the residual level of arylsulfatase in leukocytes and the age of onset. However, a correlation exists when sulfatide degradation assays are performed in cultured skin fibroblasts. Late-infantile cases are associated with null alleles and no detectable enzyme activity. The most common mutation in ARSA involves a splice in exon 2, leading to a severely truncated protein (Figure 47.2). Milder forms of the disease can be associated with missense mutations that lead to misfolding and trapping of arylsulfatase A in the endoplasmic reticulum.

SUMF1 mediates the transformation of an active site cysteine common to all sulfatases into formylglycine. Mice lacking SUMF1 display a generalized inflammatory reaction with activation of microglia and early mortality. An important feature of affected cells is the presence of excess autophagosomes which

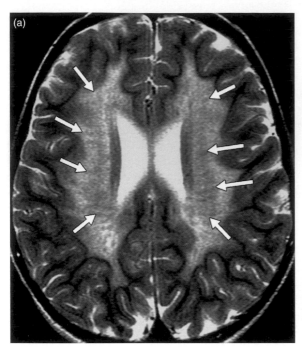
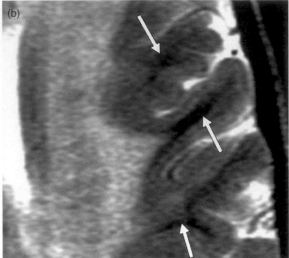

Figure 47.1 a. Four-year-old boy with metachromatic leukodystrophy who presented with gradual onset of visual and gait disorder. Axial T2-weighted MR imaging shows T2 hyperintensity within periventricular white matter of bilateral frontal and parietal lobes. There is sparing of subcortical white matter. White matter hyperintensity within corona radiata confers a tigroid appearance (arrows) due to relative sparing of perivascular white matter. b. Same image as in a magnified to show preserved subcortical white matter (arrows). Reproduced with permission from Ibrahim M et al. Inborn errors of metabolism: combining clinical and radiologic clues to solve the mystery. *AJR Am J Roentgenol.* 2014; 203(3):W315–27.

may not fuse correctly with lysosomes during normal the cell degradative cycle.

Diagnosis

Metachromatic leukodystrophy is often initially confirmed via MR imaging, which is abnormal even in presymptomatic individuals. Early, the white matter signal appears hyperintense in T2 in a tigroid pattern, particularly in the frontal, parietal, and central regions of the brain and occasionally in the corticospinal tract. This can be confused with delayed myelination. Subcortical U-fibers are spared until late in the disease course. Thalamic hypointensity has also been documented. Alternatively, diffuse brain atrophy can be the first radiological finding. Urinary sulfatide excretion is elevated in most cases and arylsulfatase A enzymatic activity absent or very diminished in white blood cells. Urine and nerve sulfatide concentration correlates with neuropathy severity. Newborn screening base on the detection of sulfatides in dried blood and urine samples by mass spectrometry is feasible.

Treatment

Hematopoietic stem cell transplantation or bone marrow transplantation has been used to treat metachromatic leukodystrophy. However, affected individuals with motor dysfunction at the time of transplantation do not benefit from this intervention. Thus, minimally symptomatic affected individuals benefit the most, with preservation of intellectual abilities in the context of a stable or deteriorating motor capacity. In these affected individuals, there is evidence of cerebral myelin recovery. Enzyme replacement via intravenous infusion is limited by reduced penetration into the central nervous system such that other more direct routes may be preferable. Lentivirus or adenovirus vehicles have been used experimentally to insert the correct gene in the nervous system. An alternative approach uses the anti-inflammatory drug simvastatin. These studies are underway.

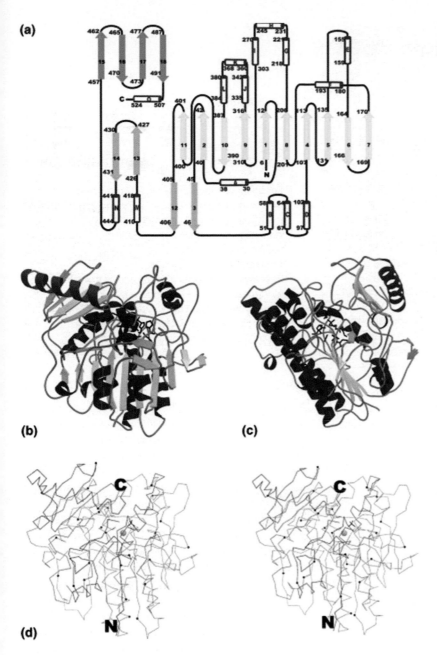

Figure 47.2 The overall fold of *Pseudomonas aeruginosa* arylsulfatase (PAS). (a) A topology diagram of the PAS structure. β strands are represented by arrows, and α helices are represented by cylinders. The first and last residue number in each secondary structural element is given. (b) A ribbon representation of the PAS structure highlighting the secondary structural elements and the calcium cation (yellow sphere) and sulfate and relevant side chains in the residues constituting the area of the active site (blue). (c) A view of the molecule rotated 90° from the view in (b). (d) A stereo view of a Ca trace of the molecule, with the color ramped from blue to red; every 20th Ca atom is marked. Reproduced with permission from Boltes I et al. 1.3 Å structure of arylsulfatase from Pseudomonas aeruginosa establishes the catalytic mechanism of sulfate ester cleavage in the sulfatase family. *Structure*. 2001; 9(6):483–91.

Bibliography

Deconinck N., Messaaoui A., Ziereisen F., et al. (2008). Metachromatic leukodystrophy without arylsulfatase A deficiency: A new case of saposin-B deficiency. *Eur J Paediatr Neurol.* Jan;12(1):46–50.

van Rappard D.F., Boelens J.J., Wolf N.I. (2015). Metachromatic leukodystrophy: Disease spectrum and approaches for treatment. *Best Pract Res Clin Endocrinol Metab.* 29(2):261–73.

Alexander Disease

An 8-year-old boy was evaluated for choking, clumsiness, and reduced IQ. He always had difficulties with dexterity, first noted at 3 years of age, but these had worsened insidiously for the past 2 years. He also had always run awkwardly such that he could not keep up with his peers. While eating a nut, he choked and had to be assisted. When he was in a recumbent position he tended to regurgitate foods that he had consumed several hours before. Swallowing became so difficult that each meal lasted 1 hour. He was previously evaluated for poor school performance and his full IQ was 72. Six months later, at 9 years of age, his speech had become unintelligible and he manifested frequent nausea. He had been falling often when ambulating. He always remained largely silent, with no spontaneous speech. Examination revealed pale optic disks and prominent glabellar and jaw reflexes. He displayed shortening of the Achilles tendons and spontaneous Babinski signs. Tendon reflexes were abnormally brisk. His muscle tone was generally increased.

Alexander Disease

Onset: Megalencephaly with aqueductal stenosis and leukodystrophy with anterior frontal and temporal lobe predilection before the second year of life. Deep white matter signal abnormality in MR images.
Additional manifestations: Combination of quadriparesis and cerebellar dysfunction and later dementia in the more common infantile form. Seizures can be prominent. Some cases have been confused with a posterior fossa tumor after biopsy.
Disease mechanism: Autosomal dominant gain of function of GFAP, encoding astrocytic glial fibrillary acid protein, which results in Rosenthal fiber inclusions with demyelination.

Testing: Genotyping by DNA sequencing and biopsy in tumor-like cases. Arg79 and Arg239 GFAP mutations are most common, with Arg239-harboring individuals following a more rapid course of deterioration
Treatment: None effective.
Research highlights: Diminished astrocytic glutamate reuptake, offering a potential therapeutic avenue using ceftriaxone analogs. Enhancement of α–B-crystallin expression as a means to disassemble GFAP aggregates.

Clinical Features

Alexander disease is a dominant demyelinating disorder that arises primarily from astrocyte dysfunction. The three predominant forms of the disorder are infantile, juvenile, and adult, which account for 25, 25, and 50 percent of cases, respectively. The infantile form presents before 2 years of age. Megalencephaly and epilepsy can be prominent, in conjunction with hydrocephalus due to aqueductal stenosis. Late stages progress to quadriparesis. The juvenile form manifests early bulbar (dysarthria, dysphagia, dysphonia) and cerebellar dysfunction and only later cognitive impairment. The adult form is associated with ataxia, quadriparesis, oculomotor dysfunction, palatal myoclonus, and late cognitive dysfunction. An alternative presentation is a posterior fossa mass that can be confused with a pilocytic astrocytoma even after biopsy. Familial cases of the disease can manifest significant variability.

Pathology

The hallmarks of the disease are focal or diffuse demyelination and Rosenthal fibers, which are astrocytic inclusions containing intermediate filaments composed of GFAP conjugated with abnormally phosphorylated and partially ubiquitinated α–B-crystallin.

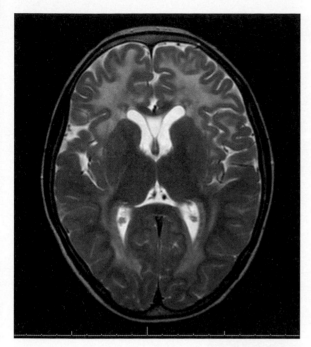

Figure 48.1 T2-weigthed MR imaging in a 9-year-old boy with Alexander disease. There is anterior predominance of white matter abnormal signal. The subcortical white matter is preserved in the temporal lobes. There is a thin corpus callosum anteriorly and mild frontal cortical atrophy.

The cerebral white matter appears yellow, granular, or cavitated, usually involving the anterior parts of the frontal and temporal lobes (Figures 48.1–48.3). The grey matter is generally normal. Rosenthal fibers are located in cell bodies and are most abundant in subependymal, subpial, and perivascular regions, with a predilection for cerebral white matter, thalamus, and striatum. Occasionally, astrocytes containing hyaline granules display nuclear atypia and mitosis, suggestive of neoplasia. Neurons usually appear preserved. Microglial activation and T cell infiltrates can also be detected.

Pathophysiology

Alexander disease results from heterozygous mutations in GFAP. The mutations are usually gain of function and involve the conserved rod domain of GFAP, resulting in overexpression (Figure 48.4). Neurons and glia contain insoluble, ubiquitinated, and pathologically phosphorylated TAR (transactive response) DNA binding protein of 43 kDa (TDP-43). Whereas mice can be used to model the disease, loss of function mutations induced in mice do not lead to disease. Glial-derived nitric oxide is a

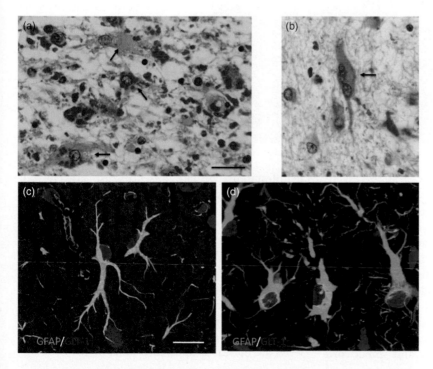

Figure 48.2 Astrocytes in Alexander disease. a,b: Enlarged, mis-shapen astrocytes in hemispheric white matter (arrows), some of which contain Rosenthal fibers (eosinophilic inclusions) in cell bodies. Other Rosenthal fibers lie in astrocyte processes. Multinucleated astrocytes are common (B). Scale bar = 20 microns. c,d: Astrocytes in the hippocampal CA1 stratum moleculare in wild type (c) and knock-in (R236H) (d) mice. Immunofluorescence for GFAP (green) and GLT-1 (red) shows enlarged, irregular astrocytes in the knock-in and an appreciable loss of GLT-1. Scale bar = 20 microns. Reproduced with permission from Messing A et al. Alexander disease. *J Neurosci.* 2012; 32(15):5017–23.

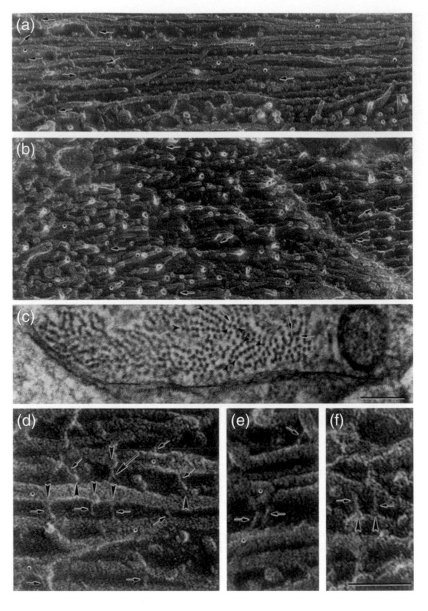

Figure 48.3 High magnification of deep-etched (a, b, d–f) and freeze-substituted (c) astrocytic processes in CA1 region in Alexander disease. They are longitudinally fractured (a, d–f), obliquely fractured (b), and cross-sectioned (c). The intermediate filaments (IFs) run parallel to each other, and they often have lateral adhesion to the neighboring ones (asterisks). This lateral assembly is clearly observed in c (between arrowheads). The laterally assembled IFs are often interconnected with filamentous cross-bridges (short arrows). The cross-bridges are uniform in structure. They are typically straight, but sometimes branched (long arrow in d). The cross-linkers often have foot-like structures, expansion at the contact with the IFs (arrowheads). (a–c) Bar, 100 nm. (d–f) Bar, 50 nm. Reproduced with permission from Miyaguchi K. Ultrastructure of intermediate filaments of nestin- and vimentin-immunoreactive astrocytes in organotypic slice cultures of hippocampus. *J Struct Biol.* 1997; 120 (1):61–8.

signaling molecule that is produced in excess in Alexander disease, triggering astrocyte-mediated neuronal degeneration. Glial cells themselves also degenerate via the cellular DNA damage response and p53. The cellular stress caused by the accumulation of GFAP may also lead to the production of inflammatory molecules and to microglial activation, as found in a mouse model of the disease. Astrocytes also show diminished glutamate transporter currents and are depolarized and not coupled to adjacent astrocytes. Mechanisms potentially responsible for the posterior fossa and spinal cord manifestations of late onset disease also include dysregulated extracellular glutamate concentration and abnormal potassium uptake via potassium channels.

Diagnosis

MR imaging illustrates leukodystrophy of anterior brain regions in infantile cases. Atrophy and signal changes of the medulla, middle cerebellar peduncle, and spinal cord are typical of late onset disease. GFAP levels are increased in cerebrospinal fluid.

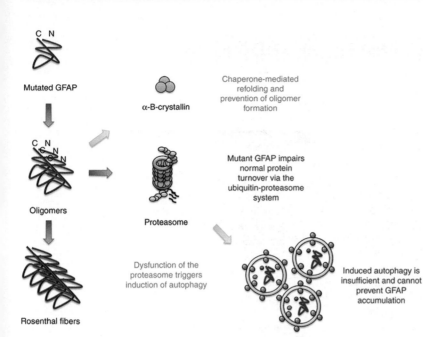

C N
Mutated GFAP

α-B-crystallin

Chaperone-mediated refolding and prevention of oligomer formation

C N
C N
C N
Oligomers

Proteasome

Mutant GFAP impairs normal protein turnover via the ubiquitin-proteasome system

Dysfunction of the proteasome triggers induction of autophagy

Induced autophagy is insufficient and cannot prevent GFAP accumulation

Rosenthal fibers

Figure 48.4 Pathological cascade of events in Alexander disease with a focus on altered protein metabolism. Accumulation of mutant glial fibrillary acidic protein (GFAP) oligomers may overwhelm the capacity of the chaperone network and proteasomal degradation with accumulating protein burden leading to further impairment of these pathways, therefore eventually creating a vicious cycle. Autophagy is induced as a compensatory action but is not sufficient to preserve protein homeostasis, which may promote cellular dysfunction and degeneration. Pathological changes in protein degradation pathways are highlighted in red, whereas compensatory changes are marked in green. Reproduced with permission from Ebrahimi-Fakhari D et al. Emerging role of autophagy in pediatric neurodegenerative and neurometabolic diseases. *Pediatr Res.* 2014; 75 (1–2):217–26.

Treatment

There is no specific treatment available for Alexander disease. Experimental treatments have included autophagy-inducing lithium. Similarly, rapamycin and its analogues can increase autophagy through inhibition of the mammalian target of rapamycin (mTOR) and have been proposed as potential treatments. Increasing expression of α-B-crystallin promotes disassembly of preformed GFAP filaments, shifting the equilibrium to smaller forms and potentially mitigating the effects of mutant GFAP on the proteasome.

Bibliography

Quinlan R.A., Brenner M., Goldman J.E., et al. (2007). GFAP and its role in Alexander disease. *Exp Cell Res.* 313(10):2077–87.

Sawaishi Y. (2009). Review of Alexander disease: Beyond the classical concept of leukodystrophy. *Brain Dev.* 31(7):493–8.

Pelizaeus-Merzbacher Disease

A girl presented during the second month of life with horizontal nystagmus and severe hypotonia. At 9 months of age, she exhibited persistently poor motor milestone development associated with ataxia of the head and trunk. Her motor abilities then improved (holding her head up at 12 months, sitting with support at 16 months and standing at 30 months), with normal psychosocial interactions and decreased nystagmus. A head MR imaging study was performed (Figure 49.1). In addition, brainstem auditory evoked potentials showed a single cochlear wave I without any subsequent recordable brain waves, suggesting a severe impairment in central conduction. At age 4 years, she continued to improve (crawling, walking with support, feeding herself, drawing a line, speaking in simple sentences). However, signs of pyramidal tract dysfunction were present in the lower limbs. The result of a repeat MR imaging study was unchanged.

Pelizaeus-Merzbacher Disease

Onset: Perinatal nystagmus.
Additional manifestations: Hypotonia and progressive spastic paraparesis with movement disorder (often including athetosis) in the first year of life. The peripheral nerves are preserved. Deep white matter signal abnormality in MR imaging studies.
Disease mechanism: X-linked recessive loss of function of oligodendrocyte-produced PLP, encoding proteolipid protein, which results in very limited myelination throughout the cerebrum. A small number of cases, who exhibit Pelizaeus-Merzbacher disease-like phenotype, is thought to be due to recessive mutations in GJC2 (gap junction protein gamma-2), which normally encodes connexin 47, another protein associated with myelin.

Testing: Genotyping of PLP1 or GJC2.
Treatment: None effective.
Research highlights: Neural precursor cell administration and dietary cholesterol to enhance trafficking of PLP.

Clinical Features

Pelizaeus-Merzbacher disease or sudanophilic leukodystrophy is an X-linked disorder of central nervous system myelin caused by mutation of the major myelin constituent proteolipid protein (PLP). The disease results in hypomyelination of the central nervous system with a predilection for the brainstem, corpus callosum and internal capsule. The common form of the disease is connatal, whereas a milder variant is associated with X-linked spastic paraplegia type 2. Affected individuals with the common form of the disease exhibit nystagmus, hypotonia, head titubation, progressive spasticity, and a movement disorder that often includes athetotic movements. Intellectual dysfunction can progress to dementia. Lifespan is shortened depending on disease severity, although survival into the seventh decade has been observed. The infantile-onset Pelizaeus-Merzbacher disease-like phenotype, also known as spastic paraplegia 44, is due to mutation of GJC2 (gap junction protein gamma 2). This mutation causes connexin 47 loss of function and slowly evolves into a form of complicated hereditary spastic paraplegia with either near-normal psychomotor development or mental retardation, dysarthria, optic atrophy, and neuropathy in adulthood.

Pathology

The brain is diminutive, with a reduction of about one half of its weight. The grey matter appears initially intact, but becomes progressively atrophied as

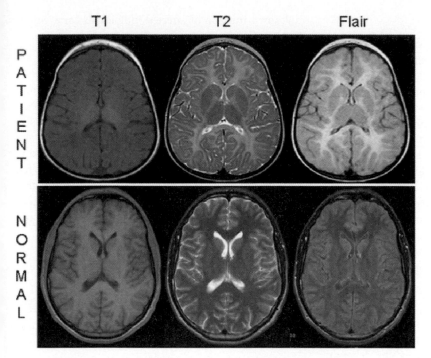

Figure 49.1 Brain magnetic resonance imaging in Pelizaeus-Merzbacher disease. Sagittal T1-weighted MR images show iso/hyposignal of the whole cerebral white matter, axial T2-weighted, and FLAIR images show diffuse hypersignal of the hemispheric white matter, internal capsule and corpus callosum in a child at 2.5 years compared to an age-matched healthy child. Reproduced with permission from Masliah-Planchon J, Dupont C, Vartzelis G, Trimouille A, Eymard-Pierre E, Gay-Bellile M, Renaldo F, Dorboz I, Pagan C, Quentin S, Elmaleh M, Kotsogianni C, Konstantelou E, Drunat S, Tabet AC, Boespflug-Tanguy O. Insertion of an extra copy of Xq22.2 into 1p36 results in functional duplication of the PLP1 gene in a girl with classical Pelizaeus-Merzbacher disease. *BMC Med Genet.* 2015 Sep 2; 16:77.

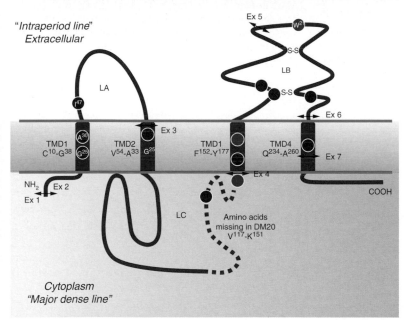

Figure 49.2 Distribution of PLP1gene mutations identified in individuals with PLP1-related disorders in relation to a model of the tetra-span proteolipid proteins, PLP, and DM20. With respect to the missense mutations included here, the amino acid residues affected by novel mutations are shown in purple, whereas residues harbouring previously reported mutations are given in green. The four predicted transmembrane domains (TMD1-4) are depicted, the first and last amino acids being indicated for each TMD. The PLP1-specific region (which is absent from DM20) is denoted by a dotted line. The locations of the two disulfide bridges (Cys184-Cys228 and Cys201-Cys220) within loop B (LB) are marked "S–S." The double arrow indicates the relative placement of the exon-exon (Ex) junctions superimposed upon the PLP1 protein. Reproduced with permission from Grossi S et al. Molecular genetic analysis of the PLP1 gene in 38 families with PLP1-related disorders: identification and functional characterization of 11 novel PLP1 mutations. *Orphanet J Rare Dis.* 2011; 6:40.

the white matter also undergoes atrophy. The degree of atrophy of the brainstem and the corticospinal tract of internal capsule correlate with clinical disease severity. U-fibers are initially spared, in the setting of gelatinous myelin distributed in a tigroid pattern (Figure 49.1). The optic nerves (but not other cranial nerves) are involved. There is astrocytic proliferation and oligodendrocytes are absent or substantially diminished in number. Perivascular macrophages are filled with lipid granules. Neuronal loss can be prominent in the substantia nigra, thalamus, and hippocampus. In the cerebellum, granule and Purkinje cells degenerate.

Pathophysiology

The PLP gene codes for two splice variants: PLP1 and DM20, which help compact the extracellular surface of myelin (Figure 49.2). Mutant PLP accumulates in the endoplasmic reticulum and induces stress. PLP mutants inhibit Golgi apparatus to endoplasmic reticulum trafficking, reducing the supply of endoplasmic reticulum chaperones and inducing Golgi fragmentation. Thus, depletion of endoplasmic reticulum chaperones induced by mutant misfolded proteins may contribute to disease pathogenesis. The *shaking pup* (shp) is a mouse model of the disease. In this mouse, oligodendrocytes exhibit delay in differentiation, increased cell death and marked distension of the rough endoplasmic reticulum. Activated microglia in the white and grey matter of transgenic mice appear before demyelination is apparent.

Diagnosis

About 2/3 of affected individuals harbor a duplication in the PLP1 gene. The remainder 1/3 exhibit deletions and point mutations and some with particularly severe forms of the disease exhibit triplications and pentuplications. MR imaging shows absence of cerebral myelin or abnormally appearing myelin. An unknown fraction of affected individuals carry mutations in GJC2 (gap junction protein gamma-2).

Treatment

Treatment of the dysmyelinated *shiverer* mouse model has included human oligodendrocyte progenitor cells or human neural precursor cells. Two observations are relevant for the dietary therapy of the disease: cholesterol promotes normal PLP trafficking and dietary cholesterol influences pathology. Mice fed a cholesterol-rich diet display restored oligodendrocyte numbers and decreased intracellular PLP accumulation in addition to increased myelin content and reduced inflammation and gliosis.

Bibliography

Hobson G.M., Garbern J.Y. (2012). Pelizaeus-Merzbacher disease, Pelizaeus-Merzbacher-like disease 1, and related hypomyelinating disorders. *Semin Neurol.* 32(1):62–7.

Masliah-Planchon J., Dupont C., Vartzelis G., et al. (2015). Boespflug-Tanguy O. Insertion of an extra copy of Xq22.2 into 1p36 results in functional duplication of the PLP1 gene in a girl with classical Pelizaeus-Merzbacher disease. *BMC Med Genet.* Sep 2; 16:77.

Rett Syndrome

A 7-year-old girl was evaluated for severe intellectual and social interactive dysfunction. Normal development was observed until the age of 6 months, after which her skills regressed and her head growth rate decreased. Loss of eye contact was observed at the age of 7 months and this was followed by a gradual lack of interaction with her environment. At age 7 years, microcephaly (head circumference 49 cm, with a normal birth circumference), short stature (120 cm), low-set ears, strabismus, repetitive hand wrestling movement, irritability, and loss of speech were noted. She had stereotypic inflexible behaviors and suffered from prominent sleep disturbances. At 15 years old she was still microcephalic (52 cm), short (145 cm) and exhibited sleep disturbances, repetitive hand wrestling movements, rigidity of hand muscles, irritability, absent speech, writing or reading, emitted guttural noises and lacked control of urinary and fecal excretion.

Rett Syndrome

Onset: Delayed acquisition of complex motor skills and loss of hand dexterity in a girl after 6–18 months of age when due to mutation of MeCP2 (methyl-CpG binding protein 2).

Additional manifestations: Acquired microcephaly. Hyperventilation, autonomic dysfunction, sleep disturbance and hand stereotypic movements followed by loss of any acquired communicative capacities. Epilepsy can appear after 3 years of age. Facial dysmorphism, early epilepsy, hypotonia, and spasticity are characteristic of CDKL5 (cyclin-dependent kinase-like 5) mutations, which may not be associated with an early period of normal development. FOXG1 (forkhead box G1) mutations also impair early development and can cause severe early epilepsy.

Disease mechanism: X-linked loss or gain of several copies of MeCP2. Females are mosaic for the causal mutation because of X-inactivation and thus can exhibit a broad range of disease severity.

Testing: Genotyping of MeCP2 (95 percent of cases), CDKL5 or FOXG1.

Treatment: None effective. Signaling mechanisms downstream of MeCP2 are being pharmacologically explored.

Research highlights: Role of transcriptional regulation by MeCP2 in mature neuron function and its restoration in mouse models of Rett syndrome.

Clinical Features

Rett syndrome is a multiform disorder that affects 1 in 12,000 girls. The common form of the disease occurs in 95 percent of Rett affected individuals and is rather stereotyped. The remainder suffer from either more severe or milder variants, most of which are also due to mutations in MeCP2, a gene expressed throughout the organism with multiple functions in the nervous system. In common Rett syndrome, motor abilities are normally acquired until disease onset at 6–18 months of age. In some cases, fine motor capacity does not develop. In others, there is loss of hand dexterity. In all of them, stereotypic hand and arm movements replace any purposeful use. There is also acquired microcephaly, which becomes more apparent with age (Figure 50.1). Epilepsy (generalized tonic-clonic and partial complex) is uncommon before 3 years of age. Neurological dysfunction can stabilize after 5 years. Scoliosis sets in by 11 years of age (Figure 50.2). Survival into the fifth decade is common. Most affected individuals evolve across four disease phases. In stage I, abnormal spontaneous movements may be noted during prolonged observation in the context of normal early psychomotor development.

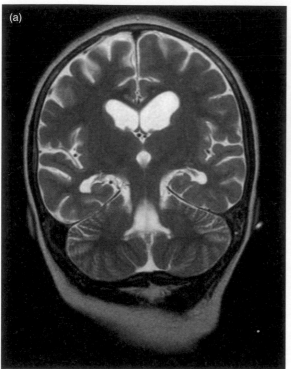

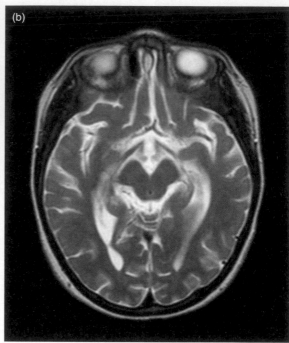

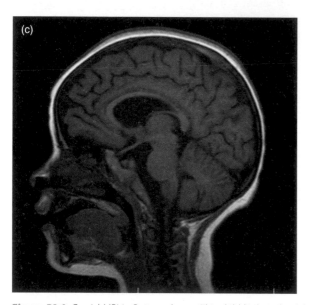

Figure 50.1 Cranial MRI in Rett syndrome. This child harbored a deletion of exons 3 and 4 in the MeCP2 gene. Coronal (a) and axial (b) T2-weighted images illustrate cortical cerebral atrophy and slight white matter signal increase. The parasaggital T1-weighted image (c) illustrates cerebral cortical atrophy allowing the visualization of fluid-filled spaces surrounding the cerebral sulci.

Stage II most often begins between the ages of 1 year and 3 years with the rapid loss of any acquired language and social interactions, loss of purposeful hand action, appearance of hand stereotypies (including wringing/squeezing, clapping/tapping, mouthing, and washing/rubbing automatisms), hypotonia, gait impairment, deceleration of head growth, respiratory abnormalities, and seizures. Inconsolable crying appears by age

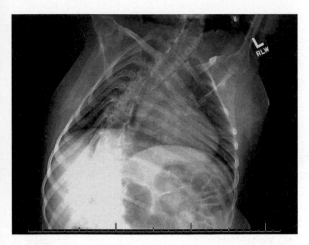

Figure 50.2 Scoliosis in Rett syndrome. There is an endotracheal tube projecting over the neck and upper chest with the tip near T2. There is a slight central interstitial prominence without focal airspace opacities. The cardiac silhouette is not enlarged. There is marked dextroconvex curvature of the thoracic spine, distorting the chest wall.

18–24 months. Stage III begins between the ages of 2 years and 10 years as a stationary phase, with some improvement in communication skills but slow motor deterioration, rigidity, and seizures. In stage IV, further motor deterioration leads to loss of the ability to walk in cases when it was achieved. The EEG is helpful in stratifying the four disease stages. It can be normal or exhibit slowing of occipital background activity in the awake state in stage I. In stage II, there is loss of non-REM sleep characteristics and focal spikes or sharp waves appear in sleep and, subsequently, also during wakefulness. In stage III, further slowing of background activity, absence of non-REM sleep characteristics, multifocal epileptiform discharges, generalized slow spike-wave, and rhythmic delta over the central regions during sleep and in the awake state are prominent. Marked slowing of background activity with delta rhythms, multifocal epileptiform activity in the awake state, and generalized slow spike-wave activity in sleep are frequent in stage IV. Sleep disturbances (night-time laughter, seizures, daytime napping) can be present at any or all stages, as are episodic apnea and/or hyperpnea. Most affected individuals are growth-retarded and wasted as the disease progresses. Death is commonly due to secondary cardiopulmonary diseases or malnutrition related to complete incapacity. In some affected individuals, sudden death is attributed to cardiopathy which manifests as prolonged QT interval, T-wave abnormalities, and reduced heart rate variability.

Males with MeCP2 mutations are born with severe encephalopathy and often die soon after birth. The disorder is said to resemble autism in a fraction of girls with mild Rett syndrome, which has been taken by some as an example of a shared disease mechanism. Such a unifying mechanism, however, has not been found and the autism phenotype has been contested. Better understood forms of the disease include a preserved-speech variant, an early-seizure variant (which can include infantile spasms) and a congenital variant.

Pathology

The most characteristic finding is diminished cerebral and somatic growth. All body organs are small for age except the adrenal gland. Encephalic weight remains stable after the 4th year, without growth nor atrophy. There is reduced melanin in the pars compacta of the substantia nigra accompanying tyrosine hydroxylase depletion. The cerebral cortex shows decreased neuronal size, dendritic arborization, dendritic spines, and pyramidal neuron numbers in the context of increased overall neuronal density. Basal ganglia and hippocampus exhibit an array of abnormalities and Purkinje cells are progressively lost. However, there is no neurodegeneration in the forebrain. Distal axonal neuropathy and muscle biopsy abnormalities have also been documented.

Subtle cerebral dysgenesis has been identified in CDKL5 (cyclin-dependent kinase-like 5) mutations in the context of heterotopias and Purkinje cell degeneration.

Hypo- or agenesis of the anterior corpus callosum in combination with acquired microcephaly has been described in FOXG1 (forkhead box G1) related disease.

Pathophysiology

The expression of the disease is determined by the pattern of inheritance of the X chromosome. Most cases are sporadic and, in some cases, females who are obligate heterozygous for a pathogenic MeCP2 mutation are normal, which is attributed to protective, highly skewed X-chromosome inactivation. MeCP2 encodes a methyl-CpG binding protein that conjugates with histone deacetylases to repress the transcription of multiple genes (Figure 50.3).

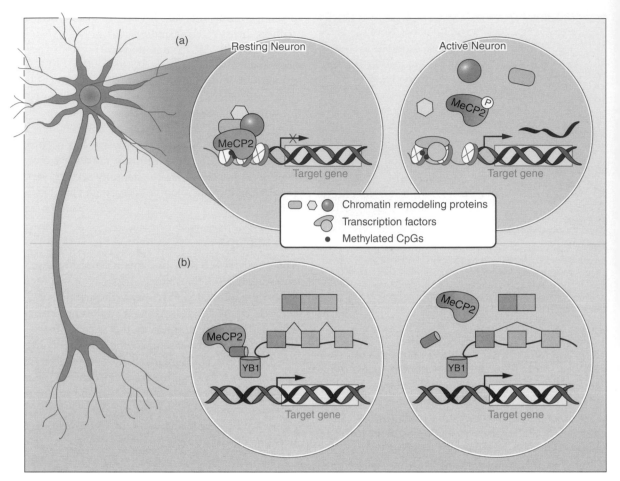

Figure 50.3 Model for MeCP2 mechanisms of action. (a) In resting neurons MeCP2 regulates gene expression by binding to methylated CpG dinucleotides and recruiting the Sin3A-HDAC corepressor complex and chromatin remodeling proteins. This leads to chromatin compaction, making the promoter inaccessible to members of the transcriptional machinery. Neuronal activity induces MeCP2 phosphorylation and leads to its release from the promoter region and dissociation of the corepressor complex. The hyperacetylated chromatin allows access to transcriptional machinery and target gene expression. (b) MeCP2 interacts with YB1 and regulates alternative splicing of target transcripts. In the absence of MeCP2, these transcripts are aberrantly spliced. Reproduced with permission from Chahrour M et al. The story of Rett syndrome: from clinic to neurobiology. *Neuron*. 2007; 56(3):422–37.

In addition, several genes are repressed in MeCP2 deficient cells, illustrating that MeCP2 is also a transcriptional activator. Thus, X-linked dominant MeCP2 loss of function leads to broadly dysregulated gene transcription (perhaps including several hundred genes) with differential impact across brain regions. Curiously, a similar mechanism appears to play out in gene multiplications.

Despite its ubiquitous expression, MeCP2 is preferentially expressed in mature neurons of the brain and located inside the cell nucleus. MeCP2 mutations also increase the expression of retrotransposons in neural precursor cells, perhaps leading to secondary

mutation during development. However, neuronal precursor proliferation and differentiation do not seem to be affected by MeCP2 deficiency. In fact, the disease can be partially recapitulated in mutant mice by inducing loss of MeCP2 in the adult brain. Analogously, overexpression of MeCP2 in mutant mice also recapitulates aspects of the disease phenotype. Controlled loss and regaining of function of MeCP2 by inducible transgenetic approaches has shown that the Rett-like phenotype can be reversed, such that neurons are not subject to irreversible damage.

Mice deficient in MeCP2 are also deficient in brain-derived neurotrophic factor (BDNF) after a

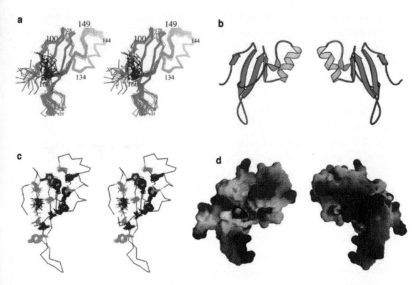

Figure 50.4 Structure of the methylated DNA binding domain from MeCP2: (a) Stereo-pair representation of a superposition of backbone (Ca) traces for the 28 structures with lowest energy out of a set of 30 calculated. (b) MOLSCRIPT representations of MBD (residues 92–164); the representation on the left is in the same orientation as in (a); the one on the right is rotated 180 degrees. (c) Stereo-pair showing the 14 side-chains which contribute to the hydrophobic core. The side-chains of the 28 accepted structures are drawn, based on a superposition of backbone atoms as shown in (a). A Ca trace of residues 92–161 of a typical structure is shown to provide orientation. The Phe side-chains are coloured blue; Leu, orange; Arg, brown; Val, red; Tyr, cyan; and Trp, magenta. (d) Molecular surface coloured by electrostatic potential (blue is positive, red is negative) at ±5 keV using GRASP. The same two views as used in Figure 3(b) are shown. Reproduced with permission from Wakefield RI et al. The solution structure of the domain from MeCP2 that binds to methylated DNA. *J Mol Biol.* 1999; 291(5):1055–65.

presymptomatic period, with a decline in BDNF correlative with Rett-like manifestations. Postnatal deletion of BDNF in forebrain excitatory neurons of normal mice is associated with Rett-like features, whereas overexpression of BDNF in MeCP2-deficient mice leads to amelioration of these features, making BDNF and its downstream molecular partners a potential therapeutic target.

Among the more than 300 mutations that have been identified, Arg133Cys, Arg294X, Arg306Cys, truncations and other point mutations are associated with relatively less severe typical and atypical Rett syndrome (Figure 50.4). In contrast, Arg106Trp, Arg168X, Arg255X, Arg270X, splice site mutations, deletions, insertions, and deletions tend to be clinically more severe.

CDKL5 expression is stimulated in early postnatal stages and in the adult brain is present in mature neurons. CDKL5 shuttles between the cytoplasm and the nucleus. Disease-causing truncations of the C terminus of CDKL5 are constitutively nuclear, suggesting that they might act as gain of function mutations in this cellular compartment. In contrast with MeCP2, CDKL5, which is a MeCP2-repressed target gene, is crucial for neuronal morphogenesis via the action of cytoplasmic signaling mechanisms. CDKL5 forms a protein complex with Rac1, a cytoplasmic regulator of actin remodeling and neuronal morphogenesis. Reduction of CDKL5 in the rat brain by in utero electroporation results in delayed neuronal migration and diminished dendritic arborization.

FOXG1, another poorly understood regulator, is a winged-helix transcription factor involved in telencephalic development. In FOXG1 null mutants, excessive Cajal-Retzius cells (the earliest born neurons, which undergo cell death during development) are produced in the cerebral cortex. These cells and their secreted gene product, reelin, are involved in neuronal migration by acting on migrating neurons and on radial glial cells.

Diagnosis

Several clinical criteria have been proposed for the diagnosis of Rett syndrome but none is helpful to identify the early stage of the disease and thus are not repeated here. None of the abnormalities in ancillary studies such as cerebrospinal fluid analysis, muscle histopathology or imaging is sufficiently specific. Thus, although it is possible to definitively diagnose Rett syndrome on clinical grounds alone, particularly in its common form after the initial stages, early-stage disease can be confirmed by genotyping.

Treatment

Epilepsy in Rett syndrome is largely treatable. Between 60% and 75% of treated Rett syndrome affected individuals achieve seizure remission after the first and second drug tried. Carbamazepine, valproate, and lamotrigine are the most frequently used drugs, although they are used on a purely empirical bases.

Based on the hypothesis that altering DNA methylation could improve global DNA methylation and thereby improve residual MeCP2 function, a trial of oral creatine has been undertaken. A statistical increase in global DNA methylation was seen. Improvement in the total and subscores of the Rett Syndrome Motor and Behavioral Assessment was observed, although it did not reach statistical significance

Because elevated opioids had been observed in the CSF of individuals with Rett syndrome, the oral opiate antagonist, naltrexone, was investigated. Although it decreased breathing dysrhythmias and had some sedating properties, its efficacy remains unclear.

A variety of drugs target mechanisms downstream McCP2. The sphingosine-1 phosphate receptor agonist fingolimod, a drug that crosses the blood–brain barrier, increases BDNF levels in cultured neurons. Insulin-like growth factor IGF-1 exerts effects on neuronal function similar to BDNF. Parenteral administration of a tri-peptide form of IGF-1 (mecasermin) is being investigated. The tricyclic antidepressant desipramine is also under study, specifically focusing on the respiratory abnormalities associated with Rett syndrome. The NMDA receptor antagonist dextromethorphan is currently in trials targeting glutamate and NMDA receptor associated neuronal toxicity and is focused on respiratory, seizure, and motor outcomes. The protein tyrosine phosphatase PTP1B is another therapeutic candidate for the treatment of Rett syndrome. The PTPN1 gene, which encodes PTP1B, is a target of MeCP2. Disruption of MeCP2 function is associated with increased levels of PTP1B. Pharmacological inhibition of PTP1B ameliorates several effects of MeCP2 disruption in mouse models of Rett syndrome.

Bibliography

Chapleau C.A., Lane J., Larimore J., Li W., Pozzo-Miller L., Percy A.K. (2013). Recent progress in Rett syndrome and MeCP2 dysfunction: Assessment of potential treatment options. *Future Neurol.* 8(1): doi:10.2217/fnl.12.79.

Gharesouran J., Khalili A.F., Azari N.S., Vahedi L. (2015). First case report of Rett syndrome in the Azeri Turkish population and brief review of the literature. *Epilepsy Behav Case Rep.* 3:15–19.

Spinal Muscular Atrophy

A 5-month-old infant was referred by his pediatrician for physical therapist evaluation with a diagnosis of hypotonia and poor motor development. According to his mother, the infant also had continual chest congestion. At 4 weeks of age, he ceased breastfeeding due to difficult latching. Within the first 2 months, the family observed decreased head control. At the evaluation, he made no attempts at antigravity movement of the head or upper or lower extremities during parent handling or transitioning to the examination room. Pulmonary exam revealed audible chest congestion and abdominal breathing. In pull-to-sit testing, he demonstrated a full head lag with no arm participation or traction present. When testing ventral suspension, the infant's head and upper and lower extremities remained below the level of the trunk. With testing vertical suspension, he was unable to stabilize the scapulae, essentially slipping through the examiner's hands. The infant required maximal assistance at the proximal trunk to maintain a sitting position and was unable to bring his head upright from a fully flexed position. Equilibrium and righting responses were absent when he was gently tilted laterally in supported sitting and vertical suspension. When placed in a prone position, the infant maintained his head rotated to the left. He was unable to turn his head to clear his nose from the surface with auditory or visual stimulus. When placed in a prone-on-elbows position, he was unable to elevate his forehead from resting on the mat table. In a supine position, neither midline head position nor antigravity reaching toward midline was observed. The infant demonstrated occasional distal movements at the feet and hands and weak bilateral grasp. He also exhibited fasciculations of the tongue.

Spinal Muscular Atrophy

Onset: Hypotonia and weakness in the first 6 months of life manifested as poor head control, weak cry, and respiratory failure in type 1 disease. In type 2, limb (leg) weakness and fasciculations manifest at 6–18 months. Type 3 individuals become symptomatic after 18 months of age.

Additional manifestations: Floppy baby syndrome. Inability to sit unsupported or to stand depending on severity. Tongue fasciculations. Nutritional and respiratory failure and susceptibility to pulmonary infections. Scoliosis and osteopenia.

Disease mechanism: Autosomal recessive loss of function of SMN1 (survival motor neuron type 1 gene) with variable compensation provided by the less efficient SMN2 analog gene. The SMN protein participates in the spliceasome, excising intron RNA to generate mature RNA inside Cajal bodies.

Testing: Electromyography shows denervation. Genotyping of SMN1 confirms 99 percent of cases.

Treatment: None effective.

Research highlights: SMN protein restoration via modulation of translation using antisense oligonucleotides and elucidation of downstream targets of SMN protein interacting with the spliceasome.

Clinical Features

Spinal muscular atrophy is a progressive disease of variable age of onset and severity that stems from spinal motor neuron cell death. Loss of muscle strength in this disease may be most evident at onset with subsequent stabilization for many years. This suggests that some disease manifestations are due to impaired development of the motor unit rather than to neurodegeneration. Spinal muscular atrophy is a frequent disease: The incidence is 1 in 10,000 live births and the carrier frequency is 1 in 50. Three forms of the disease are commonly recognized. Type 1 (Werdnig-Hoffmann disease; 45 percent of cases) includes infantile onset (first 6 months of life) and severe weakness, followed by death often before the 3rd birthday, depending on respiratory function. Type 2 (23 percent of cases) is of intermediate severity and includes children who can sit but not walk. Type 3 (Kugelberg-Welander disease; 30 percent of cases) is milder, affects older children, and is associated with normal lifespan. Intellect is preserved in all forms of the disease. Additional forms are type 0, which manifests prenatally with joint contractures and is followed by very early death and type 4, with onset in adulthood.

Type 1 affected individuals never sit without support. Infants manifest proximal and generalized axial weakness that interferes with head movements, breathing, and nutrition (Figure 51.1). Breathing is diaphragmatic rather than intercostal. Tongue atrophy and fasciculations can be prominent. Oculomotor function and intellect are preserved. Reflexes are absent. Hypotonia is profound, leading to a habitual splayed out frog-like supine posture. Some affected individuals are prone to cardiac malformation, digital vascular necrosis, and thrombosis. Survival can be prolonged well beyond the second year of life via nutritional and respiratory support.

Type 2 affected individuals manifest between 6 and 18 months of age and can usually sit unsupported by the normal expected age of 9 months. Some affected individuals learn to sit later but all eventually do. However, they never walk unaided. Weakness is most prominent in the legs. Many other disease features are shared with type 1 affected individuals

except that obesity is more common. After a period of motor decline, strength stabilizes for a prolonged time that can span many years.

Type 3 affected individuals become symptomatic after 18 months of age and most achieve the capacity to ambulate before that age. Proximal leg weakness is often associated with a Gowers sign. Ambulation is preserved even in cases with severe weakness, which may be related to the development of segmental muscular compensation. Some affected individuals exhibit limb fasciculations and calf muscle pseudohypertrophy. Respiratory function is generally preserved.

Additional forms of spinal muscular atrophy are caused by other gene mutations, but they are associated with characteristic clinical features, allowing for clear distinctions. Among these, spinal muscular atrophy with respiratory distress is a distal form with early diaphragmatic weakness. Forms with pontocerebellar hypoplasia, vocal cord paralysis, or myoclonic epilepsy have also been recognized. A potentially treatable form is Brown-Vialetto-van Laere disease, which causes deafness and cranial nerve palsies and has been associated with deficiency of a riboflavin transporter.

Pathology

There is spinal and bulbar motor neuron loss, with atrophy of the anterior roots of the spinal cord and reactive glial proliferation. Autonomic nuclei neurons are preserved, as are cortical pyramidal neurons (Betz cells) and pyramidal tracts. Motor neurons are atrophic or swollen and pale, with loss of the Nissl substance and accumulation of phosphorylated neurofilaments. Heterotopic (migratory) motor neurons are often detected, in support of the contention that this is both a degenerative and a developmental disease. Phrenic nerve motor neurons are usually preserved, probably accounting for residual diaphragmatic activity. Using the TUNEL (terminal deoxynucleotidyl transferase dUTP nick end labeling) method, fetuses 10–20 weeks old exhibit excess apoptosis, a developmental period critical for the establishment of neuromuscular synapses. The skeletal muscle can also be apoptotic. In addition, type 1 fibers can be hypertrophic in the setting of abundant atrophic fibers. In type 3 disease, myopathic changes including fiber splitting, increased density of central nuclei and of

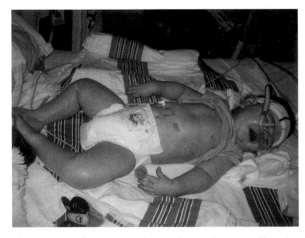

Figure 51.1 Infant with spinal muscular atrophy type 1. There is decreased head control and the child makes no attempts at antigravity movement of the head or upper or lower extremities. There is also abdominal breathing.

endomysial tissue may occur. Significant vascular bed depletion with loss of blood vessels is also seen in severe disease, both in the muscle of affected individuals and in the spinal cord of model mice.

Pathophysiology

Chromosome 5q harbors SMN1, which is responsible for most of the SMN protein produced in normal subjects. 5q also contains a duplicate gene, SMN2, which differs from SMN1 in only 5 nucleotides. This variant gene results in about 10 percent intact SMN protein production relative to SMN1 and also in a truncated protein that lacks the amino acids encoded by exon 7. The truncated protein is rapidly degraded. All individuals carry a variable number of copies of SMN2, and thus those with one or more copies (85 percent of all persons) produce variable amounts of full length SMN protein. In favorable cases, multiple copies of SMN2 act as effective disease modifiers. A common mutation in SMN1 disrupts transcription of exon 7, effectively converting the gene into SMN2. This mutation is associated with a milder phenotype. Mutations in other genes adjacent to SMN1 and SMN2 (GTF2H2 or general transcription factor IIH subunit 2; NAIP or neuronal apoptosis inhibitory protein; SERF1 or small EDRK-rich factor 1) also act as disease modifiers. The SMN protein is expressed in nucleus and cytoplasm throughout the organism, including motor neurons. It is localized in nuclear gems (gemini of coiled bodies) that associate with Cajal or coiled bodies. SMN is important for the assembly of the spliceosome, which accomplishes pre-mRNA splicing by catalyzing the removal of introns from mRNA precursors. What RNAs are affected and why this mechanism predominantly affects motor neurons is largely unknown, but RNAs consistent with hyper-activation of the endoplasmic reticulum stress pathway are increased in motor neurons, suggesting that selective activation of endoplasmic reticulum stress may underlie motor neuron death.

Diagnosis

Plasma creatine kinase is usually moderately increased. Electromyography illustrates denervation of the muscle, as does muscle biopsy. There is active and chronic denervation, reinnervation, fibrillation potentials, positive sharp waves, fasciculations, and large and prolonged motor unit action potentials with reduced recruitment. Nerve conduction responses are normal and compound muscle action potentials are reduced, in the context of normal or mildly reduced motor conduction velocities. However, these tests are rarely necessary. Genotyping for SMN1 mutations yields the diagnosis in about 95 percent of cases of spinal muscular atrophy. Most cases are associated with a homozygous deletion of exon 7. SMN2 copy number can also be assayed.

Treatment

In the absence of replacement therapies for SMN, the mainstay of the treatment remains rehabilitative, respiratory, nutritional, and orthopedic. Recurrent pneumonia, disordered sleep, dysphagia, delayed gastric emptying, poor oral and respiratory secretion clearance, decreased caloric needs are commonly associated with severe disease forms. Noninvasive ventilation combined with nutritional supplementation and reflux therapy, and sometimes gastrostomy, have resulted in increased survival for type 1 affected individuals. Gastrointestinal prokinetic agents such as metoclopramide and erythromycin are often used. Spinal fixation delays the decline in pulmonary function and helps maintain posture.

Treatments aimed at increasing SMN protein production or at ameliorating other aspects of the disease have included gabapentin, riluzole, albuterol, creatine, carnitine, valproate, hydroxyurea, and phenylbutyrate. Some are histone deacetylase (HDAC) inhibitors, which increase SMN2 transcriptional activity via inhibition of HDAC1 and HDAC2, but central nervous system penetration is not uniformly high for all of them, whereas some are broad inhibitors of other histone deacetylases and thus prone to unintended effects. High throughput drug screening has revealed that quinazoline derivatives enhance the activity of the SMN promotor. Antisense oligonucleotides delivered intrathecally aim to modify endogenous RNA processing, resulting in the conversion of SMN2 RNA into SMN1 RNA by read-through of the SMN2 gene. Small-molecule enhancers of SMN2 splicing increase full-length SMN protein and extend survival in a severe disease mouse model. Their mechanism of action is the stabilization of the transient double-strand RNA structure formed by the SMN2 pre-mRNA and U1 small nuclear ribonucleic protein (snRNP) complex in a sequence-selective manner. Gene therapy has increased SMN abundance using cDNA under the control of a promoter and encapsulated in the self-complementary adeno-associated virus serotype-9.

Bibliography

Kolb S.J., Kissel J.T. (2015). Spinal muscular atrophy. *Neurol Clin.* 33(4):831–46.

Malerba K.H., Tecklin J.S. (2013). Clinical decision making in hypotonia and gross motor delay: A case report of type 1 spinal muscular atrophy in an infant. *Phys Ther.* Jun;93(6):833–41.

Infantile Neuroaxonal Dystrophy

A 28-month-old girl was evaluated for abnormal devel-opment and gross neurological deterioration. Early motor development was somewhat delayed, but she was able to stand independently at the age of 18 months. Her social interaction and speech development were appropriate for her age at that time. She had no feeding problems from birth and was transitioned to solid foods at 5.5 months of age. Rapid global regres-sion of skills with gradually increasing hypotonia was noted from the age of 18 months. At 2 years 6 months of age she could sit only with support and expressed no words. Her feeding skills deteriorated and she could feed only on puréed food and fluids. Examination revealed marked hypotonia with head lag; her reflexes were normal with bilateral extensor responses. She had inter-rupted saccadic eye movements with intermittent nys-tagmus. Ophthalmological examination showed right-sided esotropia with pigmentary changes in the fundus. Electromyography revealed mild neurogenic abnormal-ities suggestive of motor neuron dysfunction. An MR imaging study was obtained (Figure 52.1).

Infantile Neuroaxonal Dystrophy

Onset: Delayed acquisition of motor skills between 6 and 18 months of life.

Additional manifestations: Areflexia, hypotonia, and weakness followed by ataxia, rigidity, and spasticity. Dementia. Seizures are rare. Death is common before 6 years of age.

Disease mechanism: Autosomal recessive loss of function of calcium-independent phospholipase A2 iPLA2, encoded by the gene PLA2G6. This leads to phospholipid abnormalities, impacting membrane function and signaling.

Testing: Genotyping of PLA2G6. Skin biopsy documents nerve spheroids.

Treatment: None effective.

Research highlights: Animal models of impaired phospholipid turnover.

Clinical Features

The neuroaxonal dystrophies are disorders of the central and peripheral nervous system characterized by iron accumulation and axonal swellings, the largest of which are called axonal spheroids. They are part of the neurodegeneration with brain iron accumulation class of diseases, which is discussed separately. Infantile neuroaxonal dystrophy, also known as Seitelberger's syndrome or PLA2G6-associated neurodegeneration (PLAN), is caused by mutation of the calcium-independent phospholipase A2 iPLA2 beta, encoded by the gene PLA2G6. Mutations that lead to loss of phospholipase activity are associated with infantile neuroaxonal dystrophy, whereas mutations with normal enzyme activity cause dystonia-parkinsonism type PARK14. Indi-viduals with infantile neuroaxonal dystrophy pre-sent between 6 and 18 months and experience delays in acquiring new motor and intellectual skills, such as crawling or beginning to speak. Weakness, hypotonia, and are flexia ensue. Later manifestations include spasticity, rigidity, cerebellar dysfunction, deafness, optic atrophy, and dementia. Seizures are uncommon. Survival is often limited to less than 6 years of age.

Pathology

The finding of neuroaxonal dystrophy is normal after the age of 10 years in the medial globus palli-dus, pars reticulata of the substantia nigra and in the gracile and cuneiform nuclei. In infantile neu-roaxonal dystrophy, the globus pallidus is dis-colored, the substantia nigra is depigmented and there is diffuse cerebral cortical and cerebellar atro-phy (Figure 52.1). There is widespread spheroid formation in brain and nerves, which can be detected in skin. Iron accumulates intracellularly and around blood vessels in the pallidum. There is also Purkinje cell degeneration. Widespread hyperphosphorylated tau and synuclein pathology coexists with Lewy body formation. In a *Drosophila* model of the disease, there is mitochondrial respiratory chain dysfunction, reduced ATP synthesis, and abnormal mitochondrial morphology.

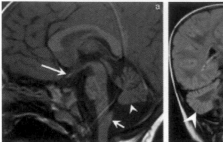
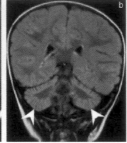

Figure 52.1 Infantile neuroaxonal dystrophy. A mid-sagittal T1-weighted magnetic resonance image (a) demonstrates marked atrophy of the inferior cerebellar vermis (arrowhead), claval hypertrophy (short arrow), and chiasmal atrophy (long arrow). A coronal fluid-attenuated inversion recovery image (b) demonstrates subtle diffuse cerebellar cortical hyperintensity (arrowheads) and widening of the cerebrospinal fluid spaces between the cerebellar folia, in keeping with cerebellar atrophy. Reproduced with permission from Solomons J et al. Infantile neuroaxonal dystrophy caused by uniparental disomy. *Dev Med Child Neurol.* 2014; 56(4):386–9.

Pathophysiology

iPLA2 beta is important for the remodeling of membrane phospholipids, significantly impacting signal transduction, cell proliferation, and apoptosis (Figure 52.2). The mechanism of iPLA2 beta deficiency may thus be mediated by abnormal plasma, organelle or vesicular membrane phospholipid composition. In infantile neuroaxonal dystrophy, a greater than 80 percent loss of phospholipase and lysophospholipase activities leads to accumulation of phospholipid substrates. The normal products of iPLA2 beta are lysophospholipids and fatty acids, which may be deficient in the disease. *O*-linked glycosylation and sialylation are also abnormal. ATP-dependent calcium responses in astrocytes are severely abnormal in a mouse model of PLA2G6 deficiency.

Diagnosis

Genetic diagnosis is available for PLA2G6 deficiency. In contrast, MR imaging studies are not universally helpful. Cerebellar atrophy is common and can be associated with variable pallidal iron accumulation, especially as the disease progresses. Additional iron deposits throughout the brain are sometimes detected by MR imaging. Claval hypertrophy with pontine atrophy may also be

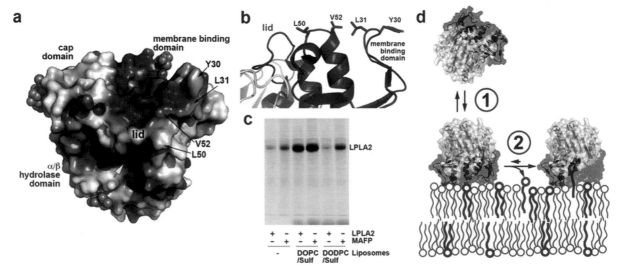

Figure 52.2 LPLA2 lysosomal phospholipase A2 membrane association. (a) Electrostatic surface potential (± 5 kT/e) of LPLA2 at pH 5. Glycosylation sites (orange spheres) would not sterically interfere with the interaction between the membrane binding domain and lipid bilayers. Yellow arrow indicates the entrance into the active site. (b) The membrane binding surface of LPLA2. (c) LPLA2 requires either MAFP modification or substrate liposomes (DOPC-sulfatide) to stably associate with liposomes in pull down assays. (d) Membrane association model. First, transient membrane binding is driven by complementary electrostatic charge and the hydrophobic patch on the membrane binding domain. Second, formation of covalent acyl intermediate tethers LPLA2 at the membrane. Reproduced with permission from Glukhova A et al. Structure and function of lysosomal phospholipase A2 and lecithin: Cholesterol acyltransferase. *Nat Commun.* 2015 Mar 2; 6:6250.

apparent. Electromyography demonstrates changes consistent with chronic denervation. Skin biopsy including sensory nerves reveals spheroid formation.

Treatment

The treatment of brain iron accumulation disorders in general is symptomatic and eventually proves ineffective. There is no specific treatment for infantile neuroaxonal dystrophy.

Bibliography

Solomons J., Ridgway O., Hardy C., et al. (2014). Infantile neuroaxonal dystrophy caused by uniparental disomy. *Dev Med Child Neurol.* 56(4):386–9.

Kurian M.A., McNeill A., Lin J.P., Maher E.R. (2011). Childhood disorders of neurodegeneration with brain iron accumulation (NBIA). *Dev Med Child Neurol.* 53(5):394–404.

Déjérine–Sottas Disease

A 10-year-old girl was the third child born to nonconsanguineous parents. She had two healthy older sisters (Figures 53.1 and 53.2). The 10-year old manifested delayed motor development, with autonomous walking not present until 24 months of age. During childhood she developed gait difficulties with clumsiness and balance problems. However, disease progression was very slow. At 10 years of age she exhibited bilateral pes cavus, scoliosis, and a broad-based gait. She had severe weakness of foot eversion without proximal muscle involvement. Her sensitivity to pinprick, touch, position, and vibration was decreased. Vibratory sensation was more severely disturbed than pain sensation in all limbs. Sensory ataxia and a Romberg sign were present. Tendon reflexes were absent and pathologic reflexes were not found. Neurologic and electrophysiologic examinations revealed that the parents and two sisters did not exhibit any distal weakness, sensory deficits, or abnormal electrophysiological findings.

Déjérine–Sottas Disease

Onset: Delayed acquisition of motor skills in infancy.
Additional manifestations: Areflexia and weakness followed by ataxia and ambulatory disability with normal intelligence. Congenital hypomyelinating neuropathy is a more severe form of neuropathy with onset at birth which is often caused by mutation in the same genes. Floppy baby syndrome and respiratory, nutritional failure are typical of the latter entity.
Disease mechanism: Autosomal dominant or recessive loss of function of one of several known genes leading to hypomyelination and insufficient remyelination.
Testing: Genotyping of several potential genes. Nerve biopsy documents hypomyelination and onion bulb formation.

Treatment: None effective.
Research highlights: The *trembler* mouse is a model of PMP22-associated disease.

Clinical Features

This disease is also known as hereditary motor sensory neuropathy type III and as Charcot-Marie-Tooth disease type 3. Déjérine–Sottas disease is a severe hypomyelinating sensor motor polyneuropathy of infantile onset that most often manifests before the age of 3 years. The most frequently mutated genes in Déjérine–Sottas disease are PMP22 (peripheral myelin protein 22), MPZ (myelin protein-zero), PRX (periaxin), and EGR2 (early growth response gene-2). Children exhibit delayed accomplishment of motor abilities in infancy in the context of normal intelligence. Some nerves are palpable against bony prominences and feel as thickened, stiff cords. Sensory ataxia and severe ambulatory impairment are common. Pes cavus and scoliosis are the rule.

A distinct entity within the same syndromic category is congenital hypomyelinating neuropathy. This disorder manifests at birth and is an important cause of severe floppy baby syndrome with early mortality. Infants experience swallowing and respiratory insufficiency. Mutations in PMP22, MPZ, PRX, and EGR2 have also been reported.

Pathology

Limb nerves are increased in size, firm, and gelatinous. Nerve biopsy illustrates hypomyelination with thin myelin sheaths surrounding many axons, large numbers of onion bulbs, or incompletely remyelinated axons, endoneurial fibrosis, and loss of axons (Figures 53.1 and 53.2).

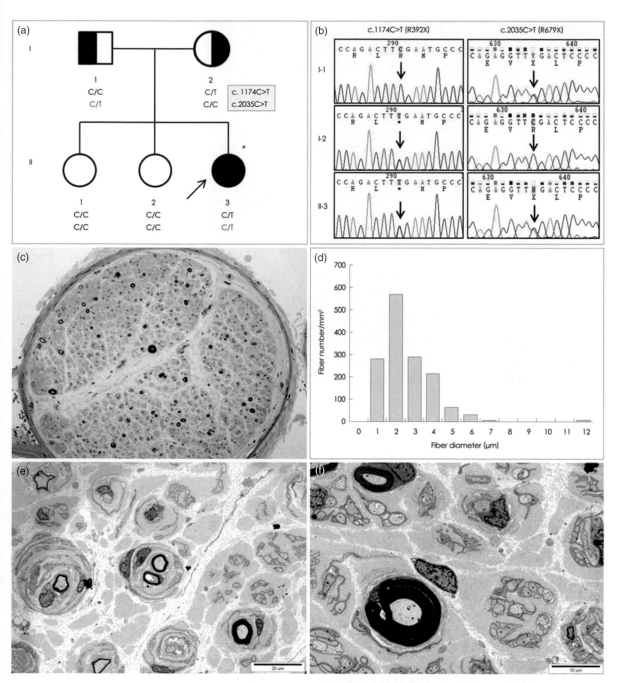

Figure 53.1 Pedigree, sequencing analysis and distal sural nerve biopsy of the proband with compound heterozygous mutations in PRX. a. Pedigree of affected individual's family. Genotypes of both PRX mutations are indicated at the bottom of each examined individual. Open symbols, unaffected; filled symbol, affected; half-filled symbols, individuals possessing only a heterozygous mutation; asterisk, whole-exome sequencing performed; and arrow, proband. b. Sequencing chromatograms from the proband and her parents. Vertical arrows indicate the mutation site. * (asterisk) and X indicate the mutation codon in I-2 and and I-1, respectively. c. Transverse semi-thin sections with toluidine blue stain (×400). Light microscopy images reveal nerve fascicles that are markedly decreased in size, diffuse subendoneurial edema, and moderately to markedly decreased numbers of myelinated fibers (MFs) of all calibers with suggestive onion bulb formation and endoneurial fibrosis. d. Histogram of the sural nerve biopsy showing a unimodal distribution pattern. The mean diameter of MF (3.14 μm) and the percentage area of MFs (1.39%) were lower than in age-matched controls. e and f. Ultrastructural micrographs by electron microscopy (×1,000) reveals findings consistent with demyelinating neuropathy, such as focally folded, uncompacted, or deteriorating myelin, irregular myelin thickness, and fragmented myelin structures in Schwann cells or nearby macrophages. Reproduced with permission from Choi YJ, Hyun YS, Nam SH, Koo H, Hong YB, Chung KW, Choi BO. Novel compound heterozygous nonsense PRX mutations in a Korean Dejerine-Sottas neuropathy family. *J Clin Neurol.* 2015; 11(1):92–6.

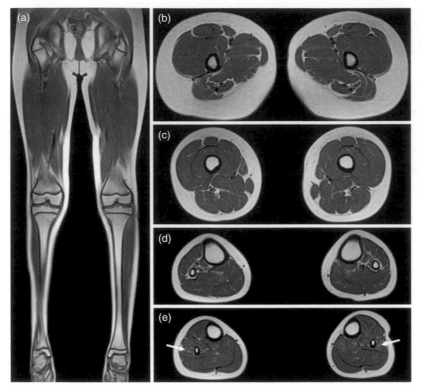

Figure 53.2 Hip, thigh, and lower calf MR imaging of the same individual as in Figure 53.1 with a PRX mutation. a. Coronal scan of lower limbs. T1-weighted images demonstrates no definite fatty or atrophic changes in hip and thigh muscles. b–e. Axial scans of lower limbs. b and c. At the thigh levels, MR images are normal. d and e. On the lower calf levels, there are mild fatty changes in distal peronei muscles (arrows), but the tibialis anterior and soleus muscles are not involved. Reproduced with permission from Choi YJ, Hyun YS, Nam SH, Koo H, Hong YB, Chung KW, Choi BO. Novel compound heterozygous nonsense PRX mutations in a Korean Dejerine-Sottas neuropathy family. *J Clin Neurol*. 2015; 11(1):92–6.

Pathophysiology

Several genes are responsible for the phenotype. Inheritance may be autosomal dominant or recessive.

PMP22 is produced primarily by Schwann cells, participating in the development and maintenance of myelin (Figure 53.3). The PMP22 gene may also be important for Schwann cell growth and differentiation. Mutations in PMP22 additionally cause the distinct disorder of hereditary neuropathy with liability to pressure palsies, which is also associated with hypomyelination.

Myelin protein-zero (MPZ) is the major structural protein of peripheral myelin, accounting for more than 50 percent of the protein present in the sheath of peripheral nerves. MPZ links adjacent lamellae, thereby stabilizing the myelin assembly. Severe mutations cause intracellular accumulation of mutant proteins, primarily within the endoplasmic reticulum.

The PRX gene encodes 2 isoforms, L- and S-periaxin, which are structural proteins expressed by myelinating Schwann cells in the peripheral nervous system. Periaxin interacts with the dystroglycan complex, linking the basal lamina to the Schwann cell cytoskeleton.

EGR2 is a transcription factor that binds to specific areas of DNA, regulating the activity of numerous genes. Thus, it is thought that ERG2 mutations disrupt the control of genes involved in myelin formation and maintenance.

Diagnosis

Cerebrospinal fluid protein is elevated and attributed to nerve root involvement. Nerve conduction is very slow and often below 10 m/s. Genotyping for several genetic defects is available. The most frequent gene mutations involve PMP22.

Treatment

Treatment for Déjérine–Sottas is supportive. In the *trembler* mouse, reduced apoptosis was detected after curcumin treatment of cells in tissue culture that express PMP22 mutants. Curcumin significantly decreases the percentage of apoptotic Schwann cells, resulting in increased number and size of myelinated

(a)

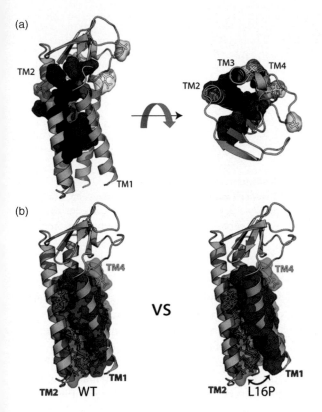

(b)

VS

Figure 53.3 Assessment of disease mutation locations in a PMP22 model. **a.** PMP22 homology model with color coding of wild-type residues mutated in neuropathies according to affected individual motor nerve conduction velocities (NCVs), with maroon having the lowest NCVs and cream representing a benign polymorphism. Note that for a number of known disease mutations, nerve conduction velocities have not been reported, such that the associated sites are not highlighted in this figure. Note also that the lone site of a severe mutation facing the lipid environment is a proline substitution (Leu71Pro) in the middle of transmembrabe domain 2, which is expected also to disrupt helical packing. **b.** Comparison of the packing interface between the wild type model and the top two L16P models, showing a reduced interface for L16P between transmembrane domain 1 and the rest of the bundle: red for transmembrane domain 1, marine for transmembrane domain 2, violet for transmembrane domain 3, green for transmembrane domain 4, and salmon for the additional contacting residue on L16P transmembrane domain 1. Reproduced with permission from Mittendorf KF et al. The homology model of PMP22 suggests mutations resulting in peripheral neuropathy disrupt transmembrane helix packing. *Biochemistry.* 2014; 53(39):6139–41.

axons in sciatic nerves in association with improved motor performance. MPZ frameshift mutations associated with severe disease also cause an intracellular accumulation of mutant proteins, primarily within the endoplasmic reticulum, which induces apoptosis. Curcumin releases the ER-retained MPZ mutants into the cytoplasm, and this is also accompanied by a lower number of apoptotic cells.

Bibliography

Choi Y.J., Hyun Y.S., Nam S.H., et al. (2015). Novel compound heterozygous nonsense PRX mutations in a Korean Dejerine-Sottas neuropathy family. *J Clin Neurol.* 11(1):92–6.

Jani-Acsadi A., Ounpuu S., Pierz K., et al. (2015). Pediatric Charcot-Marie-tooth disease. *Pediatr Clin North Am.* 62(3):767–86.

Myotonic Dystrophy

A boy came to medical attention because of abnormal language and motor development in early childhood. His birth and early development were unremarkable. In retrospect, concerns could have been raised at 9 months of age, when he first sat unsupported. He ambulated at 18 months. His overall intellectual development was judged very poor by the age of 4 years. At that time, he had no weakness and no myopathic features. There was no myotonia. He was dysarthric, with a prominent nasal voice. His full IQ at 4 years was 58 (Wechsler Preschool and Primary Scale of Intelligence). At 11 years old, his IQ had decreased to 47 (Wechsler Intelligence Scale for Children). By that time, he suffered from chronic diarrhea and exhibited a conduct disorder. He carried 2400 repeats in the 3′untranslated region of the myotonic dystrophy protein kinase gene DMPK, an expansion that he had inherited from his mother, who harbored fewer repeats.

Myotonic Dystrophy

Onset: Delayed acquisition of motor skills in infancy and decreased exercise tolerance.
Additional manifestations: Weakness (including the face), wasting and myotonia. Intelligence is usually subnormal. Congenital myotonic dystrophy causes floppy baby syndrome with respiratory and nutritional failure.
Disease mechanism: Autosomal dominant gain of function of an expanded untranslated CTG repeat in the gene that encodes dystrophia myotonica serine-threonine protein kinase (DMPK). The repeat induces the aggregation of RNA binding proteins, leading to aggregation and abnormal premRNA splicing.
Testing: Genotyping of DMPK for triplet repeat expansion.

Treatment: None effective.
Research highlights: Antisense oligonucleotides directed against the expanded repeat can restore excess protein aggregation and reduce myotonia.

Clinical Features

Myotonic dystrophy type 1 or Steinert disease is associated with progressive weakness and excessively sustained muscle contraction (myotonia) in the context of multisystem abnormalities. Its prevalence is about 10 in 100,000 individuals except in regions where a founder effect is present. These abnormalities involve the brain, eyes, and smooth muscle, and the cardiovascular and endocrine systems. Although the disease can be a prominent cause of progressive weakness in infancy, later onset and adult forms represent the most common muscular adult dystrophies. A congenital form is a frequent cause of severe floppy baby syndrome. In these cases, and for unknown reasons, the mutant myotonic gene is almost always inherited from the mother. In contrast, myotonic dystrophy type 2 is caused by mutation in a different gene, CNBP (CCHC (CysCysHisCys)-type zinc finger nucleic acid binding protein)/ZNF9 (Zinc Finger 9) and usually affects adults, except when it coexists with an additional mutation in the skeletal muscle chloride channel gene.

Myotonic dystrophy type 1 exhibits generational anticipation, with decreasing age of onset and increasing severity within the younger members of a family.

Infants with myotonic dystrophy first present to medical attention after a normal early developmental period. The age of onset is typically the second year of life. Initial manifestations include intellectual disability, speech or hearing impairment, delayed voluntary sphincter control, poor fine motor skills, and, more rarely, cardiac arrhythmia or postoperative apnea. Myotonia involves the hands, leading to decreased grip strength, with percussion myotonia often detected in the hand thenar eminence. Myotonia, however, may not be present in the infantile form of the disease. The pattern of weakness is prominent over the finger flexor and face muscles. Ptosis and dysarthria can also be present. Atrophy of the anterior neck, masseter, and temporalis muscles may be revealing. Median disease survival is 50 years.

Later onset forms of the disease and the advanced disease are also characterized by cataracts, heart block, gonadal failure, and features of the metabolic syndrome (insulin resistance and hyperlipidemia, which can be compounded by hypothyroidism). Smooth muscle dysfunction is thought to account for gastroesophageal reflux, gastroparesis, intestinal dysmotility and pseudoobstruction and anorectal dysfunction. There may be pain in skeletal muscles, which is aggravated by cold or exercise. Manifestations during pregnancy include polyhydramnios, placenta previa, miscarriage, and postpartum hemorrhage.

Pathology

Muscle nuclei are internally located in the myotonic dystrophies and can be grouped in chains. Muscle fibers are lost and replaced with fibrous and fat tissue. There are sarcoplasmic masses of disorganized myofibrils and dilated sarcoplasmic reticulum. Atrophy of type 1 muscle fibers is associated with hypertrophy of type 2 fibers. Accumulation of the protein musclebind can be detected and is useful in distinguishing myotonic dystrophy type 1 from type 2.

Pathophysiology

Myotonic dystrophy results from a dominantly heritable trinucleotide repeat (CTG) expansion in the 3' region of the dystrophia myotonica serine-threonine protein kinase (DMPK) gene. This region normally spans 4–40 copies of the trinucleotide. The tendency of the repeat to multiply increases with size. Asymptomatic carriers of the expanded repeat (often called premutation carriers) harbor 3–50 copies, whereas affected individuals carry 50 to 4000 copies. Affected children typically exhibit over 1000 repeats. The CTG tract, however, may be interrupted towards the 3' end of the repeat. Nevertheless, the serine-threonine kinase activity remains normal. The expansion of the repeat forms a hairpin and leads to a gain of function of the resulting 3' end of the mutant RNA. Excessive nuclear accumulation of this very stable mutant RNA sequesters regulatory proteins, leading to abnormal pre-mRNA splicing for several proteins including the skeletal muscle chloride channel and the insulin receptor, which are responsible for myotonia and diabetes, respectively. The expression of both molecules is dysregulated, with a preponderant expression of fetal isoforms. This results in the production of a chloride channel with reduced conductance and of an insulin receptor with decreased sensitivity to its natural ligand insulin. Additional mechanisms include the spurious translation initiation of the expanded mRNA, bidirectional transcription, aberrant DNA methylation and microRNA dysregulation.

The CTG repeat exhibits somatic instability, undergoing expansion over time and across generations. Most individuals are mosaic for different repeat lengths, with greater expansions detectable in muscle, heart, and brain.

Diagnosis

Genotyping is used for the diagnosis of myotonic dystrophy. Long-range polymerase chain reaction followed by agarose gel size-separation of the resulting DNA fragments is also used for diagnosis. However, about 5% of affected individuals carry interruptions in the 3' end of the repeat that make standard polymerase chain reaction unsuitable. A variety of polymerase chain reaction-based alternative methods is available to diagnose such affected individuals. Muscle biopsy can illustrate typical changes in affected individuals who elude DNA diagnosis.

Treatment

In addition to symptomatic supportive treatment, several drugs and other interventions are being investigated. Mexiletine, a muscle sodium channel blocker, can provide symptomatic relief of myotonia. Antisense oligonucleotides are small synthetic analogs of DNA or RNA that bind specifically to a target RNA blocking it or inducing its cleavage by the enzyme RNaseH. These oligonucleotides, which must be delivered systemically or intramuscularly, appear to be effective in a mouse model of the disease via the release of proteins from pathological aggregates, with correction of RNA splicing defects and reduction of myotonia.

Bibliography

Echenne B., Rideau A., Roubertie A., et al. (2008). Myotonic dystrophy type I in childhood Long-term evolution in patients surviving the neonatal period. *Eur J Paediatr Neurol.* 12(3):210–23.

Ho G., Cardamone M., Farrar M. (2015). Congenital and childhood myotonic dystrophy: Current aspects of disease and future directions. *World J Clin Pediatr.* 4(4):66–80.

Vici Syndrome

A group of 18 children afflicted by the same disorder was studied for the purpose of causal gene discovery. They were included in the study if four of five diagnostic criteria (callosal agenesis, cataracts, cardiomyopathy, hypopigmentation, and immunodeficiency) were fulfilled. They also exhibited marked generalized hypopigmentation relative to their ethnic background. Coarsening of facial features with full lips and macroglossia was noted in some of the older children. There was marked retinal hypopigmentation on fundoscopy. Microcephaly was either present at birth or developed over time. Failure to thrive was a common finding. Additional neural abnormalities included (in order of frequency) cerebellar and pontine hypoplasia, paucity of white matter and ventricular dilatation, heterotopias, abnormalities of the septum pellucidum, and schizencephaly. About one half of the children had died before their fourth birthday.

Vici Syndrome

Onset: Neonatal or early infantile combination of hypotonia, decreased pigmentation, and poor feeding. Dysmorphic features may be present.

Additional manifestations: Minimal neurological development with loss of rolling ability. Optic nerve hypoplasia and cataracts. Sensorineural hearing loss. Agenesis of the corpus callosum. Medication refractory seizures. Progressive skeletal and cardiac myopathy. Immune deficiency.

Disease mechanism: Vici syndrome is a disorder of autophagy. Autosomal recessive loss of function of EPG5 leads to failure of autophagosome-lysosome fusion with deficient cargo delivery to the lysosome.

Testing: No specific testing is available other than genetic assay.

Treatment: Immunoglobulin and antibiotic prophylaxis for immune deficiency.

Research highlights: EPG5 knockout mice recapitulate the autophagy defect and the skeletal muscle myopathy typical of the human syndrome.

Clinical Features

Vici syndrome is a progressive multisystem disorder caused by autosomal recessive mutation of EPG5, which encodes ectopic P-granules autophagy protein 5, a regulator of autophagy. The main features of the disease include agenesis of the corpus callosum, cataracts, oculocutaneous hypopigmentation, cardiomyopathy, and combined immunodeficiency.

There is hypopigmentation of eyes and hair. Some affected individuals exhibit facial dysmorphic features such as cleft lip or palate and micrognathia, or syndactyly. Head size is normal at birth but progresses to microcephaly. Feeding difficulties are usually noted at onset soon after birth and eventually lead to failure to thrive. Optic nerve hypoplasia and cataracts lead to poor vision with nystagmus. Sensorineural hearing loss may also account in part for developmental disability. Intellectual development is poor and seizures occur often. Children learn to roll over but do not sit independently or acquire speech. The ability to roll may later disappear. Progressive skeletal muscle myopathy is associated with hypotonia and abnormal motor development. Tendon reflexes may be absent. Cardiomyopathy may lead to progressive heart failure. Most affected individuals suffer from repetitive infections of the respiratory, gastrointestinal, and urinary systems in addition to mucocutaneous candidiasis, conjunctivitis, and sepsis. Hepatomegaly with liver dysfunction has been sometimes in association with increased glycogen storage. Death occurs at a median age of 42 months.

Pathology

Brain MR imaging demonstrates agenesis of the corpus callosum, pontine hypoplasia, reduced opercularization of the Sylvian fissures, and decreased myelination (Figure 55.1). There is also abnormal thalamic signal similar to what has been described in affected individuals with lysosomal storage disorders. The skeletal muscle displays marked fiber type disproportion, increase in internal nuclei, numerous vacuoles, abnormal mitochondria, and excess glycogen storage (Figure 55.2). There is also type I fiber hypotrophy with normally sized type 2 fibers resembling fiber type disproportion. In the nerve, almost complete absence of myelinated axons has been reported.

Pathophysiology

Autophagy involves several regulated steps, comprising from the formation of phagophores to the generation of autophagosomes, which are fused with lysosomes resulting in autolysosomes, the final structures of degradation. EPG5 deficiency results in failure of autophagosome-lysosome fusion and, ultimately, impaired cargo delivery to the lysosome. It is not known whether impaired autophagy is the

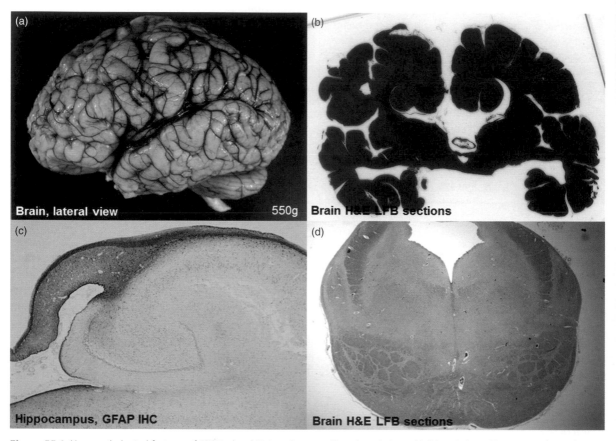

Figure 55.1 Neuropathological features of EPG5-related Vici syndrome. a. Gross lateral view of left hemisphere. Note somewhat indistinct gyral pattern, and relatively prominent sulci for age. The insula is visible, consistent with an opercularization defect, and the Sylvian fissure extends more posteriorly than normal. b. Whole-brain section stained with Luxol Fast blue/haematoxylin and eosin (LFB/H&E) at the level of the thalamus. Note the callosal agenesis, prominent temporal ventricles, and malrotated hippocampi. c. Hippocampus immunostained for glial fibrillary acidic protein (GFAP). Most notable is the diminutive size of the fornix and associated reactive gliosis. d. Transverse brainstem section at the level of the pons, stained with LFB/H&E. Note the small size of the pons, which is estimated to be less than half its normal volume. The superior cerebellar peduncles are relatively normal, as is the tegmentum, but the size of the medial lemniscus and corticospinal tracts are somewhat reduced, albeit less than the pontine grey matter. Reproduced with permission from Byrne S et al. EPG5-related Vici syndrome: a paradigm of neurodevelopmental disorders with defective autophagy. *Brain.* 2016; 139(Pt 3):765–81.

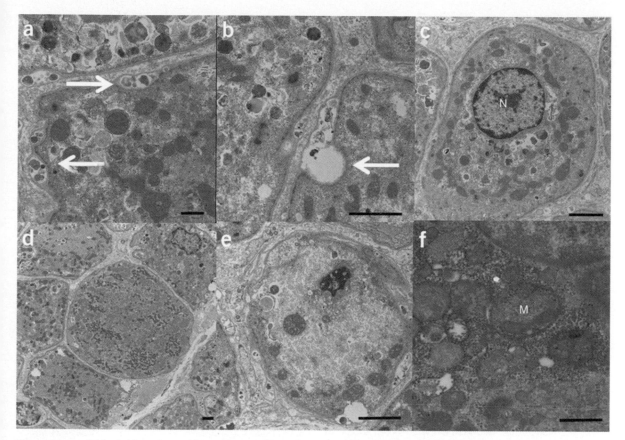

Figure 55.2 a–f. Muscle biopsy from a Vicy syndrome subject subjected to electron microscopy (transverse sections). In many fibers, there is material between the layers of basal lamina (a, arrows; scale bar, 500 nm) or overt exocytic vacuoles (b, arrow; scale bar, 2 µm). Some fibers show a single centralized nucleus (c; scale bar, 2 µm). Mitochondria are of variable size and distribution. In some fibers, they form a loop around the nucleus in the periphery of the fiber, resembling a necklace as in c; in others, they form clusters (d; scale bar, 2 µm). The appearance of cristae is often abnormal (e; scale bar, 2 µm; f; scale bar, 500 nm). N, nucleus; M, mitochondrion. Reproduced with permission from Cullup T et al. Recessive mutations in EPG5 cause Vici syndrome, a multisystem disorder with defective autophagy. *Nat Genet*. 2013; 45(1):83–7.

only consequence of EPG5 deficiency, or one expression of a generalized vesicular trafficking defect. In addition, some aspects of the syndrome may represent secondary effects of the defective autophagy such as reduced mitochondrial quality control and accumulation of defective proteins.

Diagnosis

There is no specific diagnostic assay other than genetic analysis.

Treatment

Intravenous immunoglobulin replacement and antimicrobial prophylaxis can be instituted to palliate immune deficiency.

Bibliography

Cullup T., Kho A.L., Dionisi-Vici C., et al. (2013). Recessive mutations in EPG5 cause Vici syndrome, a multisystem disorder with defective autophagy. *Nat Genet*. 45(1):83–7.

Aicardi–Goutières Syndrome

A boy was born at 35 weeks gestation with a birth weight of 2550 g (3rd percentile) and a head circumference of 33 cm (3rd percentile). On the first day of life, he developed truncal purpura due to thrombocytopenia (76000 platelets/mL). During the first weeks of life, hepatomegaly, hypersomnia and hypotonia with poor feeding were noted. At 3 months of age, the child developed episodes of irritability and insomnia accompanied by opisthotonus that evolved into dyskinesia and myoclonic seizures over the course of several weeks. Cerebrospinal fluid glucose and lactate, examined on several occasions during the first year of life were within normal limits, but lymphocyte count and interferon-α were increased. Initial EEGs showed diffuse background slowing and intermittent delta slowing over the posterior regions. At 5 years of age, bi-frontal sharp slow waves with secondary generalization appeared. At this time, seizure semiology was myoclonic with occasional tonic seizures and atypical absences. Epilepsy was managed with various combinations of antiepileptic drugs, but seizure freedom was never achieved. Computed tomography and magnetic resonance imaging findings included calcifications, white matter abnormalities with temporo-polar cystic degeneration, as well as frontal cerebral atrophy (Figure). The skin on ears, legs, feet, and hands was dry and scaly and nails were brittle. Since the age of 3 years, he presented with erythematous ulcerating lesions, also known as chilblain lesions, on fingers, heels, toes, and nose (Figure). In addition, recurrent ulcers of the oral mucosa and lips appeared. At the age of 6 years, he experienced painful swelling of his knees, elbows, and interphalangeal and metacarpophalangeal joints. At age 12 years, the child was in poor condition with severe developmental delay, spastic tetraplegia, multiple contractures, and severe scoliosis. He also continued to have dystonia and refractory epilepsy.

Aicardi-Goutières Syndrome

Onset: In 20% of cases, neonatal hepatosplenomegaly and thrombocytopenia. In 80%, severe subacute encephalopathy with irritability and feeding difficulties.

Additional manifestations: Epilepsy, developmental regression, leukoencephalopathy and cerebral calcifications. Chilblains over the fingers, toes, and ears. Intracranial vasculopathy in some forms.

Disease mechanism: Autosomal dominant or recessive in one of six causal genes. Accumulation of DNA and RNA due to deficient nuclease activity, which triggers inflammation.

Testing: Chronic cerebrospinal fluid pleocytosis and neopterin and interferon-α elevation. Characteristic interferon pattern in plasma.

Treatment: None effective.

Clinical Features

Aicardi–Goutières syndrome is an autosomal dominant or recessive disorder that affects principally the brain, the immune system, and the skin. Mutations in six genes have been identified in individuals with Aicardi–Goutières syndrome: TREX1 (three prime repair exonuclease 1), RNASEH2A (subunit A of ribonuclease H2), RNASEH2B (subunit B of ribonuclease H2), RNASEH2C (subunit C of ribonuclease H2), SAMHD1 (SAM (sterile alpha motif (SAM)) domain and HD (histidine-aspartic) domain-containing protein 1) and ADAR (double-stranded RNA-specific adenosine deaminase). Whereas most mutations are inherited recessively, TREX1-related and ADAR-related Aicardi–Goutières syndrome can be the result of a *de novo* dominant pathogenic variant.

About 20 percent newborns with Aicardi–Goutières syndrome, mainly those harboring TREX1 pathogenic variants, are born with hepatosplenomegaly, elevated blood levels of liver enzymes and thrombocytopenia and exhibit abnormal neurological development. While this combination of signs and symptoms is typically associated with response to congenital viral infection, no infection is detected in these infants.

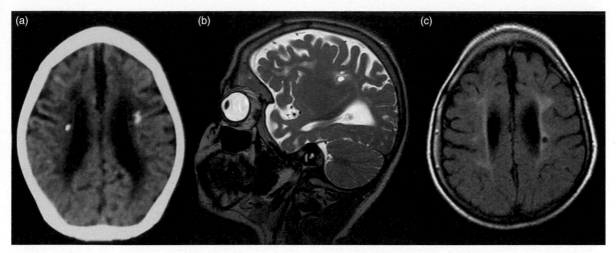

Figure 56.1 Brain imaging findings in Aicardi–Goutières syndrome. Computed tomography scans taken at the age of 1 year (a) show periventricular hypodensities with spotty calcifications around slightly dilated ventricles. Magnetic resonance imaging scans taken at 9 years of age (b: sagittal T2-weighted sequence, c: axial fluid-attenuated inversion recovery sequence) depict mild cerebral atrophy and extensive leucoencephalopathy more pronounced in the frontal lobes with a cystic vacuole on the left side. Reproduced with permission from Ramantani G et al. Aicardi–Goutières syndrome and systemic lupus erythematosus (SLE) in a 12-year-old boy with SAMHD1 mutations. *J Child Neurol.* 2011; 26(11):1425–8.

In the remainder 80 percent of cases and within the first year of life, most individuals with Aicardi–Goutières syndrome experience an episode of severe subacute encephalopathy that may last for several months. During this phase of the disorder, affected babies are usually irritable and do not feed well. They may develop intermittent fevers in the absence of infection and may have seizures. They stop developing new skills and later experience developmental regression. Growth of the brain and skull is retarded, resulting in microcephaly. In this phase of the disorder, white blood cells and inflammatory mediators can be detected in the cerebrospinal fluid. Neuroimaging reveals leukodystrophy and calcification (Figure 56.1). This encephalopathic phase of Aicardi–Goutières syndrome leaves neurological sequelae, including profound intellectual disability, spasticity, dystonia, and truncal hypotonia.

About 40 percent of individuals with Aicardi–Goutières syndrome develop painful, itchy skin lesions, located usually on the fingers, toes, and ears (Figure 56.2). These puffy, red lesions, which are called chilblains, are caused by inflammation of small blood vessels. They may be brought on or made worse by exposure to cold. Mouth ulcers may also occur.

As a result of the severe neurological problems associated with the disease, many individuals do not survive past childhood.

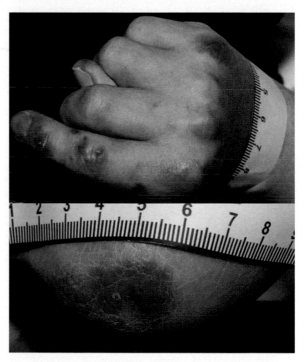

Figure 56.2 Aicardi–Goutières syndrome. Chilblain lesions on fingers and heel at age 12 years. Reproduced with permission from Ramantani G et al. Aicardi–Goutières syndrome and systemic lupus erythematosus (SLE) in a 12-year-old boy with SAMHD1 mutations. *J Child Neurol.* 2011; 26(11):1425–8.

Several special phenotypes can occur: RNASEH2B pathogenic variants are associated with a later age at presentation, lower childhood mortality, and relatively preserved intellectual function and head circumference. Milder phenotypes have also been associated with pathogenic variants in SAMHD1. ADAR-related disease resembles bilateral striatal necrosis with severe dystonia.

Pathology

There is marked microcephaly and diffuse but non-homogeneous demyelination with astrocytosis in the absence of storage or myelin breakdown. Multiple wedge-shaped microinfarcts in the neocortex and cerebellar cortex suggest microangiopathy. There are also calcific deposits in the white matter, thalami, basal ganglia and dentate nuclei, in addition to calcification of the media, adventitia, and perivascular spaces of small vessels.

Inflammation in the leptomeninges with areas of necrosis is also characteristic.

In the skin, tubuloreticular inclusions in endothelial cells have been observed in some individuals, particularly those with high circulating levels of IFN-α. On direct immunofluorescence, fine granular staining for IgM may be seen in the basement membrane. Biopsies frequently show a lymphocytic or leukocytoclastic vasculitis.

Pathophysiology

The TREX1, RNASEH2A, RNASEH2B, and RNASEH2C genes encode nucleases, which degrade DNA and RNA. Mutations in any of these genes probably result in an absent or dysfunctional nuclease. This may result in the accumulation of discarded DNA and RNA in cells. These DNA and RNA molecules or fragments may be generated during the first stage of protein transcription, replication in preparation for cell division, DNA repair, cell death and other processes. The unneeded DNA and RNA may elicit immune reactions that result in encephalopathy, skin lesions, and other features of the syndrome.

The SAMHD1 gene encodes a protein of unknown function possibly related to the immune system and inflammation.

Diagnosis

Neuroimaging reveals calcification of the basal ganglia putamen, globus pallidus and thalamus, and white matter. In particular, MR imaging shows leukodystrophic changes manifest in T2-weighted images as a hyperintense signal most commonly located around the horns of the ventricles. In severe early-onset cases, white matter changes can be prominent frontally and be associated with temporal lobe cyst formation. Progressive atrophy of the periventricular white matter and sulci is a frequent feature. Cerebellar atrophy and brain stem atrophy may be prominent.

Aicardi–Goutières syndrome is associated with an interferon signature, which is sustained over time and can thus be used to reliably identify affected individuals. Chronic cerebrospinal fluid lymphocytosis is another common feature. Typical values range from 5–100 lymphocytes/mm^3 (normal: <2 lymphocytes/mm^3). There is also increased concentration of interferon-α in the cerebrospinal fluid in addition to elevated neopterin.

Treatment

There is no effective treatment. The role of immunosuppressive agents in the treatment of Aicardi–Goutières syndrome is being studied. In the syndrome variant associated with intracranial large-vessel disease in association with mutation of SAMHD1, the typically occlusive and aneurysmal arteriopathies described may be amenable to treatment (revascularization for the former and coiling or clipping for the latter). The possible inflammatory basis of this arteriopathy suggests that additional immunosuppression may have therapeutic value.

Bibliography

Ramantani G., Häusler M., Niggemann P., et al. (2011). Aicardi-Goutières syndrome and systemic lupus erythematosus (SLE) in a 12-year-old boy with SAMHD1 mutations. *J Child Neurol.* 26(11:1425–8.

Rice G.I., Forte G.M., Szynkiewicz M., et al. (2013). Assessment of interferon-related biomarkers in Aicardi-Goutières syndrome associated with mutations in TREX1, RNASEH2A, RNASEH2B, RNASEH2C, SAMHD1, and ADAR: a case-control study. *Lancet Neurol.* 12(12):1159–69.

Infantile Andersen Disease

A girl, the first child of consanguineous parents, was born at 33 weeks of gestation by emergency cesarean section due to fetal bradycardia. She was unable to breathe, was intubated, and was administered mechanical ventilation and nasogastric feeding for the rest of her life. Birth weight was 2120 g, head circumference was 34 cm and length 46 cm. Apgar scores were 2, 5, and 7 at 1, 5, and 10 min, respectively. She manifested severe generalized hypotonia, slight knee and ankle contractures and spontaneous movements were limited to the feet. There were bilateral ptosis and roving eye movements. Tendon reflexes were present. Echocardiogram showed cardiomyopathy with ventricular hypokinesia and markedly reduced ejection fraction (25%). She required tracheostomy because of recurrent respiratory infections. She died of cardiorespiratory failure at 3 months, 16 days of age. A muscle biopsy was obtained at 1 month of age and an autopsy was also performed (Figures 57.1, 57.2 and 57.3).

Infantile Andersen Disease

Onset: Polyhydramnios and decreased fetal movement. Severe progressive neonatal hypotonia and weakness.
Additional manifestations: In the infantile form, hypoglycemia, hepatopathy and cardiomyopathy. Features of anterior horn cell disease with respiratory and nutritional failure. Death ensues in the first weeks or months of life.
Disease mechanism: Accumulation of abnormal glycogen with fewer branching points and longer outer branches due to glycogen branching enzyme deficiency.
Testing: Biopsy of accessible tissues (muscle, fibroblasts, and liver) followed by enzymatic assay.

Treatment: None effective.
Research highlights: Characterization of disparate disease forms (congenital, perinatal, juvenile and adult) due to the same enzyme deficiency.

Clinical Features

Glycogen storage disease type IV or Andersen disease, is an autosomal recessive disorder due to glycogen branching enzyme deficiency with an incidence of 1 in every 800,000 births. The clinical presentation of glycogen branching enzyme deficiency is heterogeneous. The most common branching enzyme mutations cause rapidly progressive cirrhosis and liver failure in childhood. A milder, non-progressive hepatic variant has also been described. In a few children cardiomyopathy dominates the phenotype. The neuromuscular presentations may be of variable onset (congenital, perinatal, juvenile, and adult) and in severity and include severe hypotonia in the neonatal period, multisystemic disorders with myopathy, neuropathy, and variably severe liver involvement, or late-onset neurodegenerative disease (adult polyglucosan body disease).

The fatal infantile neuromuscular variant of glycogen branching enzyme deficiency shares with Werdnig–Hoffmann disease severe hypotonia early in life, rapid deteriorating course and electromyographic findings. Some cases have been associated to polyhydramnios and decreased fetal movements. Cardiomyopathy may also be an associated feature. Fasting hypoglycemia is a typical feature of glycogen storage disease type I and III, but is rarely seen in type IV. Death typically occurs between 4 weeks and 4 months of age.

Pathology

An important disease feature are periodic acid-Schiff-positive and diastase-resistant globules in tissues from infants with profound weakness (Figures 57.1 to 57.3). These polyglucosan bodies consist of amorphous electron-dense granules and irregular branched filaments and appear to form whenever there is an imbalance between the activities of the two main enzymes of glycogen synthesis, glycogen synthase and glycogen branching enzyme, to the advantage of the former. Muscle biopsy reveals accumulation of abundant polyglucosan in muscle fibers. Electron microscopy shows accumulation of amorphous electron-dense granules and irregular branched amylopectin-like filaments (polyglucosans) in the cytoplasm, together with very electron-dense material showing a sharp and irregular contour resembling asteroid bodies.

Pathophysiology

Glycogen branching enzyme 1 is ubiquitously expressed. The enzyme catalyzes the last step in glycogen biosynthesis by attaching short glucosyl chains (about six glucosyl units in length) in α-1,6 glucosidic links to naked peripheral chains of nascent glycogen. The newly attached short branches are then elongated by the other major glycogenosynthetic enzyme, glycogen synthetase. Thus, glycogen branching enzyme

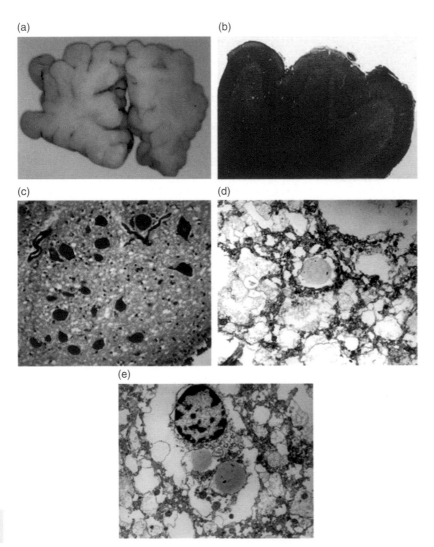

(a)

(b)

(c)

(d)

(e)

Figure 57.1 Andersen disease. Central nervous system. a. Focal cortical polymicrogyria, mainly in the right orbito-frontal cortex. b. Absence of clear lamination with protrusion of layer I into deeper layers. c. PAS-positive polyglucosan inclusions are evident in neurons of the oculomotor nuclei (PAS 400×). d. At electron microscopy (EM) polyglucosan bodies are observed in neurons in both processes and (e) perikaryon (EM 14,000× and 8800×). Reproduced with permission from Taratuto AL et al. Branching enzyme deficiency/glycogenosis storage disease type IV presenting as a severe congenital hypotonia: Muscle biopsy and autopsy findings, biochemical and molecular genetic studies. *Neuromuscul Disord*. 2010; 20(12):783–90.

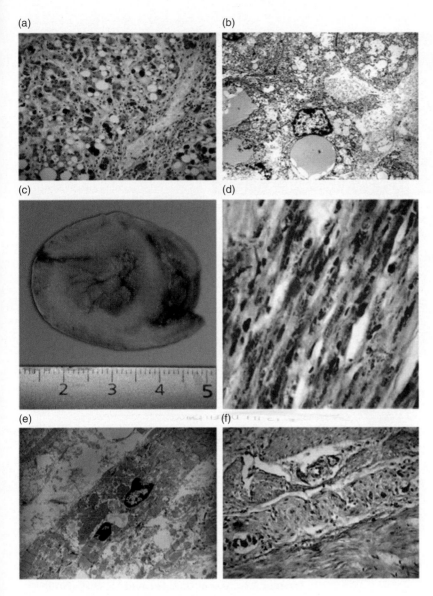

Figure 57.2 Andersen disease. Liver. **a.** Steatosis and structural disorganization, fibrosis, and extensive polyglucosan inclusions (PAS-hematoxylin 250×). **b.** Intracytoplasmic polyglucosan inclusion (EM 6000×). Heart. **c.** Hypertrophic cardiomyopathy. **d.** PAS positive, diastase resistant intracellular deposits in the myocardium (PAS 250×). **e.** Polyglucosan bodies could be disclosed in the myofibers together with enlarged mitochondria (EM 6000×). f Neurons from the myenteric plexus of the large bowel are also involved. PAS-hematoxylin 100×. Reproduced with permission from Taratuto AL et al. Branching enzyme deficiency/glycogenosis storage disease type IV presenting as a severe congenital hypotonia: Muscle biopsy and autopsy findings, biochemical and molecular genetic studies. *Neuromuscul Disord.* 2010; 20(12):783–90.

deficiency results in the accumulation of abnormal glycogen with fewer branching points and longer outer branches, an amylopectin-like structure. This abnormal glycogen, known as polyglucosan, accumulates in all tissues to various degrees.

Missense mutations in the glycogen branching enzyme gene have been identified in individuals with typical presentation, with non-progressive hepatic presentations and with adult polyglucosan body disease. None of these mutations involve the proposed catalytic sites of the enzyme, which may explain why they are associated with less severe and later-onset disease. In contrast, the mutations reported in all neonatal cases are either large deletions or frameshift mutations, which effectively abolish branching enzyme activity.

Diagnosis

The diagnosis can be established via biopsy of accessible tissues (muscle, fibroblasts, and liver) followed by enzymatic assay.

Electromyography can reveal fibrillations and positive sharp waves suggestive of a neurogenic process, or short duration polyphasic potentials suggestive of a myopathy. This is in agreement with autopsy

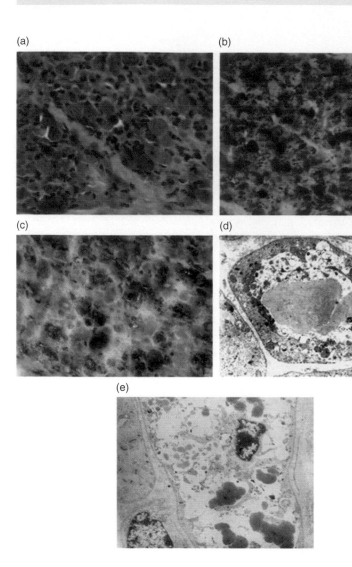

Figure 57.3 Andersen disease. Muscle biopsy. **a.** Prominent perimysial fibrosis, rounded and angulated fibers with variation in sizes within the same fascicles (H&E 250×). **b.** PAS-positive material within muscle fibers, most of which is resistant to diastase digestion (PAS-diastase 250×). **c.** Abnormal reddish material within some vacuolated fibers (Gomori trichrome 250×). **d.** and **e.** Electron microscopy shows myofibrillar degeneration and intracytoplasmic inclusions of amorphous, homogeneous or slightly granular polyglucosan bodies, some of them with higher density (**e**) (8800× EM). Reproduced with permission from Taratuto AL et al. Branching enzyme deficiency/glycogenosis storage disease type IV presenting as a severe congenital hypotonia: Muscle biopsy and autopsy findings, biochemical and molecular genetic studies. *Neuromuscul Disord.* 2010; 20(12): 783–90.

findings in which some affected individuals display marked accumulation of abnormal polysaccharide in spinal motor neurons.

Prenatal diagnosis has been achieved through determination of branching enzyme activity and DNA analysis of chorionic villi or cultured amniocytes.

Treatment

There is no effective treatment.

Bibliography

Taratuto A.L., Akman H.O., Saccoliti M., et al. (2010). Branching enzyme deficiency/glycogenosis storage disease type IV presenting as a severe congenital hypotonia: Muscle biopsy and autopsy findings, biochemical and molecular genetic studies. *Neuromuscul Disord.* 20(12):783–90.

Tay S.K., Akman H.O., Chung W.K., et al. (2004). Fatal infantile neuromuscular presentation of glycogen storage disease type IV. *Neuromuscul Disord.* 14(4):253–60.

Familial Infantile Bilateral Striatal Necrosis

A girl was born following an uneventful pregnancy and delivery at 37 weeks of gestation. Her development was normal until age 15 months, when she was evaluated because of an inability to walk alone. Examination revealed truncal hypotonicity with brisk tendon reflexes (3+). She could sit without support, crawl on all four extremities and pull herself up from a sitting to a standing position. Reevaluation was performed at 21 months. The mother reported that during the 6 months prior to the visit, the child had lost the ability to crawl. She was no longer able to do purposeful hand movements or to speak. There were signs of increasing difficulty with swallowing and weight loss. The most prominent neurologic feature was choreoathetosis of the trunk, face, and limbs. The child could not stand, and ambulated by shuffling on her buttocks; this explained the pressure sores noted on the lateral malleoli. When she was pulled from a supine to a sitting position, she showed extreme head lag. When helped to stand, she arched her head backwards in an opisthotonic posture. She could reach for an object, but her grasp was clumsy. Ten months later, gastrostomy feeding was initiated because of dysphagia and severe weight loss. At the age of 40 months, pendular nystagmus was first noted. On the last examination at 10 years, there were choreoathetoid and hemiballistic movements of the extremities with spastic quadriplegia. Although the child was bedridden and had no verbal skills, she was able to communicate nonverbally with her parents and caregivers. Sensation was normal. Optic disc examination revealed bilateral pallor of the discs. At age 11 years, she died of sepsis and cachexia.

Familial Infantile Bilateral Striatal Necrosis

Onset: 7 to 15 months of age, with dysphagia and vomiting, failure to achieve developmental milestones or motor and cognitive regression.

Additional manifestations: Choreoathetosis, dystonia, spasticity, nystagmus, optic atrophy, and mental retardation.

Disease mechanism: Mitochondrial dysfunction due to mutation of ATP6 or NDUFV1 respiratory chain genes, or nuclear pore dysfunction caused by mutation of NUP62. There is spongy degeneration of the caudate nucleus and putamen and, occasionally, of the globus pallidus.

Testing: Neuroimaging or autopsy illustrate typical morphologic disease features.

Treatment: Biotin has resulted in interruption of disease progression in some individuals and in amelioration of motor symptoms in others.

Research highlights: Elucidation of the function of nuclear pore complex proteins including NUP62, a disease causing gene.

Clinical Features

Familial infantile bilateral striatal necrosis or infantile striatal necrosis is an autosomal recessive or mitochondrial DNA disorder characterized by symmetric spongy degeneration of the caudate nucleus, putamen, and occasionally the globus pallidus, with little or no involvement of the rest of the brain. The disease differs from Leigh syndrome on several respects: later age at onset, lesser severity of symptoms, normal levels of lactate and pyruvate, and normal morphology on electron microscopy muscle biopsy studies.

Age at disease onset ranges from 7 to 15 months. At presentation, all children have typically achieved a developmental age of 5 to 6 months. Initial symptoms include sudden appearance of dysphagia and vomiting, failure to achieve developmental milestones or motor and cognitive regression. Additional early clinical features include developmental regression, choreoathetosis, dystonia, spasticity, dysphagia, failure to thrive, nystagmus, optic atrophy, and mental retardation.

Head circumference at birth may be below the second percentile. Growth charts can illustrate a steep decline in the weight curve at the start of the symptoms, with all affected children fulfilling the criteria for failure to thrive. Some children are eventually able to walk with assistance and speak several words (developmental age of 12 to 15 months). Affected children appear alert and in a responsive nonverbal state. The most prominent finding, however, is choreoathetoid movements of the face, trunk, and extremities.

Over the years, children may become bedridden and unable to perform voluntary movements. Their choreoathetosis can progress to hemiballismus combined with dystonic postures. Acquired horizontal pendular nystagmus, commonly occurring in congenital and acquired disorders of myelin, may be prominent before 5 years of age. This is later followed by optic atrophy. Seizures are rare. All affected children ultimately develop spastic quadriparesis with scissoring of the legs, hyperactive tendon reflexes, and flexor plantar responses. Late in the disease course, children are able to hear, fixate and follow eye movements and to produce a social smile when they see their parents. The prognosis is poor, with early death usually due to intercurrent infection.

Pathology

Bilateral, symmetric, hyperintense signals are fist visible in the putamina by MR imaging (Figure 58.1). Follow-up after several years may reveal further changes. The caudate nucleus and the putamen become atrophic and the putamen may exhibit low signal on T1-weighted images and a high signal on T2-weighted images, compatible with malacia of the deep gray matter. In addition, the ventricles enlarge ex vacuo. Late in the disease course, in the second decade of life, MR imaging reveals a small, residual caudate nucleus and putamen with abnormal signals. The corpus callosum is thin. There is no involvement of the brainstem, periaqueductal gray matter, centrum semiovale, cerebral peduncles, or cerebellar hemispheres, which are all lesions typical of Leigh syndrome.

Brain weight is markedly reduced. There is hydrocephalus ex vacuo, most prominent in the lateral ventricles. There is severe atrophy of the lenticular nuclei, with retention of their normal color. The characteristic bulge of the caudate nucleus into the anterior part of the lateral ventricle is absent (Figure 58.2). The cerebellum and brainstem are grossly unremarkable except for a pale substantia nigra. Microscopic examination shows prominent gliosis and severe loss of neurons throughout the caudate, putamen, globus pallidus, and claustrum. These changes are less pronounced in the globus pallidus, which exhibits a larger number of preserved neurons than the caudate and putamen. Gliosis and loss of neurons are also prominent in the substantia nigra. The thalamus, mammillary bodies, hypothalamus, locus ceruleus, and cerebellum are normal. The cerebral cortex is normal, without appreciable neuronal loss.

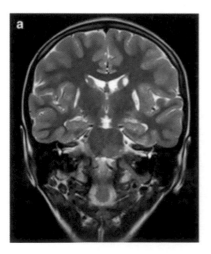
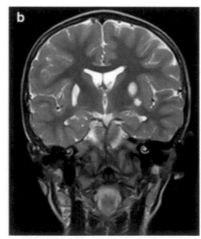

Figure 58.1 Infantile bilateral striatal necrosis. a. T2-weigthed coronal MR imaging of a 9-year-old girl demostrating symmetric cystic lesions of the putamen and caudate head. b. T2-weighted coronal MR imaging of her 5-year old sibling demonstrating bilateral lesions of the putamen resemblig those of his older sister. Reproduced with permission from Lal D et al. Homozygous missense mutation of NDUFV1 as the cause of infantile bilateral striatal necrosis. *Neurogenetics.* 2013; 14(1):85–7.

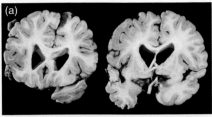
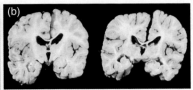
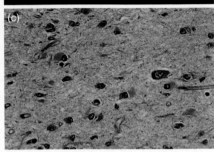

Figure 58.2 Infantile bilateral striatal necrosis. a. Coronal sections of the cerebral hemispheres. In the section on the right side, note the marked atrophy and loss of bulge of the caudate nucleus into the lateral ventricle. b. Coronal sections of the cerebral hemispheres at the level of the mamillary bodies, thalamus, and hypothalamus. c. Gliosis and neuronal loss in the putamen. Note the residual large neuron on the right side (LFB-hematoxylin-eosin, original magnification × 400). Reproduced with permission from Straussberg R et al. Familial infantile bilateral striatal necrosis: clinical features and response to biotin treatment. *Neurology.* 2002; 59(7):983–9.

Pathophysiology

Autosomal recessive mutations in NDUFV1 (a nuclear gene that encodes a complex I subunit) and NUP62 (a nucleoporin gene), and mitochondrial DNA mutations in ATP6 (which encodes part of complex V) cause familial infantile bilateral striatal necrosis. The disease mechanism can be provisionally inferred from its causal gene mutations. ATP6 and NDUFV1 mutations can be expected to impair the function of complexes V and I of the respiratory chain, respectively. The protein encoded by NUP62 belongs to the class of nucleoporins and is an essential part of the nuclear pore complex. The complex extends across the nuclear envelope, forming a gateway that regulates the flow of messenger RNA and proteins between the nucleus and the cytoplasm. Another gene encoding a protein localizing to a nuclear pore complex that causes human disease has been described previously. Mutations in the nucleoporin called ALADIN cause Allgrove (triple A) syndrome, which is characterized by adrenal insufficiency, abnormal development of the autonomic nervous system causing achalasia of the esophagus and alacrima, and late-onset progressive neurological symptoms (including cerebellar ataxia, peripheral neuropathy, and mild dementia).

Diagnosis

The diagnosis is established on a clinical and pathological or neuroimaging bases. EEG, visual evoked potentials, brainstem auditory response, electromyography, nerve conduction studies, and somatosensory evoked potentials are typically normal.

Treatment

Oral treatment with biotin has been associated with interruption of disease progression and with mild improvement in gross and fine motor capabilities in some individuals.

Bibliography

Basel-Vanagaite L., Muncher L., Straussberg R., et al. (2006). Mutated nup62 causes autosomal recessive infantile bilateral striatal necrosis. *Ann Neurol.* 60(2):214–22.

Lal D., Becker K., Motameny S., et al. (2013). Homozygous missense mutation of NDUFV1 as the cause of infantile bilateral striatal necrosis. *Neurogenetics.* 14(1):85–7.

Straussberg R., Shorer Z., Weitz R., et al. (2002). Familial infantile bilateral striatal necrosis: clinical features and response to biotin treatment. *Neurology.* 59(7):983–9.

Inherited Cobalamin Deficiency

A boy was born after an uneventful pregnancy by cesarean section due to an abnormal cardiotocography on gestational week 39. On day of life 3, he was admitted to the hospital because of feeding difficulties, absent suck reflex, weight loss of 12 percent, and hypotonia. Brain sonography, abdominal sonography, echocardiography, audiometry, and ophthalmologic examination were normal. Electroencephalography revealed mild unspecific alterations. Tandem mass spectrometry revealed elevated C3 carnitine levels in dried blood spots on day 5 of life. On follow-up the concentration of methylmalonic acid in urine was elevated (2200 mmol/mol creatinine, reference <10) as was the level of total homocysteine in serum (314 μmol/l, reference <15). The diagnosis of cobalamine Cbl-C defect was confirmed enzymatically and by mutation analysis. Enzyme studies performed on fibroblasts showed deficient methionine and serine formation when cells were grown in normal medium, compatible with the Cbl-C/D defect. In cells grown in medium supplemented with varying concentrations of hydroxocobalamin an increase of synthesis of methionine and serine was observed constituting a clear in vitro response to vitamin B12. The child was homozygous for the most frequent mutation of the MMACHC gene (Arg91Lys,fsX14).

Inherited Cobalamin Deficiency

Onset: In the early-onset infantile form, feeding difficulties, failure to thrive, somnolence, and hypotonia. In late-onset childhood or adolescence form, behavioral and psychiatric disturbances, or extrapyramidal and gait abnormalities.
Additional manifestations: Minor facial anomalies, epilepsy and progressive retinal disease. Hemolytic uremic syndrome. Megaloblastic anemia, hypersegmented neutrophils, thrombocytopenia, or pancytopenia.

Gastrointestinal dysfunction and congenital heart disease. In late-onset disease, myelopathy with progressive or relapsing-remitting course simulating multiple sclerosis.
Disease mechanism: Impaired conversion of dietary cobalamin into its two metabolically active forms.
Testing: Accumulation of homocysteine and methylmalonic acid and reduced methionine.
Treatment: Vitamin B12, betaine, and folic acid.
Research highlights: Deregulation of proteins involved in cellular detoxification, especially in glutathione metabolism, identified by proteomic analysis.

Clinical Features

The cobalamin C (Cbl-C) defect is the most common inborn error of cobalamin metabolism. Its incidence has been estimated as 1 in 100,000 live births. There are two predominant disease forms, depending on age of onset.

The clinical features of the early-onset infantile form include a multisystem disease with neurological, ocular, hematological, renal, gastrointestinal, cardiac, and pulmonary manifestations. Compared with the common forms of methylmalonic aciduria, the clinical manifestations of the Cbl-C defect are usually less acute. Affected individuals present with feeding difficulties, failure to thrive, somnolence, and hypotonia. Minor facial anomalies, such as long face, high forehead, large and low-set ears, and a flat philtrum are characteristic.

The neurological findings are severe and include hypotonia, abnormal neurological developmental, microcephaly, seizures, and hydrocephalus. Epilepsy is frequent and is characterized by partial seizures, both simple and complex, sometimes leading to convulsive status epilepticus, with a nonspecific EEG pattern. Ocular and visual abnormalities include visual inattention, nystagmus, or wandering eye movements. There may be progressive retinal disease ranging from subtle retinal nerve fiber layer loss to advanced macular and optic atrophy with salt and pepper pigmentation. Electroretinography studies indicate that, early in life, photopic and scotopic responses follow the lower limits of a normal developmental curve, progressing to attenuated or undetectable responses. Hemolytic uremic syndrome may also occur. Other cases manifest primary glomerular disease as segmental glomerulosclerosis or atypical glomerulopathy with features similar to idiopathic membranoproliferative glomerulonephritis and thrombotic microangiopathy. Megaloblastic anemia, hypersegmented neutrophils, thrombocytopenia or severe pancytopenia are the most common hematological findings. Gastrointestinal involvement manifests with vomiting, glossitis, stomatitis, atrophic gastritis and protein-losing enteropathy. Congenital heart disease may also occur and includes ventricular septal defect, pulmonary stenosis, dysplastic pulmonary valve, atrial defects and mitral valve prolapse.

The late onset form of the disease is rarer. It can manifest at any time from childhood to adulthood. In the context of milder or no hematological abnormalities, the clinical course is characterized by behavioral and psychiatric disturbances, rapid mental deterioration with confusion and disorientation, dementia, delirium, and psychosis.

Late onset disease can also present with purely neurological manifestations characterized by extrapyramidal symptoms and gait abnormalities occurring acutely or displaying a slowly progressive or relapsing-remitting course simulating multiple sclerosis. Myelopathic signs are the clinical expression of subacute degeneration of spinal cord, characterized by multifocal demyelination with vacuolation of dorsal and lateral columns, changes which are similar to adult spinal cord degeneration due to vitamin B12 deficiency. Renal disease may include chronic thrombotic microangiopathic glomerulo-nephropathy, which leads to end-stage renal failure. There is also retinal degeneration. Marfanoid features such as increased arm span, arachnodactyly, joint hyperlaxity and scoliosis have also been reported. The characteristic occurrence in late-onset cases of thromboembolic events, which are mostly localized in the great pulmonary vessels, and of spinal cord degeneration may indicate an age-dependent mechanism.

Pathology

MR imaging abnormalities in the early disease stage include hydrocephalus and diffuse supratentorial white matter swelling, followed by variable degrees of brain atrophy and white matter abnormalities. Basal ganglia lesions have also been reported.

Pathophysiology

The Cbl-C defect leads to impaired conversion of dietary cobalamin into its two metabolically active forms, methylcobalamin (MeCbl) and adenosylcobalamin (AdoCbl). MeCbl is the cofactor for methionine synthase, which catalyzes the conversion of homocysteine into methionine in the cytosol; AdoCbl is the cofactor for methylmalonyl-CoA mutase, which converts methylmalonyl coenzyme A into succinyl coenzyme A in mitochondria. The impaired activity of these two enzymes results in accumulation of homocysteine and methylmalonic acid as well as in reduced synthesis of methionine.

The gene responsible for the Cbl-C defect is MMACHC (methylmalonic aciduria and homocystinuria type C protein), which codifies the synthesis of CNCbl decyanase, an enzyme that catalyzes the decyanation reaction of CNCbl by using reducing equivalents given by cytosolic diflavin oxidoreductase, the prerequisite for CNCbl conversion into the active cofactors. The MMACHC protein also displays an alkyltransferase activity that catalyzes the dealkylation of newly internalized methylcobalamin and 5′-deoxyadenosylcobalamin, the naturally occurring alkylcobalamins that are present in the diet, in a reaction requiring glutathione transferase activity.

Diagnosis

Measurements of plasma amino acid levels and urinary organic acids are useful for diagnosis. Acylcarnitine profiling by tandem mass spectrometry demonstrates that most Cbl-C-mutated individuals exhibit increased propionylcarnitine in blood.

Treatment

The treatment includes supplementation of vitamin B12, betaine and folic acid. Pharmacological doses of vitamin B12, preferably in the form of hydroxycobalamin, are given to maximize enzyme activity. Betaine and folic acid are used to reduce homocysteine and to increase methionine levels. Betaine provides the substrate for betaine-homocysteine methyltransferase, an alternative route for the synthesis of methionine in liver, whereas folic acid enhances the remethylation pathway. Carnitine deficiency, requiring supplementation, can sometimes be observed either due to its loss in buffering intramitochondrial accumulation of methylmalonic acid or because of reduced synthesis due to low methionine availability. No proven efficacy has been demonstrated with dietary protein restriction.

Biochemical abnormalities usually improve under treatment but without reaching complete normalization. Homocysteine levels remain above normal in the majority of cases. The prognosis is poorer in early-onset individuals, who manifest an increased death rate. In early-onset disease, treatment may result in improvement of visceral and hematological signs, but in most cases has less efficacy on neurological outcome and on ocular manifestations.

Bibliography

Biancheri R., Cerone R., Schiaffino M.C., et al. (2001). Cobalamin (Cbl) C/D deficiency: Clinical, neurophysiological and neuroradiologic findings in 14 cases. *Neuropediatrics*. 32(1):14–22.

Grünert S.C., Fowler B., Superti-Furga A., et al. (2011) Hyperpyrexia resulting in encephalopathy in a 14-month-old patient with cblC disease. *Brain Dev*. 33(5):432–6.

Martinelli D., Deodato F., Dionisi-Vici C. (2011). Cobalamin C defect: Natural history, pathophysiology, and treatment. *J Inherit Metab Dis*. 34(1):127–35.

Hereditary Folate Disorders

A girl was the second child born full-term (2600 g) to a nonconsanguineous couple. She showed recurrent megaloblastic anemia induced by fever or diarrhea from 7 months of age. Intermittent limb tremor presented at 3 years of age, followed by seizures 6 months later. These seizures occurred every two months. During seizures, the girl experienced sudden loss of consciousness followed by myoclonus of her right limbs lasting for about 30 min. Electroencephalogram revealed spikes and slow waves in the left occipital and left posterior temporal regions. Cranial CT revealed intracranial calcification. Upon evaluation at age 5 years, lower-extremity weakness, difficulty in sleeping and irritability were observed. Head circumference was 47.5 cm and body weight and height 15 kg and 97 cm, respectively. General neurologic and physical examinations were normal. Blood tests showed megaloblastic anemia. Total homocysteine levels in her plasma and urine were markedly increased. Plasma folate decreased to 4.5 nmol/L (normal > 6.8 nmol/L). Plasma cobalamin levels were normal. Blood amino acids and acylcarnitine profiles showed no abnormalities. Urine organic acid profile was also normal. Folate and 5-methylterahydrofolate in cerebrospinal fluid were undetectable. Brain CT (Figure 60.1) showed symmetrical white-matter calcification of bilateral frontal, temporal, parietal and occipital lobes, and basal ganglia. Cranial MR imaging (Figure 60.1) showed leukodystrophy in bilateral parietal lobes, left occipital lobe and bilateral lentiform nucleus. Mutations in SLC46A1 were identified, confirming the diagnosis of hereditary folate malabsorption. Folinic calcium was initiated at her age of 5 years. One week later, she displayed hematological normalization. Hematological indices, folate, and total homocysteine returned to normal. One month after treatment, intermittent limb tremor and epileptic seizures disappeared. Sleeping difficulties and irritability disappeared one year after treatment. A progressive improvement in mental development

was also observed. However, leg weakness was still manifest when using the stairs.

Hereditary Folate Disorders

Onset: Infantile encephalopathy with developmental regression.
Additional manifestations: Variable. Seizures, hydrocephalus, and demyelinating lesions are most common. Anemia in some forms.
Disease mechanism: The folates act as coenzymes in one-carbon metabolism. Folate participates in the synthesis of thymidine, purines, myelin and neurotransmitters and in the metabolism of amino acids such as homocysteine, methionine, serine, and glycine.
Testing: Determination of folate and derivatives in biological fluids including cerebrospinal fluid.
Treatment: Folinic acid or the pharmacological form of 5-MTHF (mefolinate).
Research highlights: Secondary neurotransmitter synthetic abnormalities in cerebral folate deficiency syndromes.

Clinical Features

The cerebral folate disorders are associated with decreased cerebrospinal fluid concentration of folate and 5-methylenetetrahydrofolate (5-MTHF). Several heterogeneous subtypes are recognized. Five of them are discussed here.

Methylenetetrahydrofolate reductase deficiency represents an autosomal recessive defect associated with progressive encephalopathy including apnea, seizures, and hydrocephalus during the first months of life. Later, infants manifest neurological deterioration, ataxia, seizures, brain atrophy, and delayed myelination. Vascular occlusion, psychiatric manifestations, demyelinating

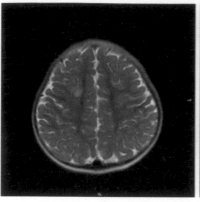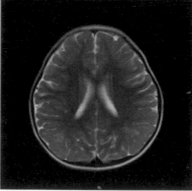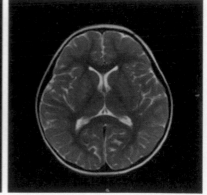

Figure 60.1 Cerebral folate deficiency. Cranial MR imaging reveals hyperintensity in bilateral parietal lobes, left occipital lobe and bilateral lentiform nucleus on T2-weighted imaging. Reproduced with permission from Wang Q et al. The first Chinese case report of hereditary folate malabsorption with a novel mutation on SLC46A1. *Brain Dev.* 2015; 37(1):163–7.

brain and spinal cord lesions are frequent in older children and in adult onset forms.

Dihydrofolate reductase deficiency is characterized by megaloblastic anemia or pancytopenia together with severe neurological abnormalities that include microcephaly, refractory seizures, learning disabilities, white matter disturbances, and cerebellar or cerebral atrophy.

Proton-coupled folate transporter (PCFT or SLC46A1) deficiency or hereditary folate malabsorption is an early onset, severe disease encompassing both blood and cerebrospinal fluid folate deficiency. The reduced availability of all forms of folate within cells results in disturbances in several folate-related reactions. Decreased nucleic acid synthesis impacts tissues with rapid turnover such as blood and epithelial cells, causing megaloblastic anemia, pancytopenia, recurrent infections, diarrhea, oral ulcers, failure to thrive and weight loss. Within the central nervous system, demyelination and intracranial calcifications are frequent, together with abnormal neurological developmental, mental retardation, seizures and motor disturbances.

FRα defect or FOLR1 deficiency is an autosomal recessive disorder of the folate receptor that manifests during infancy as psychomotor regression, ataxia, tremor, chorea, and myoclonic seizures. MR imaging shows hypomyelination in combination with acute demyelinating processes, together with cerebellar atrophy in some cases.

Autoantibodies against folate receptors have been suggested to lead to cerebral folate deficiency. In this disorder, there are circulating blocking autoantibodies directed against FRα in the choroid plexus. The clinical syndrome includes irritability, insomnia, decelerating head growth, regression, autistic traits, hypotonia, ataxia, dyskinesia, epilepsy, visual disturbances, and hearing loss during with onset in early infancy.

Pathology

There are few pathological observations available. MR imaging generally illustrates abnormal white matter signal (Figure 60.1). There may be calcifications in the white matter (Figure 60.2).

Pathophysiology

Folate is a water-soluble B vitamin comprising several vitamers, which are compounds that act as coenzymes for cellular one-carbon metabolism. Folate is essential for the synthesis of thymidine, purines, myelin, and neurotransmitters, and for the metabolism of amino acids such as homocysteine, methionine, serine, and glycine. Homocysteine remethylation to methionine leads to more than 100 methylation reactions via S-adenosylmethione, which is involved in many essential reactions. Folate deficiency is a prevalent vitamin deficiency that leads to a wide spectrum of clinical abnormalities. It has been related to megaloblastic anemia, growth retardation, congenital birth defects, pregnancy complications, osteoporosis, cancer, and several neurodegenerative and psychiatric diseases.

The brain needs a continuous supply of the active-reduced form of folate (mainly 5-MTHF) to maintain methylation reactions, as demonstrated by the fact that disorders affecting folate transport trough the choroid plexus cause severe neurological disease.

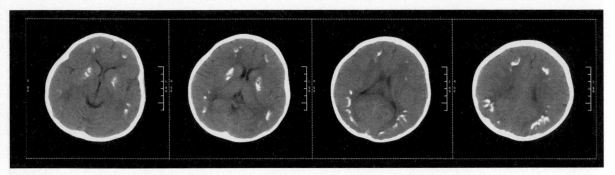

Figure 60.2 Cerebral folate deficiency. Cranial computerized tomography showing multiple high-density lesions in bilateral basal ganglia as well as frontal, parietal and occipital lobes. Reproduced with permission from Wang Q et al. The first Chinese case report of hereditary folate malabsorption with a novel mutation on SLC46A1. *Brain Dev.* 2015; 37(1):163–7.

Folate is essential for brain maturation and function, and one common feature of inherited disorders leading to cerebral folate deficiency is a disturbance in myelination. These findings reflect the importance of cerebral folate availability for the maintenance of single-carbon transfer pathways and myelin formation and turnover.

Methylenetetrahydrofolate reductase deficiency leads to impaired synthesis of 5-MTHF, the essential methyl group donor for the remethylation of homocysteine to methionine. This enzyme is expressed in several tissues, although the liver is the main source of circulating 5-MTHF. The core biochemical features include hyperhomocysteinemia, decreased plasma methionine values and severe cerebrospinal fluid 5-MTHF deficiency. Although folate transport is preserved, limited amounts of 5-MTHF are available to be transported across the choroid plexus. Hyperhomocysteinemia and profound cerebrospinal fluid 5-MTHF deficiency are the main pathophysiological mechanisms of this disease. Treatment is directed at reducing the increased homocysteine levels through betaine, pyridoxine and cobalamin, and to improve defective methylation using folinic acid

In dihydrofolate reductase deficiency, affected individuals exhibit normal serum folate and cobalamin levels with no hyperhomocysteinemia. Severe cerebral 5-MTHF deficiency is detected in all cases, similar to that observed in genetic folate transport disturbances. In this disorder, cerebral folate deficiency and megaloblastic anemia in the presence of normal serum folate excludes the possibility of defects in any of the known folate transporters. The absence of hyperhomocysteinemia indicates that the defect does not involve the methylation cycle but is probably in the DNA-synthesis arm of folate metabolism. The hypothesis that arises is that an intact intracellular folate metabolism is fundamental for maintaining sufficient cerebrospinal fluid and red blood folate levels. Affected individuals generally manifest a favorable response to oral folinic acid and improvement in both hematological and neurological signs. Cerebrospinal fluid 5-MTHF values can also be restored.

In hereditary folate malabsorption, there is an abnormal cerebrospinal fluid: serum folate ratio in the presence of severe folate deficiency (or even after folate supplementation). Treatment of these individuals with folinic acid can partially improve the clinical syndrome.

In the deficiency of the folate receptor FOLR1, there is decreased cerebrospinal fluid 5-MTHF values with normal blood folate. One explanation for the symptom-free period in this defect is that expression of FRβ in the fetal brain is greater than that of FRα, which might initially compensate for the loss of receptor function. Folinic acid therapy can ameliorate clinical signs and white matter disturbances or even reverse the phenotype if administered when the first symptoms arise.

Production of autoantibodies against folate receptors probably occurs during the first six months of life because the first clinical manifestations appear after that age and the mothers do not exhibit autoantibodies. Candidates for a possible trigger for this autoimmune reaction include the soluble folate-binding proteins in human or bovine milk because they exhibit significant amino acid sequence homology with the membrane-bound human FRα. Blocking autoantibodies have also been observed in other diseases, such as in individuals with autistic disorders and other neurological deficits. Some affected individuals with autoantibodies respond well to folinic acid therapy.

Diagnosis

Two distinct procedures are available to measure folate in biological fluids. The most common is the automated chemoimmunoluminiscence procedure for the measurement of total serum folate (which includes several folate derivatives). Another method for quantifying 5-MTHF is reverse-phase high pressure liquid chromatography with fluorescence detection.

Treatment

There are several forms of folate. The first is folic acid, which is not a natural form of the vitamin and is only found in fortified foods, supplements, and pharmaceuticals. It lacks coenzyme activity and must be reduced to its metabolically active tetrahydrofolate form. 5-formyltetrahydrofolate (or folinic acid) is a reduced form of folate that has been widely used. The pharmacological form of 5-MTHF (also known as mefolinate) has also been used. 5-MTHF constitutes the form of folate that is normally transported into peripheral tissues to be used for cellular metabolism.

Bibliography

Serrano M., Pérez-Dueñas B., Montoya J., et al. (2012). Genetic causes of cerebral folate deficiency: Clinical, biochemical and therapeutic aspects. *Drug Discov Today*. 17(23–24):1299–306.

Wang Q., Li X., Ding Y., et al. (2015). The first Chinese case report of hereditary folate malabsorption with a novel mutation on SLC46A1. *Brain Dev*. 37(1):163–7.

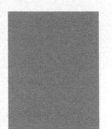

Childhood Disorders

Unverricht–Lundborg Disease

Five of eleven siblings were afflicted by the same disease. Their parents were first-degree cousins. The median age at onset of disease was three (range: 2–4) years. Early morning myoclonic jerks and action- or stimulus-sensitive myoclonus and generalized tonic–clonic seizures were noted in all the children. The median age at onset of myoclonus and generalized seizures was about 3 to 4 years. Multisegmental myoclonus and generalized status myoclonicus occurred in four of the siblings. Dysarthria and ataxia were observed in all of them at a mean age of 8 years. Frequent falls and viral infections were noted in all the children. Severe sphincter dysfunction was reported at a median age of 6 years in three of the siblings. Cognitive dysfunction was present in all, with a mean age at onset of 8 years. Three of them exhibited moderately severe learning difficulties. Spasticity and motor dysfunction were steadily progressive and affected all the children at a median age of 7–8 years.

Clinical Features

The progressive myoclonus epilepsies include several diseases characterized by myoclonus, epilepsy and progressive neurological deterioration. Unverricht–Lundborg disease, also known as Baltic myoclonus, Mediterranean myoclonus, or progressive myoclonic epilepsy type 1 is an autosomal recessively inherited disorder that represents the most common cause for progressive myoclonus epilepsy. The highest prevalence recorded in certain populations such as the Southern European and North African Mediterranean is 4 in 100,000. The highest incidence, however, occurs in Finland, with 1 in 20,000 births per year, although there may be an ancient founder mutation in some of the affected countries.

The first manifestation of Unverricht–Lundborg disease in one-half of children is myoclonic jerks with

Table 61.1 The progressive myoclonic epilepsies

Progressive myoclonic epilepsy type	Gene
Unverricht–Lundborg disease	Cystatin B (CSTB)
Lafora disease	Laforin (EPM2A) or malin (NHLRC1)
Neuronal ceroid lipofuscinosis	Various
Myoclonic epilepsy with ragged red fibers (MERRF)	Various mitochondrial DNA genes including MT-TK, MT-TL1, MT-TH, and MT-TS1
Sialidosis	Neuraminidase 1 (NEU1)

or without generalized tonic clonic seizures, which become apparent between 6 and 16 years. The myoclonic jerks are action-activated and stimulus sensitive and may be provoked by light, physical exertion, noise, or stress. They occur predominantly in the proximal muscles of the extremities and are asynchronous. They may be focal or multifocal and may generalize to a series of myoclonic seizures or even status myoclonicus characterized by continuous myoclonic jerks with impaired consciousness. In another half of children, the first symptom is tonic clonic seizures. There may also be absence, simple motor, or complex focal seizures. Some of these events might also represent poorly described myoclonic symptomatology or status myoclonicus. Epileptic seizures are relatively infrequent in the early stages of the disease and often increase in frequency during the following 3 to 7 years. Later, they may cease entirely with antiepileptic drug treatment. In rare cases, tonic–clonic seizures never occur. During the first decade following disease onset, the symptoms characteristically progress and about one-third of children become severely incapacitated. The disease displays few other symptoms. Additional neurological findings are initially absent. However, over time, recurrent, almost imperceptible myoclonus may occur. This is especially noticeable in response to photic or other stimuli (threat, clapping of hands, nose tapping, tendon percussion) or to action (movements or loud noise). Gradually, myoclonus becomes more evident. Over the years, ataxia, intentional tremor, and dysarthria develop. Individuals with Unverricht–Lundborg disease are usually mentally fit but exhibit emotional liability and depression. A mild decline in intellectual performance may also ensue over time. In some cases, the phenotype is one of progressive myoclonic ataxia without epilepsy. Pyramidal or extrapyramidal dysfunction is rare. Death follows after 40–50 years.

Pathology

The pathological findings are restricted to the brain. There are widespread nonspecific degenerative brain changes. Loss of Purkinje cells and of cerebellar granule cells with Bergmann gliosis is conspicuous. There is also neuronal loss in the medial thalamus and the spinal cord. There is loss of cortical GABA terminals. Neuronal cytoplasmic inclusions containing lysosomal proteins, cathepsin-B and CD68 have been detected. In the neuronal nucleus, TDP-43 (transactive response DNA binding protein 43) and FUS (fused in sarcoma) have also been identified.

Pathophysiology

Unverricht–Lundborg disease is due to mutations in the cysteine protease inhibitor cystatin B. All affected individuals harbor an unstable expansion of a 12-nucleotide (dodecamer) repeat (5′-CCC-CGC-CCC-GCG-3′) in the promoter region of the gene in at least one of the two altered cystatin B alleles. The majority of individuals display two expanded repeats in abnormal allele range. The expanded dodecamer repeat mutation accounts for approximately 90 percent of disease alleles throughout the world. Normal alleles comprise 2 to 3 dodecamer repeats, whereas full penetrance alleles associated with the disease phenotype contain at least 30 dodecamer repeats. The largest allele observed has been about 125 dodecamer repeats in size. The expansion results in significant downregulation of protein expression, which is likely the result of reduced promotor activity in the presence of the expansion mutation. This may be a consequence of the stable, mainly tetraplex, secondary structures that the dodecamer repeat forms under physiological conditions, resulting in disrupted spacing of promoter elements from the transcription initiation site and repression of transcription.

Cystatins form a group of homologous small molecular weight proteins of single polypeptide chain and without carbohydrate side chains or disulphide bonds. They inhibit *in vitro* several papain-family cysteine proteases, cathepsins, by tight reversible binding. Although the cysteine protease inhibitor cystatin B has been characterized in detail *in vitro*, its physiological function remains unknown.

Hippocampal brain slices prepared from mixed background CSTB-null mice are hyperexcitable, as they responded to afferent stimuli in the hippocampal CA1 region with multiple population spikes and as kainate provokes the appearance of epileptic-like activity earlier in them than in control mice. This hyperexcitability may be due to loss of synaptic inhibition.

Diagnosis

EEG background activity is slowed, particularly in the majority of affected individuals with a severe disease course, such that it was customary to expect slowing in Unverricht–Lundborg disease when distinguishing it from other myoclonic epilepsies such as juvenile myoclonus epilepsy. However, it is also recognized that EEG background activity may be normal in some individuals. The EEG abnormalities (spike-wave discharges, photosensitivity and polyspike discharges during REM sleep) are more pronounced during the initial stages of the disease, when there are usually also generalized tonic clonic seizures. EEG abnormalities tend to diminish with time in correlation with the stabilization of the clinical condition over the years.

Treatment

Benzodiazepines may reduce myoclonus. Brivaracetam, a synaptic vesicle glycoprotein 2A ligand that differs from levetiracetam in its mechanism of action, has displayed antiepileptic activity in experimental models of epilepsy and myoclonus and thus may offer benefit in Unverricht–Lundborg disease. Vagus nerve stimulator therapy reduces seizures and may significantly improve cerebellar function. Otherwise, the disease course is unrelenting.

Bibliography

Joensuu T., Lehesjoki A.E., Kopra O. (2008). Molecular background of EPM1-Unverricht–Lundborg disease. *Epilepsia*. 49(4):557–63.

Kälviäinen R., Khyuppenen J., Koskenkorva P., et al. (2008). Clinical picture of EPM1-Unverricht–Lundborg disease. *Epilepsia*. 49(4).549–56.

Saadah M., El Beshari M., Saadah L., et al. (2014). Progressive myoclonic epilepsy type 1: Report of an Emirati family and literature review. *Epilepsy Behav Case Rep*. 2:112–17.

Lafora Disease

A 14-year-old girl was evaluated for progressive myoclonus epilepsy. Her parents were third-degree relatives. She had no health problems up to age 13 years. She presented with generalized tonic-clonic seizures that began with visual auras at that time and generalized myoclonic seizures were observed in later periods. Her seizures could not be controlled despite several antiepileptic drugs. One year later, segmental myoclonus started in addition to the occipital and generalized seizures. Over time, truncal ataxia, gait impairment, dysarthria, and significant learning difficulties became manifest. Feeding difficulties, loss of the ability to walk without assistance, and dementia ultimately developed.

Lafora Disease

Onset: Headaches, Impaired school attainment, myoclonic jerks and generalized seizures between 8 and 18 years of age.
Additional manifestations: Visual hallucinations due to epilepsy or psychosis. Stimulus-related myoclonus, myoclonic absence seizures, and status myoclonicus. Pyramidal tract dysfunction. Cerebellar degeneration. Depression and dementia. Death occurs a decade after disease onset.
Disease mechanism: Loss of function of EPM2A (laforin) or EPM2B (malin). Potential glycogen synthase hyperactivation and glycogen formation with long strands and inadequate branching, and excess glycogen-bound phosphate that also distorts glycogen, rendering it insoluble.
Testing: Biopsy can show PAS-positive cytoplasmic inclusions (Lafora bodies) in multiple tissues. EEG displays slow background and spike-wave and polyspike-wave complexes early in the disease course.

Treatment: None effective. Valproate, clonazepam, and other anticonvulsants can ameliorate myoclonus and myoclonic seizures.
Research highlights: Defective autophagy, neuroinflammation, and diminished excitatory neurotransmitter reuptake.

Clinical Features

Lafora disease is an autosomal recessive, rapidly progressive myoclonic epilepsy with late childhood or early adolescent onset defined by the accumulation of Lafora bodies throughout multiple tissues. Most individuals with typical Lafora disease harbor mutations in the EPM2A gene encoding laforin or in the EPM2B (NHLRC1) gene encoding malin. A third likely genetic locus, which accounts for about 10 percent of cases, remains unidentified. The disease is characterized by medication-refractory generalized tonic clonic or visual seizures and spontaneous and stimulus-sensitive myoclonus (Figure 62.1). Onset is between 8 and 18 years of age. The first symptoms are headaches, impaired school performance, myoclonic jerks, generalized seizures and, in some cases, visual hallucinations of both epileptic and psychotic origin. Myoclonus is usually distal, erratic, triggered by light and sound stimulation, and enhanced by emotion. Myoclonus, epilepsy, and hallucinations gradually worsen and become intractable. Pyramidal tract dysfunction is common, as is late cerebellar degeneration. Affected individuals remain communicative throughout the early course of the disease except for very frequent myoclonic absence seizures. However, they often demonstrate depression. Gradually, dementia sets in and, by the tenth year following onset, affected individuals enters a state characterized by near-continuous myoclonus with absences, frequent generalized seizures, and severe dementia. A vegetative state follows. Death is frequently caused by aspiration pneumonia during status epilepticus and supervenes about a decade after disease onset.

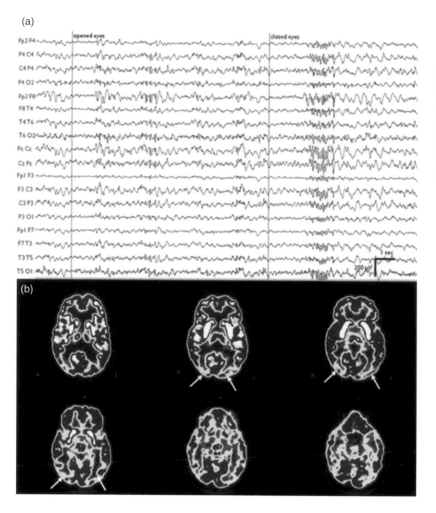

Figure 62.1 Lafora disease. a. Bipolar longitudinal electroencephalography (EEG) performed 3 days before [18] Fluorodeoxyglucose positron emission tomography (FDG-PET) and showing bursts of generalized polyspikes and polyspike-waves and slow background activity. b. Axial FDG-PET scan showing bilateral posterior heterogeneous metabolism (white arrows). Reproduced with permission from Jennesson M et al. Posterior glucose hypometabolism in Lafora disease: Early and late FDG-PET assessment. *Epilepsia*. 2010; 51(4):708–11.

An early onset Lafora disease form presents at about 5 years of age with dysarthria, myoclonus, and ataxia. These manifestations suggest late infantile variant neuronal ceroid lipofuscinosis, but children exhibit the characteristic widespread Lafora body deposition rather than ceroid lipofuscinosis. A single mutation, Phe261Leu in the gene PRDM8, induces the abnormal translocation of laforin and malin to the cell nucleus. The subsequent course of this disease variant is that of a very slowly progressive myoclonic epilepsy much more protracted than any infantile neuronal ceroid lipofuscinosis or Lafora disease, with affected individuals surviving into their fourth decade.

Pathology

Lafora bodies are dense accumulations of malformed and insoluble ovoid PAS (periodic acid-Schiff)-

positive glycogen molecules termed polyglucosans (Figures 62.2–62.3). These aggregates are 30–40 μm in size and differ from normal glycogen in that they lack the symmetric branching that allows glycogen to be soluble. The bodies consist of granular and fibrillary material composed of insoluble glycogen packed more densely in the center (Figure 62.4). They are closely associated with the endoplasmic reticulum. Lafora bodies are present in all brain regions and in most neurons, with a predilection for neuronal cell bodies and dendrites. They are not present in glia. The most affected structures are the cerebellar cortex, thalamus, globus pallidus, substantia nigra and dentate nucleus. In addition to the brain, Lafora bodies are prominent in skin, sweat glands (peripheral cells and apocrine myoepithelial cells), heart, liver, striated muscle, and spinal cord. Gradual occupation of dendrites by Lafora bodies is correlated with the onset

(a)

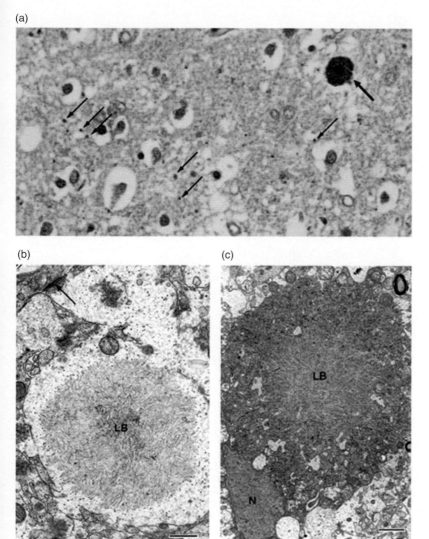

Figure 62.2 Lafora disease. Brain at autopsy. **a.** Light micrograph of the neuropil stained with periodic acid–Schiff reagent following diastase digestion. Both type I (thin arrows) and type II (thick arrow) lafora bodies (LBs) are present. **b.** Electron micrograph of a type I LB. A postsynaptic density (arrow) demonstrates the location of the LB in the dendrite. Bar equals 1 microm. **c.** Electron micrograph of a type II LB. Note that the LB occupies the majority of the cytoplasm. The nucleus (N) is pressed to the periphery of the cell. Bar equals 2 microm. Abbreviations: LB, Lafora body; N, nucleus. Reproduced with permission from Striano P et al. Typical progression of myoclonic epilepsy of the Lafora type: A case report. *Nat Clin Pract Neurol.* 2008; 4(2):106–11.

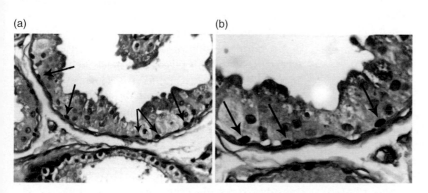

Figure 62.3 Lafora bodies on skin biopsy. **a.** Histopathologic examination of the skin biopsy taken from the axillary region reveals round-to-oval intracytoplasmic, periodic acid–Schiff-positive, diastase-resistant inclusions within the myoepithelial and acinar cells of sweat glands, corresponding to Lafora bodies (arrows). Periodic acid–Schiff stain, 200×. **b.** Lafora bodies in a magnified view (arrows). Periodic acid–Schiff stain, 400×. Reproduced with permission from de Assis Franco I et al. Mystery Case: Lafora periodic acid-Schiff inclusion bodies. *Neurology.* 2015; 85(17):e130–1.

(a)   (b)

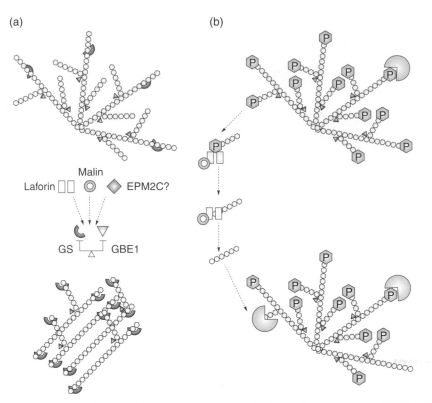

Figure 62.4 Two theories of the pathogenesis of Lafora bodies. a. Glycogen synthase (GS) (light blue) extends the growing glycogen chain in a linear manner. Glycogen brancher enzyme (GBE1) (green) branches the linear glycogen, giving the molecule its spherical shape. If the balance between extension and branching is disrupted, poorly branched glycogen, or polyglucosans, form instead of normal glycogen. Laforin, malin, and, possibly, other proteins involved in Lafora disease regulate the balance of the two enzymes, preventing polyglucosan formation. b. Glycogen is normally phosphorylated, and this hinders its degradation. Laforin (yellow) dephosphorylates glycogen. Laforin must then be removed to enable degradation to start, and this is accomplished by malin (red circle). If laforin or malin is not present, glycogen cannot be degraded and, over time, it loses its spherical structure, accumulating as polyglucosans to form Lafora bodies. Abbreviations: GBE1, glycogen branching enzyme; GS, glycogen synthase; P, phosphate. Reproduced with permission from Striano P et al. Typical progression of myoclonic epilepsy of the Lafora type: A case report. *Nat Clin Pract Neurol.* 2008; 4(2):106–11.

and then the unrelenting progression of epilepsy and other neurological symptoms. The dendritic location may be of relevance because in the other disease in which Lafora bodies are found, adult polyglucosan body disease, which is caused by mutations in the glycogen branching enzyme gene, the bodies are located in axons and affected individuals manifest myelopathy, motor neuron dysfunction, and dementia, but no epilepsy.

Pathophysiology

Lafora disease is characterized by the accumulation of insoluble ubiquitinated polyglucosan inclusions in the cytoplasm and dendrites of neurons. The two known causal genes encode a glucan phosphatase (laforin; EPM2A) and an E3-ubiquitin ligase (malin; EPM2B)

(Figure 62.5). A slowly progressive form of Lafora disease may be associated with a third locus. Of note, insoluble starch-like accumulations also form in neurons during human aging: corpora amylacea are insoluble, glucan-based aggregates that occur in brain, eye, and peripheral nervous system neurons of individuals older than 30 years.

In normal conditions, neurons contain low levels of glycogen, and this glycogen protects neurons from hypoxic stress *in vitro* and *in vivo*. The disease symptoms in Lafora disease may result from neuronal apoptosis driven by the accumulation of the cytoplasmic, hyperphosphorylated, water-insoluble Lafora body inclusions, which are normally prevented by the action of laforin. Although these inclusions occur throughout many tissues, neurons may be particularly sensitive to polyglucosan-mediated toxicity.

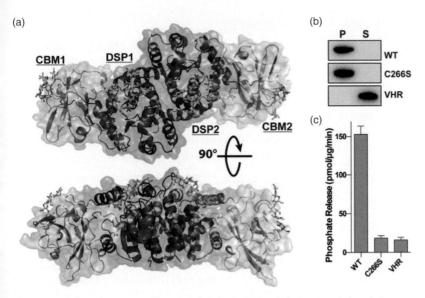

Figure 62.5 Crystal structure of human laforin bound to maltohexaose and phosphate.
a. Structure of human laforin bound to maltohexaose (green) and phosphate (orange). The laforin structure is an anti-parallel dimer with one molecule in blue and the other in red. Each molecule contains a CBM and DSP domain yielding a tetramodular CBM1-DSP1-DSP2-CBM2 structure. Maltohexaose chains are bound at the CBM and DSP domains with a single phosphate molecule located at the base of the catalytic site. b. Glycogen co-sedimentation assay to measure glycogen binding. Recombinant laforin wild-type (WT), laforin C266S, and VHR were incubated with glycogen bound to Con A agarose beads, glycogen was pelleted by centrifugation, and proteins in the pellet (P) and supernatant (S) were separated by SDS-PAGE and visualized by Western analysis. Glycogen-bound proteins are in the pellet and unbound proteins are in the supernatant. c. Specific activity of laforin WT, inactive mutant laforin C266S, and human VHR against glycogen. 100 ng of protein was incubated with 45 μg glycogen for 20 minutes. Each bar is the mean ± SEM of six replicates, P < 0.05. Reproduced with permission from Raththagala M et al. Structural mechanism of laforin function in glycogen dephosphorylation and lafora disease. *Mol Cell.* 2015; 57(2):261–72.

Two mechanistic hypotheses may explain neuronal dysfunction. In the first, the laforin–malin complex may regulate glycogen synthase. Deficiency of either protein leads to glycogen synthase hyperactivation, exceeding glycogen branching enzyme activity and resulting in the production of glycogen molecules with excessively long strands and inadequate branching. This abnormal glycogen, polyglucosan, is insoluble and can precipitate and accumulate to form Lafora bodies. The second pathogenic hypothesis is that laforin acts directly on glycogen, dephosphorylating its excess phosphate. In the absence of laforin, the excess phosphate distorts the double helices of glycogen strands and its symmetric branch pattern, both of which are necessary for its solubility. This would also lead to precipitation of abnormal glycogen and accumulation into Lafora bodies.

Autophagic impairment precedes the formation of Lafora bodies in knockout mice models. A transcription factor, FoxO3a (forkhead box O3), is a possible cause for the autophagic defect in cellular and animal models of the disease. Expression of FoxO3a and its targets Map1LC3b (microtubule associated protein 1 light chain 3 beta) and Atg12 (autophagy-related protein 12) are decreased in laforin-deficient cells and mice. FoxO3a exerts a negative control over mTOR (mammalian target of rapamycin), and its loss could result in autophagic defects in Lafora disease associated with laforin deficiency. In addition, increased innate inflammatory responses may participate in this neurodegenerative disease with polyglucosan intraneuronal deposits in a manner similar to neurodegenerative diseases with abnormal protein aggregation. Lastly, the laforin–malin complex retards the endocytic recycling of the excitatory amino acid glutamate transporter GLT-1 (EAAT2; excitatory amino acid transporter 2). Defects in this transporter lead to excitotoxicity and epilepsy, such that the epilepsy that accompanies Lafora disease may be aggravated by GLT-1 loss of function.

Diagnosis

The diagnosis of Lafora disease can be established when the characteristic PAS-positive cytoplasmic inclusion Lafora bodies are found in one or more of multiple tissues including brain, spinal cord, liver, skin, skeletal muscle, heart, and retina. Because Lafora bodies can be detected in the myoepithelial cells of the secretory acini of the apocrine sweat glands and in the eccrine and apocrine sweat duct cells, an axillary skin biopsy is often diagnostic.

EEG may also be useful for diagnosis. The EEG becomes disorganized early in the disease course and is characterized by a slow background with superimposed generalized high-voltage spike-wave and polyspike-wave complexes. Multifocal, predominantly posterior, epileptiform discharges appear in addition to generalized bursts. In the final stages of the disease, the EEG is highly disorganized and the epileptiform discharges are almost continuous.

Treatment

There is no effective treatment. The antiepileptic and antimyoclonic drug valproate remains the drug of choice. Clonazepam may also be used to treat myoclonic seizures. High-dose piracetam can be useful in the treatment of myoclonus. Levetiracetam may also be effective for both myoclonus and generalized seizures. Topiramate and zonisamide may be also used as adjuvant anticonvulsants.

Bibliography

Monaghan T.S., Delanty N. (2010). Lafora disease: epidemiology, pathophysiology and management. *CNS Drugs.* 24(7):549–61.

Poyrazoğlu H.G., Karaca E., Per H., et al. (2015). Three patients with lafora disease: Different clinical presentations and a novel mutation. *J Child Neurol.* 30(6):777–81.

Neuronal Intranuclear Inclusion Disease

A 5-year-old boy was diagnosed with hyperactivity and attention-deficit disorder and exhibited frequent temper tantrums. A gradual decline in his school performance was attributed to these behavioral problems. He soon developed "mumbled" speech, drooling, and a hand tremor. Over the 10 months prior the initial evaluation at age 5, his speech became nearly incomprehensible and was accompanied by severe psychomotor slowing. He had gained 7 kilograms in the preceding year and had a long history of constipation. Exam revealed bradykinesia and drooling. He was easily elated despite a history of depressed mood. He was attentive sitting up but fell asleep during the examination in a supine position. His speech was profoundly dysarthric, hypophonic, and poorly intelligible. Cognitive function, including immediate and short-term memory, was intact. He had inconsistent gaze evoked horizontal nystagmus and saccadic pursuit and was unable to converge. There was mild facial weakness. There was also bilateral resting and intention hand tremor enhanced by efforts to speak. The small muscles of his hands and feet were wasted, muscle tone was increased in the lower extremities and ankle clonus was elicited bilaterally. Reflexes were brisk in the lower extremities with flexor plantar responses. Arm swing was decreased while walking. Subsequently, he developed parkinsonian features comprising resting and intention hand tremor, and bradykinesia progressed to cog-wheeling rigidity and prominent postural instability with episodes of freezing. Signs of upper motor neuron dysfunction also became apparent in the upper extremities.

Neuronal Intranuclear Inclusion Disease

Onset: Behavioral impairment at ages 1 to 17 years (central nervous system form) or gastrointestinal dysfunction (autonomic form).

Additional manifestations: Multisystem degeneration, including upper and lower motor neuron signs, extrapyramidal abnormalities and cognitive decline. Autonomic failure. Cerebellar degeneration.

Disease mechanism: Accumulation of intranuclear inclusions in neurons and glia containing ubiquitin and polyglutamine.

Testing: Rectal biopsy illustrates intranuclear inclusions in neurons in the myenteric plexus.

Treatment: None effective. Levodopa may alleviate dystonia.

Research highlights: Characterization of hyaline inclusion composition.

Clinical Features

Neuronal intranuclear inclusion disease or neuronal intranuclear hyaline inclusion disease is a slowly progressive neurodegenerative disorder characterized by eosinophilic intranuclear inclusions and neuronal loss throughout the central, peripheral, and autonomous nervous systems. Most cases are sporadic, but some cases suggest autosomal dominant or autosomal recessive inheritance.

Two phenotypes have been associated with neuronal intranuclear hyaline inclusions. One group of individuals presents with neurologic involvement and the other with gastrointestinal dysfunction and other manifestations of autonomic dysfunction sometimes in association with additional neurologic symptoms. In the gastrointestinal dysfunction form, chronic intestinal pseudo-obstruction and autonomic failure have been described in individuals with intranuclear hyaline inclusions in rectal biopsies (Figures 63.1 and 63.2). Neurologic abnormalities in these subjects include impaired pupillary reaction to light, dementia with paranoid behavior and abnormal

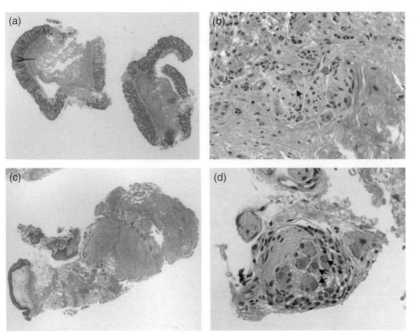

Figure 63.1 Neuronal intranuclear hyaline inclusion disease. Rectal biopsy findings showing partial-thickness intestinal wall section (a) and a single well-defined, eosinophilic hyaline inclusion within the nucleus of a ganglion cell of the submucosal (Meissner's) plexus (b) in P1. Full-thickness intestinal wall section (c) with multiple eosinophilic hyaline inclusions within the nuclei of ganglion cells of the myenteric (Auerbach's) plexus (d) in P2. (Hematoxylin-eosin stain; magnification: a and c, ×8; b and d, ×110). Reproduced with permission from Kulikova-Schupak R et al. Rectal biopsy in the diagnosis of neuronal intranuclear hyaline inclusion disease. *J Child Neurol.* 2004; 19(1):59–62.

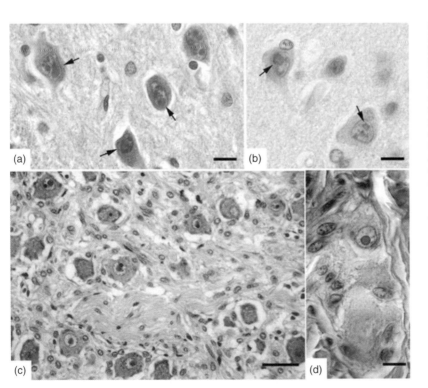

Figure 63.2 Neuronal intranuclear hyaline inclusion disease. (a) Intranuclear hyaline inclusions (arrows) are observed in almost all neurons in the red nucleus (hematoxylin and eosin staining). (b) Ubiquitin immunostaining showing ubiquitin-positive intranuclear inclusions. (c) Almost all of the dorsal root ganglia neurons contain large and well-developed intranuclear inclusions. (d) Intranuclear inclusions are observed in about 10 percent of the Meissner ganglion neurons of the stomach. Scale bar: a, b, c, d = 10 μm. Reproduced with permission from Mano T et al. Neuronal intranuclear hyaline inclusion disease with rapidly progressive neurological symptoms. *J Child Neurol.* 2007; 22(1):60–6.

development. Electroretinography is abnormal. Other affected individuals have presented with intestinal pseudo-obstruction and neurodegeneration manifesting as ataxia, dysarthria, diminished pupillary reaction to light, decreased tendon reflexes, and impaired vibratory and joint position sense.

In the primarily neurological form of the disease, the age at onset ranges from 8 months to 17 years (median 9 years). Progression is inexorable, with death occurring between 4 and 30 years (median 23 years) of age. Neurodegeneration is multisystemic, with considerable interindividual variation in the distribution of lesions. Brain imaging is usually normal until diffuse atrophy becomes manifest late in the course. Cerebellar atrophy may be observed in children with progressive ataxia. Extrapyramidal signs may be prominent and, when present, dystonia may respond to levodopa. Common associated findings include skeletal deformities (pes cavus, hammer toes, scoliosis, platybasia, spina bifida) and behavioral disturbances. The latter are often the presenting symptom in children. Seizures are not frequent early in the course, but can present later.

Pathology

The brain displays generalized atrophy with ventricular dilatation and reduced thickness of the cerebral cortex. The brainstem may also be atrophic and the substantia nigra is pale. Neuronal intranuclear inclusions occur in neurons and glia in the central and peripheral nervous systems, muscle, and adrenal tissue, without overt adrenal dysfunction. Occasionally, cardiomyocytes, adipocytes, fibroblasts, and sweat gland cells may also contain neuronal inclusions. There is neuronal loss in association with modest glial proliferation. This astrogliosis is most prominent in the substantia nigra, red nucleus, inferior olives, Purkinje cell layer, spinal anterior horn, and Clarke's dorsal nucleus. The inclusions are typically round or oval, with or without a well-demarcated halo, measure 8–15 nm, stain with eosin, display a hyaline appearance and are autofluorescent. Electron microscopy shows thin filamentous structures within the inclusions, which contain ubiquitin and polyglutamine. This polyglutamine is also found in CAG trinucleotide repeat diseases, but immunohistological staining for these repeats is characteristically weaker in neuronal intranuclear inclusion disease than in the canonical trinucleotide repeat diseases.

Pathophysiology

The pathogenesis of neuronal intranuclear inclusions has not been elucidated.

Diagnosis

The disease is often diagnosed postmortem, although it is possible to establish the diagnosis in life via rectal biopsy.

Treatment

There is no effective treatment. Levodopa may alleviate dystonia when present.

Bibliography

Kulikova-Schupak R., Knupp K.G., Pascual J.M., et al. (2004). Rectal biopsy in the diagnosis of neuronal intranuclear hyaline inclusion disease. *J Child Neurol.* 19(1):59–62.

Late Infantile Neuronal Ceroid Lipofuscinosis (Jansky-Bielschowsky Disease)

Two brothers and a sister, the children of consanguineous parents, were afflicted by the same disease. They failed a school vision test at the ages of 5-6 years. All three children subsequently developed seizures and regression of motor milestones was noted in the older two siblings. The first child was 14 years old. His vision declined rapidly after the age of 5 years. Fundus examination showed severe optic disc pallor and arteriolar attenuation. A full field electroretinogram showed severe rod-cone dysfunction. He developed seizures at the age of 7 years, and exhibited further progression in the form of recurrent myoclonic jerks and generalized tonic clonic seizures. There was progressive cognitive decline and visual impairment. He became bed-bound with very poor vision and uncontrolled seizures while on multiple anticonvulsants.

His brother was 12 years old. Fundus showed bilateral pale optic discs, severe arteriolar attenuation with diffuse pigment mottling throughout the fundus and few bony spicules. He developed seizures at the age of 7 years. He manifested slurred speech with difficulty in walking and needed assistance. Neurological examination revealed ataxia with brisk reflexes in both upper and lower limbs. MR imaging of the brain demonstrated diffuse cerebral and cerebellar atrophy.

Their sister was 8 years old. Her eye exam was similar to her younger brother's. She developed seizures at 6 years of age. MR imaging revealed mild cerebral atrophy and a normal cerebellum.

Jansky-Bielschowsky Disease

Onset: Speech impairment, hypotonia, ataxia, and epilepsy between 2 and 4 years of age.
Additional manifestations: Visual loss.
Myoclonus. Dementia. Affected children are often

bedbound by age 5 years. Death ensues in the second decade of life.
Disease mechanism: Deficiency of tripeptidyl peptidase 1, a serine-carboxyl proteinase. Accumulation of subunit c of mitochondrial ATP synthase and other storage material in dysfunctional lysosomes, which become curvilinear inclusions in neurons and other cells.
Testing: Biopsy of skin, rectum, or nerve demonstrates curvilinear inclusions, which may also be seen in lymphocytes and urine.
Treatment: None effective.
Research highlights: Targeted disruption of the TPP1 gene in mice, which replicate the human disorder.

Clinical Features

Late infantile neuronal ceroid lipofuscinosis or Jansky-Bielschowsky disease is associated with locus CLN2 of the ceroid lipofuscinoses and is caused by autosomal recessive deficiency of lysosomal TPP1 or tripeptidyl peptidase 1. As in all ceroid lipofuscinoses of young persons, the disease is characterized by progressive mental and motor decline and blindness. Disease onset occurs between the ages of 2 and 4 years and may include speech dysfunction, hypotonia, ataxia, and epilepsy. Seizures can be partial or generalized and progress gradually, as do ataxia, myoclonus, visual loss and general mental deterioration. Myoclonus may be the dominant source of disability early in the disease course until dementia sets in. Affected children are often bedbound and mute by the age of 5 years. Death ensues in the second decade of life.

Pathology

Neuroimaging demonstrates cerebral and cerebellar atrophy, with hyperintensity of the periventricular white matter on T2-weighted images. Brain weights of 500–700 g are common in the terminal stage of the disease. In addition to gross cerebral and cerebellar cortical atrophy, the white matter is atrophied and firm. There is severe neuronal loss with astrocytic gliosis and microglial activation. There is excess apoptosis as made manifest by BCL-2 (B-cell lymphoma 2) and TUNEL (terminal deoxynucleotidyl transferase dUTP nick end labeling) immunocytochemical staining. Remaining cells display distended cytoplasm containing granular storage material. Meganeurites are present in some cortical neurons but, in contrast with gangliosidoses and Niemann-Pick type C disease, ectopic dendrites are not detected. The stored material is autofluorescent under ultraviolet light and stains with PAS (periodic acid–Schiff). Immunoreactivity for subunit c of mitochondrial ATP synthase can be detected in the neuronal storage material. This material consists of curvilinear inclusions enclosed by a single unit membrane and displays acid phosphatase activity. Retinal degeneration with gliosis and neuronal loss is also characteristic. Curvilinear inclusions are also detected in rectal and skin biopsies and accumulate in sweat gland, nerves, smooth muscle, lymphocytes, and endothelial cells as well as urine.

Pathophysiology

Tripeptidyl peptidase 1 is a serine-carboxyl proteinase that cleaves tripeptides from the amino terminus of small proteins. Several peptide hormones including cholecystokinin and glucagon are substrates for the enzyme. TPP1 also initiates the degradation of subunit c of mitochondrial ATP synthase, which is a hydrophobic protein that accumulates in all the neuronal ceroid lipofuscinoses. This degradation is completed by cathepsin D. Deficiency of cathepsin D is the cause of another form of ceroid lipofuscinosis (CLN10). In addition to subunit c of mitochondrial ATP synthase, stored lysosomal material in CLN2 includes dolichol and sphingolipid activator proteins A and D. The mechanism of neuronal death involves defective autophagy. Accumulation of subunit c of mitochondrial ATP synthase may be a factor in the autophagic process since the autophagic degradation of mitochondria is mediated by this protein. In addition, the lysosomal membrane is permeabilized in CLN2, leading to lysosomal rupture and release of subunit c of mitochondrial ATP synthase to the cytoplasm, where protein aggregation mediated by p62-protein may take place.

Diagnosis

Skin or rectal biopsies can be diagnostic. EEG illustrates an occipital photosensitive response that persists until late disease stages. Electroretinography demonstrates a diminished response that eventually becomes extinguished. Visual evoked potentials are enhanced at the time when the EEG photosensitivity is prominent. They later diminished in amplitude towards the end stage of the disease. Enzyme activity testing can be performed for diagnostic purposes.

Treatment

There is no effective treatment. Among attempted therapies, human central nervous system stem cell administration, gene transfer adeno-associated vectors and cerliponase alfa, a recombinant human tripeptidyl peptidase 1 administered via intracerebroventricular injection, have been investigated.

Bibliography

Cooper J.D., Tarczyluk M.A., Nelvagal H.R. (2015). Towards a new understanding of NCL pathogenesis. *Biochim Biophys Acta*. 1852(10 Pt B):2256–61.

Patiño L.C., Battu R., Ortega-Recalde O., et al. (2014). Exome sequencing is an efficient tool for variant late-infantile neuronal ceroid lipofuscinosis molecular diagnosis. *PLoS One*. 9(10):e109576.

Juvenile Neuronal Ceroid Lipofuscinosis (Spielmeyer–Vogt Disease)

A 10-year-old girl manifested prenatal gastroschisis. Delivery was by cesarean section at 35 weeks. Development was normal except for stuttering (noted since age 3 years). Fine motor difficulties began at age 4. Abnormalities of gait, balance, coordination, and difficulties with academic performance were noted at age 6. Cognitive assessment (age 8) identified impaired visual capacity, visual memory and attention, and expressive and receptive language skills in the below-average to average range. There had been no frank loss of cognitive skills, although symptoms of cerebellar dysfunction had been progressive. She continued to ambulate and run independently with balance difficulties, but could no longer ride a bicycle. Neurologic examination was notable for scanning speech. Examination also demonstrated intermittent bilateral horizontal gaze-evoked nystagmus, saccadic breakdown of ocular pursuit, overshoot of horizontal saccades, and oculomotor apraxia. Movement abnormalities included bilateral upper extremity dysmetria, slowed fine finger movements and truncal titubation. Gait was wide-based and moderately unsteady. The child was able to stand on one foot briefly. Motor examination, reflexes, and sensory examination were normal. Brain MR imaging (age 9) demonstrated cerebellar and pontine atrophy and ill-defined T2 hyperintensity and volume loss in the posterior periventricular white matter.

Spielmeyer–Vogt Disease

Onset: Progressive visual loss between 6 and 8 years due to retinal degeneration.
Additional manifestations: Cognitive decline. Speech deterioration and seizures of variable severity. Extrapyramidal symptoms. Hallucinations and aggression. Blindness. Death occurs in the third decade of life.

Disease mechanism: Loss of function of CLN3, a lysosomal transmembrane protein. This is associated with storage of subunit c of mitochondrial ATP synthase, dolichols, and other proteins and may result from lysosome-processing defects of autophagy and phagocytosis. Apoptosis is the most likely cell death mechanism, which occurs in conjunction with neuroinflammation.
Testing: Biopsy or blood smear for the detection of granular storage material in cells.
Treatment: None effective.
Research highlights: Neuroinflammation in CLN3 null mice.

Clinical Features

Juvenile neuronal ceroid lipofuscinosis or Spielmeyer–Vogt disease is associated with locus CLN3. This autosomal recessive disorder occurs with a relatively high incidence in individuals of Scandinavian or Northern European ancestry. The term Batten disease was originally used to designate CLN3-associated disease, although it is also loosely used to refer to the neuronal ceroid lipofuscinoses in general. Onset is between 4 and 8 years of age, usually with visual loss due to progressive retinitis pigmentosa. Additional ophthalmic findings include macular degeneration, optic atrophy and blood vessel atrophy. Cognitive impairment ensues within months or a few years and this is followed by speech difficulties and epilepsy before 10 years of age. Seizures, however, can be of a variable degree of severity. Before 20 years of age, affected individuals are blind and mute. Parkinsonism is a late disease feature, as are hallucinations and aggressive behavior. Mean age at death is 25 years.

Pathology

The brain is moderately to severely atrophic. Neuronal loss is most prominent in the cerebrum and cerebellum. In the cortex, there is selective neuronal loss in layers II and V. The cell bodies of the remaining neurons are distended and include granular storage material that stains with periodic acid-Schiff. This material is autofluorescent under ultraviolet illumination and immunoreacts with subunit c of mitochondrial ATP synthase staining antibodies. Significant neuronal loss also takes place in the retina, where there is apoptosis of photoreceptors. There are conspicuous vacuolated lymphocytes. These lymphocyte inclusions are also present in neurons and resemble fingerprints. Numerous visceral tissues also display granular storage material, which may differ morphologically slightly from the neural material. In contrast with CLN2, there is no subunit c of mitochondrial ATP synthase accumulation in visceral organs. Myopathy with rimmed vacuoles has also been associated with CLN3.

Pathophysiology

The gene CLN3 encodes a lysosomal and endosomal transmembrane protein that may also be localized to the Golgi apparatus and synaptic vesicles. The function of this protein remains unclear, but it may be related to lysosomal acidification, lysosomal arginine transport, membrane fusion or vesicular transport. This may lead to lysosome processing defects affecting both autophagy and phagocytosis. The main stored material in Spielmeyer–Vogt disease is the same hydrophobic protein that accumulates in all the ceroid lipofuscinosis. In addition to this deposition of subunit c of mitochondrial ATP synthase, the enzymes tripeptidyl peptidase 1 (TPP1) and cathepsin D accumulate in stored granules. Sphingolipid activator proteins A and D and phosphorylated dolichols also accumulate in these granules.

Relatively unique to Spielmeyer–Vogt disease among the ceroid lipofuscinosis, a significant neuroimmune response occurs in the disorder.

Diagnosis

The diagnosis can be established by biopsy of accessible tissues or blood smear illustrating the characteristic lipofuscin storage in visceral cells, neurons, or lymphocytes.

Treatment

None effective. Mycophenolate mofetil, an immunosuppressant, has been investigated for its potential to reduce neuroinflammation.

Bibliography

Adams H.R., Mink J.W. (2013). Neurobehavioral features and natural history of juvenile neuronal ceroid lipofuscinosis (Batten disease). *J Child Neurol.* 28(9):1128–36.

Cárcel-Trullols J., Kovács A.D., Pearce D.A. (2015). Cell biology of the NCL proteins: What they do and don't do. *Biochim Biophys Acta.* 1852(10 Pt B):2242–55.

Dy M.E., Sims K.B., Friedman J. (2015). TPP1 deficiency: Rare cause of isolated childhood-onset progressive ataxia. *Neurology.* 85(14):1259–61.

Coenzyme Q10 Deficiency

A 35-year-old woman manifested rapid exertional fatigue beginning in early childhood. She began walking late, still required some assistance with ambulation at the age of 30 months and displayed generalized mild weakness. At age 7, she developed migraines with nausea, vomiting, and photophobia and phonophobia sometimes followed by the visual perception of colored dots. These symptoms often followed exertion. Since age 9, she had complex partial seizures of occipital origin with occasional secondary generalization. At age 15 years, she had her first episode of pigmenturia precipitated by exercise and similar episodes recurred about 20 times. She also complained of muscle pain and cramps after minimal exertion. Her examination was notable for bilateral ptosis and restricted upgaze. She also exhibited axial and proximal limb weakness with mild wasting of the shoulder muscles.

Coenzyme Q10 Deficiency

Onset: Childhood ataxia and cerebellar atrophy in the most common form.

Additional manifestations: Epilepsy, pyramidal tract dysfunction, nystagmus, and migraines in the ataxic form. Additional forms include encephalomyopathy with myoglobinuria, infantile multisystem dysfunction, myopathy, nephrotic syndrome, and multiple system atrophy.

Disease mechanism: Decreased activities of NADH: cytochrome c oxidoreductase and succinate: cytochrome c oxidoreductase of the mitochondrial respiratory chain possibly leading to decreased ATP synthesis. Increased free radical damage. Several forms of secondary coenzyme Q10 deficiency cause disease via additional mechanisms.

Testing: Muscle biopsies occasionally demonstrate mitochondrial proliferation or lipid droplets. Muscle respiratory chain activity determination can be suggestive. Direct measurement of coenzyme Q10 in skeletal muscle is definitive.

Treatment: Coenzyme Q10.

Research highlights: Elucidation of novel genes and clinical phenotypes.

Clinical Features

Coenzyme Q10 is a lipid essential for diverse metabolic processes such as the mitochondrial respiratory chain, the beta-oxidation of fatty acids and pyrimidine biosynthesis, and is also one of the principal cellular antioxidants. Its biosynthesis is still incompletely characterized, but requires the participation at least 15 genes. Mutations in eight of them (PDSS1 (prenyl-diphosphate synthase subunit 1), PDSS2 (prenyl-diphosphate synthase subunit 2), COQ2, COQ4, COQ6, ADCK3 (AarF domain containing kinase 3), ADCK4 (AarF domain containing kinase 4) and COQ9) cause primary coenzyme Q10 deficiency, a heterogeneous group of autosomal recessive disorders with variable age of onset (from birth to the seventh decade) and associated phenotypes, including an encephalomyopathy accompanied by ragged-red fibers and recurrent myoglobinuria, a severe infantile multisystem disorder with encephalopathy and neuropathy, an ataxic syndrome with cerebellar atrophy, an isolated myopathy and a steroid-resistant nephrotic syndrome. Pathogenic variants in CoQ2 are also associated with multiple system atrophy.

Secondary coenzyme Q10 deficiency may occur in diseases linked to mutations in unrelated genes such as ataxin, the electron transferring-flavoprotein dehydrogenase gene or the B-Raf proto-oncogene serine/threonine-protein kinase gene associated with cardiofaciocutaneous syndrome, or in association with mitochondrial DNA depletion, dietary insufficiency or use of statins Neonatal coenzyme Q10 deficiency is discussed with the newborn mitochondrial disorders.

Table 66.1 Primary and secondary coenzyme Q10 deficiencies

Primary coenzyme Q10 deficiencies	Secondary coenzyme Q10 deficiencies
Encephalomyopathy with myoglobinuria	Aprataxin deficiency
Infantile multisystem form	Electron transferring-flavoprotein dehydrogenase (ETFDH) deficiency
Ataxia and cerebellar atrophy	Mitochondrial DNA depletion
Myopathy	Dietary insufficiency
Nephrotic syndrome	Statin use
Multiple system atrophy	

The ataxic form of coenzyme Q10 deficiency is the most common and is the one discussed here.

In the ataxic form, all affected individuals manifest childhood-onset cerebellar ataxia as the main neurological sign, in association with profound muscle coenzyme Q10 deficiency. Additional features include pyramidal tract dysfunction, nystagmus, migraine, absence of tendon reflexes, and epilepsy. Less commonly, affected individuals manifest weakness, peripheral neuropathy, or hypergonadotrophic hypogonadism. Hypoalbuminemia and hypercholesterolemia have been noted in some individuals. A frequent clinical feature is a favorable response to coenzyme Q10 supplementation.

Pathology

In the ataxic form, all affected subjects have exhibited cerebellar atrophy in brain MR imaging studies. Morphologic and biochemical findings differ in the various clinical forms. In subjects with the encephalomyopathic, myopathic, or infantile multisystemic forms, muscle biopsies can reveal abnormal mitochondrial proliferation (ragged-red fibers or excessive succinate dehydrogenase histochemical activity) and lipid accumulation as well as reduced biochemical activities of respiratory chain enzyme complexes I+III and II+III. Muscle samples exhibit decreased coenzyme Q10 levels.

Pathophysiology

The hallmark of coenzyme Q10 deficiency syndromes is a decreased concentration of the compound in muscle or fibroblasts. Body fluid markers of mitochondrial dysfunction (lactate, pyruvate, alanine, organic acids, and coenzyme Q10) are normal in almost all cases reported. There is a variable degree of coenzyme Q10 deficiency and this leads to decreased activities of NADH:cytochrome c oxidoreductase (complex I + coenzyme Q10 + III) and succinate:cytochrome c oxidoreductase (complex II + coenzyme Q10 + III) of the mitochondrial respiratory chain. The degree of the deficiency is broad, ranging from extremely low coenzyme Q10 concentration in muscle to much milder deficiencies. It is plausible that myopathic forms of coenzyme deficiency only occur in association with decreased coenzyme Q10 levels in muscle, while individuals with predominantly brain involvement and with other severe presentations) are associated with decreased coenzyme Q10 values both in muscle and fibroblasts and perhaps in other tissues as well. Myopathic forms present a profound coenzyme Q10 deficiency in muscle homogenates and, consequently, a clear decrease in coenzyme Q10-dependent respiratory chain enzyme activities, while ataxic forms present partial deficiencies in muscle. It is likely that coenzyme Q10 cerebellar deficiency is more profound in the latter group.

Among the functional consequences of coenzyme Q10 deficiency, there is a slight to severe decrease in oxygen consumption in muscle mitochondria. A reduction in mitochondrial membrane potential in cultured skin fibroblasts from an individual with cerebellar ataxia and muscle coenzyme Q10 deficiency has also been demonstrated. These findings suggest that oxidative phosphorylation dysfunction may occur in coenzyme Q10 deficiency syndromes. An increase in free radical damage in tissues from coenzyme Q10-deficient individuals has been demonstrated.

Diagnosis

The biochemical evaluation of individuals with suspected coenzyme Q10 deficiency includes blood lactate measurement, although normal values do not exclude ubiquinone deficiency. Muscle biopsies occasionally demonstrate mitochondrial proliferation or lipid droplets, but they can be normal or display only nonspecific changes. Reduced biochemical activities of respiratory chain complexes, in particular complexes I+III (nicotinamide adenine dinucleotide–cytochrome c oxidoreductase) and complexes II+III (succinate–cytochrome c oxidoreductase) in muscle suggest coenzyme Q10 deficiency, although activities of these enzymes may be normal, particularly when the deficiency is mild. Reduction of these enzyme activities and deficiency of coenzyme Q10 in skin fibroblasts confirm ubiquinone deficiency; however, normal levels do not exclude deficiency in muscle. Direct measurement of coenzyme Q10 in skeletal muscle by high-performance liquid chromatography is the most reliable test for the diagnosis.

Treatment

Affected individuals with coenzyme Q10 deficiency manifest variable responses to coenzyme Q10 supplementation. In subjects with encephalomyopathy, muscle symptoms tend to improve after therapy. Individuals with isolated myopathy usually improved after supplementation, while those with ETFDH mutations improve only after the addition of riboflavin. In some children with the infantile multisystemic form, coenzyme Q10 supplementation has halted progression of the encephalopathy and improved the myopathy.

Bibliography

Desbats M.A., Lunardi G., Doimo M., et al. (2015). Genetic bases and clinical manifestations of coenzyme Q10 (CoQ 10) deficiency. *J Inherit Metab Dis.* 38(1):145–56.

Laredj L.N., Licitra F., Puccio H.M. (2014). The molecular genetics of coenzyme Q biosynthesis in health and disease. *Biochimie.* 100:78–87.

Sobreira C., Hirano M., Shanske S., et al. (1997). Mitochondrial encephalomyopathy with coenzyme Q10 deficiency. *Neurology.* 48(5):1238–43.

Common Mitochondrial Disorders of Children

A 10-year-old boy was evaluated for seizures. He had had a normal birth and infancy other than for having been delivered via cesarean section due to breech position. At 4 years of age, it became apparent that he was smaller and thinner than his relatives and peers and he was also easily fatigable. At age 10 years, he experienced prostration and headache followed by a generalized seizure that started on the left side of his body. The seizure resolved, leading to persistent headache and lethargy for several hours. One month later, a second seizure took place and this was followed by recurrent monthly seizures. In almost every case, the seizures were preceded by headache and vomiting. When examined, he was small and frail and displayed ptosis, upgaze palsy and a Gowers sign when rising from the floor. Reflexes were diminished and his left arm and leg were minimally weak (both at "50 percent strength," he felt). CT scanning of the head revealed putaminal calcifications. Blood lactate was 8.6 mM. He harbored mitochondrial DNA mutation A3243G at 73 percent abundance in blood, causative of MELAS. Over the next decade, he manifested almost annual events consisting of subacute hemiparesis and visual loss with seizures. MR imaging documented large, ill-defined hemispheric lesions each time that progressed to brain atrophy. In two occasions, the seizures evolved to epilepsia partialis continua of the left foot, which lasted for weeks. He became gradually demented. His mother was small, almost deaf and had manifested hypothyroidism and gestational diabetes. Her own mother had died at 75 years of age from a progressive neurological illness after major neurological event in her middle age.

Common Mitochondrial Disorders of Children

Onset: Any age, with pleomorphic manifestations.
Additional manifestations: Mitochondrial diseases can affect any organ depending on

mutation type. Brain, nerve, muscle, and heart are prime targets and are usually affected, at least to some degree, in most individuals.
Disease mechanism: Respiratory chain insufficiency leading to energy failure is often invoked. Secondary tricarboxylic acid cycle block due to excess NADH. Excess reactive oxygen species production and consequent molecular damage. Dysregulation and induction of apoptosis. Decreased nitric oxide production.
Testing: Lactate can be elevated in serum. Muscle biopsy can be normal or illustrate characteristic histological and histochemical abnormalities, in addition to providing a source of tissue for enzymatic diagnosis.
Treatment: None effective.
Research highlights: Non-invasive MR based methods for the interrogation of human brain and muscle metabolism *in vivo*.

Clinical Features

Mitochondrial diseases arise from mutation of the nuclear or the mitochondrial genomes. Often, nuclear DNA mutations cause more severe disease and manifests earlier in life than mitochondrial DNA-associated mutations. Many of the characteristic manifestations of canonical mitochondrial diseases are variable. This is probably due to the degree of tissue expression (or heteroplasmy) or abundance of the mutant mitochondrial DNA responsible for the disease. Some mitochondrial diseases have been described in other chapters. Several affect single complexes of the respiratory chain (Figure 67.1) whereas most involve more than one complex. Only the most common mitochondrial disorders are summarized here.

MELAS, mitochondrial encephalomyopathy, lactic acidosis, and stroke-like episodes, is characterized by predominantly parietal and occipital stroke-like events

Table 67.1 Common mitochondrial diseases of children

Childhood mitochondrial disorders	Frequent manifestations
MELAS, mitochondrial encephalomyopathy, lactic acidosis, and stroke-like episodes	Stroke-like events Ragged-red fiber myopathy Epilepsy Cardiomyopathy
MERFF, myoclonic epilepsy with ragged-red fibers	Myoclonus Epilepsy Cerebellar ataxia Myopathy
LHON, Leber's hereditary optic neuropathy	Subacute visual loss Dystonia Wolff-Parkinson-White syndrome
CPEO, chronic progressive external opthalmoplegia	Progressive external ophthalmoplegia Ptosis Myopathy
NARP, neurogenic weakness with ataxia and retinitis pigmentosa	Neuropathy Ataxia Retinitis pigmentosa
MNGIE, mitochondrial neurogastrointestinal encephalomyopathy	Progressive external ophthalmoplegia Gastrointestinal dysmotility Neuropathy Myopathy
Kearns-Sayre syndrome (Figure 67.2)	Progressive external ophthalmoplegia Elevated cerebrospinal fluid protein Heart block Cerebellar ataxia
Leigh syndrome	Encephalomyopathy Lactic acidemia
Pearson syndrome	Sideroblastic anemia Exocrine pancreatic failure Renal tubular failure
Alpers-Huttenlocher syndrome	Hepatopathy Epilepsy

in association with elevated cerebrospinal fluid and serum lactate. The stroke-like episodes may develop abruptly and resolve near completely in the course of weeks, only to recur in a similar or different cerebral region. Because the topography of MELAS lesions does not conform to well-demarcated vascular territories, the usual vasculoocclusive mechanisms are unlikely. This, however, does not exclude vasculopathy as an important disease mechanism. The first disease sign may be cardiac pre-excitation or Wolff-Parkinson-White syndrome. Infantile and childhood development may be normal or minimally abnormal until frank disease onset. Deafness, migraines, diabetes, and intestinal dysmotility and pseudo-obstruction are common (Figure 67.3). Neuropathy can be a late manifestation. Cardiomyopathy is often present but rarely lethal. Neuroimaging reveals sizeable, resolving gray and white matter lesions that eventually lead to generalized

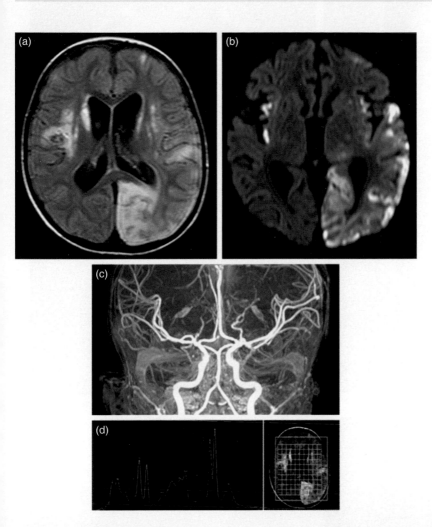

Figure 67.1 Isolated complex IV deficiency. **a**. Axial FLAIR MR imaging shows abnormal hyperintensity signal lesions in basal ganglia and left cortical occipital and parietal lobes, brain atrophy, and ventriculomegaly. **b**. Diffusion-weighted MR imaging shows restricted diffusion at the same location. **c**. Magnetic resonance angiography shows no vascular occlusion or stenosis. **d**. Magnetic resonance spectroscopy with lactate peak in the cortex. Reproduced with permission from Longo MG et al. Brain imaging and genetic risk in the pediatric population, part 1: inherited metabolic diseases. *Neuroimaging Clin N Am*. 2015; 25(1):31–51.

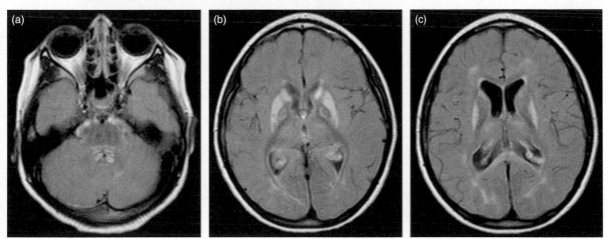

Figure 67.2 Kearns-Sayre syndrome. **a–c**. Axial FLAIR MR imaging shows symmetric and bilateral hyperintensity signal in the white matter, basal ganglia, thalamus, and midbrain. Reproduced with permission from Longo MG et al. Brain imaging and genetic risk in the pediatric population, part 1: inherited metabolic diseases. *Neuroimaging Clin N Am*. 2015; 25(1):31–51.

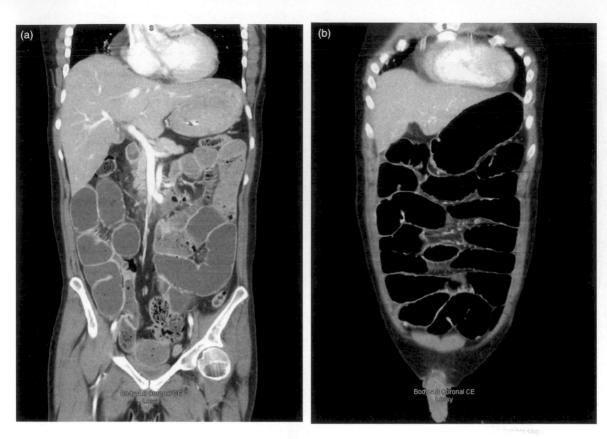

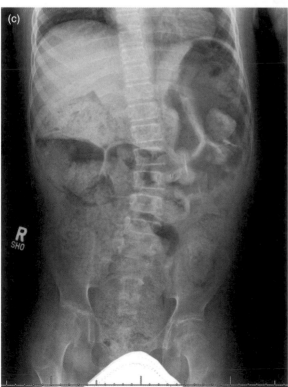

Figure 67.3 MELAS. **a** and **b**. Computerized tomography of a 33 year old man with MELAS associated with mutation A3243G at 76% heteroplasmy in blood. There is significant dilation of the bowel in an obstructive or pseudobstructive pattern. This was part of his terminal disease exarcerbation. **c**. Abdominal X ray of a 13-year-old child with MELAS associated with mutation A3243G at 88 percent heteroplasmy in blood. Abundant stool is noted in the bowel in an impaction pattern. The boy had never experienced intestinal pseudoobstruction.

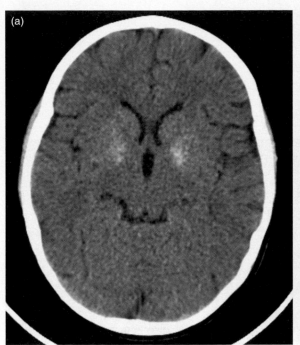 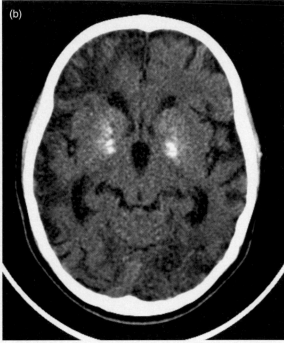

Figure 67.4 MELAS. Axial CT scan of the same child as in Figure 67.3.C. a. Image taken at the time of the fist metabolic infarct. There is effacement of the parietal and occipital sulci, suggestive of infarction. There are pallidal calcifications. There is also mild diffuse cerebral atrophy. b. Image obtained 4 years later. Calcifications have increased. The sequelae of nultiple infacts are visible throughout the hemispheres.

cerebral atrophy (Figures 67.4 to 6). There may be calcification of the basal ganglia. The most common mutation in the mitochondrial genome is A3243G. This substitution also causes maternally inherited diabetes and deafness, and chronic progressive external ophthalmoplegia.

Myoclonic epilepsy with ragged-red fibers or MERRF leads to progressive myoclonus, focal and generalized epilepsy, and myopathy. Age at onset is variable, but MERRF is common in childhood and adolescence. Sensorimotor neuropathy compounds cerebellar dysfunction and both result in ataxia. Proximal limb weakness can be pronounced and be accompanied by wasting. The dorsal root ganglia and posterior spinal columns can degenerate, aggravating neuropathic proprioceptive deficits. Pyramidal tract dysfunction may also be prominent, with spasticity, brisk tendon reflexes and Babinski signs. Seizures are common and there is photosensitive myoclonus in many affected individuals. There may also be a dorsal lipoma at the base of the neck. Wolff-Parkinson-White pre-excitation syndrome and cardiomyopathy can also occur. Many affected individuals have been previously diagnosed with Ramsay Hunt syndrome

(dyssynergia cerebellaris myoclonica). A common causative mutation is substitution A8344G in the mitochondrial DNA.

Leber's hereditary optic neuropathy or LHON presents in young adults with sequential bilateral visual failure. Teleangiectasia of the retinal artery and optic atrophy ensue. The disease displays male predominance. Three mutations in genes that encode complex I of the respiratory chain account for most cases: A3460G in MTND1, G11778A in MTND4 and T14484C in MTND6. Only 50% of males and 10 percent of females harboring a pathogenic mutation develop the disease, indicating that other factors participate in pathogenesis.

Chronic progressive external ophthalmoplegia or CPEO is characterized by slowly progressive ophthalmoparesis and ptosis. Age of onset is variable. Affected individuals may exhibit marked asymmetry as the ophthalmoparesis progresses. The disease often manifests as diplopia in early stages. Later, proximal weakness and fatigue ensue. The gene defect is most often either a single mitochondrial DNA deletion or multiple mitochondrial DNA deletions due to mutations in nuclear DNA genes involved in

255

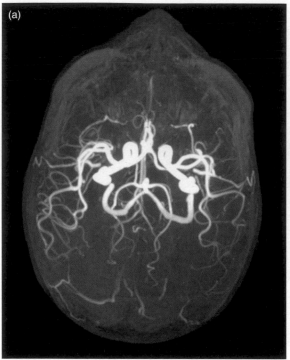

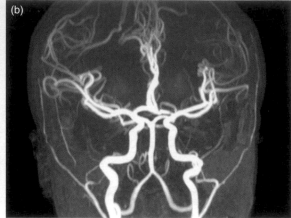

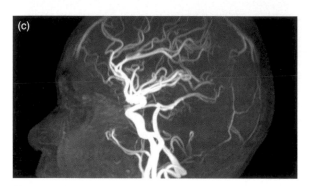

Figure 67.5 MELAS in the same child as the previous figure. Axial (a), coronal (b), and saggital (c) views of a magnetic resonance angiogram. MRA is normal in this disease, indicating a nonobstructive blood flow pattern. This pattern does not exclude vasculopathy of the vessel wall.

mitochondrial DNA replication and maintenance. The mechanism of inheritance in these cases is either autosomal dominant or autosomal recessive. Both dominant and recessive forms of chronic progressive external ophthalmoplegia can be caused by mutation of polymerase gamma (POLG). Mutations in POLG are associated with parkinsonism, psychiatric disorders, neuropathy, or deafness. Chronic progressive external ophthalmoplegia may also be part of complex syndromes such as MELAS, MERRF, SANDO (sensory ataxic neuropathy with dysphagia and ophthalmoplegia), and MIRAS (mitochondrial recessive ataxia syndrome)

Neurogenic weakness with ataxia and retinitis pigmentosa or NARP includes abnormal neurological development or dementia, retinitis pigmentosa, ataxia, epilepsy, and sensory neuropathy. The most common mutation involves nucleotide 8993 of the mitochondrial DNA, which is part of the ATP6 gene, a determinant of the complex V ATPase. Some cases of Leigh syndrome have been attributed to this mutation.

Pathology and Diagnosis

Neuroimaging techniques may be suggestive but are rarely diagnostic. In some mitochondrial diseases, lactate is often elevated in blood, as may be alanine.

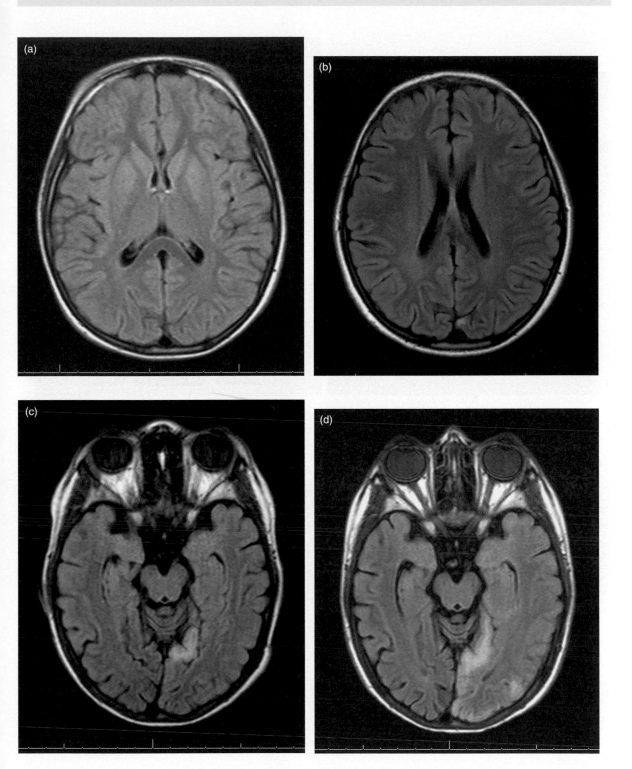

Figure 67.6 MELAS in the same individual as the previous figure. a to i illustrate disease progression. Axial FLAIR magnetic resonance images. Images taken at each of 9 clinically significant events. a: Normal MR imaging at onset at 10 years of age with seizures. b–i: MRI at ages (in years/months) 10/0, 10/7, 10/9, 10/9 1/2, 10/11, 11/4, 11/5, 12, 14. Clinical event included focal neurological deficits and seizures of progressively decreasing severity. The boy was severely demented by 14 years of age.

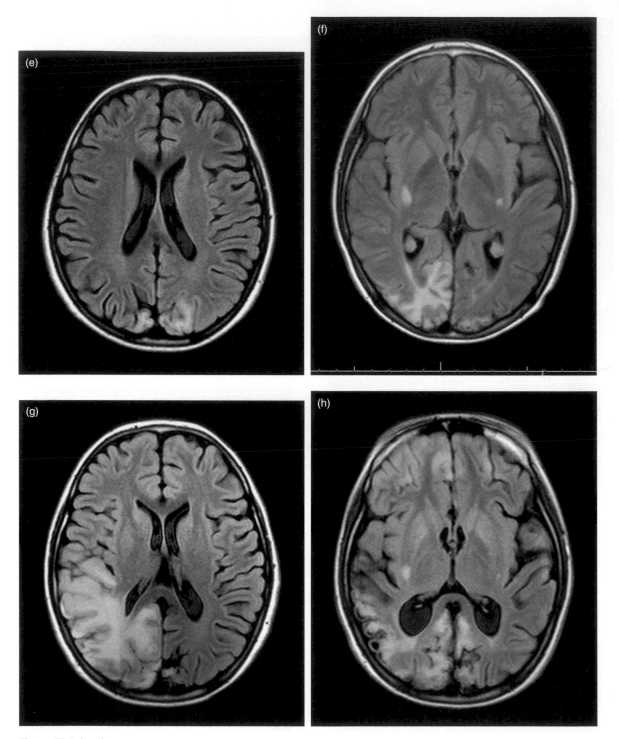

Figure 67.6 (cont.)

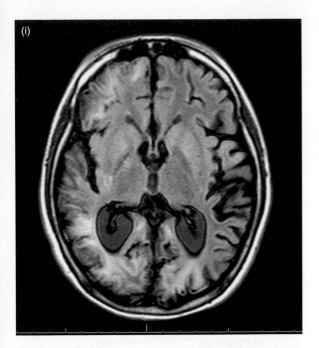

(i)

Figure 67.6 (*cont.*)

Muscle biopsy provides the best tissue to confirm a mitochondrial disease. Histochemical features often correlate with specific syndromes and facilitate the selection of biochemical and genetic studies. Ragged-red fibers indicate subsarcolemmal mitochondrial accumulation and nearly always indicate a combination defect of respiratory complexes I and IV. Increased punctate lipid within myofibers is a regular feature of Kearns-Sayre and PEO, but not of MELAS and MERRF. Total deficiency of succinate dehydrogenase indicates a severe defect in complex II; total absence of cytochrome-c-oxidase activity in all myofibers correlates with a severe deficiency of complex IV. The selective loss of cytochrome c oxidase activity in scattered myofibers, particularly if accompanied by strong succinate dehydrogenase staining in these same fibers, is evidence of mitochondrial cytopathy and often of a significant mitochondrial DNA mutation, though it is not specific for complex IV disorders. Ultrastructural analysis by electron microscopy may provide evidence of mitochondrial cytopathy in axons and endothelial cells as well as myocytes. Abnormal axonal mitochondria may contribute to neurogenic atrophy of muscle, a secondary chronic feature. Quantitative determinations of respiratory chain enzyme complexes, with citrate synthase as an internal control, confirm the histochemical impressions or may be the only evidence of mitochondrial disease. Skin biopsy may be useful for the determination of mitochondrial ultrastructure in smooth erector pili muscles and axons.

Pathophysiology

A central function of mitochondria is the production of energy through oxidative phosphorylation, which is carried out by the electron transport chain complexes located in the inner mitochondrial membrane. In addition to energy production, mitochondria are essential for calcium homeostasis and normal apoptosis. Mutations in mitochondrial DNA or in mitochondria-related nuclear genes result in defective electron transport complex function and, potentially, in energy failure, although this is more often suggested than demonstrated. Further consequences of mitochondrial dysfunction may include excessive reactive oxygen species formation, aberrant calcium handling, and apoptotic dysregulation.

Additionally, due to the impairment in oxidative phosphorylation, NADH cannot be utilized, such that NADH:NAD ratio increases, which results in inhibition of the tricarboxylic acid cycle. Pyruvate, which produced through glycolysis, is increased due to tricarboxylic acid cycle inhibition. Both elevated pyruvate and NADH:NAD ratio result in a shift of the equilibrium of lactate dehydrogenase toward the production of lactate from pyruvate. Lactate can then accumulate, causing systemic acidosis.

During oxidative phosphorylation, a faction of all available oxygen is partially reduced and converted into reactive oxygen species (superoxide and hydrogen peroxide). These species can be toxic to the cell, but they also participate in diverse signaling mechanisms. Reactive oxygen species are generated mainly at complexes I and III of the respiratory chain. Under normal conditions, they are scavenged by various enzymes, including the mitochondrial superoxide dismutase and glutathione peroxidase. The generation of reactive oxygen species is stimulated by inhibition of complex I and III. Moreover, inhibition of complexes IV or V also results in increased reactive oxygen species production indirectly, since the accumulation of reduced coenzyme Q10 is an inducer of reactive oxygen species production by complex I. Increased reactive oxygen species production can result in protein, lipid, and DNA damage, which may potentially lead to further cellular dysfunction. The Fe–S cluster-containing enzymes including complexes I and III are highly sensitive to this type of oxidative damage, such that their damage may result in additional respiratory chain inhibition.

Mitochondria also regulate apoptosis. Supermolecular channels, the mitochondrial permeability transition pores, open in response to several intracellular stimuli, resulting in increased mitochondrial inner membrane permeability. Apoptosis is initiated when the inner mitochondrial membrane becomes permeable, releasing several toxic mitochondrial proteins into the cytosol, including cytochrome c. These proteins activate latent forms of caspases, resulting in apoptosis.

Nitric oxide (NO) deficiency may also occur in mitochondrial diseases. This may be due to impaired NO production and to postproduction sequestration. Impaired NO production can result from endothelial dysfunction, decreased availability of the NO precursors arginine and citrulline or impaired NO synthase activity. Postproduction NO sequestration may occur due to increased cytochrome c oxidase and shunting of NO into reactive nitrogen species formation.

Treatment

There is no effective therapy for mitochondrial disorders. Several cofactor supplementations have been tried, but with minimal data supporting any benefit. Coenzyme Q10 (ubiquinone) supplementation for individuals with coenzyme Q10 deficiency may result in significant clinical improvement. EPI-743, a parabenzoquinone which is an analog of coenzyme Q10, may improve some clinical outcomes in children with some mitochondrial diseases. Creatine monohydrate supplementation can improve exercise capacity in some affected individuals. Combination therapy using creatine monohydrate, coenzyme Q10, and lipoic acid can be beneficial in individuals with mitochondrial cytopathies in lowering lactic acidemia and in improving strength. Supplementation with riboflavin has been associated with improvement in a few individuals with complex I deficiency myopathy. B vitamins and antioxidants such as alpha lipoic acid, vitamin E, and vitamin C all have been used in mitochondrial disorders, but there is very limited evidence of any effect.

Bibliography

El-Hattab A.W., Scaglia F. (2016). Mitochondrial cytopathies. *Cell Calcium*. pii:S0143–4160(16) 30021–5.

Sarnat H.B., Marín-García J. (2005). Pathology of mitochondrial encephalomyopathies. *Can J Neurol Sci.* 32(2):152–66.

Acute Necrotizing Encephalopathy

A 2-year, 7-month-old girl was admitted to the hospital for a 4 day history of mild fever, lethargy, and vomiting due to a presumed viral infection. She became acutely encephalopathic and developed brain stem and pyramidal signs. Computed tomography of her brain was normal. A lumbar puncture was not performed, but liver function tests were normal. An EEG showed slow-wave activity consistent with encephalopathy and no epileptiform discharges. Magnetic resonance imaging (Figure 68.1) showed lesions compatible with acute disseminated encephalomyelitis. Because of this diagnosis, she was given 30 mg/kg of intravenous methylprednisolone once daily for five days. She improved and was discharged from the hospital on a four week tapering course of oral prednisolone. She made a good initial recovery at two months, and at the age 3.3 years she had residual upper motor neuron signs in her right leg.

One and a half years later, her younger sister, aged 1 year and 4 months, presented with a brief history of diarrhea, vomiting and a generalized tonic clonic seizure. On assessment, she was encephalopathic (Glasgow coma scale 7), dysarthric with poor axial tone and upper motor neuron signs in the limbs. Meningoencephalitis was suspected. Lumbar puncture showed a white cell count of $5 \times 10^6/L$, elevated protein of 1.25 g/l, and normal lactate of 1.2 mmol/l. MR imaging (Figure 68.1) was also abnormal and consistent with acute disseminated encephalomyelitis. She also received methylprednisolone (30 mg/kg) for five days followed by a three week oral course of oral prednisolone. She made a good recovery at 1 month and at the age of 1.8 years she had returned to her pre-disease state.

Acute Necrotizing Encephalopathy

Onset: Following a febrile illness, depressed consciousness, focal neurological deficits, and seizures around 3 years of age.

Additional manifestations: Recurrent forms exist. MR imaging lesions in the thalamus and other widespread structures including the brainstem and spinal cord. Elevated cerebrospinal fluid protein without pleocytosis. The disease resembles acute disseminated encephalomyelitis.

Disease mechanism: Autosomal dominant mutation of RANBP2, which encodes the nuclear pore component of RAN Binding Protein 2. Blood brain barrier dysfunction with cytokine toxicity.

Testing: MR imaging and cerebrospinal fluid profile are characteristic.

Treatment: Steroids may shorten recovery.

Research highlights: Role of dysfunctional RANBP2 in energy metabolism in neurons when the cell is challenged by acute infection.

Clinical Features

Acute necrotizing encephalopathy or acute infection-induced encephalopathy is characterized by rapidly progressive and severe brain dysfunction associated with seizures and coma occurring after common viral infections such as influenza and parainfluenza. Some of the clinical and radiological features of acute disseminated encephalomyelitis can be mistaken for acute necrotizing encephalopathy at an early stage, as when a child presents with encephalopathy, focal neurological deficits, and perhaps seizures (Figure 68.1). When there is a familial predisposition for recurrent acute necrotizing encephalopathy, the modified designation type 1 is used. Acute necrotizing

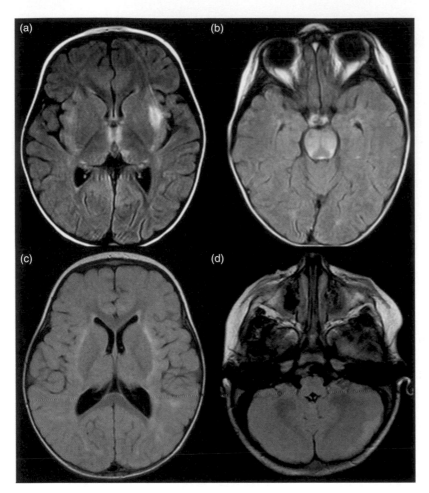

Figure 68.1 Acute necrotizing encephalopathy in two cases. MR images of cases 1 (a + b) and 2 (c + d). T2 FLAIR images of case 1 (a, b) and 2 (C,D). Neuroimaging of case 1 reveals increased signal in the left insular (a) and brainstem, particularly the midbrain bilaterally extending into the pons (b). In case 2, high signal within bilateral external capsules (c) and left cerebellar gray matter (d) is identified. Reproduced with permission from Singh RR et al. RANBP2 mutation and acute necrotizing encephalopathy: 2 cases and a literature review of the expanding clinico-radiological phenotype. *Eur J Paediatr Neurol.* 2015; 19(2):106–13.

encephalopathy type 1 can be inherited in autosomal dominant fashion and is associated with mutations in the gene RANBP2, which encodes the nuclear pore component of RAN Binding Protein 2. There have also been cases of familial and recurrent acute necrotizing encephalopathy without RANBP2 mutation.

The median age of onset of acute necrotizing encephalopathy type 1 is 3 years (range 5 months–36 years). The disease usually affects younger children following a febrile illness and presents with encephalopathy, focal neurological deficits and, occasionally, seizures. Magnetic resonance imaging illustrates increased T2 signal in both thalami in about 80 percent of cases. Other supportive MR imaging features include symmetrical multifocal lesions in periventricular white matter, internal capsules, basal ganglia, brainstem, and cerebellum. The genetically determined form of the disease (type 1) is perhaps associated with more widespread lesions (including spinal cord lesions) than generic acute necrotizing encephalopathy. The outcome of children with both generic and type 1 acute necrotizing encephalopathy is variable.

Pathology

The pathological features of the disease have only been inferred through MR imaging. There are most often symmetric, multifocal lesions of the thalamus. There may also be lesions in the periventricular white matter, internal capsule, putamen, brainstem or cerebellum. In some cases, there is symmetric involvement of medial temporal lobes, insular cortex, amygdala-hippocampus complex, claustrum, or external capsule. Brainstem involvement can be seen in 75 percent of affected individuals. Spinal cord involvement and cerebellar changes can also occur.

Pathophysiology

Mutations in RANBP2, which encodes the nuclear pore component of RAN Binding Protein 2, are associated with acute necrotizing encephalopathy. RAN is a small GTP-binding protein of the RAS superfamily that is associated with the nuclear membrane and may control a variety of cellular functions through its interactions with other proteins. The RANBP2 gene encodes a large RAN-binding protein localized in the nuclear pore complex. The protein is a giant scaffold nucleoporin implicated in the Ran-GTPase cycle. The encoded protein directly interacts with the E2 enzyme UBC9 (ubiquitin-conjugating enzyme 9) and enhances SUMO1 (small ubiquitin-like modifier 1) transfer from UBC9 to the SUMO1 target SP100. The gene is partially duplicated in a gene cluster that lies in a region prone to recombination on chromosome 2q.

Most cases of acute necrotizing encephalopathy type 1 harbor RANBP2 mutation Thr585Met. RAN Binding Protein 2 participates in energy metabolism of neuronal cells. Dysfunction of the RANBP2 nuclear pore leads to energy failure when the cell mechanisms are challenged by acute infection. Mutations in RANBP2 thus merely predispose to the clinical syndrome of acute necrotizing encephalopathy. The development of acute necrotizing encephalopathy requires a triggering factor; most commonly a viral infection. Influenza A, influenza B, parainfluenza, human herpesvirus 6, varicella, *Mycoplasma pneumoniae* and the diphtheria, tetanus, and pertussis (DTP) vaccination have all triggered acute necrotizing encephalopathy. In the absence of direct invasion of the nervous system by viruses, the disease is induced by mediators of peripheral inflammation causing disruption of the blood–brain barrier. A plausible consequence of this disruption is the elevated cerebrospinal fluid protein, which is accom-panied by a relative absence of pleocytosis. Disruption of the blood–brain barrier is also supported by the neuroimaging findings of thalamic lesions showing concentric lamellar changes with peripheral high absolute diffusion coefficient, probably reflecting vasogenic edema, low absolute diffusion coefficient in the intermediate zone indicating cytotoxic edema, and high absolute diffusion coefficient in the center representing hemorrhage and necrosis. Hypercytokinemia has also been documented. The preferential passage of proteins and absence of significant leukocyte trafficking into the cerebrospinal fluid can help distinguish acute necrotizing encephalopathy from other encephalitides including acute disseminated encephalomyelitis.

Diagnosis

Several clinical findings, in addition to MR imaging, facilitate the diagnosis. An increase in serum transaminases is variably present. An absence of cerebrospinal fluid pleocytosis ($>5 \times 10^6$ cells/L) and an increase in protein (>0.45 g/L) are common.

Treatment

Early treatment with steroids provides the best outcome for individuals who do not manifest brainstem lesions.

Bibliography

Singh R.R., Sedani S., Lim M., et al. (2015). RANBP2 mutation and acute necrotizing encephalopathy: 2 cases and a literature review of the expanding clinico-radiological phenotype. *Eur J Paediatr Neurol.* 19(2):106–13.

Gaucher Disease

A boy, the older of two siblings, was born to nonconsanguineous parents. His sister was healthy. Development was normal until a first, sleep-related, generalized tonic–clonic seizure occurred at the age of 11 years. He had had a previous, isolated, and brief episode of dysarthria. EEG showed posterior spikes and spike-and-wave discharges. He was given phenobarbital and was seizure free for the following 8 months. At age 12 years, visual seizures appeared, described as brief, multicolored sparkling perceptions. Generalized tonic-clonic seizures recurred, and the child became ataxic, especially on awakening, because of mild action myoclonus. In the following months, his seizures became intractable. Myoclonus, dysarthria, and ataxia also became progressively worse. Examination revealed mild hypotonia. Tendon reflexes and ocular fundi were normal. Ocular motility also was normal. His intellectual quotient (Wechsler Intelligence Scale for Children) was within the average range. Moderate hepatomegaly was observed. At age 14 years, cognitive deterioration became apparent, and worsening of action myoclonus and ataxia made standing impossible. There was no anemia, thrombocytopenia, bone pain, or supranuclear ophthalmoplegia.

Gaucher Disease

Onset: Congenital, infantile, or childhood hepatosplenomegaly with progressive neurological deterioration.
Additional manifestations: Skeletal destruction with avascular necrosis and pathological fractures. Thrombocytopenia and anemia. Myoclonus. Horizontal supranuclear gaze palsy. Bulbar dysfunction such as strabismus and dysphagia. Parkinsonism. Type II is more severe than type III disease, whereas type I is rarely associated with a neurological disorder.

Disease mechanism: Glucosylsphingosine, a byproduct of glucosylceramide, accumulates in visceral organs and brain. Release proinflammatory cytokines by Gaucher cells or microglia with neuroinflammation.
Testing: Enzymatic assay in blood or solid tissue samples.
Treatment: Enzyme replacement alleviates visceral manifestations.
Research highlights: Chaperones that stabilize the active enzyme conformation.

Clinical Features

Gaucher disease is caused by autosomal recessive mutations in the GBA1 gene encoding the lysosomal hydrolase β–glucosidase (glucosylceramidase beta),

Table 69.1 Clinical features of Gaucher disease forms

Gaucher disease types	Principal characteristics
I Non-neuronopathic	Adulthood Hepatosplenomegaly Skeletal abnormalities
II Acute neuronopathic	Infancy Hepatosplenomegaly Progressive neural dysfunction
IIIa Chronic neuronopathic	Progressive neural dysfunction Myoclonus Dementia
IIIb Chronic neuronopathic	Horizontal supranuclear gaze palsy Visceral dysfunction Skeletal abnormalities
IIIc Chronic neuronopathic	Horizontal supranuclear gaze palsy Less visceral involvement
Parkinsonian	Typical Parkinson's disease

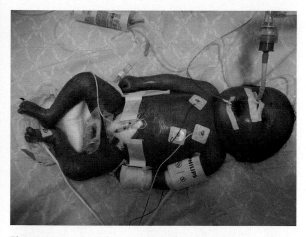

Figure 69.1 Neonatal presentation of Gaucher disease demonstrating hydrops, peeling, and shiny skin. Reproduced with permission from BenHamida E et al. Perinatal-lethal Gaucher disease presenting as hydrops fetalis. *Pan Afr Med J.* 2015; 21:110.

which lead to progressive glycolipid storage in macrophagic and, in some cases, neural cells. Three forms that represent a broad clinical continuum are recognized.

Type I Gaucher disease is a non-neurological adult (and occasionally childhood) disorder characterized by hepatosplenomegaly with anemia and thrombocytopenia and destructive skeletal disease.

Type II Gaucher disease is associated with infantile hepatosplenomegaly and progressive neurological deterioration. Oculomotor abnormalities are often the first symptom, including strabismus and horizontal supranuclear gaze palsy. Additional manifestations of brainstem dysfunction include dysphagia and stridor. Stimulus-induced myoclonus can be prominent. The myoclonus is usually cortical in origin and may be associated with dystonia. Most

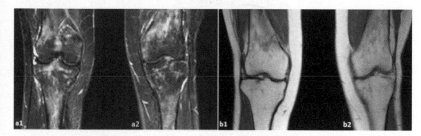

Figure 69.2 Skeletal involvement in Gaucher disease. Thirty-one-year-old female, first diagnosed with Gaucher disease type 1 at the age of 14 years. TIRM sequence (a1, a2) and T1-TSE sequence (b1, b2). The a1 and b1 panels show follow-up MR images and a2 and b2 panels show the baseline MR images for the epiphysis area. There is stable infiltration of the epiphysis area (area 6). Reproduced with permission from Laudemann K et al. Evaluation of treatment response to enzyme replacement therapy with Velaglucerase alfa in patients with Gaucher disease using whole-body magnetic resonance imaging. *Blood Cells Mol Dis.* 2016; 57:35–41.

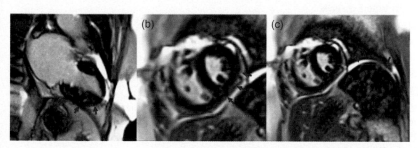

Figure 69.3 Cardiac infiltration in Gaucher disease. Cardiac MR imaging with late gadolinium enhancement (LGE). Inversion recovery sequences 10 min after administration. Panel a: Long axis view of the left ventricle (LV). Greyish and patchy intramyocardial areas interspersed in the LV inferior wall are compatible with myocardial interstitial fibrosis secondary to Gaucher cells nodular infiltration at this level (arrows). Panel b: Left ventricle short axis view at the mid-ventricular level. Patchy LGE is present in both inferior and inferolateral segments (arrow). Panel c: Prominent hepatomegaly due to Gaucher cells storage. A characteristic patchy LGE is observed (arrow), due to the infiltrative interstitial fibrosis secondary to the scattered deposit of sphingolipids. Reproduced with permission from Solanich X et al. Myocardial infiltration in Gaucher disease detected by cardiac MRI. *Int J Cardiol.* 2012; 155(1):e5–6.

affected children die within two years of disease onset. A severe neonatal form is associated with ichthyotic skin (collodion baby) or hydrops fetalis (Figure 69.1).

Gaucher disease type III is of intermediate severity between types I and II, with neurological manifestations occurring later in the disease course. Seizures may occur, but they are usually medication-sensitive. In type IIIa, myoclonus and dementia dominate the clinical syndrome. In type IIIb, neurological abnormalities consist primarily of horizontal supranuclear gaze palsy in the context of severe visceral and skeletal abnormalities (Figures 69.2 and 69.3). Type IIIc is characterized by horizontal supranuclear gaze palsy, cardiac valve calcification, and corneal opacity with little visceral manifestations.

Lastly, affected adults with and carriers of Gaucher disease may develop Parkinson's disease. This is most common in type I disease.

Pathology

There is massive infiltration of visceral macrophages with glucocerebroside (Gaucher cells) in all disease types (Figures 69.4 and 69.5). This infiltration is particularly severe in liver and spleen, leading to hepatosplenomegaly. Infiltration of the bone marrow with Gaucher cells may lead to pathological fractures and avascular necrosis. Bone disease is more pronounced in splenectomized individuals. The cytoplasm of Gaucher cells is wrinkled and stains with periodic acid-Schiff. Glucocerebroside accumulates in curved or twisted tubular structures.

In the brain, type I disease can be associated with Gaucher cell infiltration of the leptomeninges and perivascular regions. In individuals with type I disease and parkinsonism, there are α-synuclein inclusions similar to Lewy bodies in the hippocampus.

In type II disease with severe manifestations there is marked Gaucher cell infiltration with neuronal degeneration and gliosis. Neurodegeneration is most prominent in the cerebellar nuclei, brainstem, and hypothalamus. In the cerebral cortex, infiltration by Gaucher cells is most prominent in the occipital cortex. Neurons may also contain typical tubular inclusions.

The neuropathology of type III disease is similar but less severe than that of type II. In cases of myoclonus, selective degeneration of the cerebellar dentate nucleus and dentatorubrothalamic pathway has been documented.

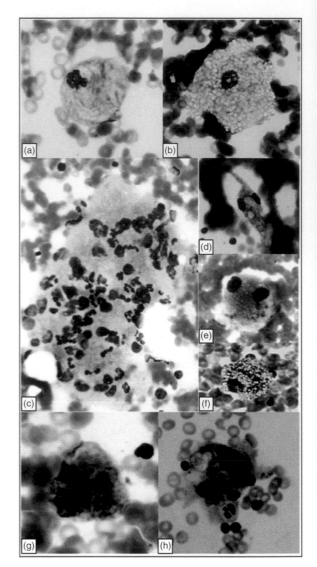

Figure 69.4 Gaucher cells showing typical (a) and atypical (B–H) morphology. a. Typical Gaucher cell (GC) with fibrillary cytoplasm and an eccentric placed nucleus; b. GC with foamy cytoplasm and almost central nucleus; c. A syncytium of GCs with phagocytosed neutrophilic granulocytes; d. GC with cytoplasmic projections and two nuclei; e. GC with two nuclei and thrombophagocytosis; f. Foamy GC with hemosiderin grains; g. GC with erythrophagocytosis; h. GC with phagocytosis of erythroblasts, neutrophilic granulocytes, an eosinophilic granulocyte and some unidentified nucleated cells. Bone marrow smears, May-Grünwald Giemsa staining. Reproduced with permission from Markuszewska-Kuczynska A et al. Atypical cytomorphology of Gaucher cells is frequently seen in bone marrow smears from untreated patients with Gaucher disease type 1. *Folia Histochem Cytobiol.* 2015; 53(1):62–9.

Pathophysiology

Glucosylceramide is the stored product in all organs in Gaucher disease (Figure 69.6). However, the affected brain contains only relatively small amounts

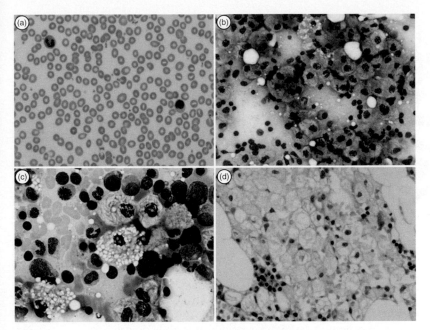

Figure 69.5 Gaucher cells. Microscopic examination of (a) peripheral blood (×400, Wright-Giemsa stain) and (b) bone marrow aspiration (×400, Wright-Giemsa stain). (c) Atypical Gaucher cell with vacuolations and typical Gaucher cell with a "wrinkled tissue pattern" on bone marrow aspirate smear (×1,000, Wright-Giemsa stain). (d) Bone marrow biopsy specimen presenting with several Gaucher cells (×400, Hematoxylin & Eosin stain). Reproduced with permission from Rim JH et al. Clinical Utility of Bone Marrow Study in Gaucher Disease: A Case Report of Gaucher Disease Type 3 With Intractable Myoclonic Seizures. *Ann Lab Med.* 2016; 36(2):177–9.

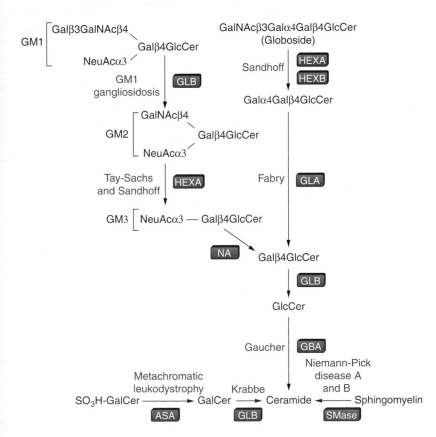

Figure 69.6 Sphingolipid metabolism. The enzymes that catalyse the catabolism of one metabolite to another are shown in red, and the diseases that result from defects of these enzymes are shown in blue. ASA, arylsulphatase A; GBA, β-glucocerebrosidase; GLA, a-galactosidase; GLB, β-galactosidase; HEXA, β-hexosaminidase A; HEXB, β-hexosaminidase B; NA, neuraminidase; SMase, acid sphingomyelinase. Reproduced with permission from Platt FM. Sphingolipid lysosomal storage disorders. *Nature.* 2014; 510(7503):68–75.

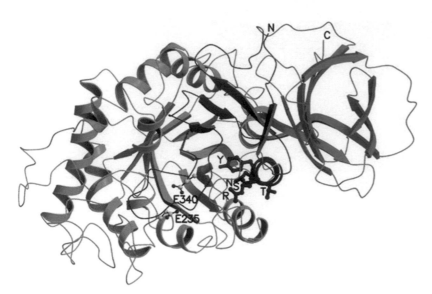

Figure 69.7 Glucosylceramidase beta mutations in Gaucher disease. A cluster of mutations in a-helix 7 that cause Gaucher disease. Transparent ribbon diagram showing the three domains of acid-ß-glucosidase. Helix 7 is shown in red. The amino acids on this helix that are mutated in Gaucher disease (Arg359, Tyr363, Ser366, Thr369, and Asn370) are shown as red balls and sticks. Glu235 and Glu340 (the active-site residues) are shown with carbon atoms as yellow balls and oxygen atoms as red balls. Reproduced with permission from Dvir H et al. X-ray structure of human acid-beta-glucosidase, the defective enzyme in Gaucher disease. *EMBO Rep.* 2003; 4(7):704–9.

of glucosylceramide. Glucosylsphingosine, a byproduct of glucosylceramide, on the other hand, accumulates in all visceral organs and brain. Whereas visceral glucosylsphingosine levels exhibit little correlation with disease severity, brain levels are closely related to the extent of neurodegeneration. Glucosylsphingosine may reach toxic concentrations in neural cells, accumulating in type II brain to a greater extent than in type III brain. The highest level of glucosylsphingosine deposition occurs in hydrops fetalis.

In addition, Gaucher cells release proinflammatory cytokines. In the brain, it is plausible that neuronal glucosylceramide accumulation may lead to microglial activation, which then releases inflammatory cytokines that promote neuronal death.

The most common mutation in glucosylceramidase beta is Asn370Ser, which is associated with nonneuronopathic type I disease (Figure 69.7). Mutations Lys444Pro and Asp409His occur in individuals with neurological manifestations. In addition, other less frequent mutations account for relatively selective symptom specificity.

Diagnosis

Auditory evoked potentials gradually deteriorate as the disease progresses. Somatosensory evoked potentials, particularly in individuals with myoclonus, exhibit increased amplitude.

Enzyme testing can be performed in blood cells and other readily accessible tissues.

Treatment

Splenectomy normalizes platelet count and hemoglobin levels but eventually leads to more severe skeletal complications. Blood transfusions have also been used. Bone marrow transplantation alleviates the visceral manifestations of the disease but does not influence the rate of neurological decline.

Enzyme replacement is the treatment of choice for type III disease, but it is not effective in type II. However, this therapy does not impact neurological manifestations. Pharmacological chaperones such as ambroxol are active site competitive inhibitors that penetrate brain tissue and induce the normal conformations of glucocerebroside, which may thus regain normal activity and lysosomal localization.

Bibliography

Filocamo M., Mazzotti R., Stroppiano M., et al. (2004). Early visual seizures and progressive myoclonus epilepsy in neuronopathic Gaucher disease due to a rare compound heterozygosity (N188S/S107L). *Epilepsia.* 45(9):1154–7.

Mistry P.K., Belmatoug N., vom Dahl S., et al. (2015). Understanding the natural history of Gaucher disease. *Am J Hematol.* 90 Suppl 1:S6–11.

Niemann–Pick Type C Disease

A 24-year-old man was evaluated following a 12-year history of obsessive-compulsive disorder. His main complaint was now a 2-year history of slowly progressive leg clumsiness associated with repeated falls, frequently occurring during soccer practice. Following a normal birth from a twin pregnancy, he developed splenomegaly for which several diagnostic tests were undertaken. At the age of 12 years, he manifested intrusive recurrent and persistent thoughts that caused significant distress and anxiety. At the age of 21 his symptoms worsened, with the appearance of persecutory delusions and magical thinking (e.g., he believed that his thoughts could prevent his parents from being harmed by strangers). Examination revealed laconic and sluggish speech. Neuropsychological evaluation revealed global cognitive deficits, in particular in short- and long-term verbal memory, working memory, and executive functions. He exhibited vertical gaze supranuclear ophthalmoplegia, more pronounced during down gaze, with full horizontal ocular movements. He manifested a Romberg sign with a broad-based ataxic gait. Strength and tone were normal. Tendon reflexes were hyperactive in the lower limbs, with bilateral ankle clonus. Sensory examination was unremarkable. He also displayed moderate bilateral limb dysmetria at the finger-to-nose and heel-to-shin tests.

Niemann–Pick Type C Disease

Onset: Intellectual disability, fine motor incoordination and ataxia in late infantile and juvenile cases. Transient neonatal cholestasis with jaundice in one half of cases.

Additional manifestations: Seizures, dystonia, cataplexy, and supranuclear vertical gaze palsy. Psychosis or progressive dementia in older individuals.

Disease mechanism: Autosomal recessive mutations in NPC1 or NPC2 lead to impaired cholesterol trafficking with accumulation in the neuronal cell body and deficiency elsewhere. Neuroinflammation and disrupted neurosteroid synthesis.

Testing: Elevation of free cholesterol in cultured fibroblasts by staining with filipin or determination of the rate of cellular cholesterol esterification.

Treatment: None effective. Miglustat is aimed to inhibit glycolipid synthesis.

Research highlights: Intracerebral administration of cyclodextran to bind cholesterol.

Clinical Features

Individuals with Niemann–Pick type C and D disease are often considered to suffer from the same disorder for reason of simplicity. Indeed, Niemann–Pick type D disease is circumscribed to individuals of Nova Scotian descent and overlaps significantly with the more common Niemann–Pick type C disease. Niemann–Pick types A and B are discussed separately.

Niemann–Pick type C disease is characterized by mild hepatosplenomegaly and profound neurological dysfunction caused by autosomal recessive mutation of one of two genes, NPC1 and NPC2. The disease is associated with abnormal intracellular cholesterol-sphingolipid trafficking. The age of presentation is variable and the initial symptoms may be hepatic, neurological, or psychiatric. The most common forms are late infantile and juvenile with neurological onset and hepatosplenomegaly. The first symptoms are reduced scholastic performance due to intellectual disability, fine motor incoordination, and ataxia. Seizures, dystonia, cataplexy, and supranuclear vertical gaze palsy (downward, upward, or both) follow. Prolonged neonatal cholestasis with jaundice and

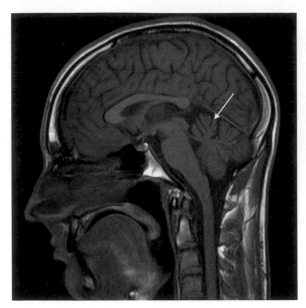

Figure 70.1 MR imaging in Niemann–Pick disease type C showing mild vermian cerebellar atrophy (arrow). The MR brain appearances in Niemann–Pick type C are non-specific and occur in several different ataxias. Reproduced with permission from Kheder A et al. Niemann–Pick type C: a potentially treatable disorder? *Pract Neurol.* 2013; 13(6):382–5.

progressive hepatosplenomegaly may occur in about one half of these affected individuals, but follows a benign course with resolution in 2–4 months. About 10 percent of affected infants, however, exhibit rapid progression of liver dysfunction and die before 6 months without any neurological manifestations. Older individuals, including adults, may manifest psychosis or progressive dementia. In them, organomegaly and supranuclear gaze palsy may be absent.

Pathology

Neuroimaging may reveal cerebral or cerebellar atrophy in association with white matter hyperintensity on T2-weighted images (Figure 70.1). The cerebral cortex is atrophic and contains swollen neurons with inclusions. The basal ganglia, thalamus, brainstem, and spinal cord are prominently affected (Figure 70.2). In the cerebellum, lipid deposition occurs in Purkinje cells and cells of the dentate nucleus. Neuronal storage is more prominent in young disease cases with rapid progression. Stored material predominantly consists of gangliosides GM2 and GM3 and cholesterol (Figure 70.3). Swollen axon hillocks called meganeurites and ectopic neurites are frequent throughout the brain, as are axonal spheroids. These spheroids are particularly prominent in

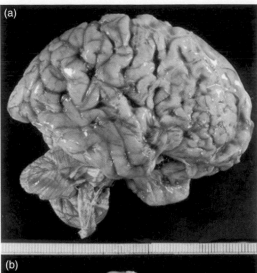

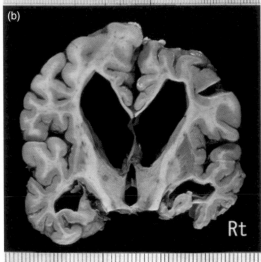

Figure 70.2 Gross neuropathological findings in Niemann–Pick disease type C. (a) Lateral aspect of the brain. Note marked atrophy of the frontal and temporal lobes. (b) Coronal sections of the cerebral hemisphere exhibit marked atrophy of the deep white matter with thinning of the corpus callosum, atrophy of the frontal and temporal cortices, hippocampus, parahippocampal region, thalamus and hypothalamus, accompanied by dilatation of the lateral and third ventricles. The Sommer's sectors of hippocampi bilaterally exhibit brownish discoloration. The superior temporal gyri are relatively spared compared with the middle and inferior temporal gyri. Reproduced with permission from Chiba Y et al. Niemann–Pick disease type C1 predominantly involving the frontotemporal region, with cortical and brainstem Lewy bodies: an autopsy case. *Neuropathology.* 2014; 34(1):49–57.

Purkinje cells. Neurofibrillary tangles are also commonly found, particularly in slowly progressive forms of Niemann–Pick type C disease. α-synuclein can be demonstrated in swollen neurons and in glia. There is

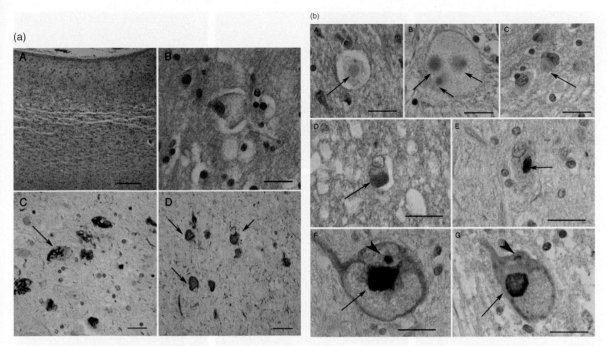

Figure 70.3 Microscopic neuropathological findings in the case from Figure 70.2. A. (**a**) Severe neuronal loss and gliosis of the cortex of the medial aspect of the precentral gyrus. Advanced degeneration with a laminar necrosis-like appearance is evident in the middle layers of the cortex. HE stain. (**b**) Swollen storage neurons distended with accumulated lipids in the cortex of the medial aspect of the precentral gyrus. HE stain. Neurofibrillary tangles (NFTs) are frequently seen in the (**c**) CA1 pyramidal cells (Gallyas-Braak silver stain) and (**d**) neurons of the frontal cortex (AT8 immunohistochemistry). Storage neurons often contain NFTs (arrows). Bars: (a) 200 μm; (b–d) 20 μm. B. Additional microscopic findings. Occurrence of Lewy bodies (LBs) in the cerebral cortex and brainstem. (a) A cortical LB (arrow) formed in lipid-filled cytoplasm of a neuron in the frontal cortex. HE stain. (b) LBs (arrows) in a swollen storage cell of the midbrain. HE stain. (c) Cortical LB (arrow) in an amygdala neuron with minimal lipid storage. HE stain. (d–g) LBs (arrows) were immunohistochemically stained for (d, frontal cortex) a-synuclein, (e, frontal cortex) ubiquitin, (f, midbrain) HDAC6 and (g, midbrain) p62/SQSTM1. (f and g, arrowheads) Marinesco bodies were also immunohistochemically stained with anti-HDAC6 and anti-p62/SQSTM1 antibodies. Bars: 20 μm. Reproduced with permission from Chiba Y et al. Niemann–Pick disease type C1 predominantly involving the frontotemporal region, with cortical and brainstem Lewy bodies: an autopsy case. *Neuropathology*. 2014; 34(1):49–57.

neuronal and glial apoptosis. There is also release of proinflammatory cytokines.

The spleen is infiltrated by foam cells that contain cholesterol, phospholipids, and glycolipids. Both Kuppfer cells and hepatocytes are involved. In the infantile presentation, hepatic vacuolization is associated with cholestasis and giant cell formation, a phenomenon called giant cell hepatitis. Sea-blue histiocytes containing basophilic granules are found in the bone marrow and resemble foam cells. Sea-blue histiocytes accumulate in the splenic red pulp and within hepatic sinusoids. Pulmonary involvement has been documented in infantile cases with NPC2 mutations.

Pathophysiology

The NPC1 and NPC2 proteins are involved in cholesterol egress from late endosomes and lysosomes. The

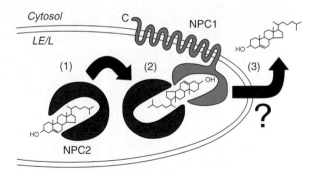

Figure 70.4 Potential mechanism for NPC1/NPC2-mediated cholesterol export from late endosomes/lysosome (LE/L). (1) NPC2 (soluble protein) binds unesterified cholesterol in the LE/L with the iso-octyl chain in the binding pocket, an event that may be enhanced by bis(monoacylglycero)phosphate. (2) NPC2 transfers cholesterol to the N-terminal loop of NPC1 (a multi-pass membrane protein) which binds cholesterol with the hydroxyl group in the binding pocket. (3) Cholesterol is exported from LE/L by an unknown mechanism. Reproduced with permission from Peake KB et al. Defective cholesterol trafficking in Niemann–Pick C-deficient cells. *FEBS Lett*. 2010; 584(13):2731–9.

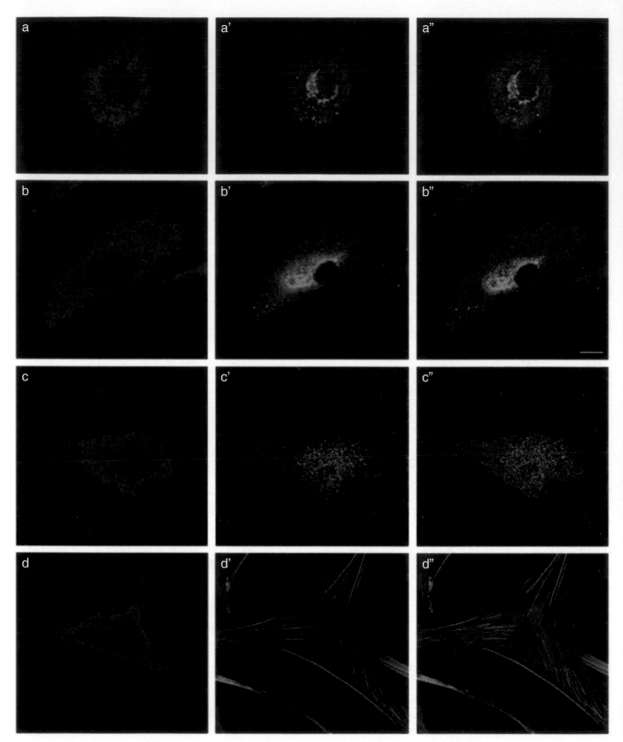

Figure 70.5 Negligible co-immunostaining of perfringolysin O fused with glutathione S-transferase (GST-PFO)-positive structures and other organelles in NPC cells. The GST-PFO probe detects cholesterol deposits. (a–d) Distribution of GST-PFO-positive structures, (a'–d') patterns of staining by antibodies directed against golgin-84 (a'), PDI - an endoplasmic reticulum marker (b'), anti-PMP70 – a peroxisomal marker (c') and phalloidin labeling actin filaments (d'). (a"–d") merging of the corresponding pairs of images displays traces of the yellow color indicating different localization of GST-PFO-positive structures and the examined proteins. Scale bar, 20 μm. Reproduced with permission from Kwiatkowska K et al. Visualization of cholesterol deposits in lysosomes of Niemann–Pick type C fibroblasts using recombinant perfringolysin O. *Orphanet J Rare Dis*. 2014; 9:64.

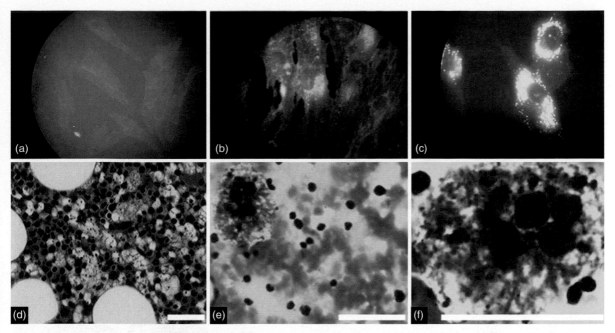

Figure 70.6 Cells obtained from a fibroblast culture (skin biopsy) in Niemann–Pick type disease showing the presence of intracellular lipid accumulation observed with filipin staining: normal control with clear negative fluorescence (a); "variant" pattern with moderated fluorescence in Case 2 (b); and typical pattern with cholesterol-filled perinuclear vesicles typically strongly fluorescent in Case 3 (c); bone marrow biopsy showing foamy cells with hematoxilin-eosin staining in Case 1 (d); bone marrow aspiration reveals sea blue histiocites with May-Grümwald-Giemsa staining, or Niemann–Pick cells in Case 3 (e, f). Bar=50μm. Reproduced with permission from Lorenzoni PJ et al. Niemann–Pick disease type C: a case series of Brazilian patients. *Arq Neuropsiquiatr.* 2014; 72(3):214–8.

cholesterol that accumulates in Niemann–Pick type C disease derives primarily from extracellular cholesterol associated with low-density lipoprotein (Figure 70.4). NPC2 may bind unsterified cholesterol in the late endosome or lysosome and transfers it to the membrane-associated NPC1 for facilitated egress out of the organelle. Therefore, dysfunction of NPC1 or NPC2 is similarly followed by accumulation of unsterified cholesterol in neurons (Figures 70.5 and 70.6). Excess cell body cholesterol is the counterpart of reduced cell processes cholesterol such as that found in the axon. There is also compensatory stimulation of cholesterol synthesis by the liver, probably exacerbating neuronal cholesterol storage. The accumulation of GM2 and GM3 gangliosides and neutral sphingolipids may occur via a similar blockade of egress followed by compensatory increases in glycosphingolipid synthesis. Additional secondary effects include abnormal production of neurosteroids and activation of neuroinflammation.

Functionally important residues involved in interactions with cholesterol have been identified (Figure 70.7).

Diagnosis

Brainstem auditory evoked potentials reveal a delay, with absence of acoustic reflexes. The diagnosis can be established by demonstrating an elevation of free cholesterol in cultured fibroblasts by staining with filipin or by determining the rate of cellular cholesterol esterification.

Treatment

There is no effective treatment. Substrate reduction has employed miglustat, an inhibitor of glycolioid synthesis, which has been utilized with some success in affected individuals and mouse models. Cyclodextrans have been employed to extract cholesterol from the membrane of neural cells via

273

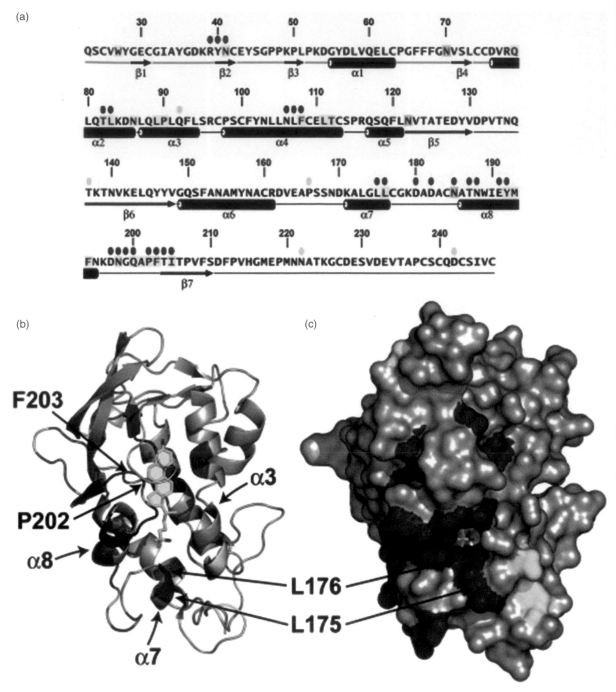

Figure 70.7 Location of functionally important residues in NPC1. (a) Amino acid sequence of NPC1(NTD) with functionally important residues highlighted. Blue ovals denote residues that exhibit decreased binding of cholesterol and 25-hydroxycholesterol by >75% when mutated to alanine. Red ovals denote residues that exhibit decreased transfer of cholesterol to liposomes by >70% when mutated to alanine. Cyan ovals denote naturally occurring mutations in patients with NPC1 disease. Residues that line the binding pocket are shaded yellow. N-linked glycosylation sites that were eliminated are shaded green. The secondary structure of NPC1 is indicated below the sequence. (b and c) Ribbon diagram (b) and surface representation (c) of NPC1, showing the positions of functionally important residues. Bound 25-hydroxycholesterol is shown as a stick model in green. Color coding is the same as in (a). The locations of the Leu175, Leu176, Pro202, and Phe203 residues are denoted by arrows. Reproduced with permission from Kwon HJ et al. Structure of N-terminal domain of NPC1 reveals distinct subdomains for binding and transfer of cholesterol. *Cell.* 2009; 137(7):1213–24. .

direct administration to the brain. Cholesterol-lowering agents, bone marrow transplantation, and dietary restriction of cholesterol have met with little success.

Bibliography

Benussi A., Alberici A., Premi E., et al. (2015). Phenotypic heterogeneity of Niemann–Pick disease type C in monozygotic twins. *J Neurol.* 262(3):642–7.

GM2 Gangliosidoses

A 19-month-old girl was evaluated for globally abnormal development. The infant's father was the maternal uncle of the infant's mother and the maternal great-grandparents were uncle and niece. The infant was able to roll at 3 months of age, but she did not sit independently until 10 months. At 9 months, she displayed axial hypotonia. By 15 months, she could wave, pull to stand, and walk with both hands held. She used a pincer grasp at 9 months and ate finger foods at 15 months. At 19 months, she was not walking, even with support, and had stopped sitting, standing, or waving. She started saying "mama" and "dada" indiscriminately at 9 months; at 15 months, she used 5 words appropriately. At 19 months, the infant had ceased to say any words. Her length had dropped from the 60th to the 20th percentile, her weight from the 25th to the 5th percentile. Her head circumference was still within the normal range at the 25th percentile. Examination at 19 months revealed a markedly increased startle response, inability to fix and follow, diffuse hypotonia, mild hyperreflexia, and flexor plantar responses. She had no organomegaly. Funduscopic examination showed bilateral optic nerve pallor and cherry-red spots.

GM2 Gangliosidosis

Onset: Progressive psychomotor retardation in infancy or childhood in Tay-Sachs disease. Additionally, mild hepatosplenomegaly in Sandhoff disease.
Additional manifestations: Hypotonia, poor head control and hyperacusis with an exaggerated startle reflex. Cherry red spots. Megalencephaly, seizures and myoclonus. In adult forms, psychoses, cerebellar degeneration, and anterior horn cell disease dominate the phenotype.
Disease mechanism: Loss of function of lysosomal hexosaminidase leading to storage of gangliosides

predominantly in neurons. This results in aberrant neurite formation, neuronal dysfunction, and apoptosis.
Testing: Hexosaminidase assay of serum or leukocytes. Pseudodeficiency may occur depending on assay substrate.
Treatment: None effective.
Research highlights: Localized gene transfer to the cerebellum or striatum in mice arrests disease progression in these regions.

Clinical Features

The GM2 gangliosidoses are neuronal storage disorders is caused by deficiency of lysosomal hexosaminidases. Three disease variants are associated with deficiency of this class of enzymes: Tay-Sachs disease, AB variant, and Sandhoff disease. All of them can manifest at any age from infancy to adulthood.

Tay-Sachs disease is caused by hexosaminidase A deficiency and most commonly presents as an infantile disorder that occurs with greatest frequency among Ashkenazi Jews. After a normal period of early postnatal life, infants first manifest progressive psychomotor retardation. This is followed by hypotonia, poor head control, and hyperacusis with an exaggerated startle reflex. There is poor fixation on visually interesting objects. Fundoscopy reveals macular cherry red spots caused by lipid deposition in the bipolar ganglion cells of most of the retina. Megalencephaly and seizures appear later in the disease course, in association with myoclonus. By 4 years, children die blind in a vegetative state. Later-onset forms later in childhood or adulthood are milder. In the juvenile form, affected individuals first manifest gait or speech dysfunction between 2 and 7 years of age. There is subsequent psychomotor regression with loss of speech and ambulatory capacity. Death occurs before the ages of 10 and 15 years. In late-onset forms, psychiatric disorders affect as many as 40 percent of

Tay-Sachs individuals. They also develop ataxia and progressive cognitive and ambulatory difficulty and, eventually, incapacity. Anterior horn cell disease is common. Particularly frequent is difficulty using stairs. Dysarthria and broken saccadic pursuit are also common, as is marked cerebellar atrophy. Macular cherry red spots are not common in this disease form. These individuals typically only reach the sixth decade of life.

Sandhoff disease does not exhibit any ethnic predominance. Disease manifestations are often indistinguishable from Tay-Sachs disease except for the presence of hepatosplenomegaly and occasional cardiomegaly in infants. In addition, and in contrast with Tay-Sachs disease, N-acetylglucosamine oligosaccharides are characteristically excreted in the urine in Sandhoff disease. Infants with Sandhoff disease usually die before 5 years of age. Late-onset variants have also been recognized.

AB variant GM2 gangliosidosis clinically resembles other forms of GM2 gangliosidosis. Onset is typically between 6 and 9 months with psychomotor deterioration and an exaggerated startle response.

Pathology

The pathology is limited to the nervous system in Tay-Sachs disease and AB variant. In early-onset Tay-Sachs disease, the brain is initially atrophic during the first 12–14 months. Subsequently, brain weight increases between 14 and 24 months, until marked enlargement becomes apparent after 25 months (Figure 71.1). Brain consistency is rubbery and firm. The white matter is translucent and the grey-white junction becomes blurred. Optic nerves, cerebellum, and brainstem are atrophied. Neural cells show massive storage, with distension of the cytoplasm and relegation of the Nissl material to the periphery. Meganeurite and ectopic dendrite formation similar to GM1 gangliosidosis is conspicuous. The neuronal cell body is packed with concentric lamellar lipid inclusions measuring 1 μm in diameter. These inclusions contain GM2 ganglioside, cholesterol, phospholipids, and proteins. Demyelination is severe and accompanied by an astrocytic, microglial, and macrophagic reaction resembling leukodystrophy. In the cerebellum, there is loss of Purkinje and

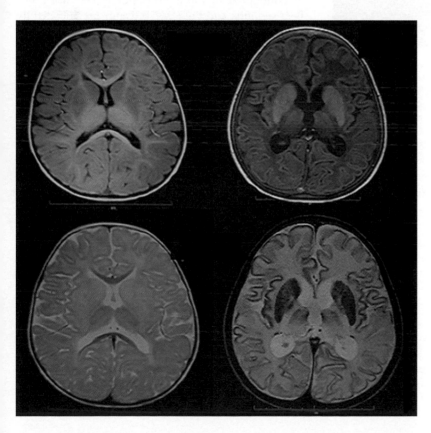

Figure 71.1 Sequential MR imaging in Tay-Sachs disease in a girl aged 14 months and 4 years and 5 months. Reproduced with permission from Posso Gomez LJ et al. Clinical, biochemical, and molecular findings in a Colombian patient with Tay-Sachs disease. *Neurología*. 2016. pii: S0213-4853(16):7–4.

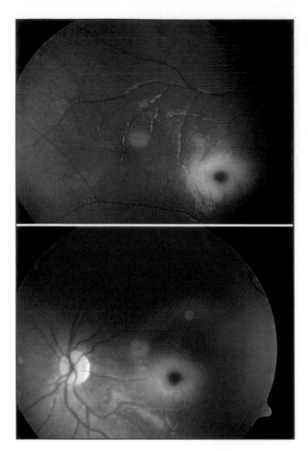

Figure 71.2 Cherry red spot in Tay-Sachs disease in a 19-month-old male child. Reproduced with permission from Aragão RE et al. "Cherry red spot" in a patient with Tay-Sachs disease: case report. *Arq Bras Oftalmol.* 2009; 72(4):537–9.

granular cells. There are swellings or spheroids in Purkinje cell axons. The cell bodies of other Purkinje cells are distended and some display apoptosis. Neuronal storage can also be detected in ganglion cells of the retina, autonomic ganglia, dorsal root ganglia, and myenteric plexus (Figure 71.2).

The pathology of infantile Sandhoff disease resembles Tay-Sachs disease except that the cerebral stored material contains much greater concentrations of ceramide trihexoside (Figures 71.3 and 71.4). In Sandhoff disease, visceral storage is present in liver, pancreas, spleen, and kidney and is represented by vacuolated hepatocytes and pancreatic acinar cells. Periodic-acid Schiff positive Kupffer cells in hepatic sinusoids and in the renal tubular epithelium and histiocytes in the spleen germinal centers are common.

Pathological findings in AB variant gangliosidosis are also similar to the other two variants but include zebra bodies in some cortical neurons. In addition, heterogeneous inclusions are present in astrocytes, oligodendrocytes, and microglia.

Pathophysiology

Gangliosides are complex glycolipids that contain ceramide linked to monosaccharide and sialic acid residues (Figure 71.5). GM2 gangliosides and its sialic acid derivative GA2 are normally degraded by the concerted action of the lysosomal enzyme beta-hexosaminidase A and its cofactor GM2-activator protein (Figure 71.6). The normal beta-hexosaminidase enzyme complex consists of two major isoenzymes, beta-hexosaminidase A and B, one minor isozyme S, and the GM2 activator protein. The isozymes are formed by combinations of two subunits, alpha and beta. Hexosaminidase A is a heterodimer composed of alpha and beta subunits, whereas hexosaminidase B is a homodimer of two beta subunits. The minor form, hexosaminidase S is a homodimer of the alpha subunit. The alpha and beta subunits and the GM2 activator are encoded by three distinct genes. Deficiency of any of these genes results in disrupted GM2 degradation. In Tay-Sachs disease, hexosaminidase A is genetically defective, but hexosaminidase B is intact. In Sandhoff disease, which results from genetic deficiency of the beta subunit, the activity of both hexosaminidase A and B is deficient. As a result, sphingolipid and glycolipids cannot be degraded normally and unusual sphingoglycolipids such as globoside additionally accumulate in visceral organs. The GM2 activator protein is necessary for the degradation of GM2 ganglioside. Deficiency of the GM2 activator in AB variant closely resembles beta-hexosaminidase A deficiency despite normal enzyme activity.

Normally, GM2 ganglioside exists in very small quantities in normal mature brain as part of synthetic and degradative reactions in the Golgi apparatus and the lysosome, respectively. Excess lysosomal ganglioside storage may lead to the redistribution of ganglioside to other areas of the neuron and to dysregulation of complex ganglioside synthesis. This may be associated with abnormal plasma membrane signaling and ectopic dendrite formation. The resulting abnormalities in neuronal connectivity

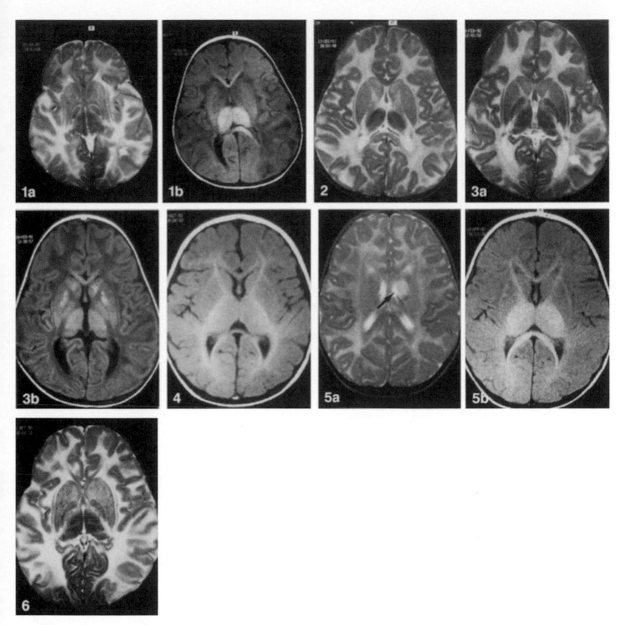

Figure 71.3 MR imaging in Sandhoff disease. 1a, b. Subject 1, aged 19 months, a Axial T2-weighted section. Increased signal bilaterally in the temporal and parieto-occipital white matter, b Axial imaging shows high signal in the thalamus. Note normal myelineation of anterior and posterior parts of corpus callosum. 2. Subject 1, at 24 months of age. Axial imaging as in la shows advancing, diffuse high signal in the white matter. Note the focal high signal in the posterior limb of the internal capsules and the low signal from the thalamus. 3a, b. Subject 1, at 27 months of age. a as 1 a. High signal areas in the white matter of the frontal and parietal lobes are more extensive, b Axial image shows new focal areas of high signal in the head of the caudate nucleus and globus pallidus on both sides. Note loss of the high signal in the thalamus. 4, Subject 2 at 9 months of age, when clinically presymptomatic. Axial image shows no abnormality. 5 a,b. Subject 2 at age of 15 months, a Axial image shows abnormal high signal in white matter, especially in the occipital and temporal lobes. Circumscribed high signal is seen in left globus pallidus (arrow). b Axial image shows increased signal in the thalamus and corpus callosum. Note loss of myelin signal in the optic radiations. 6. Subject 2 at the age of 23 months. Axial T2-weighted image shows that the high signal lesions have spread to the frontal white matter. Reproduced with permission from Koelfen W et al. GM-2 gangliosidosis (Sandhoff's disease): two year follow-up by MRI. *Neuroradiology*. 1994; 36(2):152–4.

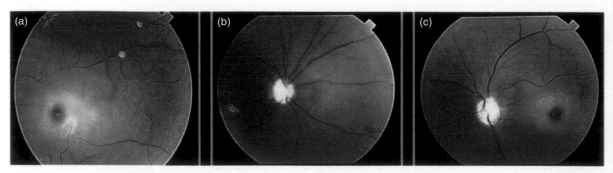

Figure 71.4 Ocular fundus photographs in Sandhoff disease. Right eye shows a cherry red spot in the macula and a pale optic disc (**a, b**). Left eye also shows a cherry red spot in the macula and a pale optic disc (**c**). Reproduced with permission from Yun YM et al. A case report of Sandhoff disease. *Korean J Ophthalmol.* 2005; 19(1):68–72.

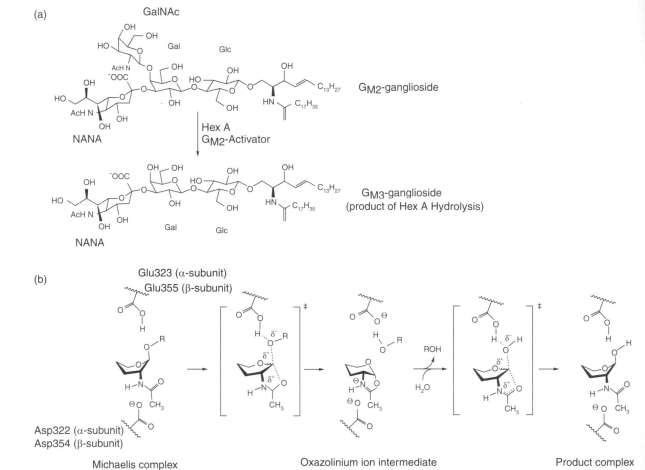

Figure 71.5 Proposed catalytic mechanism for hexosaminidase A (Hex A). (**a**) Hydrolysis of the GM2 ganglioside by Hex A results in the loss of GalNAc to produce a GM3 ganglioside. (**b**) Proposed catalytic mechanism for Hex A showing substrate-assisted catalysis. αGlu323 in the α-subunit and βGlu355 in the β-subunit act as the general base, while αAsp322 in the α-subunit and βAsp354 in the β-subunit act to orient the C2-acetamido group into position for nucleophilic attack and subsequently stabilizes the oxazolinium ion intermediate. The hydroxyl residues and C6 have been removed from the pyranose ring of the substrate for clarity. The exact positions for these groups have not been determined. Reproduced with permission from Lemieux MJ et al. Crystallographic structure of human beta-hexosaminidase A: interpretation of Tay-Sachs mutations and loss of GM2 ganglioside hydrolysis. *J Mol Biol.* 2006; 359(4):913–29.

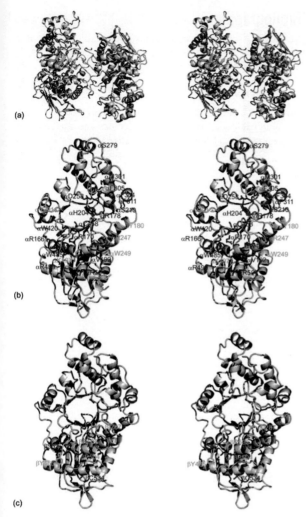

Figure 71.6 Known mutations of hexosaminidase A (Hex A) contributing to Tay-Sachs and Sandhoff disease. (a) Stereo view of a ribbon representation of Hex A (wheat), with residues known to disrupt Hex A activity: acute to sub-acute, red; chronic, green; asymptomatic, cyan. (b) A stereo view of the a-subunit of Hex A and residues associated with Tay-Sachs disease. (c) A stereo view of the β-subunit and residues associated with Sandhoff disease. Reproduced with permission from Lemieux MJ et al. Crystallographic structure of human beta-hexosaminidase A: interpretation of Tay-Sachs mutations and loss of GM2 ganglioside hydrolysis. *J Mol Biol.* 2006; 359(4):913–29.

may result in the extensive neural dysfunction typical of the disease. The generation of the byproduct lyso-ganglioside GM2 may also lead to neuronal toxicity. In addition to these potential mechanisms, neuroinflammation may contribute to neuronal dysfunction and degeneration. Lysosomal storage in GM2 gangliosidosis is accompanied by deposition of α-synuclein.

Diagnosis

Neuroimaging reveals early decreased T2-weighted MR imaging signal in the thalamus and basal ganglia. Later in the disease course, cortical atrophy and ventricular dilatation become apparent, as does cerebellar degeneration. The cerebral white matter can be abnormally intense in a patchy distribution.

The GM2 gangliosidoses may be definitively diagnosed by hexosaminidase assay of serum or leukocytes. Total hexosaminidase activity is obtained and hexosaminidase B activity is determined after heat inactivation of hexosaminidase A. Hexosaminidase A activity is thus calculated as the difference in activity between these two assays. In Tay-Sachs disease, total hexosaminidase activity is diminished, whereas hexosaminidase B activity is normal or elevated. In Sandhoff disease, hexosaminidase A and B activities are both decreased and *N*-acetylglucosamine oligosaccharides are detectable in the urine. A state of pseudodeficiency can arise when hexosaminidase is assayed using an artificial rather than the natural substrate. In such cases, hexosaminidase assay is falsely positive. This occurs with two genetic variants of the enzyme. In addition, false positive results may be obtained using the plasma of pregnant individuals or during contraceptive use. The cause of this phenomenon is the existence of another hexosaminidase (P) that is not heat-labile. This results in an overall reduction of the calculated residual activity for hexosaminidase A. Performing the assay in white blood cells, which lack hexosaminidase P, eliminate this source of error.

Treatment

There is no effective treatment. Hematopoietic stem cell transplantation has been used in infantile GM2 gangliosidosis and has prolonged survival. In the juvenile form, presymptomatic hematopoietic stem cell transplantation has proven ineffective in terms of ultimate outcome. Enzyme replacement therapy is not considered feasible via intravenous infusion due to impermeability of the blood–brain barrier. Substrate reduction therapy has exploited the capacity of miglustat to inhibit glucosylceramide synthetase, which could be followed by a reduction in glycosphingolipid synthesis. However, this agent has been ineffective in terms of neurological progression in the juvenile form of the disease. Pyrimethamine acts as a chaperone of mutant hexosaminidase A by binding to the active site of hexosaminidase B, stabilizing the complex, and has been tested in the adult form of the disease, resulting in increased enzymatic activity, although side effects are significant. Intracranial injection of recombinant adeno-associated viral vectors into mice with Sandhoff disease prolongs survival. Localized gene transfer to the cerebellum or striatum in mice has also arrested disease progression in these regions and resulted in symptom amelioration.

Bibliography

Kenney D., Wickremasinghe A.C., Ameenuddin N., et al. (2014). A 19-month-old girl of South Indian parents presented to a general pediatric clinic for evaluation of global developmental regression. *Semin Pediatr Neurol.* 21(2):88–9.

Sandhoff K., Harzer K. (2013). Gangliosides and gangliosidoses: Principles of molecular and metabolic pathogenesis. *J Neurosci.* 33(25):10195–208.

Mucopolysaccharidoses

An 8-year-old boy was evaluated for swollen legs and enlarged abdomen of 8 months duration with progressive difficulty breathing for 4 months. His parents noticed an abnormal facial appearance when he was about 3 years old, described as prominent forehead, protruding eyes and enlarged jaw with thickened skin. He had also manifested snoring and recurrent ear discharge, with resultant hearing impairment. There had been a regression in language development as he could no longer communicate in sentences, which he was previously able to do. Examination revealed a large head with frontal bossing and caput quadratum, low set ears, depressed nasal bridge, up-turned nose, enlarged jaw, protruding tongue, short neck, and short stubby digits. He had an inspiratory stridor, was centrally cyanotic and had pitting edema up to the thigh and sacrum. His height was 98 cm (81% of expected). He had joint stiffness with the forearms slightly flexed at elbow joints. He also manifested tachycardia. There was a grade III pansystolic murmur. He was tachypneic and had transmitted sounds in the chest. The abdomen was distended with an umbilical hernia and there was also tender hepatosplenomegaly and ascites. Echocardiography showed mitral valve prolapse with severe regurgitation, moderate pericardial effusion, and severe pulmonary hypertension. He died two months later.

Mucopolysaccharidoses

Onset: Infantile or childhood skeletal and facial deformities with abnormal intellectual development in some forms.
Additional manifestations: Accumulation of glycosaminoglycans in visceral tissues, heart and joints. Short stature. Hydrocephalus. Compressive myelopathy. Carpal tunnel syndrome. Obstructive sleep apnea. Cardiac valvular insufficiency. Intellectual development ranges from normal to progressively declining.
Disease mechanism: Mechanical disruption of some structures. Substrate mimicry with activation of apoptosis and inflammation.
Testing: Determination urinary glycosaminoglycan levels and types followed by specific enzymatic determination in fibroblasts.
Treatment: Hematopoietic stem cell transplantation and enzyme replacement therapy for some forms.
Research highlights: Activation of signaling cascades by glycosaminoglycan byproducts.

Clinical Features

The mucopolysaccharidoses are caused by deficiency of specific lysosomal enzymes responsible for the degradation of mucopolysaccharides (glycosaminoglycans) (Figure 72.1). This results in the progressive accumulation of mucopolysaccharidoses and gangliosides in various tissues and in the excretion of partially degraded mucopolysaccharidoses in urine, including dermatan sulfate, heparin sulfate, keratan sulfate, and chondroitin sulfates. The brain is affected in several of these disorders. All of the mucopolysaccharides share a progressive course, multisystem involvement with organomegaly, dysostosis multiplex and joint deformity, corneal opacification, hearing loss, abnormal facies, and cardiovascular dysfunction. Accumulation of dermatan sulfate in Hurler, Hunter, Maroteaux–Lamy, and Sly syndromes is associated with prominent skeletal abnormalities, whereas deposition of heparan sulfate in Hurler, Hunter, and Sanfilippo syndromes correlates with progressive intellectual disability.

Mucopolysaccharidosis type I arises from α-L-iduronidase deficiency and is associated with three clinical syndromes (Hurler, Hunter–Scheie, and Scheie

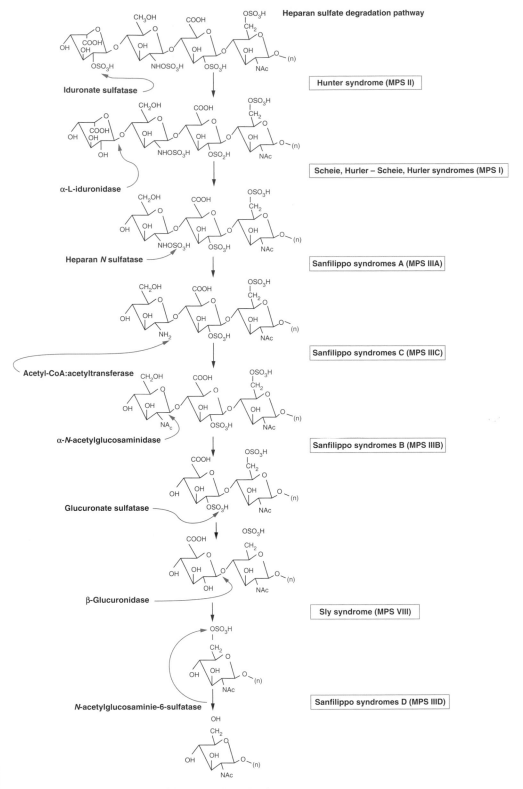

Figure 72.1 Schematic diagram of the mucopolysaccharidoses.

Table 72.1 The muchopolisaccharidoses

Mucopolysaccharidosis	Designation	Enzyme defect	Inheritance
Hurler	IH	α-L-iduronidase	Autosomal recessive
Hurler–Scheie	IHS	α-L-iduronidase	Autosomal recessive
Scheie	IS	α-L-iduronidase	Autosomal recessive
Hunter	II	Iduronosulfate sulfatase	X-linked recessive
Sanfilippo A	IIIA	Sulfamidase	Autosomal recessive
Sanfilippo B	IIIB	α-N-acetylglucosaminidase	Autosomal recessive
Sanfilippo C	IIIC	Acetyl coenzyme A α-glucosaminide N-acetyltransferase	Autosomal recessive
Sanfilippo D	IIID	N-acetylglucosamine-6-sulfate sulfatase	Autosomal recessive
Morquio A	IVA	N-acetylgalactosamine-6-sulfate sulfatase	Autosomal recessive
Morquio B	IVB	β-galactosidase	Autosomal recessive
Maroteaux–Lamy	VI	N-acetylgalactosamine-4-sulfate sulfatase	Autosomal recessive
Sly	VII	β-glucuronidase	Autosomal recessive
Hyaluronidase deficiency	IX	Hyaluronidase	Autosomal recessive

diseases) that are almost indistinguishable before 1 year of age. Hurler disease is the prototypic mucopolysaccharidosis (Figures 72.2 and 72.3). Children with Hurler disease appear normal at birth, but coarse facies develops after 6 months and is usually recognized between 9 and 18 months. Hepatosplenomegaly and umbilical hernias may also be noticeable. Repetitive upper airway infections, otitis media and tonsillar hypertrophy are common. Hearing becomes impaired. Kyphosis is initially mild but later progresses to a characteristic gibbus in the setting of short stature. In some children, cardiomyopathy and heart failure are the presenting manifestation. Corneal opacifications may appear in the first year of life. The ability to sit, walk, and speak is gradually lost over time with as the syndrome evolves to severe mental retardation. Ultimate disability leads to a bedbound state in which the child is severely ill. Death usually ensues before 10 years.

In Hurler-Scheie syndrome, there are skeletal abnormalities characterized by joint deformity, small stature, and a small thorax, as well as corneal opacification and hepatosplenomegaly. In some children, mitral valve insufficiency leads to premature mortality. Compression of the spinal cord by mucopolysaccharide has been documented. Neurological involvement, however, is milder.

Scheie syndrome is at the milder end of the mucopolysaccharidosis type I spectrum. Children attain normal height and intellect. There is no coarsening of the facies and dysostosis and joint contractures are mild. The presenting complaint may be decreased vision after the age of 5 years due to corneal opacification or carpal tunnel syndrome.

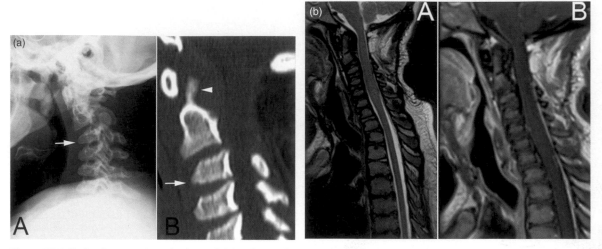

Figure 72.2 Hurler disease. **a.** Lateral radiograph (a) and sagittal computerized tomography (b) show hypoplastic cervical vertebrae with pathognomonic "inferior beaking" (arrows). Previous posterior cervical decompression and characteristic hypoplasia of the odontoid process (arrowhead) is seen. **b.** Sagittal T2 (A) and contrast-enhanced MR imaging T1 (B) sequences show expansion of the cervical cord, with no identifiable mass lesion or syrinx. Reproduced with permission from Grech R et al. Hurler syndrome (Mucopolysaccharidosis type I). *BMJ Case Rep.* 2013; 2013. pii: bcr2012008148.

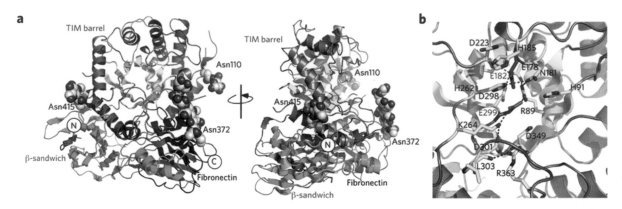

Figure 72.3 α-L-iduronidase (IDUA). (a) Two views (related by a 90° rotation) of the complete apo-IDUA molecule. The TIM barrel is in slate blue with the central eight strands of the β-barrel in yellow. Three of the six possible N-glycosylation sites have electron density for the attached sugar residues; Asn110 has a single N-acetylglucosamine (NAG); Asn372 has five saccharide residues (Man3NAG2), and Asn415 has a single NAG. The β-sandwich domain is represented in green. The C-terminal type III fibronectin-like domain is represented in red. (b) A close-up view of the active site of IDUA. The carbon atoms of the nucleophile, Glu299 and the general acid/base Glu182 are in magenta. Other residues that are proposed to be of importance in substrate binding and the catalytic mechanism have the following color scheme: yellow, carbon atoms; red, oxygen atoms; blue, nitrogen atoms. The residues involved in substrate binding are Arg363, Asp349, His91, and Asn181. Arg89 and Lys264 provide a positively charged environment that ensures a depressed pK_a for the carboxyl group of Glu299. Reproduced with permission from Bie H et al. Insights into mucopolysaccharidosis I from the structure and action of α-L-iduronidase. *Nat Chem Biol.* 2013; 9(11):739–45.

There are two forms of Hunter syndrome: one severe with encephalopathy and the other milder (Figures 72.4 to 72.8). Both are heritable in X-linked recessive form although some female cases have been documented. The general phenotype is similar to that of Hurler syndrome with some exceptions: there is no corneal opacification in Hunter syndrome but there is hearing loss. There is also a macular rash over arms, shoulders and thighs. In the milder disease form, affected individuals manifest carpal tunnel syndrome, heart failure or airway obstruction as they age. They may survive until the fifth decade.

Four genetically distinct forms of Sanfilippo syndrome are recognized (Figures 72.9 to 72.10). They all

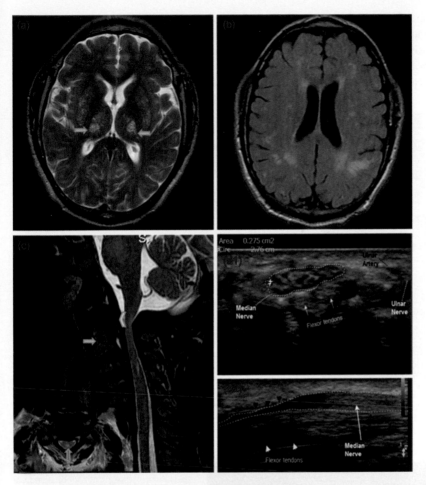

Figure 72.4 Hunter disease. Brain MR imaging showing characteristic honeycomb-like appearance of basal ganglia and thalami (arrows in panel **a**; axial T2 sequence) with diffuse white-matter hyperintensities (panel **b**; axial FLAIR sequence). Cervical MRI (panel **c**; sagittal T2 sequence) depicts dens subluxation (arrow) and periodontoid tissue thickening (arrowhead) causing spinal canal stenosis. Peripheral nerve sonography discloses marked median nerve enlargement [panel **d1**; B-mode sonography transverse plane: right median nerve cross-sectional area: 0.275 cm^2 (normal values < 0.11 cm^2)] and nerve-compression under flexor retinaculum at the carpal tunnel (arrowheads panel **d2**; B-mode sonography longitudinal plane). Reproduced with permission from Tsivgoulis G et al. Neuroimaging findings in Hunter disease. *J Neurol Sci.* 2014.

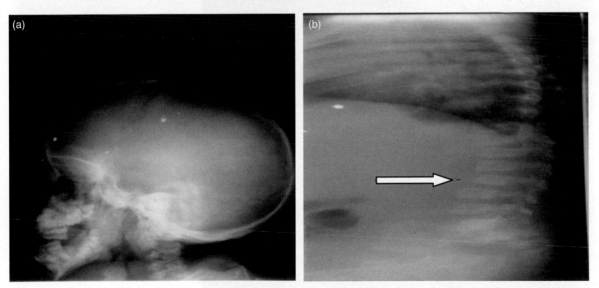

Figure 72.5 Skeletal abnormalities in Hunter disease. **a.** Lateral skull X-ray showing a widened J-shaped sella turcica. **b.** Anterior beaking of L3 vertebra (white arrow) with reduction in the vertical height and posterior displacement. Reproduced with permission from Rasheeedah I et al. Challenges in the management of mucopolysaccharidosis Type II (Hunter's Syndrome) in a developing country: A case report. *Ethiop J Health Sci.* 2015; 25(3):279–82.

share several important mild phenotypic features such as facial abnormalities, gingival hyperplasia, hepatosplenomegaly, and disostosis multiplex. The dominant clinical manifestation is hyperactivity and other forms of severe behavioral disturbance between

the age of 2 and 8 years, followed by mental retardation and later deterioration until death ensues in the second decade of life. In all four forms there is excretion of heparan sulfate without dermatan sulfaturia. Sanfilippo A is the most common form, whereas Sanfilippo C represents the mildest form.

In Morquio syndrome, skeletal dysplasia and short stature are prominent in the absence of neurological involvement. Corneal clouding is present in about one-half of cases. Hepatosplenomegaly is usually mild. There may be aortic insufficiency, sleep apnea and cor pulmonale obstructive. Cervical myelopathy may develop as a result of an unstable hypoplastic odontoid process.

Maroteaux–Lamy syndrome resembles Hurler syndrome except for a lack of mental retardation. The principal neurological manifestations may be hydrocephalus, atlantoaxial subluxation, and entrapment neuropathy. There is also a broad range of disease severity. Urinary excretion of dermatan sulfate is characteristic.

In Sly disease, intellectual impairment, short stature, hepatosplenomegaly, and disostosis are common, resembling Hurler syndrome. However, the phenotype is broad and also includes hydrops fetalis. Granulocytes may display coarse metachromatic granules.

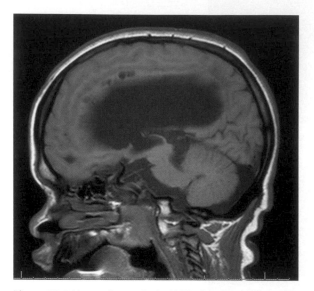

Figure 72.6 Hunter disease. Sagittal MRI of a 9-year-old boy with Hunter disease. The ventricular system is dilated, highlighting a thinned corpus callosum, which contains small cysts.

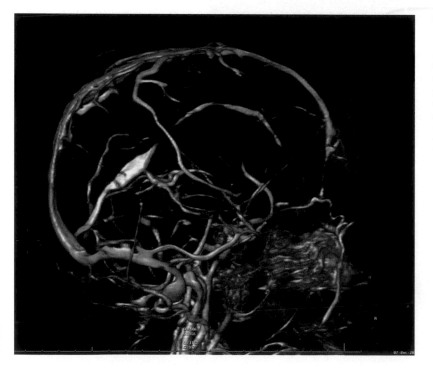

Figure 72.7 Cranial venous circulation in Hunter disease. Contrast-enhanced MR venography shows absence of the left transverse sinus, focal narrowing of the rigth transverse sinus at the junction with the sigmoid sinus. There is also segmental narrowing of the straight sinus and inferior sagittal sinus. These abnormalities are probably related to mucopolisaccharide deposition leading to venous narrowing and increased intracranial pressure.

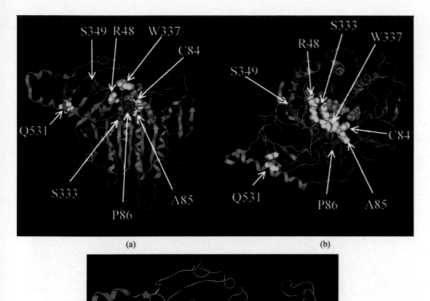

Figure 72.8 Location of mutated residues in a tertiary structural model of iduronate-2-sulfatase. (a, b) The active site centre, Cys84 residue, is shown as yellow spheres, and the other active site residues are shown as orange spheres. The residues related to the severe clinical phenotype are shown in red and those related to the attenuated clinical phenotype are shown in cyan. (c) The deleted C-terminal fragment, Gln531-Pro550, in Gln531X mutant protein is indicated as yellow. Reproduced with permission from Sukegawa-Hayasaka K et al. Effect of Hunter disease (mucopolysaccharidosis type II) mutations on molecular phenotypes of iduronate-2-sulfatase: enzymatic activity, protein processing and structural analysis. *J Inherit Metab Dis*. 2006; 29(6):755–61.

Hyaluronidase deficiency is associated with painful periarticular soft tissue masses, short stature, and normal intelligence.

Pathology

In all mucopolysaccaridosis syndromes, there is widespread accumulation of glycosaminoglycans, resulting in structural abnormalities (Figure 72.11). There are clear cells with distended cytoplasm containing multiple large clear vacuoles associated with fibrosis in visceral organs. The leptomeninges are fibrotic and this may lead to hydrocephalus. The cerebral perivascular spaces in the white matter are dilated and contain fibrous tissue. There is also neuronal storage with neuronal loss, gliosis, and microglial activation. Many of the pathological changes have been best characterized in type I mucopolysaccharidosis. There is

meganeurite and ectopic dendrite formation. The neuronal storage material stains with periodic-acid Schiff and contains GM2 and GM3 gangliosides and unsterified cholesterol, with the two gangliosides existing in different pools. These gangliosides are organized in zebra bodies, which contain multilamellar structures. Purkinje cells are diminished in number and those surviving are dilated with fusiform expansions of their dendrites.

Pathophysiology

Extracellularly accumulating mucopolysaccharides may lead to non-physiologic activation of signal transduction receptors, triggering inflammation. Glycosaminoglycan breakdown products resemble lipopolysaccharide, and this may lead to activation of the toll-like receptor TLR4. Accordingly,

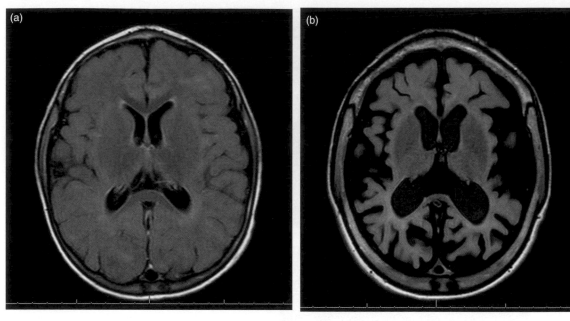

Figure 72.9 MR imaging in Sanfilippo disease. a: A FLAIR image obtained at 5 years of age is near normal, with some increased white matter signal. b: The FLAIR image at 14 years shows diffuse cerebral atrophy and thickening of the calvarium.

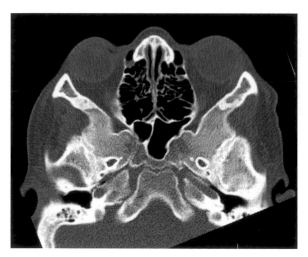

Figure 72.10 Sanfilippo disease in a 11-year-old boy. There is thickening of the cranial bones and small septations in the maxillary sinuses.

glycosaminoglycan storing chondrocytes display higher nitric oxide levels and secrete proinflammatory cytokines such as IL-1β, TNF-α, and TGF-β. Nitric oxide and cytokines induce the expression of matrix metalloproteases which through their proteolytic activity may contribute to cartilage degeneration.

TLR4 stimulation also leads to alterations of ceramide levels in stimulated cells. Since ceramide is a proapoptotic signaling molecule, this contributes to the increased apoptosis of chondrocytes in mucopolysaccharidosis models. In contrast, in synovial fibroblasts of mucopolysaccharidosis, it was the prosurvival lipid sphingosine-1-phosphate that is elevated. This proliferative lipid explains that no apoptosis is present in synovial fibroblasts, but rather an increased proliferation.

In Hurler syndrome, accumulation of heparan sulphate is not restricted to lysosomes but also occurs in the extracellular matrix. Glycosaminoglycans bind various growth factors. In some cases glycosaminoglycans act as growth factor reservoirs and as coreceptors in signal transduction. Heparan sulphate oligosaccharides accumulating extracellularly in Hurler syndrome interfere with the binding of the fibroblast growth factor FGF-2 to its receptor and impair signal transduction through this cascade. This reduces the survival promoting activity of FGF-2 and may explain the increased rate of apoptosis characteristic of cells from Hurler individuals. FGF-2 acts proliferatively and protectively on a number of cell types among which are neurons and neuronal precursor cells. Thus, it is conceivable that impaired signaling through the FGF-2-FGF receptor/heparan sulphate complex in Hurler syndrome contributes to neurodegeneration.

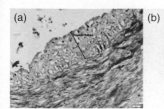
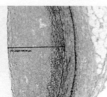
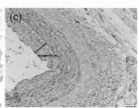

Figure 72.11 Coronary arteriopathy in mucopolysaccharidoses. (a–c) Intimal thickening (bars) is identified within the epicardial coronary arteries of patients with (a) MPS IIIA (thickness 80 μm) (Alcian blue, 40×), (b) MPS IIIC (thickness 597 μm) (Verhoeff's elastic tissue stain counterstainedwith van Gieson's connective tissue stain, 10x), and (c) MPS VI (thickness 75 μm) (Alcian blue, 20×). Reproduced with permission from Braunlin E et al. Unexpected coronary artery findings in mucopolysaccharidosis. Report of four cases and literature review. *Cardiovasc Pathol.* 2014; 23(3):145–51.

Diagnosis

The measurement of urinary glycosaminoglycan levels is a useful screening test. A positive result is very suggestive, but false-negative results are common. False-negative results occur because of a lack of sufficient sensitivity in the various assays and because of dilute samples. In normal subjects, urinary glycosaminoglycan excretion varies with age, with greater values found during the first years of life, followed by a slow and constant decrease thereafter. About 90 percent of the glycosaminoglycan content in normal urine consists of chondroitin-4 and -6 sulphate, with the remaining being heparan sulfate. Most individuals with mucopolysaccharidosis exhibit higher glycosaminoglycan excretion in urine compared with age-matched normal subjects; however, as not all affected individuals display a frank elevation of total excretion, an accurate diagnosis requires a full profile including both quantitative and qualitative analysis. The presence of specific glycosaminoglycans can suggest the mucopolysaccharidosis subtype and may direct the appropriate enzyme analyses. For example, high amounts of heparan sulphate or keratan sulfate define mucopolysaccharidosis III and IV, respectively.

The diagnosis of mucopolysaccharidosis can be confirmed by enzyme activity testing. Testing for related diseases, such as multiple sulphatase deficiency and mucolipidosis, both of which share clinical features with mucopolysaccharidosis, is appropriate. Enzyme activity typically is measured in leukocytes or cultured fibroblasts. For many types of mucopolysaccharidosis, enzyme activity can also be measured from a dried blood spot.

Treatment

Hematopoietic stem cell transplantation is the treatment of choice for individuals with severe forms of mucopolysaccharidosis type I. Transplantation before the age of 2 years (which often heralds the onset of irreversible neurological decline), alters the natural history of the disease. Treated subjects no longer appear coarse; airway and cardiac muscle function improves and the progressive cognitive difficulties are prevented. Corneal opacification, heart valve lesions, and skeletal dysplasia, however, are resistant to therapy such that many individuals receive orthopedic interventions for spinal deformity, hip dysplasia, and genu valgum. It is unknown which of the other mucopolysaccharidoses may be suitable for hematopoietic stem cell transplantation. In mucopolysaccharidosis I, enzyme replacement therapy can be used as an adjunct to hematopoietic stem cell transplantation. In this disease, early diagnosis and treatment are important for outcome, although some aspects of the disease such as the dysostosis multiplex are resistant to treatment. Generation of antibodies to the recombinant proteins, however, is common and this may limit efficacy in some individuals. For mucopolysaccharidosis III and IV, hematopoietic stem cell transplantation has not proven to be a successful therapy, although intravenous or intrathecal enzyme replacement therapy could be used.

Bibliography

Ballabio A., Gieselmann V. (2009). Lysosomal disorders: from storage to cellular damage. *Biochim Biophys Acta.* 1793(4):684–96.

Cimaz R., La Torre F. (2014). Mucopolysaccharidoses. *Curr Rheumatol Rep.* 16(1):389.

Lehman T.J., Miller N., Norquist B., Underhill L., Keutzer J. (2011). Diagnosis of the mucopolysaccharidoses. *Rheumatology (Oxford).* 50 Suppl 5:v41–8.

Rasheeedah I., Patrick O., Abdullateef A., et al. (2015). Challenges in the management of mucopolysaccharidosis Type II (Hunter's syndrome) in a developing country: A case report. *Ethiop J Health Sci.*; 25(3):279–82.

Mucolipidoses

A 13-month-old girl was evaluated for abnormal psychomotor development, dysmorphism, and dilated cardiomyopathy. She was born via cesarean section at 41 weeks because of failure of delivery progression. At 2 months of age, she preferred to maintain her hands fisted, which prompted several evaluations. She lost interest in eating and was placed on nasogastric feedings at 4 months of age. Cardiomegaly was noted on a chest X ray at that time. The infant smiled at 3 months and sat unsupported at 10 months, but did not roll over. At 13 months, she did not take steps but could get around on a walker. She was well aware of her surroundings and of familiar people. She placed objects in her mouth using either hand. Mother and relatives believed she was performing at an 8-month-old level. She displayed coarsening of the face, with flattened supraorbital ridges, prominent coronal suture, flattened nasal bridge, anteverted nostrils, and a broad philtrum. A cranial bruit was perceptible. There was a pansystolic murmur and the liver was palpable two fingers below the rib cage. Shoulders were narrowed and depressed and arms were slightly rotated anteriorly. The span of the metacarpus was shortened and the digits terminated in short and stubby phalanges. Head circumference was 45 cm, just above the 25th percentile. There was uneven wearing of both of her shoes, more marked on the anterior third of the sole and the tips symmetrically. Tone was excessively increased, superimposed on a limited range of motion on the (in order of severity) shoulder, ankle, knee, and carpal joints. Feet were held in plantar flexion. Reflexes were overactive, also in the upper extremities, with cross adductor leg reflexes and two-joint spread. There was extension of the reflex sensory field and delayed relaxation of muscle after a jerk. Ankle jerks were also strikingly brisk. Babinski signs were noted. She died of a myocardial infarction while in preparation for hematopoietic stem cell transplantation.

Mucolipidoses

Onset: Infantile or childhood cognitive and motor developmental failure with abnormal facial and skeletal features.

Additional manifestations: Four types of mucolipidosis exist. Dysostosis multiplex. Cardiopathy. Cerebral palsy in slowly progressive cases. Hepatosplenomegaly and umbilical hernias.

Disease mechanism: In types II and III, defective targeting of enzymes to the lysosome. In type IV, dysfunctional ion channel function with impaired lysosomal acidification.

Testing: In types II and III, the enzymatic activities of different lysosomal hydrolases are severely decreased in fibroblasts, whereas they are markedly increased in serum or cell culture medium.

Treatment: None effective.

Research highlights: Regulation of the rate of lysosomal metabolism by mucolipin function.

Clinical Features

The four mucolipidoses are characterized by the accumulation of lipids and glycosaminoglycans without mucopolysacchariduria. Mucolipidosis type I is also known as sialidosis and is described separately.

Mucolipidosis type II or I-cell disease is designated after the fibroblast inclusions that are typical of the disorder. These fibroblasts are thus also known as inclusion cells. Disease features include coarse features similar to Hurler syndrome, dysostosis multiplex, and progressive intellectual deterioration. Hepatosplenomegaly and umbilical hernias are common, as is kyphoscoliosis. These features are seen earlier than in Hurler syndrome. There is a small thorax and joint movements are restricted. The tongue is large, with gingival hyperplasia. Corneal opacification. There is also aortic insufficiency and cardiomegaly, sometimes accompanied by coronary artery

Table 73.1 The mucolipidoses

Mucolipidosis	Gene	Defective protein
II or I-cell disease	GNPTAB	α-β subunit of UDP-*N*-acetylglucosamine-1-phosphotransferase
IIIA or pseudo Hurler polydystrophy	GNPTAB	α-β subunit of UDP-*N*-acetylglucosamine-1-phosphotransferase
IIIC	GNPTG	γ subunit of UDP-*N*-acetylglucosamine-1-phosphotransferase
IV	TRPML1	Mucolipin-1 or transient receptor potential cation channel, mucolipin subfamily 1

stenosis due to vascular deposition of lipid and mucopolisaccharide. Death ensues in the first decade of life, usually following cardiorespiratory failure.

Mucolipidosis type III is an attenuated form of type II and is heterogeneous. Most affected individuals exhibit mild learning impairment, short stature, cardiac valve lesions, and skeletal disease primarily affecting the hips and shoulders as well as the spine. Prolonged survival is common.

Mucolipidosis type IV is more common among Ashkenazi Jews. Affected individuals manifest motor impairment, severe mental retardation, retinal degeneration, corneal clouding, iron deficiency anemia, and gastric achlorhydria associated with probably reactively elevated blood gastrin levels. Spasticity, hypotonia and the inability to walk independently are common among such children and typically begin during early childhood. Neurologic symptoms are sometimes recognized in infants, presenting as the delayed achievement of major gross motor accomplishments. In most individuals, the development of language and motor functions never progresses beyond the 12–15 months level. Prolonged survival is common as well.

Pathology

Magnetic resonance imaging studies may reveal a dysgenic corpus callosum, white matter dysmyelination, decreased signal intensity in the basal ganglia and cerebellar atrophy. Cerebellar atrophy typically occurs in older individuals with mucolipidosis IV.

The principal feature of mucolipidosis II and III is the presence of intracytoplasmic membrane-bound vacuoles in fibroblasts and lymphocytes. These cells can be found in numerous tissues such as skin, conjunctiva, lymph nodes, spleen, gingiva, heart, and bone. There is also vacuole formation in Schwann cells, perineural cells, endothelial cells, pericytes, myocardiocytes, and renal tubular cells. There is no neuronal storage and neural cell changes are very limited. There is only granular deposition in reticular formation cells of the brainstem and in anterior spinal horn cells. These granules have the structure of zebra bodies. Neurons may also contain lipofuscin.

Pathophysiology

Mucolipidosis type II is caused by mutations in the gene encoding the enzyme UDP-*N*-acetylglucosamine: lysosomal hydrolase N-acetylglucosamine-1-phosphotransferase. This enzyme is responsible for catalyzing the initial step in the synthesis of the mannose-6-phosphate recognition marker that targets newly produced enzymes to the lysosomes. The defect thus resides in the targeting of enzymes to the lysosome. There is deficiency of multiple lysosomal enzymes, which are elevated in plasma or in cell culture medium. The enzyme is a hexameric protein with composition α2β2γ2. The α and β subunits are encoded by the GNPTAB gene, while the γ subunit is encoded by the GNPTG gene. Mutations in GNPTAB can result in both mucolipidosis type II and type III phenotypes whereas mutations in GNPTG are only associated with a mucolipidosis type III phenotype.

Mucolipidosis type IV is caused by mutations in the TRPML1 (also known as mucolipin 1 or MCOLN1) gene, which encodes a transient receptor potential (TRP) protein. Mucolipin is a cation channel that may conduct Fe^{++}, Mn^{++}, Ca^{++}, Na^+, and K^+ ions that is regulated by Ca^{++}. The ion specificity of the channel may be determined by association with a regulatory protein. Most molecules that traffic through the lysosomal compartment are delayed in mucolipidosis type IV cells, either due to a primary transport defect, or secondarily because they are protected from delivery by the excess storage. The disease is also associated with a defect in autophagy.

Diagnosis

The diagnosis of mucolipidosis relies on the use of blood screening tests followed by specific enzyme assays. All of these disorders can be detected pre-natally. In mucolipidosis II and III, multiple enzyme deficiencies occur, but the diagnosis is suggested by finding a gross elevation of enzyme activity of a number of lysosomal enzymes in body fluids such as plasma or urine.

Plasma gastrin level is elevated in mucolipidosis type IV.

Treatment

There is no effective treatment. Hematopoietic stem cell transplantation for mucolipidosis type II is associated with low survival due to cardiovascular complications likely due to disease progression. Neurologic outcome is also poor.

Because in mucolipidosis type IV mutant muco-lipin 1 may cause lysosomal over-acidification via non-selective channel dysfunction, molecules with lysosomal regulatory activity have been tested. Basic chemical compounds such as nigericin, which is a proton antiport channel and chloroquine, a weak base, could lower lysosomal pH and rescue normal lysosomal degradation. However, this approach did not lead to a reduction in cultured fibroblast inclusions.

Bibliography

Lund T.C., Cathey S.S., Miller W.P., et al. (2014). Outcomes after hematopoietic stem cell transplantation for children with I-cell disease. *Biol Blood Marrow Transplant.* 20(11):1847–51.

Wakabayashi K., Gustafson A.M., Sidransky E, et al. (2011). Mucolipidosis type IV: An update. *Mol Genet Metab.* 104(3):206–13.

Wraith J.E. (2013). Mucopolysaccharidoses and mucolipidoses. *Handb Clin Neurol.* 113:1723–9.

Fucosidosis

A boy, the second child of second-cousin parents, was normal until 2 years of age, when all of his developmental acquisitions gradually evolved into abnormality. At 4 years of age, he manifested significant speech difficulties, displayed poor social interactions and moved very slowly. His face had become somewhat coarse and his skeleton was abnormal with mild dysostosis multiplex visible on X-rays (vertebral beaking, shallow acetabuli, and a J-shaped sella). At age 12, he had deteriorated significantly. He was no longer able to speak or walk without assistance and was irritable. His coarse facial features had now become prominent, with edematous eyelids, anteverted, prominent nostrils, thickened lips, a shallow philtrum, and gingival hypertrophy. He also manifested short stature. There was no organomegaly. X rays now showed mild hypoplasia of the medial distal radius and mild cortical thinning of the metacarpal bones. Brain MR imaging showed symmetric periventricular white matter high intensities contrasting with low intensities on the basal ganglia on T2 weighed images.

Fucosidosis

Onset: Infantile or childhood psychomotor abnormalities with coarse facial features.
Additional manifestations: Hypotonia followed by rigidity. Dystonia, spasticity, tremor and dementia, culminating with disconnection from the environment. The skin is thick and children sweat excessively. There may be gallbladder dysfunction. There is also dysostosis and hepatosplenomegaly.
Disease mechanism: Lysosomal α-L-fucosidase deficiency leads to accumulation and excretion of glycoproteins and glycolipids.
Testing: Assay of α-L-fucosidase in serum, leukocytes, and cultured skin fibroblasts. Normal

individuals may exhibit low serum fucosidase activity.
Treatment: None effective.
Research highlights: Bone marrow transplantation in dogs spontaneously affected by the disorder.

Clinical Features

Fucosidosis is an autosomal recessive lysosomal storage disorder characterized by deficient glycoprotein degradation due to mutations in the gene FUCA1, which encodes α–L-fucosidase. The clinical course is variable. The term type I fucosidosis is sometimes used to refer to a severe progressive neurological disorder that usually leads to death before 5 years of age. Type II fucosidosis encompasses a milder phenotype that becomes symptomatic in childhood with survival into the third decade of life.

In the severe infantile form, affected individuals manifest psychomotor retardation and hypotonia. Later in the disease course, rigidity develops, together with dystonia, spasticity, tremor, and dementia, culminating with the disconnection from the environment. The skin is thick and children sweat excessively. There may be gallbladder dysfunction. There is also dysostosis and hepatosplenomegaly.

In the later onset type II form, children manifest cognitive deterioration in the second year of life. There is coarsening of facial features, dysostosis, and dwarfism. Angiokeratoma corporis diffusum is characteristic of this form. The disease is slowly progressive and may be associated with seizures.

Pathology

Neuroimaging demonstrates abnormalities in the thalamus (decreased MR imaging signal intensity), pallidum, internal capsule, and other areas of the supratentorial white matter. The brain may be atrophic or enlarged, depending on disease stage. Cerebellar atrophy has also been documented.

There is cytoplasmic vacuolation in numerous cell types in the liver, spleen lymph nodes, endocrine glands, nerve, brain, conjunctiva, and fibroblasts. These vacuoles are complex structures bound by a membrane and including reticular material and lamellar inclusions.

The brain may be atrophied or megaencephalic. Storage vacuoles are prominent in neurons and glia. There is neuronal loss in the thalamus, dentate nucleus, and Purkinje cell layer. The remainder neurons display enlarged cytoplasm containing vacuoles. The white matter exhibits gliosis and demyelination. Rosenthal fibers may be abundant.

Pathophysiology

Fucosidosis is caused by lysosomal α-L-fucosidase deficiency. L-fucose is a ubiquitous constituent of oligosaccharides, keratan sulfate, glycolipids and glycoproteins. L-fucose residues exist attached to the terminal nonreducing position of oligosaccharide chains. The enzyme is involved in the cleavage of terminal fucose linked $\alpha 1-2$ to a galactose residue and of fucose linked $\alpha 1-3$, $\alpha 1-4$, or $\alpha 1-6$ to an N-acetylglucosamine residue on glycoproteins and glycolipids. In fucosidosis, large quantities of these compounds accumulate and are excreted in the urine.

In the brain, the principal material stored is oligosaccharide. There is a major accumulation of glycolipids expressing blood group antigens (H, X) in liver. In the urine, the most abundant abnormal species include fucose-containing oligosaccharides and glycopeptides. These glycopeptides are characterized by the presence of $\alpha 1-6$-linked fucose to a chitobiose core. The major glycopeptide, a glycoasparagine Fuc($\alpha 1-6$) GlcNAc$\beta 1$-Asn present in urine corresponds to the linkage region of the oligosaccharide. The large amount of glycopeptides excreted is unique to fucosidosis and can be explained by the steric inhibition of the glycosylasparaginase by the fucose residue; the nonfucosylated glycoasparagines are normally processed and only fucosylated glycoasparagine and oligosaccharides without $\alpha 1-6$ linked fucose residue accumulate.

α-L-fucosidase is a tetramer including four identical subunits processed from a precursor polypeptide. Abnormalities of enzyme posttranslational processing have been identified in affected individuals, as has been enzyme absence and rapid degradation. Approximately 6 percent of healthy individuals exhibit very low serum enzyme activity with normal leukocyte and tissue activity. This trait is inherited in Mendelian fashion.

Diagnosis

α-L-fucosidase deficiency can be demonstrated in serum, leukocytes, and cultured skin fibroblasts.

Treatment

Bone marrow transplantation has led to increase enzyme levels and improved psychomotor performance, but has not been systematically evaluated.

Bibliography

Kılıç E., Kılıç M., Ütine G.E., et al. (2014). A case of fucosidosis type II: Diagnosed with dysmorphological and radiological findings. *Turk J Pediatr*. 56(4).430–3.

Michalski JC, Klein A. (1999). Glycoprotein lysosomal storage disorders: Alpha- and beta-mannosidosis, fucosidosis and alpha-N-acetylgalactosaminidase deficiency. *Biochim Biophys Acta*. 1455(2–3):69–84.

Willems P.J., Seo H.C., Coucke P, et al. (1999); Spectrum of mutations in fucosidosis. *Eur J Hum Genet*. 7(1):60–7.

Mannosidoses

A 2-year-old girl was evaluated for developmental regression. She exhibited dysmorphic features, which consisted of coarse facial features, a short anteverted nose, a flattened nasal bridge, and prominent epicanthal folds. She was macrocephalic, with a head circumference of 52.2 cm (> 97th percentile). Her weight and length were appropriate for age. Examination showed firm hepatomegaly of 8 cm and a splenomegaly of 4 cm. She also displayed fixed thoraco-lumbar kyphoscoliosis. She exhibited sterterous respiration due to upper airway obstruction. She manifested global hypotonia and brisk tendon reflexes. Power grading of muscles was 4/5 in all her limbs. She could no longer walk or express herself in meaningful words. She was only able to sit, her speech was limited to babbling, she did not follow single-step instructions, and she used an immature pincer grasp. There was diffuse osteopenia with a coarse trabecular pattern suggesting marrow infiltration on radiographs of the long bones. Auditory brainstem evoked responses indicated no identifiable peaks at 90 decibels bilaterally, consistent with a profound high frequency hearing loss. MR imaging and liver biopsy results are shown below.

Mannosidoses

Onset: Childhood psychomotor regression with dysmorphic features in the severe form and speech and hearing dysfunction in the milder form. Some children are born with ankle equinus or develop hydrocephalus in the first year of life.
Additional manifestations: Cognitive deterioration and recurrent psychosis. Deafness. Dysostosis multiplex. Hepatosplenomegaly. Immune dysfunction leading to recurrent infection. Children usually die between 3 and 12 years of age. In the mild form, ataxia and tremor. Destructive arthropathy.

Disease mechanism: Deficiency of hydrolases results in the multi-systemic accumulation of undegraded glycoprotein material in lysosomes. Oligomannosides residues bind to interleukin-2 receptors, disturbing immune responses.
Testing: Vacuoles in bone marrow smears and in lymphocytes. Elevated urinary secretion of mannose-rich oligosaccharides.
Treatment: None effective.
Research highlights: Spontaneous and mouse models of α-mannosidosis replicate features of the human disorder.

Clinical Features

α- and β–mannosidosis are autosomal recessive lysosomal storage disorders characterized by lysosomal accumulation of mannose-containing oligosaccharides. α-mannosidosis is caused by mutations in the gene MANB (or MAN2B1), whereas β–mannosidosis is associated with mutations in MANB1.

α-mannosidosis occurs in 1 of 500,000 live births. There are two forms of α-mannosidosis: a severe type 1 and a milder type 2, although there is significant overlap. Type I is characterized by severe and progressive psychomotor deterioration, dysmorphic features including a large head with prominent forehead, rounded eyebrows, flattened nasal bridge, macroglossia, widely spaced teeth, prognathism and a short neck, dysostosis multiplex with scoliosis and deformation of the sternum, hepatosplenomegaly and deafness with childhood onset (Figure 75.1). These manifestations resemble mucopolysaccharidosis. Gingival hyperplasia due to macrophage accumulation is prominent. Some children are born with ankle equinus or develop hydrocephalus in the first year of life. There is significant immune dysfunction with propensity to infection. Post-immunization levels of antibody are decreased, suggesting impaired ability to produce specific antibodies after antigen presentation.

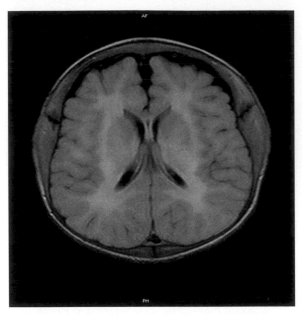

Figure 75.1 MR imaging in type I alpha mannosidosis. Axial fluid-attenuated inversion recovery showing marked calvarial thickening with extensive white matter hyperintensities. Reproduced with permission from Govender R et al. Alpha-mannosidosis: A report of 2 siblings and review of the literature. *J Child Neurol.* 2014; 29(1):131–4.

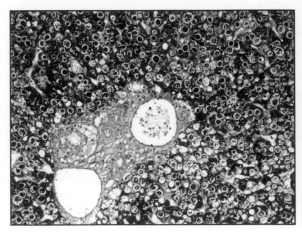

Figure 75.2 Type I alpha-mannosidosis in a case from Figure 75.1. Liver biopsy showing extensive showing extensive glycogen accumulation within the cytoplasm of the hepatocytes. Reproduced with permission from Govender R et al. Alpha-mannosidosis: A report of 2 siblings and review of the literature. *J Child Neurol.* 2014; 29(1):131–4.

A serum factor inhibits phagocytosis. Children usually die between 3 and 12 years of age.

Type 2 α-mannosidosis manifests in early adolescence with speech and hearing dysfunction, ataxia, and tremor. Immune dysfunction is also common. Intellectual disability can be mild. All affected individuals are mildly or moderately mentally retarded with an IQ of 60–80, with a declining tendency over later decades. Some individuals learn to speak late, often in the second decade of life. Because of their poor ability to speak combined with sensorineural hearing loss, affected individuals score generally better in nonverbal tests. Psychiatric symptoms occur in 25% of adults and include acute and recurrent attacks of confusion, sometimes with anxiety, depression, or hallucinations. Periods of psychosis usually last 3 to 12 weeks, followed by a long period of hypersomnia and sometimes loss of abilities, such as difficulty speaking or inability to read. Survival to adulthood is common. Over time, from the second to the fourth decade of life, affected individuals may develop destructive polyarthropathy.

β–mannosidosis is more rare and heterogeneous. Hearing loss, frequent infections, intellectual disability, and behavioral disorders including Tourette

syndrome are its most common manifestations. Angiokeratoma corporis diffusum and spinocerebellar ataxia at age 20 to 30 years have been documented.

Pathology

The pathology of α- and β–mannosidosis has been studied in spontaneous animal models. Human pathological reports have been limited. The main feature of α-mannosidosis is the accumulation of cytoplasmic vacuoles in many cell types, some of which contain large granules (Figure 75.2). The tissues most affected include the bone marrow and neutrophils and lymphocytes. These vacuolated cells are nonspecific, since they can also be seen in mucopolysaccharidosis, mucolipidosis, sialidosis, and galactosialidosis. The vacuoles contain periodic acid-Schiff-staining material, which is diastase resistant.

In the human brain, changes in α-mannosidosis include dilatation of nerve cells with empty cytoplasm in the cerebral cortex, brainstem and spinal cord. There is little neuronal storage in the basal ganglia. There is neuronal loss in the cerebral cortex and myelin loss and gliosis in the white matter. In the cerebellum, there is loss of Purkinje and granule cells. There may be focal dilatation of Purkinje cell dendrites, with scant cytoplasmic storage.

The ultrastructure of the accumulating vacuoles is characterized by a single membrane encircling loosely dispersed reticulogranular material. They may also contain stacks of membranes. In the feline model of α-mannosidosis, the vacuoles contain GM2 and GM3 gangliosides.

There is limited information about pathological changes in β–mannosidosis. In the skin, there is cytoplasmic vacuolation in endothelial cells, fibroblasts, eccrine sweat glands, and keratinocytes.

Pathophysiology

During normal catabolism, glycoproteins are digested by proteinases and glycosidases within lysosomes. These enzymes degrade glycoproteins into fragments small enough to be excreted or transported to the cytosol for reutilization. Lack or deficiency of such hydrolases results in the multi-systemic accumulation of undigested material in the lysosomes. Consequently, the lysosomes dilate, resulting in impairment of various cellular functions.

Lysosomal α-mannosidase is an exoglycosidase that cleaves the α-mannosidic linkages during the ordered degradation of N-linked oligosaccharides (Figure 75.3). The mature lysosomal MAN2B1 enzyme is a dimer. MAN2B1 post-translationally modified in the endoplasmic reticulum by N-glycosylation and disulfide bond formation. The enzyme has the capacity to cleave α(1 → 2), α(1 → 3) and α(1 → 6) mannosidic linkages found in high mannose and hybrid type glycans. The catalysis is activated by zinc and involves the reaction nucleophile Asp196. The same reaction mechanism is common to the five mammalian α-mannosidases that are part of glycoside hydrolase family.

Missense mutation c.C2248T, resulting in the replacement of arginine with tryptophan at amino acid position 750 (Arg750Trp), appears to be frequent among mannosidosis individuals, as it has been reported in most European populations studied, accounting for more than 30 percent of all disease alleles.

The bases for the immune dysfunction typical of the disease are less clear. Oligomannosides with five and six mannose residues bind to interleukin-2 (IL-2) receptors, disturbing IL-2-dependent responses. IL-2 activates T-, B-, and NK (natural killer) cells. It can therefore be speculated that blockage of this receptor is one mechanism causing immune deficiency. In a mouse model, alpha-mannosidase II deficiency reduces complex-type N-glycan branching and induces an autoimmune disease similar to human systemic lupus erythematosus, with induction of antinuclear antibodies with reactivity towards histones, Sm antigens, and DNA.

Diagnosis

Light microscopy or transmission electron microscopy demonstrates vacuoles in bone marrow smears and in lymphocytes obtained from blood. Detection of elevated urinary secretion of mannose-rich oligosaccharides by thin-layer chromatography or high performance liquid chromatography is suggestive. Mannosidase activity can be documented in serum, leukocytes, cultured fibroblasts, and other tissues. In affected individuals, acid α-mannosidase enzyme activity in peripheral blood leukocytes is 5%–15% of normal activity. Prenatal testing may be performed by analysis of acid α-mannosidase enzyme activity in fetal cells obtained by chorionic villus sampling at 10–12 weeks gestation or by amniocentesis at 15–18 weeks.

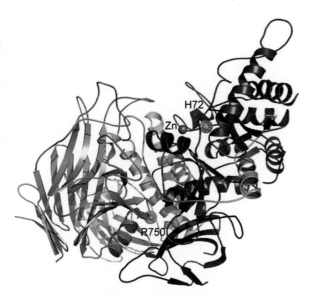

Figure 75.3 The 3-dimensional structure of lysosomal α-mannosidase. Peptides are coloured a-red, b-orange, c-yellow, d-green and e-blue. The active site is denoted by a Zn^{++} ion. Two mutant sites are displayed, demonstrating the effect of mutations His72Leu affecting Zn^{++} coordination in the actives site and the prevalent mutation Arg750Trp which is likely affecting peptide e-d interaction. Reproduced with permission from Malm D et al. Alpha-mannosidosis. *Orphanet J Rare Dis.* 2008; 3:21.

Treatment

There is no well-studied effective treatment. Bone marrow transplantation in the first decade of life has led to intellectual function stabilization with improvement in adaptive skills and verbal memory in some subjects, together with an amelioration of recurrent infection rates. Enzyme replacement therapy has been performed in a knockout mouse model and in a naturally occurring guinea pig model. There was reduction in storage material in almost all tissues in both models. Zinc therapy has been effective in an individual carrying a mutation interfering with zinc coordination in the enzyme active site.

Bibliography

Borgwardt L., Lund A.M., Dali C.I. (2014). Alpha-mannosidosis – A review of genetic, clinical findings and options of treatment. *Pediatr Endocrinol Rev.* 12 Suppl 1:185–91.

Malm D., Nilssen Ø. (2008). Alpha-mannosidosis. *Orphanet J Rare Dis.* 3:21.

GM1 Gangliosidosis

Two brothers presented with psychomotor regression in early childhood. Although the first brother walked independently at 18 months of age, his gait was unsteady because of increased muscle tone. By 18 months of age, he stopped saying "bye-bye" or "hi" and became unable to stand up from a sitting position. At 2 years of age, his finger dexterity remained poor. He received a normal brain magnetic resonance imaging study at that time. His motor and cognitive functions continued to deteriorate, and he exhibited a developmental quotient of 36 at age 3 1/2 years. At 4 years of age, he started to manifest refractory seizures. His brother become easily tired and to have a clumsy gait at 18 months of age. His mother recalled that his motor function was best between 18 months and 2 years of age, and he used approximately 50 words. By the age of 2 years, his finger dexterity had worsened. By 3 years of age, he easily stumbled, fell, and required assistance walking. His speech deteriorated, with reduced spontaneous speech and echolalia. His motor and cognitive functions progressed, and he barely walked with support and only had 10 words at 7 years of age. He developed refractory seizures. He exhibited constant dystonia, equinus feet, frequent myoclonus, and Babinski signs. At age 12 years, he was not communicative and manifested continuous dystonic posturing, requiring a wheelchair for locomotion.

GM1 Gangliosidosis

Onset: Progressive psychomotor dysfunction by 6 months of age in the infantile form. Facial and bone abnormalities can be recognized at birth. Progressive dysarthria, gait difficulties or dystonia in adults.
Additional manifestations: Progressive spasticity and epilepsy. Hepatosplenomegaly. Disostosis multiplex with spinal cord compression. Death is often due to infections.
Disease mechanism: Deficiency of GM1-degrading β-galactosidase. Accumulation of lyso-GM1 ganglioside may be responsible for neuronal degeneration. Accumulation of sialoglycolipid GM1 may also lead to apoptosis. Neuroinflammation.
Testing: Assay of β-galactosidase in fibroblasts, white blood cells, or serum. Enzymatic pseudodeficiency may occur.
Treatment: None effective.
Research highlights: Enzyme active site inhibitors as potential therapy.

Clinical Features

Autosomal recessive deficiency of lysosomal acid β-galactosidase causes GM1 gangliosidosis and Morquio disease type B. Morquio disease type A is a mucopolisaccharidosis and is discussed elsewhere, whereas Morquio type B disease is a skeletal and connective tissue disorder.

There are three forms of GM1 gangliosidosis, which are characterized by accumulation of the sphingolipid GM1 ganglioside: infantile, juvenile and chronic or adult. All of them are primary neurological disorders.

Infantile GM1 gangliosidosis leads to progressive flaccidity, hepatosplenomegaly, dysmorphic facies with depressed nasal bones, corneal opacification, macular cherry-red spots and lumbar kyphosis. Onset is before 6 months of age, although facial and bone abnormalities may be recognized at birth. In some cases, there is hydrops fetalis. There is progressive spasticity and epilepsy. The disease is rapidly progressive and children survive only several years. In the end stage, children become deaf and blind and cease to respond to stimuli. Death is usually due to infections.

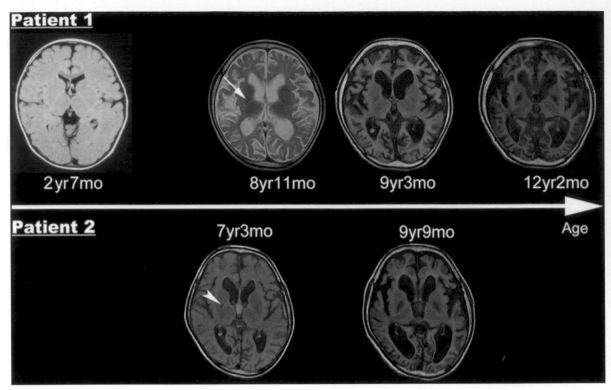

Figure 76.1 Serial neuroimaging in GM1 gangliosidosis. MR imaging in subjects 1 and 2 reveals progressive diffuse cerebral atrophy. In subject 1, fluid-attenuated inversion recovery (FLAIR) image at age 2 years and 7 months was normal. A T2-weighted image at 8 years 11 months revealed significant cerebral atrophy with barely noticeable hypointense signals in the globi pallidi (arrow). The cerebral atrophy and paramagnetic signals in the basal ganglia became more pronounced on the subsequent FLAIR images at 9 years 3 months and 12 years 2 months. In subject 2, a FLAIR image at 7 years 3 months revealed marked cerebral atrophy with minimal hypodensity in the globi pallidi (arrowhead). The cerebral atrophy and the paramagnetic signals became more apparent on the subsequent FLAIR image at 9 years 9 months. Reproduced with permission from Takenouchi T et al. Paramagnetic signals in the globus pallidus as late radiographic sign of juvenile-onset GM1 gangliosidosis. *Pediatr Neurol*. 2015; 52(2):226–9.

The juvenile form of the disease manifests after one year of age and is associated with milder neurological dysfunction. Systemic involvement may be absent. Survival usually exceeds the first decade of life.

The adult or chronic form of GM1 gangliosidosis is more variable. Onset may be from late childhood to adulthood. Slowly progressive dysarthria, gait difficulties, dystonia, and other extrapyramidal manifestations are common. There is mild cognitive impairment. The visceral and ocular features typical of the other forms are absent. Skeletal disostosis may lead to spinal cord compression.

Pathology

Computed tomography and MR imaging demonstrate increased thalamic density (increased signal in T1-weigthed images and decreased signal in T2-weigthed images) and decreased white matter density, which are features common to many lysosomal diseases (Figure 76.1). As the disease progresses, diffuse cerebral atrophy and ventricular enlargement become apparent. Loss of myelin can be prominent.

Hepatosplenomegaly and disostosis are not features of the juvenile or adult chronic forms. Infiltration by storage cells is present in spleen, lymph nodes, hepatic sinusoids, and bone marrow. The storage material is water soluble. The cytoplasm of renal glomerular cells is vacuolated. Cardiomyopathy with infiltration of myocardiocytes and mitral valve has been documented. Vacuoles are also present in sweat glands, skin fibroblasts, and lymphocytes. The cytoplasmic vacuoles contain fine filamentous or tubular structures.

The brain is firm. There are enlarged neurons with cytoplasmic storage material throughout brain, brainstem, cerebellum, and spinal cord. These cells are also visible in dorsal root ganglia, autonomic ganglia, and myenteric plexus. Neurons contain little or no periodic acid-Schiff-staining material, whereas glial cells are rich in it. This material also contains unsterified cholesterol and can thus be stained with filipin. The inclusions display the ultrastructural features of membranous cytoplasmic bodies and are similar to those found in GM2 gangliosidosis, although they primarily contain GM1 ganglioside. There is meganeurite formation in cortical pyramidal neurons. They are accompanied by ectopic dendritic spines and neurites, which is also typical of other lysosomal disorders with primary or secondary ganglioside accumulation. The cerebral white matter displays a paucity of myelin with axonal degeneration, gliosis, and macrophage infiltration. There is deficiency of proteolipid protein and myelin basic protein in the white matter and decreased numbers of oligodendrocytes. There is also atrophy of the caudate nucleus, which contains a paucity of neurons, most of which display storage.

Pathophysiology

Inherited defects of the GM1-degrading β-galactosidase cause GM1-gangliosidoses. At the biochemical level, the clinical heterogeneity is paralleled by a variation of the extent and the pattern of glycolipid accumulation and by different degrees of residual catabolic activities detected in cultured fibroblasts. Complete or nearly complete loss of GM1 catabolic activity results in the fatal infantile form of this storage disease. Mutations that allow the production of proteins with some residual catabolic activity give rise to protracted clinical forms sometimes described as late infantile, juvenile, or chronic diseases. The nonspecific and versatile GM1 degrading β-galactosidase occurs as part of a lysosomal multi-enzyme complex that contains sialidase, cathepsin A (or protective protein) and N-acetylaminogalacto-6-sulfate sulfatase. Due to changes of the substrate specificity of human mutants, inherited defects of GM1-β-galactosidase may also lead to accumulation of galactose containing keratan sulfate and oligosaccharides as part of the Morquio syndrome type B phenotype (mucopolysaccharidosis IV B).

The main storage compounds characteristic of gangliosides GM1 and GM2 are preferentially synthesized in neuronal cells. Ganglioside catabolism proceeds in stepwise fashion at the surface of luminal intralysosomal vesicle and membrane structures. These are rich in anionic bis(monoacylglycero)phosphate, which attracts polycationic proteins, glycosidases and sphingolipid activator proteins to the ganglioside-containing membrane surfaces in the acidic intralysosomal environment. Whereas GM1 hydrolyzing β-galactosidase binds to these anionic surfaces, it does not attack the membrane bound ganglioside substrate in the absence of membrane perturbing lipid binding and transfer proteins. Hydrolysis of vesicle-bound GM1 by lysosomal ganglioside β-galactosidase needs the presence of GM2AP (ganglioside GM2 activator protein) or saposin B. Anionic lipids such as bis(monoacylglycero)phosphate in the GM1 carrying vesicles stimulate GM1 hydrolysis efficiently.

As a result of lysosomal dysfunction, there is accumulation of lyso-GM1 ganglioside, which may be responsible for neuronal degeneration. Accumulation of sialoglycolipid GM1 in the endoplasmic reticulum may also lead to neuronal loss via apoptosis. In addition, there is neuroinflammation.

Diagnosis

The diagnosis of GM1 gangliosidosis may be suspected in individuals with characteristic clinical, neuroimaging, radiographic, and biochemical findings. GM1 gangliosidosis can be diagnosed by assay of β-galactosidase in fibroblasts, white blood cells, or serum using artificial substrates. Pseudodeficiency can occur and thus molecular analysis is recommended. Vacuolated lymphocytes may suggest GM1 gangliosidosis. Individuals with a suggestive phenotype but normal enzyme activity on standard assays may have activator protein deficiency, which requires specialized assays including tissue biopsy with lipid analysis. Electron microscopy of the biopsy may show characteristic multilamellar cytoplasmic bodies in both GM1 and GM2 gangliosidoses. Dysostosis multiplex may be found in infantile GM1 gangliosidosis; organomegaly may be confirmed by abdominal ultrasound, computed tomography or MR imaging. CT of the brain illustrates increased density of the basal ganglia in infantile GM1 gangliosidosis and MR imaging usually demonstrates diffuse white matter

303

changes. There may also be subtle changes in the basal ganglia.

Treatment

Treatments have included bone marrow transplantation, gene therapy, and substrate reduction.

Allogenic bone marrow transplantation has been followed by normalization of white blood cell β-galactosidase levels in the setting of continued neurological deterioration.

Imino sugars that inhibit ganglioside biosynthesis have been investigated in rodents and have resulted in a reduction of ganglioside accumulation in the brain, suggesting that substrate deprivation therapy may be a potential early intervention for GM1 gangliosidosis.

Adeno associated virus-mediated neonatal gene delivery by intracerebroventricular injection has been followed by enzymatic recovery. It results in a widespread appearance of the absent β-galactosidase activity in the murine brain and a normalization of glycosphingolipid levels.

The chemical chaperone N-octyl-4-epi-β-valienamine has been used to stabilize the mutant β-galactosidase protein, achieving restoration of enzyme activity. Oral treatment of mice carrying the mutant gene results in an increase in enzyme activity, reduction in cerebral GM1 ganglioside content and prevention of neurological deterioration. However, this therapy can only be effective in individuals with some level of β-galactosidase expression.

Bibliography

Brunetti-Pierri N., Scaglia F. (2008). GM1 gangliosidosis: review of clinical, molecular, and therapeutic aspects. *Mol Genet Metab.* 94(4):391–6.

Sandhoff K., Harzer K. (2013). Gangliosides and gangliosidoses: Principles of molecular and metabolic pathogenesis. *J Neurosci.* 33(25):10195–208.

Takenouchi T., Kosaki R., Nakabayashi K., et al. (2015). Paramagnetic signals in the globus pallidus as late radiographic sign of juvenile-onset GM1 gangliosidosis. *Pediatr Neurol.* 52(2):226–9.

77

Chapter

Fabry Disease

A 16-year-old male presented with right hypoacusia, tingling in hands and feet and burning plantar pain, which worsened in hot weather and with physical activity. He displayed asymptomatic peri-umbilical lesions since his first years of life, which had been progressing in number and size for the last 3 years. On examination, he displayed erythematous-violaceous papules of keratotic sur-faces, grouped on the upper limbs, paravertebral, paraumbilical, inguinal, scrotum, and penile regions, right thigh and knees. He also exhibited right sensorineural hearing loss, cornea verticillata, and proteinuria.

Fabry Disease

Onset: Acroparesthesia at 6 years of age in males and at 9 years of age in manifesting females.
Additional manifestations: Gastrointestinal disturbance. Cardiopathy with arrhythmia and heart failure. Cornea verticillata. Angiokeratomas of the lower trunk. Proteinuric renal failure. Hearing impairment and paroxysmal vertigo. Recurrent stroke. Symptoms in manifesting female heterozygotes are more variable. Attenuated forms of the disease exist, often manifesting as cardiopathy.
Disease mechanism: X-linked recessive decrease in α-galactosidase A activity to less than 25–30 percent of the normal level, leading to endothelial dysfunction, proliferation, and stenosis.
Testing: Decreased enzyme activity in plasma, dried blood spots, or leukocytes. Increase in cell, organ, plasma, or urinary sediment of globotriaosylceramide.
Treatment: Enzyme replacement therapy.
Research highlights: 1-deoxygalactonojirimycin, a competitive inhibitor of α-galactosidase A, results in stabilization of the native residual enzyme and increased in catalysis.

Clinical Features

Fabry disease is an X-linked recessive disorder caused by deficiency of the lysosomal enzyme α-galactosidase A. In males, its incidence is 1 in 50,000, although milder forms of the disease that present later in life may be more common.

Males experience symptoms at an earlier age and with a higher prevalence than females. The median age of symptom onset in males is 6, whereas it is 9 years in females. The first symptom in males is usually acroparesthesia or episodic neuropathic pain manifesting as burning pain of the hands and feet. Hypohidrosis and heat intolerance are also common in the early stage of the disease. Angiokeratomas appearing as small, raised, non-blanching dark-red spots are common, although they are not specific for Fabry disease (Figure 77.1 and 77.2). Diffuse angio-keratomas are typically located in the lower trunk and genital region but may also be present on the palms, around the mouth, lips, and umbilicus. Vortex kerato-pathy or cornea verticillata is the most frequent ocular sign, occurring in over 70 percent of males and females (Figure 77.3). Retinal vessel tortuosity and cataracts are also common and occur more frequently in males (Figure 77.4). The presence of vascular tortu-osity is correlated with disease severity in children and may represent a more severe phenotype. Ophthalmo-logical signs may be present in children before the onset of other manifestations, but do not usually result in visual impairment. Abdominal pain, episodic nausea and vomiting, abdominal bloating, and alter-nating constipation and diarrhea may be related to dysmotility due to autonomic dysfunction. Hearing difficulty and paroxysmal vertigo are also observed. In adulthood, proteinuric renal failure, recurrent strokes and progressive cardiomyopathy, arrhythmias and valvular disease may lead to early death. Cardio-vascular manifestations include hypertension, coron-ary disease, arrhythmias, valvular abnormalities, heart failure, and sudden death (Figure 77.5). Bradycardia

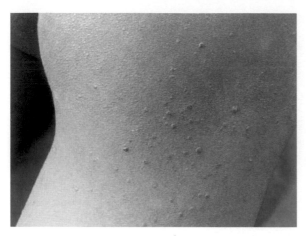

Figure 77.1 Fabry disease. Multiple discrete reddish brown papular lesions of angiokeratoma. Reproduced with permission from Jayavardhana A et al. Angiokeratoma corporis diffusum. *Indian Pediatr.* 2015; 52(2):175.

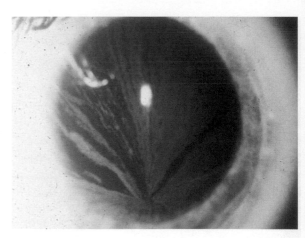

Figure 77.3 Fabry disease in a female with cornea verticillata. Reproduced with permission from Spada M et al. Cornea verticillata and Fabry disease. *J Pediatr.* 2013; 163(2):609.

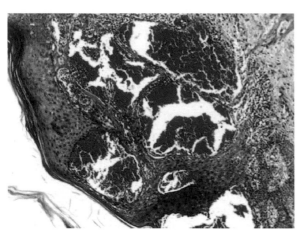

Figure 77.2 Microscopic examination of a lesion from the case in Figure 77.1. Biopsy of the papular lesion showing multiple dilated capillaries and hyperkeratosis of overlying epidermis. Reproduced with permission from Jayavardhana A et al. Angiokeratoma corporis diffusum. *Indian Pediatr.* 2015; 52(2):175.

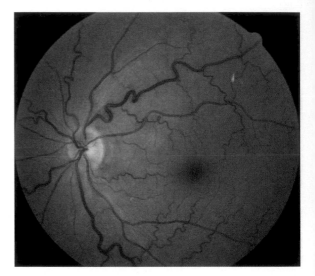

Figure 77.4 Retinal blood vessel tortuosity in a 22- year-old female with Fabry disease. Reproduced with permission from Morier AM et al. Ocular manifestations of Fabry disease within in a single kindred. *Optometry.* 2010; 81(9):437–49.

and conduction system abnormalities are possibly related to abnormal accumulation of glycolipids in the lysosomes of conduction tissues, whereas hypertrophy and fibrosis provides a substrate for persistent conduction abnormalities and ventricular arrhythmias. Sudden cardiac death may be related to bradyarrhythmias or tachyarrhythmias.

Symptoms in manifesting female heterozygotes are more variable but display the same severity as in males, including acroparesthesias, progressive proteinuric renal insufficiency, cardiac disease with rhythm and conduction disturbances, and progressive hypertrophic cardiomyopathy as well as stroke.

Attenuated forms of the disease are recognized, with cardiopathy being the most common manifestation. In addition, individuals with attenuated disease tend to exhibit higher enzyme activity and a more protracted disease natural history than individuals with the common disease form.

Pathology

The most prominent magnetic resonance imaging finding is white matter lesions of progressive severity. Hyperintensity in the pulvinar visible on T1-weighted

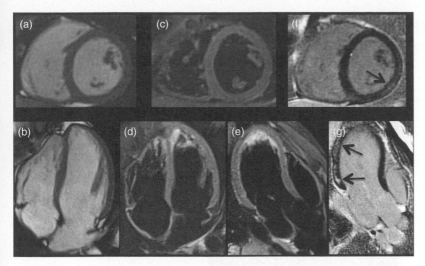

Figure 77.5 Cine and late gadolinium enhancement (LGE) cardiac MR images of a Fabry disease individual at baseline. Panel **a** and **b**: cine (steady-state free precession sequence) of short-axis (**a**) and 4-chamber (**b**) view showing normal left ventricular wall thickness. Panel **c**, **d**, and **e**: T2-weighted short-TI inversion-recovery fast spin-echo image of short-axis (**c**), 4-chamber (**d**) and 3-chamber (**e**) view showing the absence of myocardial edema. Panel **f** and **g**: contrast-enhanced inversion recovery gradient echo image of short-axis (**f**) and 3-chamber (**g**) view showing LGE involving the inferolateral wall with intramyocardial distribution (black arrow). Reproduced with permission from Sechi A et al. Myocardial fibrosis as the first sign of cardiac involvement in a male patient with Fabry disease: report of a clinical case and discussion on the utility of the magnetic resonance in Fabry pathology. *BMC Cardiovasc Disord.* 2014; 14:86.

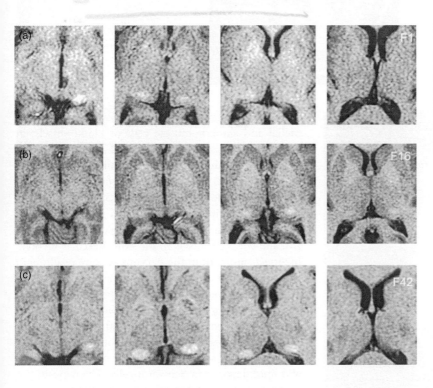

Figure 77.6 Fabry disease. Serial, axial T1-weighted MR images (5-mm sections) demonstrate a range of pulvinar hyperintensities. **a** and **b**, Mild to moderate abnormality. **c**, Marked abnormality. Reproduced with permission from Moore DF et al. Increased signal intensity in the pulvinar on T1-weighted images: a pathognomonic MR imaging sign of Fabry disease. *AJNR Am J Neuroradiol.* 2003; 24(6):1096–101.

images is also common and may represent calcification (Figures 77.6 and 77.7). This pulvinar sign is specific to Fabry disease and is found in males with cardiac signs and severe renal involvement. There is also tortuosity and dilatation of the large vessels, including increased basilar artery diameter. Strokes are not uncommon (Figure 77.8).

There is widespread deposition of glycosphingolipids in many tissues. These deposits are birefringent under polarized light and appear as Maltese crosses.

307

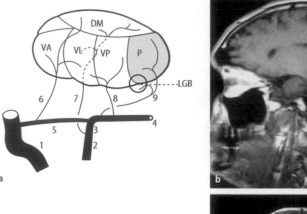

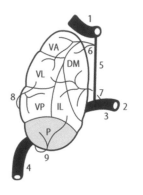

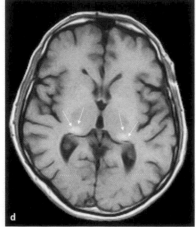

Figure 77.7 The pulvinar in Fabry disease. **a.** Schematic diagram of lateral view of the thalamus and its vascularization; the dorsal yellow part corresponds to the pulvinar. **b.** T1 sagittal image showing a slight hyperintensity (yellow arrows) in the pulvinar area of a 46-year-old male Fabry individual. **c.** Schematic diagram of dorsal view of the thalamus and its vascularization from above; the dorsal yellow part corresponds to the pulvinar. **d.** T1 axial image showing a well-defined symmetric hyperintensity (yellow arrows) of both pulvinar nuclei of a 46-year-old male Fabry individual. Reproduced with permission from Burlina AP et al. The pulvinar sign: frequency and clinical correlations in Fabry disease. *J Neurol.* 2008; 255(5):738–44.

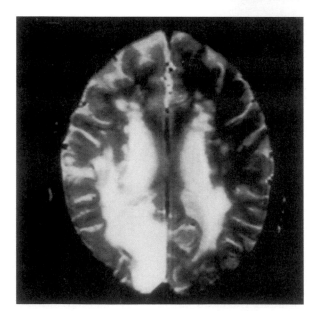

Figure 77.8 Axial T2-weighted MR images from a Fabry individual shows typical periventricular hyperintensities and a posterior circulation stroke. Reproduced with permission from Crutchfield KE et al. Quantitative analysis of cerebral vasculopathy in patients with Fabry disease. *Neurology.* 1998; 50(6):1746–9.

The lipids are predominantly deposited in the endothelial and smooth muscle cells of blood vessels, in eccrine sweat glands, pituitary and renal glomerular epithelial cells and tubules. The resulting swollen vascular endothelial cells are accompanied by endothelial proliferation and luminal obstruction with thrombus formation, leading to ischemia and infarction. There is also aneurysm formation in the retina and conjunctiva and teleangiectasias in the skin. Vascular involvement is prominent in the nervous system, resulting in ischemia and infarction and in nerve abnormalities. There is also lipid deposition in leptomeningeal cells and in neurons of the amygdala, hypothalamus, hippocampus, entorhinal cortex and brainstem. Storage in astrocytes is also conspicuous. In the nerve, there is loss of myelinated and unmyelinated axons and lipid deposits in Schwann cells. The deposits are composed of concentric lamellar structures.

Pathophysiology

Fabry disease is caused by mutations in the GLA gene that decrease α-galactosidase A activity to less than

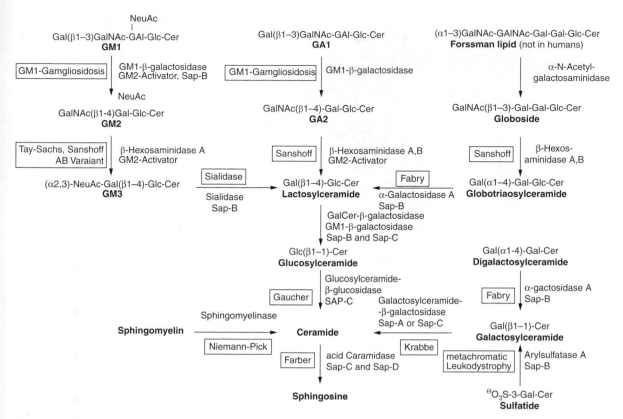

Figure 77.9 Degradation of selected sphingolipids in lysosomes. The eponyms of individual inherited diseases are given. Activator proteins required for the respective degradation step in vivo are indicated. Variant AB, AB variant of GM2 gangliosidosis (deficiency of GM2-activator protein); Sap, saposin. Reproduced with permission from Kolter T et al. Sphingolipid metabolism diseases. *Biochim Biophys Acta.* 2006; 1758(12):2057–79.

25–30 percent of the normal level (Figure 77.9). Individuals with the common form of Fabry disease display very low, if any, residual enzyme activity Deficiency of α-galactosidase A results in the inability of cells to catabolize glycosphingolipids with terminal α-D-galactosyl residues. As a result, there is progressive accumulation of globotriaosylceramide and related glycosphingolipids in the plasma and in lysosomes of the vascular endothelium of various tissues.

In addition to vascular dysfunction and stenosis, other factors influence the vasculopathy typical of the disease. Genotypes of polymorphisms G-174C of interleukin-6, G894T of endothelial nitric oxide synthase, factor V G1691A mutation (factor V Leiden), and the A-13G and G79A of protein Z are all associated with the presence of probable ischemic cerebral lesions on brain MR imaging.

Newly synthesized α-galactosidase A protein traverses the rough endoplasmic reticulum, where it receives N-linked oligosaccharide side chains (Figure 77.10). Subsequently, it passes through the Golgi apparatus, where the oligosaccharide side chains undergo a series of posttranslational modifications. There, it receives the mannose-6-phosphate recognition marker. α-galactosidase A bearing mannose-6-phosphate marker, which binds to the mannose-6-phosphate receptor in the trans-Golgi network, is packed into clathrin-coated vesicles and transported to endosomes. Due to the low pH present in this cellular compartment, the receptor–ligand complexes dissociate and α-galactosidase A is delivered to lysosomes. α-galactosidase A which does not receive the mannose-6-phosphate recognition marker in the Golgi apparatus is secreted. This extracellular α-galactosidase A can bind to plasma membrane located mannose-6-phosphate receptors, which mediates its endocytosis and transport to the lysosomes.

Diagnosis

In males, the diagnosis is achieved by screening for deficient or absent α-galactosidase A activity in

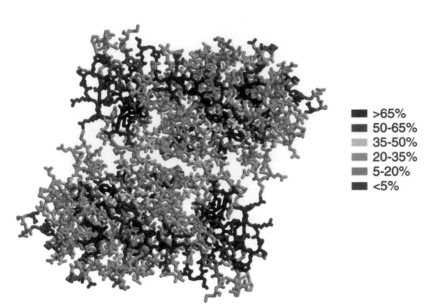

Figure 77.10 α-galactosidase (a-GAL) mutation hotspots colored by mutation frequency. The a-GAL bonds are colored according to frequency of point mutation in the neighborhood of each residue (see Experimental procedures), from highest (red) to lowest (blue), and the a-galactose ligand is in white. The high frequency of mutation around the active site suggests that minor perturbations in the vicinity of the active site reduce the catalytic activity of the enzyme and lead to Fabry disease. Note that the active site of the enzyme can be identified from only the Fabry disease mutation data and the polypeptide fold. Reproduced with permission from Garman SC et al. Structural basis of Fabry disease. *Mol Genet Metab.* 2002; 77(1–2):3–11.

>65%
50-65%
35-50%
20-35%
5-20%
<5%

plasma, dried blood spots, or leukocytes. The diagnosis is aided by the demonstration of an increase in cell, organ, plasma, or urinary sediment of globotriaosylceramide, typically arising from lysosomes.

In female heterozygotes, α-galactosidase A activity and globotriaosylceramide levels may be within the normal range.

Treatment

Several interventions are used to treat severe disease manifestations. For end-stage renal involvement of Fabry disease, renal dialysis and renal transplantation are recommended. In individuals with supraventricular rhythm disturbances, anticoagulant treatment may be initiated. A cardiac pacemaker is used in individuals with higher degrees of atrioventricular block. For advanced congestive heart failure, heart transplantation may be performed, as the intrinsic enzyme production within the graft can prevent reoccurrence of disease.

Enzyme replacement in children reduces pain. Two forms of α-galactosidase A are available: agalsidase alfa and agalsidase beta. They are functionally indistinguishable, with comparable specific activities and glycosylation patterns. Infused α-galactosidase A can bind to plasma membrane located mannose-6-phosphate receptors, which mediates its endocytosis and transports to the lysosomes. Agalsidase beta

administration may be reinstated in affected individuals who develop IgE antibodies or skin test reactivity to the recombinant enzyme.

A recombinant adeno-associated viral vector encoding human α-galactosidase A has been injected into the portal vein or into the right quadriceps muscle of Fabry mice. This leads to elevated enzyme levels and reduction in storage material.

Chemical chaperones are small molecules that bind to mutant enzyme proteins and assist in their correct folding, maturation, and trafficking to their functional site, such as the lysosomes. Oral administration of 1-deoxygalactonojirimycin, a competitive inhibitor of α-galactosidase A, to transgenic mice expressing human Arg301Gln α-galactosidase A has yielded higher α-galactosidase A activity in tissues.

A modified α–N-acetylgalactosaminidase with α-galactosidase A-like substrate specificity has also been produced. The enzyme displays the ability to catalyze the degradation of 4-methylumbelliferyl-α–D-galactopyranoside and can cleave storage material accumulated in cultured fibroblasts.

Bibliography

Ellaway C. (2016). Paediatric Fabry disease. *Transl Pediatr.* 2016; 5(1):37–42.

Silva L.B., Badiz T.C., Enokihara M.M., et al. (2014). Fabry disease: Clinical and genotypic aspects of three cases in first degree relatives. *An Bras Dermatol.* 89(1):141–3.

Hartnup Disease

An 8-year-old boy was evaluated for seizures. He could walk without support at age 18 months and spoke meaningful words at age 4 years. At age 5 years, he was diagnosed with moderate mental retardation (with an intelligence quotient of 47). In addition, he received methylphenidate for attention-deficit hyperactivity disorder. At age 8 years, he experienced several episodes of generalized tonic seizures. An electroencephalogram was normal, although cranial magnetic resonance imaging revealed abnormal peritrigonal T2 hyperintensity, with volume loss and diffuse thinning involving the body and splenium of the corpus callosum (Figure 78.1). Phenobarbital was prescribed and the seizures ceased. His weight (24 kg), height (119.6 cm), and head circumference (50 cm) were in the 10th–25th, 5th, and 10th–25th percentile ranges, respectively. On the basis of his medical history and the findings of the urinary amino acid analysis, Hartnup disorder was suspected. 3 months later, he developed pellagra on the bilateral knee-joint area, which disappeared with the introduction of niacinamide. His mental retardation and hyperactivity, however, did not improve.

which encodes the sodium-dependent and chloride-independent transporter B⁰AT1.
Testing: Excessive amino aciduria.
Treatment: High-protein diet, sunlight protection, and avoidance of photosensitizing drugs. Nicotinamide supplements and tryptophan-rich diet.
Research highlights: Measurement of altered neutral amino acid transport *in vitro* due to disease-associated mutations.

Clinical Features

Hartnup disease is an autosomal recessive aminoaciduria characterized by abnormal renal and gastrointestinal transport of neutral amino acids (tryptophan, alanine, asparagine, glutamine, histidine, isoleucine, leucine, phenylalanine, serine, threonine, tyrosine, and valine). The prevalence is approximately 1 in 30,000, but most cases are asymptomatic other than for a skin rash or diarrhea in infancy. Individuals with Hartnup disorder tend to manifest smaller body height and weight than their siblings. Renal aminoaciduria is the hallmark of the disorder because of the variability of other symptoms, such that most individuals are diagnosed by urine amino acid analysis. The clinical symptoms of Hartnup disorder are similar to pellagra or niacin deficiency. This vitamin deficiency is characterized by photosensitive dermatitis. Advanced pellagra is accompanied by depressive psychosis and diarrhea. Clinical symptoms in Hartnup disease usually appear in childhood (3–9 years of age), but sometimes manifest as early as 10 days after birth, or as late as early adulthood. Symptomatic subjects usually exhibit skin photosensitivity (a pellagra-like skin eruption), progressive neurological symptoms (intermittent cerebellar ataxia, spasticity, abnormal motor development, tremor, headaches, and hypotonia) and psychiatric symptoms (anxiety, emotional instability, delusions,

Hartnup Disease

Onset: Childhood skin photosensitivity, progressive neurological dysfunction (intermittent cerebellar ataxia, spasticity, abnormal motor development, tremor, headaches, and hypotonia) and psychiatric symptoms (anxiety, emotional instability, delusions, and hallucinations).
Additional manifestations: Infantile diarrhea. Mental retardation. Ocular abnormalities. Exacerbations can occur after sunlight exposure or stress and remit spontaneously.
Disease mechanism: Abnormal renal and gastrointestinal transport of neutral amino acids due to mutation of the gene SLC6A19,

and hallucinations). Ocular manifestations may occur (double vision, nystagmus, photophobia, and strabismus). Intellectual deficits have also been described. Exacerbations occur most frequently in the spring or early summer after sunlight exposure. Symptoms may also be triggered by fever, drugs, or stress. These manifestations progress over several days and last for 1–4 weeks before spontaneous remission occurs.

Pathology

The gastrointestinal mucosa and submucosa appear completely normal as does the kidney. Histochemical studies of muscle biopsy specimens may show considerable type II fiber atrophy.

The brain is usually reduced in weight. It is diffusely atrophic, with considerable enlargement of the subarachnoid space. The cortical gyri are reduced in size but normal in configuration. The cerebrum shows diffuse and symmetric enlargement of the ventricular system. There is prominence of the cortical U fibers and pallor of the underlying white matter, most pronounced in the optic radiations (Figure 78.1). The cerebellar folia are atrophic. Throughout the

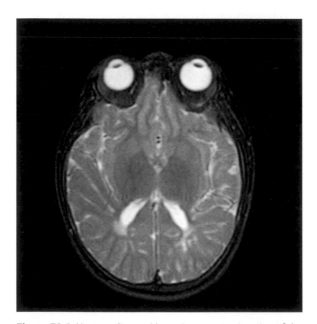

Figure 78.1 Hartnup disease. Magnetic resonance imaging of the brain illustrating abnormal peritrigonal T2 hyperintensity with volume loss and diffuse thinning, involving the body and splenium of the corpus callosum. Reproduced with permission from Cheon CK et al. Novel mutation in SLC6A19 causing late-onset seizures in Hartnup disorder. *Pediatr Neurol.* 2010; 42(5):369–71.

cerebral cortex there is a diffuse loss of neurons. This is most apparent in the occipital lobes. The neuronal loss is not associated with gliosis or distortion of the laminar cortical architecture. The remaining neurons appear normal, although the cells are darker and smaller on Nissl stain than those of age-matched controls. The cerebral white matter appears normal with the exception of the geniculocalcarine tracts. In this area, there is loss of axons and myelin and intense gliosis. The lateral geniculate nuclei are reduced in size. There is loss of their normal laminar architecture, neuronal loss, and intense gliosis. The optic nerves and tracts show loss of axons and myelin. Marked loss of Purkinje cells is evident in the cerebellum as is prominence of Bergmann glia. Occasional degenerating Purkinje cells, axonal bodies, and dendritic swellings are present. The granular layer is thinned in proportion to the overall severe generalized atrophy.

Pathophysiology

Hartnup disorder is caused by mutations in the SLC6A19 gene. SLC6A19 encodes a sodium-dependent and chloride-independent neutral amino acid transporter termed B^0AT1 (denoting a transporter for neutral amino acids (0) with broad specificity; the upper case is used to indicate Na^+-dependence), which is expressed predominately in proximal renal tubules and intestinal epithelium. The aminoaciduria of Hartnup disease is restricted to neutral amino acids, although slightly elevated amounts of glutamate may also be found. Particularly relevant are the increased amounts of tryptophan, pointing to a lack of tryptophan reabsorption. The biochemical basis of the skin rash is not understood, but in Hartnup disorder it responds to niacin supplementation, suggesting that the reduced availability of tryptophan is a likely cause for the skin rash. In addition, reduced amounts of the histidine metabolite urocanic acid have been reported in the skin of pellagrins. This compound is important for the absorption of ultraviolet light in normal skin and histidine transport is impaired in Hartnup disorder. Mammalian skin can convert L-tryptophan into melatonin. Melatonin exerts skin protective effects and is a regulator of skin function and structure.

The mechanism of encephalopathy is also unclear. Serotonin levels in the brain correspond to levels of tryptophan in blood because the Km of tryptophan hydroxylase, the rate limiting step of serotonin biosynthesis, is greater than tryptophan concentrations in the brain or the circulation. As a result, tryptophan and its metabolite 5-hydroxytryptophan may be related to cerebellar ataxia. It is unknown whether abnormal plasma levels of other neurotransmitter precursor amino acids, such as tyrosine or histidine may contribute to neurological symptoms. However, it has been noted that clinical symptoms are more likely to occur in individuals with low plasma amino acid levels.

Toxic bacterial degradation products of tryptophan may also be involved in the pathogenesis of Hartnup disease. Bacterial degradation products of tryptophan such as indol-compounds (indoxyl sulfate, indole acetic acid, indolylacetyl glutamine) and other amino acids have been identified in the urine of individuals with Hartnup disorder, demonstrating that they are absorbed in the intestine and distributed throughout the body. The occurrence of these bacterial degradation products were the first evidence that amino acid transport is impaired in the intestine. However, their contribution to the disease remains uncertain.

Diagnosis

The diagnosis can be established via analysis of urinary amino acids. Oral tryptophan loading consistently results in lower plasma tryptophan levels, but the intestinal transport of other amino acids is not consistently abnormal.

Treatment

Symptomatic subjects benefit from a high-protein diet, sunlight protection, and avoidance of photosensitizing drugs. Treatment includes nicotinamide supplements. Some affected individuals may respond to a tryptophan-rich diet.

Bibliography

Bröer S. (2009). The role of the neutral amino acid transporter B0AT1 (SLC6A19) in Hartnup disorder and protein nutrition. *IUBMB Life*. 61(6):591–9.

Cheon C.K., Lee B.H., Ko J.M., et al. (2010). Novel mutation in SLC6A19 causing late-onset seizures in Hartnup disorder. *Pediatr Neurol*. 42(5):369–71.

Tahmoush A.J., Alpers D.H, Feigin R.D., et al. (1976). Hartnup disease: Clinical, pathological, and biochemical observations. *Arch Neurol*. 33(12):797–807.

Schindler Disease

A boy was the younger of two affected brothers. He was slightly more developmentally impaired than his older brother, as he was never able to crawl, stand from a sitting position, or learn any words. The frank onset of the disease was signaled by generalized seizures, which began at 8 months and occurred five times over the next 6 months. Maximal development was achieved at 15 months of age. Thereafter, the child experienced rapid regression. He developed strabismus, nystagmus, optic atrophy, muscular hypotonia, and frequent myoclonic movements. By 3 to 4 years of age, he exhibited profound psychomotor impairment and spasticity, was immobile, displayed a decorticate posture and cortical blindness, and little, if any, contact with his environment. At 4 ½ years old, he manifested decorticate posturing, marked flexion contractures of the joints, and frequent myoclonus. He had a head circumference that was −1 SD for height, a height at the 3rd percentile, and a weight below the 3rd percentile for age. Further examination revealed symmetric hyperreflexia, spasticity with distal muscular hypotonia and proximal muscle hypertonia, rigidity, reduced muscle mass and bilateral optic atrophy. His developmental skills were at the newborn level.

Schindler Disease

Onset: In type I (infantile) disease, ambulatory disturbance with maximum motor and intellectual development at 15 months of age.
Additional manifestations: Type I: neuroaxonal dystrophy, progressive psychomotor deterioration with myoclonus, spasticity, epilepsy, optic atrophy, and blindness and decorticate posturing. Type II: adult onset angiokeratoma corporis diffusum, neuroaxonal degeneration, lymphedema, and intellectual impairment.
Disease mechanism: Autosomal recessive loss of function of α–N-acetylgalactosaminidase.

Coinciding mutations in the unrelated calcium-independent phospholipase A2 gene PLA2G6 may cause the infantile neuroaxonal dystrophy phenotype seen in Schindler disease.
Testing: Urinary oligosaccharide analysis and enzyme testing in plasma and cells.
Treatment: None effective.
Research highlights: Knockout mice replicate features of the human disorder, with lysosomal storage in the nervous system and spheroid formation.

Clinical Features

Schindler or Kanzaki disease is caused by autosomal recessive lysosomal α–N-acetylgalactosaminidase deficiency (also known as α-galactosidase B) and is characterized by tissue accumulation and urinary excretion of glycopeptides and oligosaccharides containing α–N-acetylgalactosaminyl residues. The clinical manifestations of the disorder are heterogeneous, with three forms recognized.

Type I Schindler disease leads to early onset infantile neuroaxonal dystrophy. There are three stages to the disease. First, there is normal development in the first 9–12 months of life. Then, in the second year of life, intellectual dysfunction becomes apparent, followed by rapid regression with exaggerated startle responses, clumsy gait, and falls. Lastly, there is increasing neurological dysfunction resulting in severe cognitive dysfunction, epilepsy, myoclonus, spasticity, optic atrophy, and blindness and decorticate posturing. Maximal development may be achieved at 15 months of age.

Type II Schindler disease is associated with adult onset angiokeratoma corporis diffusum, neuroaxonal degeneration of the nerve, lymphedema, and intellectual impairment. The angiokeratoma resembles Fabry disease in distribution and appearance. The lesions are small, deep-red to purple maculopapules ranging from 1 to 3 mm scattered across the axillae, breasts, lower abdomen, groin, and upper thighs. Teleangiectasias can be present on the lips and in the conjunctivae and oropharyngeal mucosa. In one individual, there was opacification of the corneal epithelial layer, which differed from the cornea verticilata typical of Fabry disease and moderate cardiomegaly in the context of normal neurological performance.

Type III Schindler disease is a milder, intermediate childhood form ranging from epilepsy with intellectual impairment in infancy to a syndrome with predominantly behavioral dysfunction with ritualistic behavior, inattention, and hyperactivity.

Pathology

There is no visceral pathology. Electron microscopy of leukocytes, secretory cells of sweat glands, myelinated axons of cutaneous nerves, and cultured fibroblasts from type I and type II individuals shows inclusions with lamellar, fibrillary, vesicular, or granular material in single-membrane bound organelles. These inclusions do not stain with periodic acid-Schiff in light microscopy studies.

Type I disease is the best characterized. MR imaging reveals atrophy of the cervical spinal cord, brainstem, and cerebellum. There are diminutive optic and other cranial nerves. Brain atrophy may extend to the supratentorial white matter and cortex. Positron emission tomography illustrates decreased accumulation of fluorodeoxyglucose in regions of brain atrophy.

In type II disease, lacunar infarctions have been identified by MR imaging of adults.

The microscopic features of the disease are those of infantile neuroaxonal dystrophy. There are abundant spheroids with straight or curved clear clefts in the cerebral cortex. These spheroids appear more prominently in GABAergic neurons and contain tubulovesicular and lameliform arrays. Ultrastructural studies of rectal mucosa from type I individuals have illustrated tubulovesicular material accumulation in some axons of the myenteric plexus.

Pathophysiology

Mutations in the gene coding α–N-acetylgalactosaminidase (NAGA) cause Schindler disease (Figure 79.1). The NAGA gene is homologous to α–galactosidase A gene, which is deficient in Fabry disease, suggesting

evolution from a common ancestral gene. Few of the known mutations causative of Schindler disease alter the enzyme active site. The mechanism of these mutations is likely destabilization of enzyme conformation leading to reduced stability.

There may be a relation between spheroid formation and an unrelated gene, thus casting doubt between the causal role of NAGA deficiency in neuroaxonal dystrophy. Spheroids are seen in Schindler disease, but in only a subset of children. Mutations in the calcium-independent phospholipase A2 gene PLA2G6 cause infantile neuroaxonal dystrophy. This disorder is characterised by progressive motor and sensory impairment, with pathological evidence of distended axons or spheroids in the central and peripheral nervous systems. On the basis of their common clinical and pathological features and the proximity of PLA2G6 to NAGA on chromosome 22, mutations in PLA2G6 might account for the childhood neurodegenerative phenotype that occurs in a subset of individuals with Schindler disease. Thus, deficiency of NAGA may account for the biochemical phenotype, whereas defective PLA2G6 may underlie the neurodegenerative disease, which is clinically and pathologically indistinguishable from that of individuals with common infantile neuroaxonal dystrophy.

Diagnosis

In type I Schindler disease, the EEG shows diffuse brain dysfunction, with multifocal spikes and spike wave complexes. There is increased β and δ activity over central and parietooccipital areas. Brainstem auditory, visual, and evoked potentials exhibit decreased amplitudes or delayed responses. Electroretinogram shows increased voltages. Nerve conduction velocities are diminished.

In type II disease, there is a marked decrease in nerve conduction amplitude with preserved velocity. Electromyography is normal.

The diagnosis of Schindler disease can be suggested by urinary oligosaccharide analysis. There is excretion of glycopeptides containing terminal and internal α–N-acetylgalactosaminyl residues. Enzymatic assay in plasma, leukocytes, cultured lymphoblasts, and fibroblasts is confirmatory. Excessive lysosomal storage of α–N-acetylgalactosamine containing material can be demonstrated in cultured

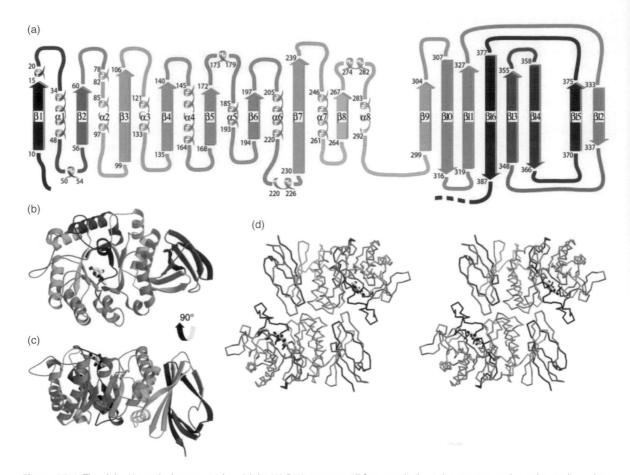

Figure 79.1 The alpha-*N*-acetylgalactosaminidase (alpha-NAGAL) structure. All four panels show the structure with a color gradient along the amino acid sequence, from the N terminus (blue) to the C terminus (red). (a) A topology diagram shows the secondary structure of the monomer. Domain 1 (on the left) contains alternating strands and α helices, while domain 2 (on the right) contains an antiparallel sheet. (b and c) Ribbon diagrams of the polypeptide fold, as seen from the top and rotated 90°. Domain 1 is on the left in these two panels. The α-GalNAc ligand is shown as bonds colored by atom type. (D) A stereo diagram of the α-carbon trace of the α-NAGAL dimer. The ligand is shown as in (b) and (c). Reproduced with permission from Garman SC et al. The 1.9 Å structure of alpha-N-acetylgalactosaminidase: Molecular basis of glycosidase deficiency diseases. *Structure.* 2002; 10(3):425–34.

fibroblasts using a lectin specific for α–*N*-acetylgalactosamine residues. Prenatal diagnosis can be achieved in chorionic villi or cultured amniocytes.

Treatment

There is no treatment at present. However, a potential treatment has been identified by the realization that Schindler disease is a protein folding disorder in many cases. The iminosugar 2-acetamido-1, 2-dideoxy-D-galactonojirimycin can function as an enzyme chaperone that stabilizes the enzyme in catalytic conformation, as it blocks the active site.

Bibliography

Desnick R.J., Wang A.M. (1990). Schindler disease: An inherited neuroaxonal dystrophy due to alpha-N-acetylgalactosaminidase deficiency. *J Inherit Metab Dis.* 13(4):549–59.

Rudolf J., Grond M., Schindler D., et al. (1999). Cerebral glucose metabolism in type I alpha-N-acetylgalactosaminidase deficiency: An infantile neuroaxonal dystrophy. *J Child Neurol.* 14(8):543–7.

Westaway S.K., Gregory A., Hayflick S.J. (2007). Mutations in PLA2G6 and the riddle of Schindler disease.*J Med Genet.* 44(1):e64.

Chapter 80

X-linked Adrenoleukodystrophy

A 9-year-old boy manifested vision difficulties while in school (Figures 80.1 and 80.2). At first, this was noticeable to his teachers and parents but not to himself. His handwriting first increased in size and later became "decomposed" or poorly organized. When writing, his sentences had adequate grammatical content but his choice of characters was abnormal. Within 3 months, he experienced a brief generalized tonic-clonic seizure. Within 6 months, he exhibited poor memory and poor hearing ability. After 2 years, his scholastic performance had gradually deteriorated to the point where education had to be abandoned. His memory continued to deteriorate and became limited to daily events only. In a further 6 months, he could barely perceive light. He manifested recurrent seizures, but they were well controlled with an anticonvulsant. His exam was notable for very diminished alertness. He could only perceive light. His pupils were dilated to 7 mm and reacted to light sluggishly, with a consensual reflex. There was significant spasticity and scissoring when he attempted walking, which was not possible. His plantar responses were extensor.

X-linked Adrenoleukodystrophy

Onset: Insidiously progressive visual or auditory failure at ages 4 to 10 in X-linked adrenoleukodystrophy. Gait disturbance in adult adrenomyeloneuropathy.

Additional manifestations: Disease progression with vegetative state or death within 5 years. Occasionally, a spontaneous arrest of cerebral disease has been observed. There is also a slowly progressive axonopathy. Females may rarely manifest the disease. Isolated or associated Addison disease may occur.

Disease mechanism: X-linked dysfunction of the peroxisomal transporter ATP-binding cassette subfamily D member 1, which mediates the import of very long-chain fatty acid (VLCFA) coenzyme A esters across the peroxisomal membrane. Neuroinflammation.

Testing: VLCFA accumulate in plasma, leucocytes, and fibroblasts from affected individuals.

Treatment: Allogeneic hematopoietic stem cell transplantation can arrest inflammatory cerebral demyelination but does not impact neuropathy.

Research highlights: Identification of other factors contribute to the phenotype including the two homologs of ABCD1 ABCD2, and ABCD3.

Clinical Features

X-linked adrenoleukodystrophy is the most common inherited peroxisomal disorder. The combined incidence of hemizygotes (all phenotypes) plus heterozygous female carriers is 1 in 16,800 newborns. The disease is caused by deficiency of the peroxysomal transporter ABCD1, which leads to two distinct, relatively common clinical syndromes: X-linked adrenoleukodystrophy and adrenomyeloneuropathy. In addition, Addison's disease without neurological involvement, and a form of adrenomyeloneuropathy in females are less frequently observed.

Sixty percent of male individuals with ABCD1 deficiency develop rapidly progressive inflammatory cerebral demyelination. The onset of inflammation is most common in children aged 4 to 10 years. The inflammatory demyelination starts most often in the midline of the corpus callosum and progresses relentlessly outward as a symmetric, confluent lesion in both hemispheres (Figure 80.1). This coincides with a progressive neurologic decline with auditory and visual loss, leading to a vegetative state or death within 3–5 years (Figure 80.2). Occasionally, a spontaneous arrest of cerebral disease has been observed. There is also a slowly progressive axonopathy affecting sensory ascending and motor descending spinal

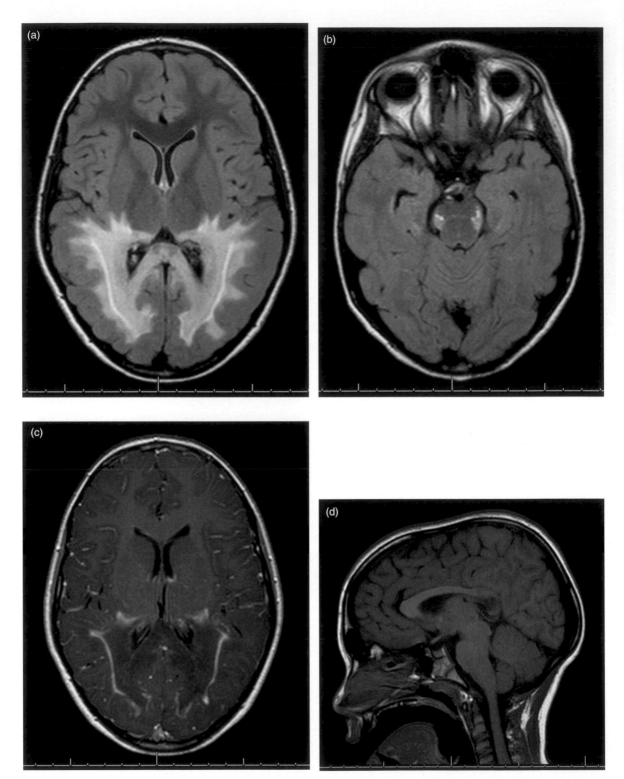

Figure 80.1 MR imaging abnormalities in X-linked adrenoleukodystrophy near disease onset. The changes represented in a–e are described in the text.

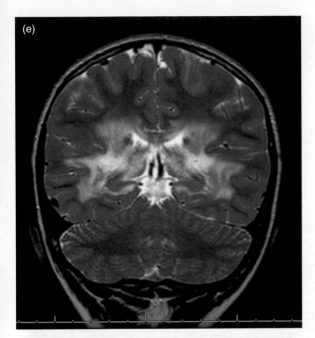

(e)

Figure 80.1 (*cont.*)

cord tracts with full penetrance in men and 65 percent in heterozygous women by the age of 60 years.

Progressive axonopathy represents the main clinical feature of adrenomyeloneuropathy in males, with onset usually between 20 and 30 years and in heterozygous females with onset between 40 and 50 years. The initial symptoms include progressive stiffness and weakness of the legs, impaired vibration sense in the lower limbs, sphincter disturbances and impotence as well as alopecia. About 66 percent of male adrenomyeloneuropathy individuals, but less than 5 percent of female individuals, exhibit adrenocortical insufficiency or Addison's disease. Abnormal MR imaging signals of white matter in the centrum ovale, pyramidal tracts in the brainstem, and internal capsules have frequently been observed in AMN, but no gadolinium enhancement is present, indicating an intact blood–brain barrier and the absence of an acute inflammatory process.

Adrenal insufficiency or Addison's disease is characteristic of X-linked adrenoleukodystrophy or adrenomyeloneuropathy and peroxisome biogenesis disorders, but can also manifest in isolation from these syndromes. It usually presents with cutaneous hyperpigmentation, hyponatremia and, more rarely, hypoglycemia. Affected individuals may exhibit a prolonged recovery from general anesthesia as the first indication of adrenal insufficiency.

About 50 percent of women heterozygous for ABCD1 mutations develop an adrenomyeloneuropathic syndrome in their late adult years. The principal manifestations are spasticity and bladder dysfunction. Neuropathic pain with dysesthesia is common, but adrenal insufficiency is rare.

Pathology

Brain MR imaging demonstrates demyelination with prolongation of T1 and T2 relaxation times. Early involvement of corpus callosum (splenium or genu), pyramidal tracts within brain stem or internal capsules, is characteristic. The localization of the demyelinating lesions within the parieto-occipital junctions and the frontal lobes can be correlated with neuropsychological deficits.

The cerebral cortex is grossly intact but myelin is replaced by gray-to-brown tissue. There is progressive degeneration of the cerebral white matter, with demyelinating lesions that are confluent, generally symmetric and show either a caudorostral progression starting from initial parieto-occipital involvement (65 percent) or a rostrocaudal progression starting frontally (35 percent). The corpus callosum, optic pathways, and posterior limbs of the internal capsules are characteristically involved in the occipital forms, with the arcuate U fibers being often spared. In this parieto-occipital form, demyelination usually starts in the splenium of corpus callosum and then extends into the parieto-occipital white matter. In the rostrocaudal progressing forms, demyelination either starts in the genu of corpus callosum and then extends, or it starts in pyramidal tracts in the internal capsules and extends to the centrum ovale (frontal), progressing to the anterior parts of the brain. The white matter of the cerebellum is also affected, although less extensively than the white matter of the cerebrum. The cerebral cortex, cerebellar cortex, and deep cerebellar nuclei, and grey matter of the brain stem are largely spared.

Three histopathological zones with a spatiotemporal sequence can be defined. The first zone or peripheral edge, in which destruction of myelin occurs initially, contains scattered periodic-acid Schiff-positive and sudanophilic macrophages, but axons are spared. It is closely followed by a second zone in which there are many lipid-laden macrophages with lamellar inclusions and some surviving myelinated axons. The third zone in the center of

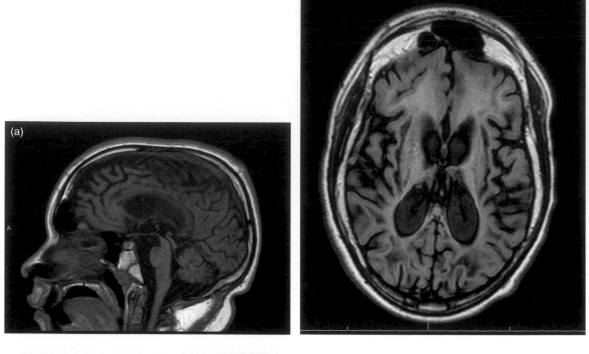

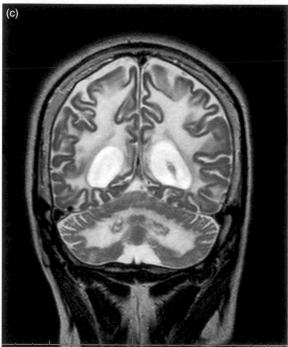

Figure 80.2 MR imaging in advanced stage X-linked adrenoleukodystrophy. Same subject as in Figure 80.1 5 years later. The child remained in a vegetative state at that time.

the lesion consists of a dense mesh of glial fibrils with absence of oligodendroglia, myelin sheaths and very often axons. Cavitated areas and calcium deposits can be present in the third zone, reflecting usually an advanced state of the lesion, although it can also be a relative early event based on magnetic resonance imaging, reflecting that a long initial non-inflammatory period, usually asymptomatic, entered an active phase of neuroinflammation becoming symptomatic.

Myelin and axon loss is accompanied by perivascular and infiltrating macrophages containing granular and lamellar inclusions which are more abundant at the sites of active degeneration than in older degenerating areas. Infiltration and perivascular accumulation of macrophages and mononuclear cells, mostly lymphocytes, is seen between the first and the second zone. This infiltrate resembles that observed in multiple sclerosis and experimental allergic encephalomyelitis. The perivascular cuffs include a T- and B-cell response typical of a cellular immune response. Inflammation tends to be found behind the active edge of demyelination. The B-cell component of the perivascular cuff is also not prominent. Myelin and axon stains reveal loss of myelin, myelin varicosities, loss of axons and occasional small axonal enlargements containing amyloid precursor protein (APP) and synaptophysin, suggesting impaired axonal transport. A few macrophages may also be seen in apparently spared zones of the white matter, indicating early degeneration of myelin and axons. Reactive microglia is present in active demyelinating lesions with infiltration of B and T lymphocytes. Loss of oligodendrocytes and reactive astrocytes is found in the demyelinated areas of the white matter. There are inflammatory infiltrates at the border of the lesions of the white matter behind the active demyelinating front. A few inflammatory infiltrates can also be encountered in the deep demyelinated areas. Inflammatory cells are CD4+ and CD8+ T lymphocytes, some of them containing granzyme B, and rare B lymphocytes. Plasma cells are rarely encountered. Importantly, CD8+ lymphocytes are seen in white matter areas distant from the lesions.

Pathophysiology

The ABCD1 gene encodes the peroxisomal transporter ATP-binding cassette subfamily D member 1, which mediates the import of very long-chain fatty

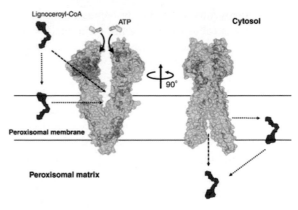

Figure 80.3 A hypothetical model of substrate transport by the peroxisomal ABC transporter. Substrate (lignoceroyl-CoA) enters putative substrate-binding pocket of the ABC transporter from cytosol and/or leaflet of the lipid bilayer facing cytosol. ATP binds to the nucleotide binding domain, causing a large conformational change of the ABC transporter. The substrate is released into the lumen of peroxisome and/or the leaflet facing lumen of peroxisome. Reproduced with permission from Morita M et al. Peroxisomal ABC transporters: Structure, function and role in disease. *Biochim Biophys Acta.* 2012; 1822(9):1387–96.

acid (VLCFA) coenzyme A esters across the peroxisomal membrane (Figure 80.3). Dysfunction of ABCD1 results in impaired degradation of VLCFA in peroxisomes and leads to their accumulation in various tissues and body fluids. While accumulation of VLCFA may directly contribute to the demyelination in adrenomyeloneuropathy, the mechanism by which VLCFA are involved in X-linked adrenoleukodystrophy is not understood.

Saturated, unbranched VLCFA (with a fatty acyl-chain length of ≥ 22 carbons) are degraded in the peroxisomal matrix by the sequential reactions of the enzymes acyl-coenzyme A oxidase 1, D-bifunctional protein and either peroxisomal β-ketothiolase 1 or sterol carrier protein x) of the β-oxidation pathway. In X- linked adrenoleukodystrophy, saturated VLCFA, in particular C26:0, accumulate in tissues and body fluids serving as a diagnostic marker.

The VLCFA that accumulate in the disease are only partly absorbed from the diet, with the majority resulting from endogenous synthesis through elongation of long-chain fatty acids. Thus, dietary restriction of VLCFA does not lower plasma C26:0 levels in affected individuals. As a result of the impaired VLCFA degradation due to the deficient import of VLCFA-coenzyme A into peroxisomes, the synthesis of VLCFA is enhanced.

The demyelination typically begins in the center of the corpus callosum, where the white-matter fiber bundles are the most tightly packed, and spreads outward into the periventricular white matter. The initiation of cerebral demyelination may be related to the amount of VLCFA in complex lipids, such as phosphatidylcholines, sulfatides or gangliosides. Oligodendrocytes derived from induced pluripotent stem cells of individuals with X-linked adrenoleukodystrophy accumulate more VLCFA than those derived from adrenomyeloneuropathy.

Polymorphisms in genes involved in the different pathways, through which excess levels of VLCFA are redistributed into various lipid species, may influence the initial phase of cerebral demyelination. This later evolves to rapidly progressive inflammatory demyelination, including breaching of the blood–brain barrier with invasion by mononuclear cells (which are predominantly macrophages, many of which contain myelin degradation products). The lesion progresses rapidly in a parieto-occipital distribution in about 80 percent of cases or in a fronto-parietal distribution in the remaining 20 percent of cases. Lysophosphatidylcholine with incorporated VLCFA can lead to microglial activation and apoptosis. Thus, microglial dysfunction may contribute to neuroinflammation and possibly alter the neurovascular unit. Elevated levels of proinflammatory chemokines (IL-8, IL-1ra, MCP-1, MIP-1b) have been observed in the cerebrospinal fluid of X-linked adrenoleukodystrophy individuals and correlate with MR imaging severity. Areas where the blood–brain barrier is disrupted exhibit infiltration of T cells, mostly CD8 cytotoxic T cells (α/β TCR positive) and, less frequently, B cells into morphologically unaffected white matter. Cytolysis, rather than apoptosis, is the mode of oligodendrocytic death.

The observation that within one family or even among monozygotic twins the same mutation can lead to different phenotypes suggests that, in addition to the primary mutation in the ABCD1 gene, other factors contribute to the phenotype. In addition to ABCD1, its two homologs ABCD2 (ALDRP) and ABCD3 (PMP70) are also located in the peroxisomal membrane. Upon overexpression, both of these homologs might compensate for a dysfunctional ABCD1. A further explanation for the lack of compensation in vivo may be different affinities toward VLCFA. Different substrate preferences were suggested for ABCD1-3: straight-chain VLCFA for ABCD1,

unsaturated VLCFA for ABCD2, and branched-chain fatty acids, dicarboxylic acids, and bile acid precursors for ABCD3. Furthermore, the ABCD family of transporters exists in dimers form in the membrane. Heterodimers or ABCD1 with ABCD2 and ABCD3 may be formed. As chimeric heterodimers of ABCD1 and ABCD2 are functional, this would raise the possibility of different substrate preferences for such heterodimers.

Diagnosis

VLCFA accumulate in plasma, leucocytes, and fibroblasts from affected individuals independently of phenotype. Thus, an elevated level of VLCFA represents the standard for the diagnosis of X-linked adrenoleukodystrophy, but does not predict the phenotype or progression of disease. VLCFA are elevated in all male affected individuals regardless of age, disease duration, metabolic status or clinical symptoms. The most frequently used diagnostic parameter is the concentration of total C26:0 (saturated fatty acid with 26 carbon atoms) after hydrolysis. Alternatively, the ratio of C26:0/C22:0 or C24:0/C22:0 can be used because C22:0 remains unchanged or is even slightly reduced in plasma samples.

While the measurement of total C26:0 is highly specific in male affected individuals, measurement of VLCFA can only detect about 85 percent of heterozygous female carriers. Thus, additional mutation analysis of the ABCD1 gene is necessary for proper identification of heterozygous affected females.

One diagnostic pitfall is that plasma VLCFA levels depend on dietary intake of VLCFA. To circumvent this, cultured skin fibroblasts were used to confirm the diagnosis. Today, other cells, like leukocytes, provide an alternative. Although other peroxisomal disorders can usually be excluded by measuring phytanic acid and plasmalogen levels, confirmation of the X-linked adrenoleukodystrophy diagnosis by ABCD1 mutation analysis is advisable, especially in subjects with atypical symptoms or when stem cell transplantation is considered.

The sequence-based analysis of the ABCD1 gene is complicated by the presence of several nonfunctional pseudogenes on different chromosomes. Five pseudogenes are assigned to chromosomal regions 2p11 (two copies), 10p11, 16p11 and 22q11. They all consist of exons 7–10 of the ABCD1 gene and are derived from one ancestral duplication, probably to chromosome 2, which was followed by further duplications in a process termed pericentromeric plasticity. As these pseudogenes show a high degree of sequence homology to the original ABCD1 gene, special care must be taken in the analysis of genomic DNA. Therefore, sequencing primers specific for the ABCD1 gene have been designed for conventional sequence analysis.

Treatment

Allogeneic hematopoietic stem cell transplantation (HSCT) is the only therapeutic approach that can arrest inflammatory cerebral demyelination when performed at an early stage of disease. In contrast to HSCT performed for lysosomal diseases, there is no cross-correction of other cell types after HSCT in X-linked adrenoleukodystrophy because ABCD1, as a peroxisomal membrane protein, cannot be released. The mechanism of stem cell transplantation-mediated arrest of the brain inflammation in X-linked adrenoleukodystrophy is not clear. However, the success of HSC gene therapy indicates that only partial correction of the HSC progeny is necessary to halt cerebral disease. After the transplantation procedure, demyelinating lesions continue to expand, usually for 12–18 months, before progression is arrested.

Hematopoietic stem cell transplantation does not impact the non-inflammatory axonopathy. Therefore, it is not a therapeutic option for adrenomyeloneuropathy subjects without inflammatory involvement.

Bibliography

Ferrer I., Aubourg P., Pujol A. (2010). General aspects and neuropathology of X-linked adrenoleukodystrophy. *Brain Pathol.* 20(4):817–30.

Kemp S., Berger J., Aubourg P. (2012). X-linked adrenoleukodystrophy: Clinical, metabolic, genetic and pathophysiological aspects. *Biochim Biophys Acta*; 1822(9):1465–74.

Wiesinger C., Eichler F.S., Berger J. (2015). The genetic landscape of X-linked adrenoleukodystrophy: Inheritance, mutations, modifier genes, and diagnosis. *Appl Clin Genet.* 8:109–21.

Pantothenate Kinase Deficiency

A 5 ½-year-old girl first raised concern when she displayed a tendency to stand on her tiptoes. She walked at 18 months, but exhibited frequent falls. At 2 ½ years she was also intellectually delayed, but continued to make developmental progress. At 5 years of age she developed severe generalized dystonia, initially affecting her limbs and progressing to her trunk after 4 weeks, and subsequently to her mandibular and orolingual musculature after 4 months. She displayed difficulty with upgaze, with pyramidal signs with brisk reflexes, clonus at the ankles, and extensor plantar responses. Fundoscopy revealed mottled changes. Her cognition progressively deteriorated and she lost expressive speech. Within 3 months of the onset of dystonia, she was in status dystonicus and remained bed-bound for months with severe episodes of opisthotonic posturing resulting in respiratory compromise. She was managed with specially placed pillows to support her neck and pelvis to prevent excessive back arching, facial oxygen, and sedatives.

Testing: Acanthocytosis is evident in 8 percent of affected individuals. Oculomotor abnormalities aid in the diagnosis.
Treatment: None permanently effective. Deep brain stimulation reduces dystonia and enhances intellectual performance for as long as 42 months.
Research highlights: Decreasing mouse brain coenzyme A levels leads to a reduction in motor coordination, resembling pantothenate kinase-associated neurodegeneration.

Clinical Features

Pantothenate kinase deficiency, pantothenate kinase-associated neurodegeneration, or Hallervorden-Spatz disease is an autosomal recessive disorder associated with cerebral basal ganglia iron deposition with a prevalence of 2 in 100,000. This syndrome is best understood in the broader context of the seven other neurodegenerative syndromes with prominent brain iron accumulation (NBIA). These diseases are characterized by the convergence of neurodegeneration, extrapyramidal symptoms, and basal ganglia iron deposition. Only pantothenate kinase-associated neurodegeneration will be discussed here.

The onset of pantothenate kinase-associated neurodegeneration is typically in childhood. An early onset form presents in the preschool years. Affected children typically exhibit abnormal motor development followed by gait impairment with falls related to dystonia, rigidity, or spasticity. The dystonia and other pyramidal and extrapyramidal abnormalities leads to wheelchair confinement within 10–15 years. There is a stepwise decline in function over the course of several weeks followed by relative stability. The dystonia is severe and debilitating. In many cases, it affects the orobuccolingual and limb muscles. Eating dystonia is characteristic. Limb dystonia can be painful and lead to fractures. Infections and surgical procedures may precipitate status dystonicus, with

Pantothenate Kinase Deficiency

Onset: Preschool gait dysfunction and falls in the early onset form. Language and psychiatric disturbances in the school age or older individual.
Additional manifestations: Dystonia, rigidity, and spasticity that lead to wheelchair confinement within 10–15 years. Parkinsonism. Supranuclear gaze palsy and abnormal saccades. Adie's pupil. There is stepwise decline. Psychiatric abnormalities include obsessive-compulsive disorder, psychosis, and personality disorders.
Disease mechanism: Mitochondrial dysfunction resulting from autosomal recessive PANK2 mutations, leading to neurodegeneration.

Table 81.1 Neurodegenerative syndromes with brain iron accumulation (NBIA)

Syndrome	Disease symbol	Gene	Protein
Pantothenate kinase-associated neurodegeneration or Hallervorden-Spatz disease	NBIA type 1	PANK2	Pantothenate kinase 2
PLA2G6 associated neurodegeneration (PLAN). Infantile neuroaxonal dystrophy	NBIA type 2	PLA2G6	Phospholipase A2 group VI
FA2H-associated neurodegeneration	FAHN	FA2H	Fatty acid 2 hydrolase
Mitochondrial membrane associated neurodegeneration	MPAN	C19ORF12	C19orf12
Kufor-Rakeb disease	PARK9	ATP13A2	Lysosomal ATPase
Aceruloplasminemia		Ceruloplasmin	Ceruloplasmin
Neuroferritinopathy		FTL	Ferritin light chain
Static encephalopathy of childhood with neurodegeneration in adulthood (SENDA)		Unknown	Unknown

pain, fever, diaphoresis, autonomic dysfunction, and rhabdomyolysis with renal failure. Juvenile onset parkinsonism is another feature of pantothenate kinase-associated neurodegeneration. Among the parkinsonian features, there is marked rigidity, freezing of gait when crossing thresholds, bradykinesia, postural instability with falls and action tremor (rather than resting tremor). Supranuclear gaze palsy and abnormal saccades may also be observed. Adie's pupil, with sectoral paresis of the iris and pupillary irregularity may be observed. There is pigmentary retinopathy with flecked retinas that progress to bull's eye maculopathy. This is associated with night blindness and visual field constriction. Spasticity due to pyramidal tract dysfunction and dysarthria are common. Progressive dementia is milder than in other disorders. Chorea and ballism may also occur, but seizures are rare.

A later onset form of pantothenate kinase-associated neurodegeneration presents in school age, adolescence, or adulthood. These individuals are more prone to language and psychiatric disturbances. Among the language manifestations are pallilalia, tachylalia, tachylogia, and dysarthria. Psychiatric dysfunction manifests as depression, psychosis, anxiety, obsessive-compulsive traits, and other personality disorders. These later onset individuals experience a slower disease progression and milder extrapyramidal manifestations. Intellect is relatively preserved.

Pathology

Neuropathological abnormalities are mostly circumscribed to the globus pallidus. The "eye-of-the-tiger" sign, a medial area of hyperintensity within a hypointense globus pallidus, is the characteristic MR imaging feature of pantothenate kinase-associated neurodegeneration, although this sign may be detected in normal individuals (Figure 81.1). The diagnosis should not rely solely on this sign, as it may be not always apparent early and very late in the disease course. In addition, although the majority of individuals with PANK2 mutations exhibit this radiological sign, it is not pathognomonic for pantothenate kinase-associated neurodegeneration. There are individuals with PANK2 mutations without this radiological sign; conversely, the "eye-of-the-tiger" sign is also observed in multiple systems atrophy, neuroferritinopathy, and progressive supranuclear palsy. Some individuals with PKAN may also exhibit hypointensity of the substantia nigra. The occurrence of central hyperintensity in the globus pallidus reflecting edema and gliosis precedes the surrounding hypointensity reflecting iron accumulation. This supports the hypothesis that iron accumulation is a secondary event, which may however predominate later during the disease course. Abnormal iron deposits eventually develop in virtually all pantothenate kinase-associated neurodegeneration subjects and may even predate the clinical symptoms.

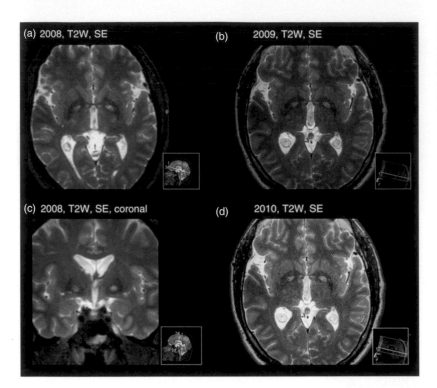

(a) 2008, T2W, SE

(b) 2009, T2W, SE

(c) 2008, T2W, SE, coronal

(d) 2010, T2W, SE

Figure 81.1 Eye-of-the-tiger sign in a healthy adult. 48-year old male who participated in a biomarker study on Huntington's disease as a healthy control subject. Reproduced with permission from van den Bogaard SJ et al. Eye-of-the-tiger-sign in a 48 year healthy adult. *J Neurol Sci.* 2014; 336(1–2):254–6.

Brown discoloration of the basal ganglia due to excessive iron deposition is noted at autopsy. Histochemical staining with Perls' method reveals granular iron deposits scattered throughout the neuropil and within microglial cells and astrocytes of the globus pallidus and substantia nigra pars reticulate (Figure 81.2). Similar concretions and spheroid bodies (focal axonal swellings) occur in the subthalamic nucleus of Luys and within the cerebral gray and white matter. Although pantothenate kinase-associated neurodegeneration cases exhibiting various pathological changes in peripheral blood lymphocytes have been reported, these have not been documented in genetically-confirmed disease.

Pathophysiology

Iron participates in cytokinesis, myelination, electron transport, antioxidant enzyme activity and biogenic amine metabolism. Iron participates in cellular redox reactions by reducing H_2O_2 to the highly cytotoxic hydroxyl radical (Fenton catalysis) or by behaving as pseudoperoxidase activity that activates nontoxic compounds (e.g., catechols) into toxic free radical intermediates. Various characteristics of nervous tissue render it vulnerable to iron- and redox-related

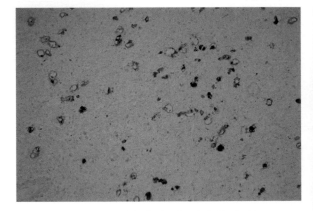

Figure 81.2 Iron stain of the brain of an individual with pantothenate kinase deficiency illustrating diffuse granules with iron deposits in the globus pallidus. Reproduced with permission from Lee CH et al. Phenotypes and genotypes of patients with pantothenate kinase-associated neurodegeneration in Asian and Caucasian populations: 2 cases and literature review. *Scientific World Journal.* 2013; 2013:860539.

damage, including the robust flux of molecular oxygen in normally-respiring neural tissues, the excessive generation of reactive oxygen species by ineffective mitochondria in aging post-mitotic neurons, the susceptibility of the brain to lipid peroxidation accruing from its high cholesterol and unsaturated fat (C20:5, C22:6) content, the abundance of oxidizable (e.g., dopamine, kynurenine) and potentially-excitotoxic (glutamate) neurotransmitters, and a relative paucity of antioxidant defenses.

Cerebral endothelial cells bind circulating diferric transferrin and the resulting complexes are internalized. After dissolution of the complexes within endothelial endosomes, apotransferrin is recycled to the

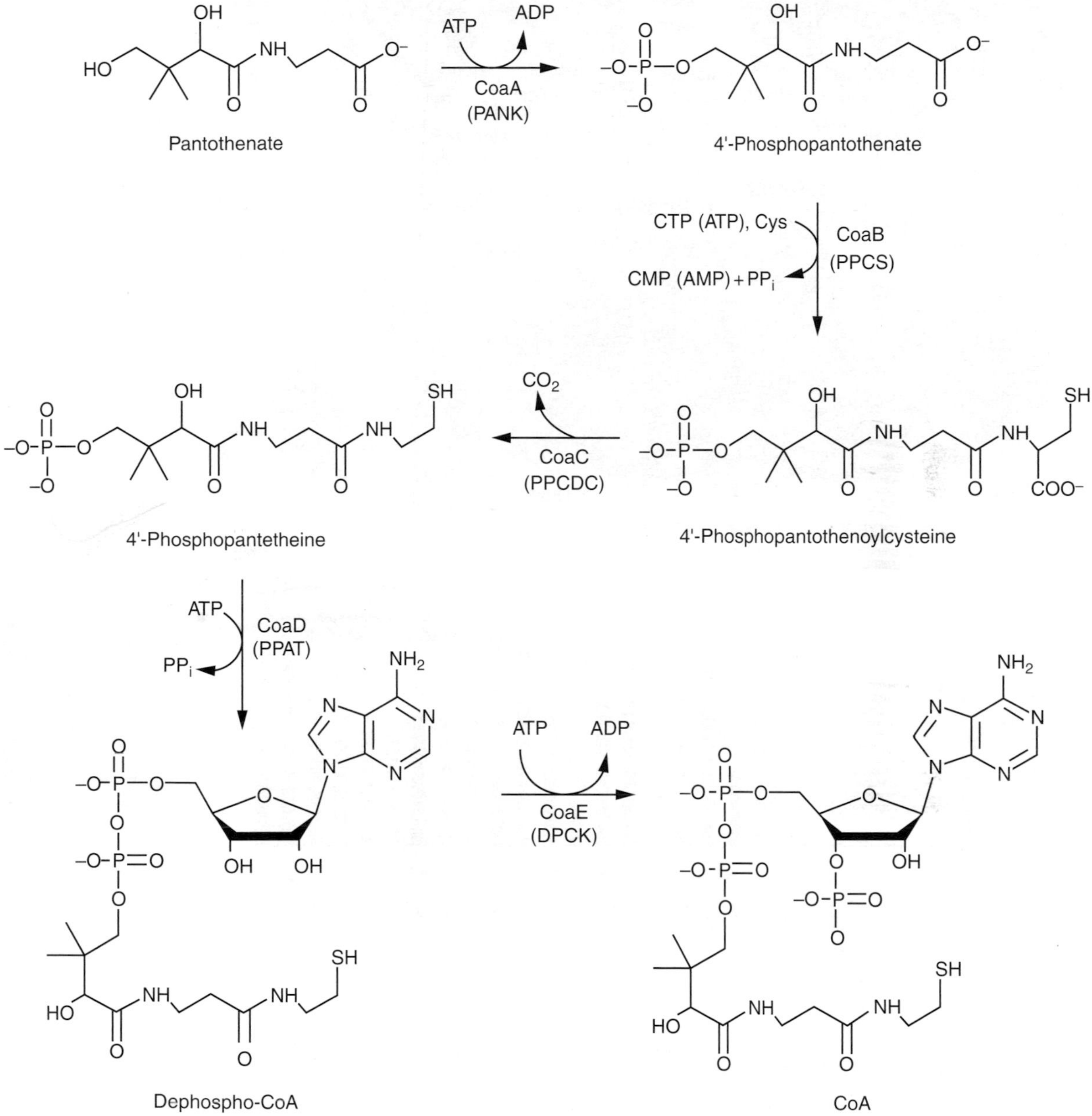

Figure 81.3 Coenzyme A (CoA) biosynthetic pathway. Pantothenate (vitamin B5) is first phosphorylated to 4′-phosphopantothenate by pantothenate kinase (CoaA), then condensed with cysteine and decarboxylated to form 4′-phosphopantetheine. These two reactions are catalyzed by the 4′-phosphopantothenoylcysteine synthase (CoaB) and 4′-phosphopantothenoylcysteine decarboxylase (CoaC) domains of a bifunctional enzyme in prokaryotes and by two distinct proteins in eukaryotes. 4′-Phosphopantetheine is subsequently converted to dephospho-CoA by phosphopanthetheine adenylyltransferase (CoaD) and phosphorylated by dephospho-CoA kinase (CoaE) at the 3′-OH of the ribose to form CoA. The CoaD and CoaE activities are associated with two separate enzymes in prokaryotes and plants but fused in a bifunctional enzyme, also termed the CoA synthase, in mammals. Alternative substrates and enzyme names in eukaryotes are indicated in brackets. Reproduced with permission from Leonardi R et al. Coenzyme A: back in action. *Prog Lipid Res.* 2005; 44(2–3):125–53.

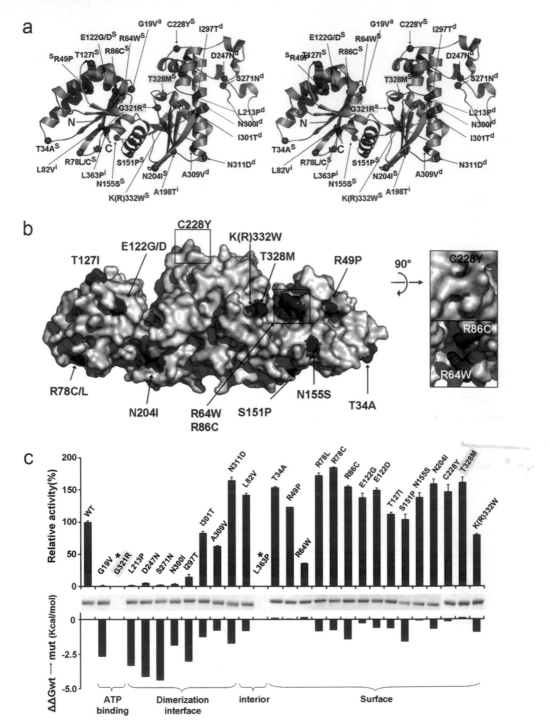

Figure 81.4 Mapping of pantothenate kinase deficiency (PKAN)-linked PanK2 mutations onto the PanK3 structure and characterization of PanK3 mutant proteins. **a**, stereo view of the PanK2 mutations mapped onto the PanK3 monomer structure. Each mutation site is marked as a red sphere. The locations of the mutation sites are labeled (a = ATP binding, d = dimerization interface, i = interior, and s = surface) and the top two frequently observed mutations in PKAN individuals are highlighted in yellow. **b**, PanK2 surface mutations mapped onto PanK3 dimer. The surface mutation sites are shown in red. The inset shows close-up views of PanK3-(R64W), -(R86C), and -(C228Y) corresponding to PanK2-(R264W), -(R286C), and -(C428Y) with a 90° rotation. **c**, relative activities and thermodynamic characterizations of PanK3 mutant proteins corresponding to the PKAN-associated PanK2 mutations. Top histogram (blue) shows the kinase activities of PanK3 mutant proteins relative to the wild-type. Each bar represents the mean of at least three independent measurements. Error bars show S.D. Bottom histogram (red) indicates denaturation free energy differences (ΔΔG) between wild-type PanK3 and its mutant proteins. SDS-PAGE is shown between the two histograms. Insoluble mutant proteins are marked with an asterisk. Reproduced with permission from Hong BS et al. Crystal structures of human pantothenate kinases. Insights into allosteric regulation and mutations linked to a neurodegeneration disorder. *J Biol Chem.* 2007; 282(38):27984–93.

blood and iron is exported across the abluminal membrane, likely via ferroportin, to the interstitial space. Despite this regulation, iron progressively accumulates in the brain with age and a portion of the metal in the brain parenchyma and cerebrospinal fluid remains redox-active. Within the normal human brain, iron is preferentially sequestered in the basal ganglia, hippocampus, certain cerebellar nuclei, and other, largely subcortical, brain regions.

The PANK2 enzyme contains a mitochondrial targeting sequence and is localized to mitochondria in the human brain. Mitochondrial dysfunction may result from PANK2 mutations, leading to neurodegeneration. PANK2 catalyzes the phosphorylation of pantothenate (vitamin B5) in the coenzyme A biosynthetic pathway (Figures 81.3 and 81.4). Coenzyme A participates in adenosine triphosphate synthesis and fatty acid and neurotransmitter

metabolism. Phosphopantothenate, the product of the PANK2 reaction normally condenses with cysteine in the next step of the pathway. Cysteine has been reported to accumulate in the globus pallidus of persons diagnosed with Hallervorden–Spatz syndrome. The excessive tissue cysteine, an amino acid with iron-chelating properties, may mediate the regional accumulation of iron in these individuals. Moreover, in the presence of transition metals, cysteine undergoes rapid autoxidation yielding reactive oxygen and sulfur species, which may promote oxidative neuronal injury in the basal ganglia of affected subjects and associated extrapyramidal symptoms.

Diagnosis

Acanthocytosis is present in 8 percent of affected individuals. Electroretinogram can demonstrate subclinical

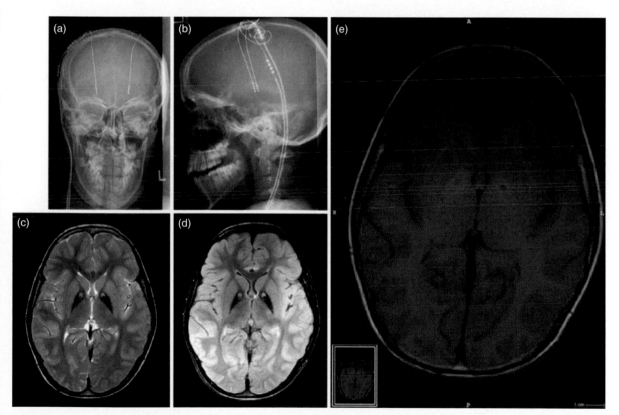

Figure 81.5 Deep brain stimulation for the treatment of pantothenate kinase deficiency. a, b X-ray pictures of the positioning of the electrodes. c T2-weighted MRI scan showing clear iron accumulation in the globus pallidus. d T2-FLAIR-weighted image also showing iron accumulation in the globus pallidus. The MRI scans show a typical eye-of-the-tiger sign. e Positioning of the electrode (red marks) as obtained by computer tomographic scans projected on the MR image. Reproduced and modified with permission from Mückschel M et al. Deep brain stimulation in the globus pallidus compensates response inhibition deficits: evidence from pantothenate kinase-associated neurodegeneration. *Brain Struct Funct*. 2016; 221(4):2251–7.

retinopathy in a significant proportion of individuals. Ocular motility studies show hypometric slowed saccadic eye movements. Ophthalmological examination also reveals sluggish pupillary reactions with sectoral iris paralysis and partial loss of the pupillary ruff. The MR imaging features are characteristic.

Treatment

Apart from symptomatic treatment, deep brain stimulation targeting the globus pallidus may be effective. Small-scale studies of individuals with pantothenate kinase-associated neurodegeneration suggest that deep brain stimulation can improve spasticity and dystonia and reduce disability, with a sustained benefit of up to 42 months in some cases. There may also be improved performance on cognitive testing in children with PANK2 disease following deep brain stimulation.

Bibliography

Hayflick S.J. (2014). Defective pantothenate metabolism and neurodegeneration *Biochem Soc Trans.* 42(4):1063–8.

Zolkipli Z., Dahmoush H., Saunders D.E., et al. (2006). Pantothenate kinase 2 mutation with classic pantothenate-kinase-associated neurodegeneration without "eye-of-the-tiger" sign on MRI in a pair of siblings. *Pediatr Radiol.* 36(8):884–6.

Ataxia Teleangiectasia

A 17-year-old girl was evaluated for unsteadiness of gait and of limb action. She had a normal early development. She was able to walk at 11 months of age and developed sphincter control at 24 months of age. However, at age 2 years, she held her head in an unusual posture with poor balance. She did improve somewhat during early childhood and her disability remained static, prompting some of her neurologists to believe that she suffered from a "static encephalopathy." However, she continued to experience an insidiously progressive course culminating at 9 years of age, at which point she needed to use a walker. One year ago, at age 16, she resorted to using a wheelchair for traveling long distances. Examination of the head revealed teleangiectasias. There were some on conjunctiva and some over the nasal bridge and ears. Eye movements were abnormal with nystagmus, much more pronounced on intentional gaze, and ocular motor dyspraxia. For example, in order to gaze laterally, she would either close her eyes or thrust her head vertically in order to reset gaze. A similar abnormality was observed with up and down gaze except that her eye movements were associated also with rotatory nystagmus. Movement checking was quite impaired, with rebounding. Rapid alternating movements were disabled due to ataxia. There was an element of dystonia and there were also subtle myoclonic jerks throughout the upper extremities. There was also chorea when attempting a hand grasp. The lower extremities were not as affected, with the girl being rather ataxic and slightly dystonic. Reflexes were nearly absent at the ankles. There was diminished temperature sensation in her lower extremities to the mid-thigh as well as diminished vibratory sensation in the lower extremities. There was dysmetria, past-pointing, and severe ataxia in the upper extremities. There was also some hesitation before the initiation of movement, felt to be a mild form of dyspraxia. Gait was quite impaired and she was able to take a few steps as long as there was two hand support provided by either people or objects.

She could not approximate her feet while standing. This resulted in significant unsteadiness.

Ataxia Teleangiectasia

Onset: Gait deterioration due to ataxia at 4 years of age. This is followed by several years of stabilization before further progression.

Additional manifestations: Dysphagia, dystonia, intention tremor, neuropathy, oculomotor apraxia. Teleangiectasia. Immunoglobulin IgG4 and immune deficiency. Radiosensitivity. Carcinogenesis. Premature aging. Metabolic syndrome. Growth retardation. Death ensues after the third decade of life.

Disease mechanism: Autosomal recessive loss of function of ataxia teleangiectasia mutated (ATM), a protein kinase with several roles including DNA damage repair.

Testing: Elevated α-fetoprotein levels in blood. Radiosensitivity assay of cultured lymphoblasts.

Treatment: None effective. Intravenous immunoglobulin can be used for frequent and severe infections.

Research highlights: Antisense morpholino oligonucleotides to redirect and restore normal splicing in the ATM gene.

Clinical Features

Ataxia teleangiectasia is an autosomal recessive disorder due to mutation of the gene ataxia teleangiectasia mutated (ATM), which encodes a multi-functional protein kinase, with an incidence of about 1 in 50,000 people. The disorder represents a genome instability syndrome. The first disease manifestation develops at about 4 years of age and consists of slowly progressive gait ataxia. Extrapyramidal dysfunction manifests as dystonia and intention tremor. Oculomotor abnormalities include apraxia, strabismus and nystagmus. Swallowing and articulation of speech are often

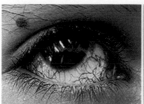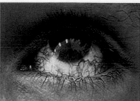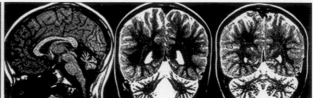

Figure 82.1 Ataxia teleangiectasia. Nine-year-old boy who presented gait difficulties since age two-years-old. Left figures: bilateral ocular telangiectasias. Right figures: MR (sagittal T1 and coronal T2) images showing cerebellar atrophy. Reproduced with permission from Sauma L et al. Ataxia telangiectasia. *Arq Neuropsiquiatr.* 2015; 73(7):638.

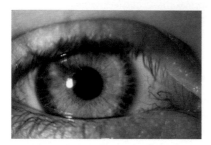

Figure 82.2 Telangiectasia of the conjunctiva in a 3-year-old girl with ataxia teleangiectasia. Reproduced with permission from Hosking KA et al. Ataxia telangiectasia in a three-year-old-girl. *Pediatr Neurol.* 2014; 50(3):279–80.

abnormal and facial expression is limited. Dysfunctional swallowing is often associated with a nutritional problems as well as unapparent aspiration, which may precipitate or aggravate lower respiratory tract infections. Absent tendon reflexes and peripheral neuropathy are common, but develop later than the other neurological manifestations. Oculocutaneous telangiectasia appear at various ages, usually in the conjunctivae and sometimes on the ears, anterior neck or face (Figures 82.1 and 82.2).

Immunodeficiency is also characteristic of ataxia-teleangiectasia. IgA, IgE, and various IgG subclasses are reduced and a diminished lymphocyte count is common, affecting B and T but not natural killer cells, often in the context of impaired antibody responses to immunizations. The thymus is typically vestigial, as are the gonads. Another prominent feature is cancer predisposition, with most malignancies being lymphoreticular of both B cell and T cell origin, including non-Hodgkin's lymphoma, Hodgkin's lymphoma, and several forms of leukemia. A wide range of carcinomas has been reported in individual cases, especially among older individuals.

Many children with ataxia-teleangiectasia grow at a diminished rate and puberty is often delayed. This may be the consequence of an endocrine defect or a primary growth defect compounded by swallowing impairment. Some individuals manifest insulin-resistant diabetes. Adolescents exhibit health problems that are typically not seen until late middle age or later. This includes fatty liver, steatohepatitis, fibrosis, or cirrhosis. There is also an increased incidence of dyslipidemia and diabetes. These abnormalities, together with elevated levels of C-reactive protein, suggest a metabolic syndrome.

The expected life span of affected individuals has recently increased, with most living beyond 25 years. Some have survived into their sixth decade. In older individuals, pulmonary failure, with or without identifiable infections, is a major cause of failing health and death. Life-threatening lymphocytic infiltration of the lung has been reported.

Female carriers display a fourfold increased risk of cancer, largely due to a two- to threefold increased risk of breast cancer, but are mildly radiosensitive, such that the safety of routine X-ray mammography has been questioned.

A related disorder, ataxia teleangiectasia-like disease, is clinically similar to mild ataxia teleangiectasia. This disease is caused by hypomorphic mutations in the MRE11 (meiotic recombination 11) gene, which encodes the MRE11 nuclease. MRE11 is part of the MRE11-RAD50 (DNA repair protein 50)-NBS1 (Nijmegen breakage syndrome 1 or Nibrin) (MRN) complex, which constitutes a DNA double strand break sensor. The phenotypic similarity between mild ataxia teleangiectasia and this syndrome may be due to the dependence of ataxia teleangiectasia mutated activation by double stranded breaks on the MRN complex (Figure 82.3).

Pathology

There is loss of occipital cortex pyramidal cells, and Lewy bodies and moderate nerve cell loss in

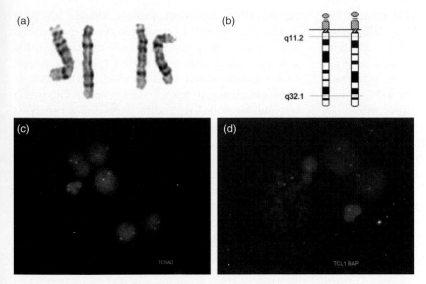

Figure 82.3 Cytogenetic and molecular cytogenetic findings in ataxia teleangiectasia. Panel **a**: two GTG-banded partial karyotypes of the inv(14) (on the right side of either pair). Panel **b**: Ideograms showing the putative breakpoints in 14q11.2 and 14q32.1. Panel **c**: FISH (fluorescence *in situ* hybridization) analysis showing interphase nuclei with a clear split of the red and green signal indicating a chromosomal breakpoint. Panel **d**: FISH analysis with a TCL1 break-apart probe showing interphase nuclei with a clear split of the red and green signal flanking the TCL1 locus indicating a chromosomal breakpoint. Colocalised red/green signals indicate an intact TCL1 locus. Metaphase analysis shows the TCL1 break to be caused by an inv(14). Reproduced with permission from Bartsch O et al. A girl with an atypical form of ataxia telangiectasia and an additional de novo 3.14 Mb microduplication in region 19q12. *Eur J Med Genet.* 2012; 55(1):49–55.

the substantia nigra. There are also vascular changes throughout the cerebrum. Hemosiderin scarring in the frontal lobe white matter, the parietal operculum, the subcortical area of the occipital lobe, and the capsula externa has been reported. Scarring has also been observed in the white matter of the precentral and post-central gyrus, together with moderate cortical gliosis of the central and parietal gyri. In the basal ganglia, there is glial scarring and demyelination.

The cerebellar pathology includes atrophy of the frontal and posterior vermis and of the hemispheres, particularly in the middle and superior peduncles. Loss of Purkinje cells and loss or reduction of granular cells, especially in the anterior cerebellar vermis, is a hallmark of the disease. Abnormal nuclear and dendritic arborizations in Purkinje neurons have also been reported. There is a small dentate nucleus, large inferior olivary nucleus venules, and cell loss. There are also reduced myelinated fibers in the nervus hypoglossus and enlarged venules in the cerebellar meninges. In some cases, glial nodules in pyramidal tracts and the medial lemnisci and gracile nuclei have been observed. Sectional demyelination of the pons and midbrain in the brachia conjunctiva and pontis has also been reported. Other pathological findings include neuroaxonal dystrophy in the medulla oblongata tegmentum, particularly in the gracilis and cuneatus nuclei. Nuclei of the 5th, 6th, 7th, and 12th cranial nerves also display neuronal loss and gliosis.

Pathology in lower motor neurons of the spinal cord is found in subjects that live past their third decade. There is spinal dorsal tract demyelination and fibrillary gliosis, especially in the cervical area and the cuneate and gracile fascicles. Proximal spinal root demyelination and fibrosis, focal necrosis in the anterior spinal cord and abnormal grey matter structures in the cervical and lumbar spinal cord have also been reported. Demyelination of the lateral corticospinal tracts and gliosis of the anterior funiculi has been documented. Anterior horn cell degeneration has also been observed. The dorsal root ganglia may be affected. Extensive myelin and axonal loss has been noted in the sural, anterior tibial, femoral and sciatic nerves, and cervico-brachial and lumbosacral plexus.

Pathophysiology

Individuals with the severe form of ataxia teleangiectasia are homozygous or compound heterozygous for null ATM alleles. The corresponding mutations usually lead to truncation of the ATM protein and subsequently to its loss due to instability of the truncated derivatives. A smaller portion of the mutations create amino acid substitutions that abolish ATM catalytic activity. ATM is a protein kinase with many roles. This large polypeptide harbors a PI3 (phosphatidyl inositol 3) kinase signature within its carboxy-terminal catalytic site, but displays the catalytic activity of a serine-threonine protein kinase. This motif is characteristic of a protein family of which ATM is a member: the PI-3 kinase-like protein kinases. This family also contains the mTOR (mammalian target of rapamycin) protein, which regulates many signaling pathways in response to nutrient levels, growth factors and energy balance; the catalytic subunit of the DNA-dependent protein kinase, which is involved in the NHEJ (non-homologous end joining) pathway of double stranded break repair and other genotoxic stress responses; SMG-1 (phosphatidylinositol 3-kinase-related kinase), which participates in nonsense-mediated mRNA decay; and ATR, which responds to stalled replication forks and a variety of DNA lesions that lead to the formation of single-stranded DNA, including deeply resected double stranded breaks.

An important function of ATM, and one associated with its most vigorous activation, is the mobilization of the complex signaling network that responds to double stranded breaks in the DNA (Figure 82.4). These lesions are induced by exogenous

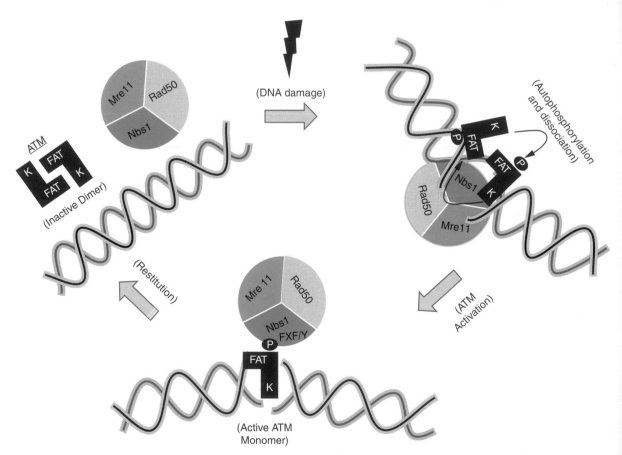

Figure 82.4 Activation of the ATM protein at the site of DNA damage. MRN (Meiotic Recombination Protein-11(Mre11)/Rad50/Nijmegen Breakage Syndrome-1 (Nbs1)) complex acts as a sensor and mediates the recruitment of ATM to the double strand breaks. ATM is recruited as an inactive dimer to the site of double strand break by binding to the C-terminus FXF/Y motif of Nbs1 protein. Following the recruitment of ATM to double stranded breaks, kinase domain of each ATM molecule phosphorylates its counterpart within the ATM dimer at the serine-1981 position in the FAT ([F]/ATR [A]/TRAAP [T]) domain. This phosphorylation causes the dissociation of ATM dimer turning them into kinase-active monomers. Reproduced with permission from Guleria A et al. ATM kinase: Much more than a DNA damage responsive protein. *DNA Repair (Amst).* 2016; 39:1–20.

DNA breaking agents or endogenous reactive oxygen species and are an integral part of physiological processes including meiotic recombination and the rearrangement of antigen receptor genes in the adaptive immune system. Double stranded breaks are repaired via nonhomologous end-joining or homologous recombination repair.

ATM may support other DNA repair pathways that respond to various genotoxic stresses, among them single-strand break repair and base excision repair, which restores ubiquitous nuclear and mitochondrial DNA damage caused by endogenous agents. ATM involvement in these processes is based on its ability to phosphorylate proteins. In this way, ATM also takes part in resolving non-canonical DNA structures that arise in DNA metabolism and in regulating other aspects of genome integrity such as nucleotide metabolism, the response to replication stress and resolution of the conflicts that may arise between DNA damage and the transcription machinery.

Cells from ataxia teleangiectasia individuals exhibit chromosomal instability and sensitivity to ionizing radiations and radiomimetic chemicals. This sensitivity results from a defect in the cellular response to DNA double strand breaks, whose principal mobilizer is the ATM protein. In addition, these cells are also moderately sensitive to other DNA damaging agents.

Lymphocyte cultures from affected individuals often contain clonal translocations that mainly involve the loci of the T-cell receptor and immunoglobulin heavy-chain genes, pointing to a defect in the maturation of these genes via V(D)J (variable, diversity, and joining) and class-switch recombination in the adaptive immune system. Such clones usually herald the onset of malignancy and expand as malignancy progresses. Cultured cell strains exhibit elevated rates of chromosome end associations and reduced telomere length.

Diagnosis

Laboratory findings in ataxia teleangiectasia include elevation of serum alpha fetoprotein and serum carcinoembryonic antigen. There may be deficiency of immunoglobulin subclasses, particularly IgG4. A 7;14 chromosome translocation is identified in 5%–15% of cells in routine chromosomal studies of peripheral blood of affected individuals in which lymphocytes have been stimulated with phytohemagglutinin (Figure 82.3).

There are several more direct in vitro assays for the diagnosis of ataxia teleangiectasia. Radiosensitivity assay in cultured lymphoblasts is diagnostic. This colony survival assay determines the survival of affected individual-derived lymphoblastoid cells following irradiation with 1.0 Gy. Intracellular ATM protein assayed by immunoblotting is severely depleted in most affected individuals. This is the most sensitive and specific test for establishing a diagnosis. Flow cytometric methods that measure ATM-dependent phosphorylation of ATM substrates, such as ATM itself, may also be used. The serine/threonine kinase activity of ATM protein can also be assessed using immunoblotting of cell lysates and antibodies to phosphorylated ATM targets.

The FC (flow cytometry)-pSMC1 (proteasome 26S subunit, ATPase 1) assay utilizes flow cytometry to measure the intranuclear phosphorylation of SMC1 protein (encoded by SMC1A). This assay reports a clear distinction of ATM heterozygotes from normal individuals and homozygotes.

Treatment

There is no effective treatment. Clinical radiosensitivity in the form of severe and adverse response to X-irradiation is well documented and should lead to a limitation in the use of radiation. Intravenous immunoglobulin replacement therapy can be administered to individuals with frequent and severe infections and decreased IgG levels. Basal ganglia dysfunction may respond to L-DOPA derivatives, dopamine agonists and, occasionally, to anticholinergics.

The antioxidant 5-carboxy-1,1,3,3-tetramethylisoindolin-2-yloxyl (CTMIO) reduces the rate of cell death of Purkinje cells in ATM-deficient mice and enhances dendritogenesis to normal levels. The likely mechanism of action of CTMIO is a reduction in oxidative stress, which is protective against both tumor progression and the development of neurological abnormalities. Thus, antioxidants have potential in ataxia telangiectasia.

Aminoglycosides achieve read-through expression of functional ATM protein in the particular case of stop-codon mutations. Aminoglycoside antibiotics bind to the internal loop of helix 44 of the 16S ribosomal RNA subunit, the decoding site, inducing a local conformational change that compromises the integrity of the codon–anticodon proofreading and allow translation through an otherwise terminating codon. However, this requires the use of aminoglycosides at concentrations that are toxic to cells.

Bibliography

Sahama I., Sinclair K., Pannek K., et al. (2014). Radiological imaging in ataxia telangiectasia: A review. *Cerebellum*. 13(4):521–30.

Shiloh Y., Lederman H.M. (2016). Ataxia-Telangiectasia (A-T): An Emerging Dimension of Premature Ageing. *Ageing Res Rev*. pii:S1568–1637(16)30078–2.

Taylor A.M., Lam Z., Last J.I., et al. (2015). Ataxia telangiectasia: More variation at clinical and cellular levels *Clin Genet*. 87(3):199–208.

Chapter 83

Friedreich Ataxia

A girl presented at the age of 7 years to the cardiology clinic for evaluation of a heart murmur. The murmur had been incidentally detected by her primary care provider at a well-child visit. She had never been able to keep up with her peers in terms of endurance. She also displayed difficulties with motor coordination. Examination revealed mild impairment of saccadic eye movements. There was mild weakness distally in the lower extremities. She had high foot arches and flexed toes at rest bilaterally. Tendon reflexes were absent at the knees and ankles. She was able to rise easily from the floor. Tandem gait was mildly difficult, as was walking on her heels, although she was able to walk on her toes. A Romberg sign was present. Sensory examination was normal. Thoracolumbar scoliosis was noted. Echocardiography revealed hypertrophic cardiomyopathy.

Friedreich Ataxia

Onset: Progressive ataxia of gait and limbs between 7 and 25 years of age.
Additional manifestations: Absent lower limb reflexes, Babinski signs, and diminished upper limb sensory nerve action potentials with normal motor conduction velocities and dysarthria. Scoliosis, lower limb pyramidal tract dysfunction and weakness, large fiber sensory loss in the lower limbs, and abnormal electrocardiogram. Diabetes mellitus.
Disease mechanism: Autosomal recessive loss of function of the frataxin gene due to a noncoding GAA expansion.
Testing: Genotyping for expansion size. Direct DNA sequencing for point mutations in a minority of individuals.
Treatment: None effective.
Research highlights: Treatment development with antioxidants, iron chelators, and histone deacetylase inhibitors.

Clinical Features

Friedreich ataxia is due to mutations in the FRDA gene, which encodes the protein frataxin, a molecule involved in the assembly of mitochondrial iron-sulfur clusters. Friedreich ataxia is the commonest genetic ataxia in Caucasian populations, accounting for about one-third of recessive ataxias, with a frequency of approximately 1 in 40,000 and a carrier rate of about 1 in 100.

The main features of the common form of Friedreich ataxia include age of onset after 7 but before 25 years, progressive ataxia of gait and limbs, absent lower limb reflexes, Babinski signs, and diminished or absent upper limb sensory nerve action potentials with normal motor conduction velocities (> 40 m/s) within the first 5 years of symptom onset, and dysarthria after at least 5 years of symptoms (Figure 83.1). Additional features present in the majority of affected individuals include scoliosis, lower limb pyramidal tract dysfunction and weakness, absent upper limb reflexes, large fiber sensory loss in the lower limbs, and abnormal electrocardiogram (Figure 83.2). Phenotypic variants exist, however, with lower limb hyporeflexia, spasticity, or chorea. In addition to dorsal root ganglionopathy, there is dentate nucleus involvement, resulting in a combination of sensory and cerebellar ataxia. There may be macrosaccadic oscillations superimposed on smooth pursuit and saccadic eye movements, scoliosis (which may occasionally be the presenting feature), relatively spared cerebellar volume with an atrophic spinal cervical cord and superior cerebellar peduncle, and EKG-repolarization abnormalities (T-wave inversion) in approximately 70 percent of affected individuals. Electrocardiography is more sensitive to detect cardiac involvement than echocardiography, although the latter can demonstrate the evolution from concentric hypertrophy to dilatation. Diabetes mellitus or impaired glucose tolerance occurs in one-third of affected individuals.

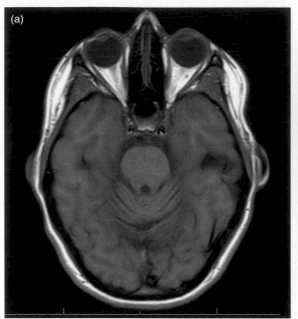
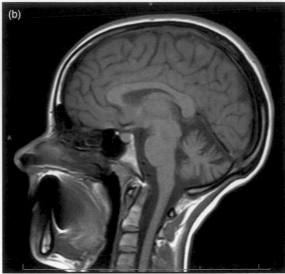

Figure 83.1 Cerebellar degeneration in a 27-year-old woman with Fridreich ataxia.

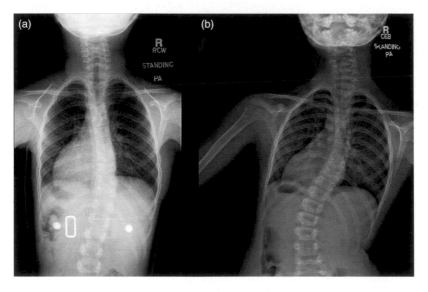

Figure 83.2 Thoracolumbar scoliosis and hypertrophic cardiomyopathy in a 7-year-old girl with Fridreich ataxia. Reproduced with permission from Dhamija R et al. A 7-year-old girl with hypertrophic cardiomyopathy and progressive scoliosis. *Semin Pediatr Neurol.* 2014; 21(2):67–71.

Reduced visual acuity by optic neuropathy and hearing loss are occasionally manifest. Most individuals become wheelchair-dependent before their third decade. Death in the fourth decade was commonly due to myocardial failure. However, treatment of cardiac disease and diabetes has resulted in a greater life expectancy.

Several disease variants are recognized. In Friedreich ataxia with retained reflexes, the reflexes may be pathologically brisk, with spasticity. The clinical syndrome may resemble complicated hereditary spastic paraparesis with ataxia. The age of onset tends to be later (e.g., in the third decade) than in common Friedreich ataxia.

Late-onset Friedreich ataxia and very late-onset Friedreich ataxia are designations used when first symptoms occur at > 25 and > 40 years, respectively. Heart disease is often mild or absent in these disease forms.

Acadian Friedreich ataxia is typical of the Cajun (French) population of North America. It is milder than typical Friedreich ataxia and is rarely accompanied by cardiomyopathy.

Pathology

Reduced levels of frataxin in Friedreich ataxia are associated with defects of iron-sulfur cluster biosynthesis, mitochondrial iron accumulation in heart and dentate nucleus, and increased susceptibility to oxidative damage. The main pathological findings are loss of large sensory neurons in the dorsal root ganglia and degenerative atrophy of the posterior columns of the spinal cord, contributing to symptoms of progressive ataxia, weakness, and sensory deficit. There is also pathological involvement of non-neuronal tissues, with hypertrophic cardiomyopathy and diabetes mellitus.

There is selective vulnerability of several types of motor and sensory neurons. Early in the course of disease, the primary large myelinated sensory neurons of the dorsal root ganglia degenerate, resulting in an axonal neuropathy. The efferent components of these neurons enter the spinal cord, where they either synapse in the Clark nucleus, which conveys sensory inputs to the cerebellum, or ascend via the dorsal columns to synapse in the gracile or cuneate nuclei in the caudal medulla, which relay sensory information to both the ipsilateral cerebellum and the contralateral sensory cortex. The degeneration of the efferent components of the dorsal root ganglia sensory neurons produces atrophy of the dorsal columns, the spinocerebellar tract nuclei and their outputs to the cerebellum and cortex. This degeneration results in impairment of proprioception and vibration and accounts for the sensory ataxia. Other sensory neurons, including those of the auditory and visual systems may also degenerate.

Motor neurons are also vulnerable in Friedreich ataxia, particularly those originating from the primary motor cortex descending as the lateral corticospinal tracts of the spinal cord. Degeneration of these neurons results in atrophy of the corticospinal tracts, which leads to upper motor neuron weakness. The combined atrophy of the dorsal columns and corticospinal tracts of the spinal cord in Friedreich ataxia is characteristic. Within the cerebellum, there is atrophy of the dentate nucleus, which results in the loss of cerebellar outputs.

The heart first displays myocyte hypertrophy, particularly in the left ventricular wall and septum, followed by loss of myocytes and progressive replacement by connective tissue. End-stage cardiac disease results in dilatation of the heart with contractile failure and iron deposition in the surviving myocardial cells.

Pathophysiology

The most common mutation in Friedreich ataxia is an expansion of a GAA triplet repeat in intron 1, which destabilizes the mRNA, resulting in a reduction of frataxin levels. Unaffected individuals harbor up to 43 GAA repeats. Pathogenic expansions range from approximately 70 to $\geq 1,000$, with the smaller expansions typically seen in late-onset and very late-onset affected individuals. The amount of residual frataxin produced from an expanded allele is inversely proportional to the repeat expansion length, such that the size of the smaller expanded allele correlates with disease severity. About 2 percent of affected individuals harbor a point mutation instead of an expansion on one allele, such that direct DNA sequencing can be fruitful in a subject with a typical clinical picture and one expanded allele. No individuals with point mutations in both alleles have been described.

The effect of the GAA repeat expansion is to decrease expression of the ubiquitously expressed mitochondrial protein frataxin. However, asymptomatic carriers produce about 50 percent frataxin levels compared to unaffected individuals. Therefore, drugs that induce frataxin expression, at least to the levels of healthy carriers, may be beneficial. The frataxin gene spans 95 kb of genomic DNA and contains seven exons, 1–5a, 5b, and 6. The first five exons are transcribed to produce a 210 amino acid major isoform of frataxin but, rarely, exon 5b can be transcribed by alternative splicing to produce a 171 amino acid protein. In addition, there are two tissue-specific transcript variants, encoding two isoforms of frataxin that lack the mitochondrial targeting sequence and are therefore different from the canonical transcript.

The functions of frataxin remain unclear. Studies focusing on iron binding and aggregate formation suggest that frataxin may act as a ferritin-like scavenger that keeps iron in a bio-available form. Clues on the function of proteins often arise after identification of interacting partners. Two such frataxin partners include hscA and hscB, two chaperone proteins involved in the synthesis of Fe-S clusters in proteobacteria, suggesting the participation of frataxin in this machinery. It has also been suggested that frataxin interacts with ferrochelatase, the enzyme that catalyzes the final step of heme biosynthesis by inserting the ferrous ion into porphyrin. In addition, frataxin may interact with mitochondrial aconitase, subunits of complex II of the mitochondrial respiratory chain, and several chaperones (GRP75 (75 kDa glucose-regulated protein), Ssc1 (supersecreting 1)). Lastly, the identification of interactions between frataxin and iron–sulfur cluster components has led to different hypotheses on the level of involvement of the frataxin protein in these metabolic reactions such that frataxin may be the iron donor which helps to solubilize and transport iron to the cluster biogenesis machine.

Diagnosis

Testing for Friedreich ataxia requires only a polymerase chain reaction in approximately 98 percent of affected individuals (those without a point mutation).

Treatment

There is no effective treatment. The pathology of Friedreich ataxia is very similar to that of ataxia with vitamin E deficiency, which is treated with vitamin E supplements. Taken together with the evidence of oxidative damage in Friedreich ataxia, it is plausible that antioxidants be considered as a therapy. However, lipid-soluble antioxidants such as the short-chain coenzyme Q analog idebenone and compound A0001 ([alpha]-tocopheryl quinone), related to both coenzyme Q and vitamin E have proved ineffective in advance-phase clinical investigations.

Other interventions are under investigation. The concerted action of the iron chelator desferrioxamine combined with a mitochondrion-permeate ligand, pyridoxal isonicotinoyl hydrazone, prevents *in vivo* cardiac iron loading and limits hypertrophy in the MCK (muscle creatine kinase)-Fxn-KO mouse model without overt cardiac depletion of iron or toxicity. Deferiprone is another iron chelator that

may act by removing excess redox-active iron from mitochondria.

Human recombinant erythropoietin increases frataxin levels in cultured cells, providing the rationale for clinical testing. However, the only controlled trial that used human recombinant erythropoietin proved negative. A similar molecule, carbamylated erythropoietin, which does not induce erythropoiesis but preserves the ability to upregulate frataxin in vitro, is under investigation.

Induction of frataxin expression has been obtained in cultured cells and animal models using a family of histone deacetylase inhibitors acting on the chromatin changes triggered by GAA repeat expansions, justifying the investigation of these compounds.

Pharmacological stimulation of antioxidant defenses has been explored. The PPAR-γ (peroxisome proliferator-activated receptor gamma) agonist, pioglitazone, induces the expression of enzymes involved in mitochondrial metabolism, including superoxide dismutase (SOD). Testing in a "knockin-knockout" mouse model of Friedreich ataxia and affected individual fibroblasts revealed that pioglitazone upregulates SOD2 in the cerebellum and spinal cord. Pioglitazone is being evaluated in clinical trials.

The transcriptional silencing of the frataxin gene by GAA repeat expansion is accompanied by histone hypoacetylation, consistent with a heterochromatin-mediated repression mechanism. Some histone deacetylase inhibitors can reverse frataxin silencing in lymphocytes from affected individuals. This treatment increases frataxin protein expression in the mouse brain and increases mitochondrial aconitase activity, thus providing the basis for further investigation.

Bibliography

Dhamija R., Kirmani S. (2014). A 7-year-old girl with hypertrophic cardiomyopathy and progressive scoliosis. *Semin Pediatr Neurol.* 21(2):67–71.

Pastore A., Puccio H. (2013). Frataxin: A protein in search for a function. *J Neurochem.* 126 Suppl 1:43–52.

Storey E. (2014). Genetic cerebellar ataxias. *Semin Neurol.* 34(3):280–92.

Bassen–Kornzweig Disease

Chapter 84

A 21-year-old male initially presented with chronic diarrhea and difficulty walking at 12 months of age. Examination at the age 21 years showed a static and kinetic cerebellar syndrome with dysarthria and nystagmus, deep sensory disturbances, absent tendon reflexes, pes cavus, hammer toes (Figure 84.1), Achilles tendon shortening and scoliosis. Fundoscopy revealed retinitis pigmentosa. He had also manifested to thrive (height: −3 standard deviations from the mean, weight: −4 SD).

Bassen–Kornzweig Disease

Onset: Fat malabsorption with steatorrhea, vomiting, abdominal distension and failure to thrive the neonatal period.

Additional manifestations: Childhood progressive retinitis pigmentosa and spinocerebellar ataxia. Acanthocytosis, anemia, hyperbilirubinemia, hemolysis, and coagulopathy due to vitamin K deficiency. Hepatomegaly, increased aminotransferases and steatosis, which can progress to steatohepatitis, fibrosis, and cirrhosis.

Disease mechanism: Autosomal recessive mutations in the microsomal triglyceride transfer protein (MTTP) gene.

Testing: Very low plasma concentrations of triglyceride and cholesterol and undetectable levels of LDL and apoB.

Treatment: Vitamin A and E and dietary fat restriction.

Research highlights: Knockout mice replicate the human phenotype with retinal degeneration and ataxia.

Clinical Features

Vitamin E, a fat-soluble antioxidant, circulates in the blood in lipoprotein particles and serves as a free radical scavenger that protects polyunsaturated fatty acids from lipid peroxidation. In two related disorders, abetalipoproteinemia and ataxia with vitamin E deficiency, deficiency of vitamins E and A occurs, resulting in a progressive ataxic neuropathy with retinopathy.

Abetalipoproteinemia, also known as Bassen–Kornzweig syndrome, is caused by autosomal recessive mutations in the microsomal triglyceride transfer protein (MTTP) gene (Figures 84.1 and 84.2). MTTP encodes MTP, which forms a heterodimer with the protein disulfide isomerase (PDI), facilitating the transfer of lipids onto nascent apoB by a shuttle mechanism. Deficiency of MTP targets the apoB for degradation, preventing the secretion of triglyceride-rich lipoproteins, including chylomicrons and very low density lipoproteins. Mutations in MTTP may

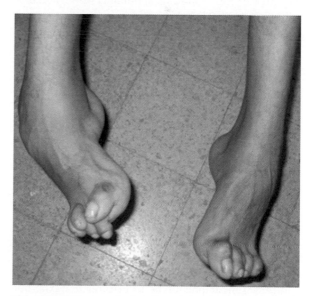

Figure 84.1 Pes cavus in abetalipoproteinemia. Reproduced with permission from Hammer MB et al. Clinical features and molecular genetics of two Tunisian families with abetalipoproteinemia. *J Clin Neurosci.* 2014; 21(2):311–15.

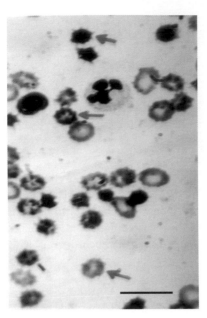

Figure 84.2 Leishman stained acanthocytes from the peripheral blood of the subject in Figure 84.1 (scale bar = 10 μm). Reproduced with permission from Hammer MB et al. Clinical features and molecular genetics of two Tunisian families with abetalipoproteinemia. *J Clin Neurosci.* 2014; 21(2):311–15.

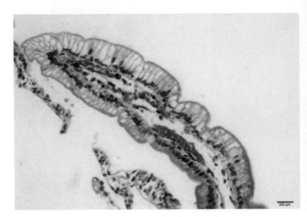

Figure 84.3 Intestinal lining abnormalities in abetalipoproteinemia. Tall villi and fine vacoulation of entrocytes. Crypts are unremarkable and there is mild infiltration of lymphoplasma cells and some eosinophils (3–16/HPF) in lamina propia alongside edema. Reproduced with permission from Rashtian P et al. A Male Infant with Abetalipoproteinemia: A Case Report from Iran. *Middle East J Dig Dis.* 2015; 7:181–4.

disrupt MTP abundance, prevent its association with PDI, or affect its ability to transfer lipids. Fat malabsorption is a cardinal feature of abetalipoproteinemia with steatorrhea, vomiting, abdominal distension and failure to thrive observed in the neonatal period, and later in life, with progression to retinitis pigmentosa and spinocerebellar ataxia (Figure 84.3). Acanthocytosis, decreased erythrocyte survival with anemia, hyperbilirubinemia, hemolysis and coagulopathy due to vitamin K deficiency may also occur. Liver abnormalities include hepatomegaly, increased aminotransferases and steatosis, which can progress to steatohepatitis, fibrosis and cirrhosis. Neuromuscular features of abetalipoproteinemia include progressive loss of tendon reflexes, vibratory sense and proprioception, weakness, and, eventually, ataxia. Ophthalmological findings include the loss of night or color vision and an atypical pigmentation of the retina, which can lead to visual field constriction and may eventually result in blindness.

Ataxia with vitamin E deficiency presents with a clinically similar phenotype to Friedreich ataxia, but serum concentrations of vitamin E are diminished. Most affected individuals are from North Africa, where it represents a common cause of ataxia. Like Friedreich ataxia, age at onset is before 20 years but, in contrast, decreased visual acuity or retinitis pigmentosa may occur early in the disease. Cardiomyopathy is less common than in Friedreich ataxia. Affected individuals also manifest more head titubation and less neuropathy in the context of a slower disease course. The disease is caused by mutation of the α-tocopherol transfer protein. The α-tocopherol transfer protein mediates the incorporation of vitamin E into circulating lipoproteins, with mutations in the gene resulting in reduced delivery to the nervous system. Supplementation with vitamin E interrupts disease progression or even ameliorates ataxia. A mouse model has been developed that exhibits late-onset head tremor, ataxia, and retinal degeneration, all of which are amenable to vitamin E supplementation. The disease mechanism may involve increased oxidative damage.

Pathology

In abetalipoproteinemia, the liver manifests accumulation of large quantities of lipid droplets in hepatocytes with intact lobular architecture and no fibrosis in early disease stages.

Abnormalities of nerve include reduced numbers of large myelinated fibers and myelin remodeling due to axonal dysfunction. In muscle, variation in fiber size, rounding of fibers, degenerative and vacuolar changes, necrosis, phagocytosis and central nucleation are present to a varying degree. These histologic features are diagnostic of a primary myopathic process, but may also be observed during the course of chronic denervation. There are also numerous granules in the muscle fibers. These granules have tinctorial characteristics of ceroid pigments (strong affinity for basic dyes, periodic acid-Schiff positive before and after diastase digestion, and acid-fast properties). Furthermore, they demonstrate green-yellow autofluorescence under ultraviolet light, resembling ceroid pigment.

The changes that occur in skeletal muscle during vitamin E therapy have not been reported except in one case of abetalipoproteinemia, when a repeat muscle biopsy showed improvement in several histologic abnormalities.

Pathophysiology

In abetalipoproteinemia, very low plasma concentrations of triglyceride and cholesterol (under 30 mg/dl) and undetectable levels of low density lipoproteins (LDL) and apoB result from mutations in the microsomal triglyceride transfer protein (MTP) gene. MTP lipidates nascent apoB in the endoplasmic reticulum to produce very low density lipoproteins (VLDL) and chylomicrons in the liver and small intestine, respectively (Figures 84.4 and 84.5). Unlipidated apoB is targeted for proteasomal degradation, leading to the absence of apoB containing lipoproteins in the plasma (and thus to markedly reduced levels of LDL-C and triglycerides). VLDL production is inhibited. Reduced triglyceride export from the liver leads to hepatic steatosis. Additionally, lack of MTP-facilitated lipidation of chylomicrons in the small intestine causes lipid accumulation in enterocytes with associated

malabsorption, steatorrhea, and diarrhea. The malabsorption and diarrhea lead to failure to thrive during infancy. In addition, there is deficiency of fat-soluble vitamins, including vitamin E. This leads to retinitis pigmentosa, spinocerebellar degeneration with ataxia

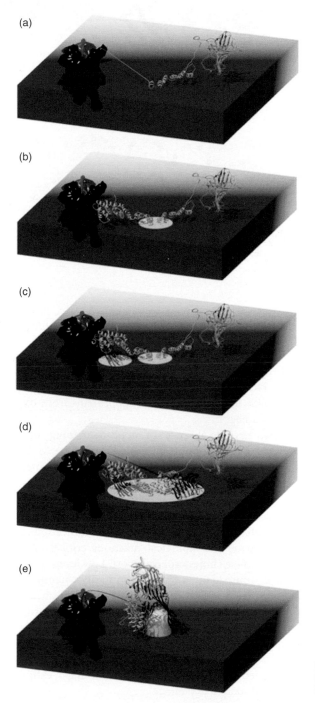

(a)

(b)

(c)

(d)

(e)

Figure 84.4 Model of apoB triacylglycerol (TAG) recruitment. a, after translocation of the β-barrel domain (green) through the translocon (black), lipid binding to the ER membrane (shaded black box) is initiated by the binding of helices 6 and 8 from the helical domain (cyan). b, as more helices are expressed, TAG molecules are recruited to the binding site (yellow patches). c and d, when the C-sheet (red) and A-sheet (blue) are expressed, they displace the C- and N-terminal portions of the a-helical domain. This increases the Π of the membrane. e, to relieve the pressure, the protein remodels the membrane into a lens that is enlarged by TAG synthesis and forms a TAG-rich "bud" to which H6 and the A- and C-sheets are bound. Finally, the β-barrel domain binds the A-sheet to form the lipovitellin-like final conformation of the βa1 domain. Reproduced with permission from Mitsche MA et al. Surface tensiometry of apolipoprotein B domains at lipid interfaces suggests a new model for the initial steps in triglyceride-rich lipoprotein assembly. *J Biol Chem.* 2014; 289(13):9000–12.

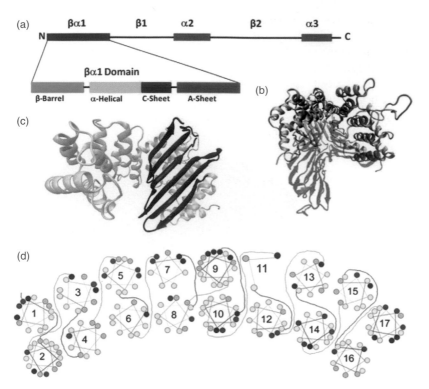

Figure 84.5 a, apolipoprotein B has five putative superdomains. The βα1 superdomain of apoB has four domains as follows: the β-barrel (green); α-helical domain (cyan); C-sheet (red); and A-sheet (blue) (4). b, homology model of the ßα1 superdomain of apoB based on the structure of lamprey lipovitellin. c, α-helical domain and C-sheet are in contact in the model, where the C-terminal half of the α helical domain is shielded from the lipid by the C-sheet. d, helical wheel diagram of all 17 helices in the α helical domain illustrates the variety of amphipathic cross-sections. Helices are labeled 1–17. The circles indicate amino acid residues with the following color scheme: yellow, hydrophobic; gray, neutral; blue, positively charged; red, negatively charged; magenta, proline or glycine. Reproduced with permission from Mitsche MA et al. Surface tensiometry of apolipoprotein B domains at lipid interfaces suggests a new model for the initial steps in triglyceride-rich lipoprotein assembly. *J Biol Chem*. 2014; 289(13):9000-12.

and vitamin K deficiency, which can precipitate bleeding. The lipid-soluble antioxidant vitamin E (α-tocopherol) circulates in the blood with cholesterol and triglyceride in lipoprotein particles and serves as a free radical scavenger that protects polyunsaturated fatty acids in membranes and lipoproteins from oxidative damage.

Due to the absence of apoB-containing lipoproteins in abetalipoproteinemia, plasma lipids are almost entirely carried in high density lipoprotein (HDL) particles, which are reduced in number and are qualitatively abnormal, with an excess of cholesterol esters and a deficit of phospholipids and polyunsaturated fatty acids. Oxidative modification of HDL impairs the biological functions critical to its role in reverse cholesterol transport. Low levels of fat-soluble antioxidant vitamins, primarily vitamin E, and the distinct HDL composition found in abetaliporoteinemia influence HDL oxidation. Subjects with low LDL-cholesterol have decreased total serum antioxidant activity and lower thiol concentrations compared to a high LDL-cholesterol group. This suggests that abetalipoproteinemia subjects may exhibit increased oxidative damage.

Diagnosis

Abetalipoproteinemia is characterized by very low plasma concentrations of triglyceride and cholesterol (under 30 mg/dl) and undetectable levels of LDL and apoB.

Acanthocytosis of red blood cells on peripheral blood smears is a distinguishing feature. The determination of acanthocytosis in peripheral blood smears may fail in a standard setting. Automated blood counts usually reveal an elevated number of hyperchromic erythrocytes. A more sensitive and specific method for the detection of acanthocytes uses a 1:1 dilution with physiological saline followed by phase contrast microscopy.

Treatment

Supplementation with vitamin E and A from a young age can prevent the development of neurological or retinal features. Additional treatment measures include a low-fat diet and supplementation with essential fatty acids.

Plasma markers of oxidative damage and antioxidant capacity after therapeutic vitamin E supplementation are normal in abetalipoproteinemia subjects: plasma carbonyl levels (a marker of protein oxidative damage) and HDL lag phase and oxidizability rates are normal, providing no evidence for increased oxidative capacity in individuals with abetalipoproteinemia receiving high-dose vitamin E and A supplements. In contrast, there is increased oxidative capacity in abetalipoproteinemia subjects, as evidenced by increased urinary F2-isoprostanes, a marker of *in vivo* lipid peroxidation.

Bibliography

Burnett J.R., Hooper A.J. (2015). Vitamin E and oxidative stress in abetalipoproteinemia and familial hypobetalipoproteinemia. *Free Radic Biol Med.* 88(Pt A):59–62.

Hammer M.B., El Euch-Fayache G., Nehdi H., et al. (2014). Clinical features and molecular genetics of two Tunisian families with abetalipoproteinemia. *J Clin Neurosci.* 21(2):311–15.

Levy E. (2015). Insights from human congenital disorders of intestinal lipid metabolism. *J Lipid Res.* 56(5):945–62.

Chapter 85

Vanishing White Matter Disease

A 2 ½-year-old-girl lost the ability to run and jump over the course of several days following a minor fall. She was born via cesarean section due to cephalopelvic disproportion. She had accomplished all her intellectual and motor development either ahead of her peers or on time. By 3 years of age, she was irritable and displayed considerable unsteadiness of limb action, signifying ataxia. Slurred speech appeared several weeks later and her sentences became simplified, containing only two or three words such that she resorted to pointing at objects for many of her interactions. Examination at 3 years old revealed macrocephaly (head circumference greater than the 95th percentile), lax knee and elbow joints, increased distal limb tone, abnormally brisk reflexes with unsustained ankle clonus and Babinski signs. Her gait was ataxic and her stance broad-based. Three months later, her gait had deteriorated, with significant spasticity. Two febrile illnesses of unknown cause led to significant gait decompensation. Sustained ankle clonus appeared. DNA sequencing of the EIF2B5 gene revealed two heterozygous mutations.

Research highlights: Aberrant activation of the unfolded protein response restricted to the oligodendroglial and astroglial cells.

Clinical Features

Childhood ataxia with central hypomyelination or vanishing white matter disease is an autosomal recessive disorder caused by mutations in any of the genes encoding the five subunits of eukaryotic translation initiation factor eIF2B.

Children with vanishing white matter disease usually present with prominent ataxia, mild spasticity, and relatively spared cognition. The course is progressive, with episodic deterioration triggered by infections, head trauma or other sources of acute stress. These episodes consist of hypotonia, irritability, vomiting and seizures evolving to depressed consciousness or unexplained coma. Recovery from each episode is slow and incomplete. Seizures and optic atrophy may develop. The presence of macrocephaly is variable, although progressive macrocephaly has been described. Adolescents and adults exhibit a milder course. Neurologic symptoms may include ataxia, gait abnormality with mild spasticity, seizures, complicated migraine, cognitive or psychiatric dysfunction. In females, ovarian failure may precede or coexist with neurologic symptoms, giving raise to the term ovarioleukodystrophy. Stress-induced episodes of deterioration are less common than in young children. More severe forms, including prenatal and neonatal presentations, have also been described. For example, Cree encephalopathy is a severe variant of leukoencephalopathy with vanishing white matter.

Pathology

MR imaging findings are characteristic in the childhood form, but are variable in later-onset forms. Diffuse symmetric cerebral white matter changes are

Vanishing White Matter Disease

Onset: Prominent childhood ataxia with mild spasticity and relatively spared cognition.

Additional manifestations: Episodic deterioration triggered by infections, head trauma or other stresses. Episodes consist of hypotonia, irritability, vomiting and seizures evolving to depressed consciousness or unexplained coma. Recovery from each episode is incomplete. Seizures, optic atrophy and macrocephaly may develop.

Disease mechanism: Autosomal recessive loss of function of eIF2B, which is involved in the regulation of the first steps of protein synthesis.

Testing: MR imaging is specific. Elevated cerebrospinal fluid glycine and decreased asialotransferrin.

Treatment: None effective.

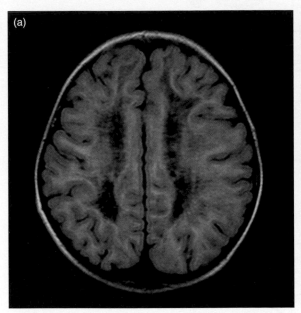

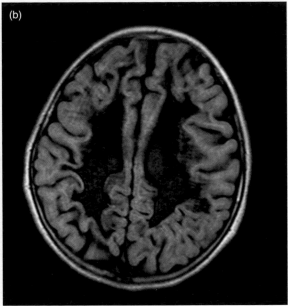

Figure 85.1 Vanishing white matter disease in a girl. a: FLAIR MR image at 2 years of age. b: FLAIR MR image at 7 years of age. The child harbored a homozygous mutation in the gene EIF2B5.

present early, with sparing of the subcortical U fibers, outer corpus callosum, internal capsules, and anterior commissure (Figure 85.1). Progressive cystic degeneration results in replacement of the white matter by cerebrospinal fluid. Within the cystic regions, radial stripes extend from the ventricular wall to the subcortical region. The gray matter is spared. Cerebellar atrophy develops later in the disease course.

External examination of the brain is unrevealing except in infants and younger children in whom there usually is swelling of the brain and flattening of the gyri. Cerebral atrophy with enlargement of subarachnoid spaces and lateral ventricles is rarely observed in children but is common in adults. The white matter appears grayish and partly gelatinous or cystic. White matter rarefaction is more prominent in deep cerebral areas. Grey matter structures including the cerebral cortex, basal ganglia, and brainstem nuclei appear macroscopically normal.

Microscopically, the U fibers are often affected, whereas the outer rim of the corpus callosum, anterior commissure, fornix, optic tracts, internal capsules, and intrinsic fibers of the thalami are less severely affected. In the mesencephalon, the cerebral peduncles are generally intact. In the pons, the ventral trigeminothalamic and central tegmental tracts may be affected. The deep cerebellar white matter shows discoloration that is most marked in the hilus of the dentate nucleus. Discoloration is also observed in the hilus of the inferior olivary nucleus, pyramids and corpus restiforme. There is more marked myelin loss in the spinocerebellar tracts, lateral and anterior corticospinal tracts and the anterolateral fascicles containing the spinoreticular and spinothalamic tracts.

Histopathologic and immunohistochemical findings support the inclusion of the disease among the orthochromatic sudanophilic leukoencephalopathies. Myelin stains of affected white matter show paucity of myelin sheaths and the remaining sheaths appear thinned and dispersed by vacuoles, giving rise to a spongiform appearance. The amount of myelin breakdown products appears disproportionately mild compared with the severity of the myelin lesions. The number of axons in the white matter is decreased, which is usually commensurate with the decrease of myelin. The degree of reactive gliosis is limited. Only moderate numbers of macrophages and microglial cells are seen and T and B lymphocytes are absent. Around cavitated areas and in less affected regions, an increased cellular density is observed. This increased cellular density has been ascribed to oligodendrocytes. Oligodendrocytic loss via apoptosis may predominate in infants and younger children, whereas in older individuals with long-standing disease, antiapoptotic

347

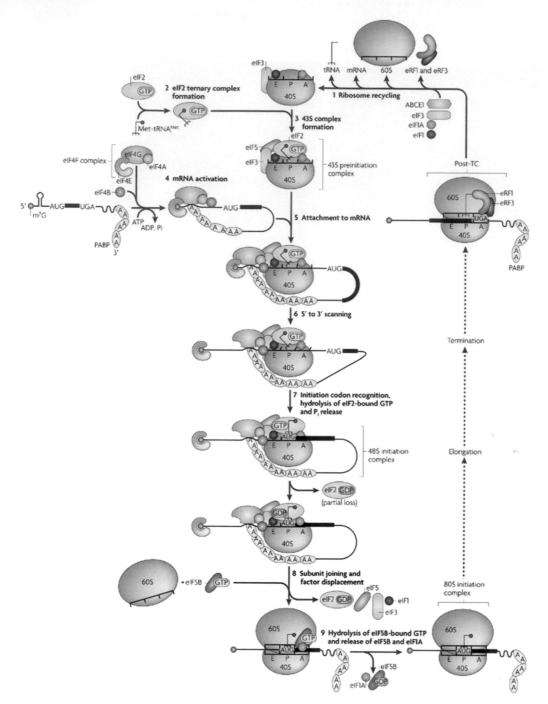

Figure 85.2 The canonical pathway of eukaryotic translation initiation is divided into eight stages (2–9). These stages follow the recycling of post-termination complexes (post-TCs; 1) to yield separated 40S and 60S ribosomal subunits, and result in the formation of an 80S ribosomal initiation complex, in which Met-tRNAMeti is base paired with the initiation codon in the ribosomal P-site and which is competent to start the translation elongation stage. These stages are: eukaryotic initiation factor 2 (eIF2)–GTP–Met-tRNAMeti ternary complex formation (2); formation of a 43S preinitiation complex comprising a 40S subunit, eIF1, eIF1A, eIF3, eIF2–GTP–Met-tRNAMeti and probably eIF5 (3); mRNA activation, during which the mRNA cap-proximal region is unwound in an ATP-dependent manner by eIF4F with eIF4B (4); attachment of the 43S complex to this mRNA region (5); scanning of the 5′ UTR in a 5′ to 3′ direction by 43S complexes (6); recognition of the initiation codon and 48S initiation complex formation, which switches the scanning complex to a "closed" conformation and leads to displacement of eIF1 to allow eIF5-mediated hydrolysis of eIF2-bound GTP and Pi release (7); joining of 60S subunits to 48S complexes and concomitant displacement of eIF2–GDP and other factors (eIF1, eIF3, eIF4B, eIF4F and eIF5) mediated by eIF5B (8); and GTP hydrolysis by eIF5B and release of eIF1A and GDP-bound eIF5B from assembled elongation-competent 80S ribosomes (9). Translation is a cyclical process, in which termination follows elongation and leads to recycling (1), which generates separated ribosomal subunits. The model omits potential 'closed loop' interactions involving poly(A)-binding protein (PABP), eukaryotic release factor 3 (eRF3) and eIF4F during recycling (see Supplementary information S5 (box)), and the recycling of eIF2–GDP by eIF2B. Whether eRF3 is still present on ribosomes at the recycling stage is unknown. Reproduced with permission from Jackson RJ et al. The mechanism of eukaryotic translation initiation and principles of its regulation. *Nat Rev Mol Cell Biol.* 2010; 11(2):113–27.

mechanisms may allow the proliferation of persisting oligodendrocytes, thus accounting for the increase in their numbers.

Pathophysiology

The protein complex eIF2B is involved in the regulation of the first steps of protein synthesis (Figure 85.2). It consists of 5 subunits, termed α through ε (Figure 85.3). Subunit ε is catalytic, whereas subunits α through δ are regulatory. In eukaryotes, translation initiation is a multistep process, in which the interplay of the mRNA, initiator methionyl-tRNA (tRNAi Met), the ribosomal subunits, and several multiple translation initiation factors (eIFs), ensures start of the translation process at the AUG start codon of the mRNA. One of the first steps in this initiation process involves the formation of a ternary complex consisting of tRNAi Met, eIF2, and GTP, which binds to the ribosome. On recognition of the start codon of the

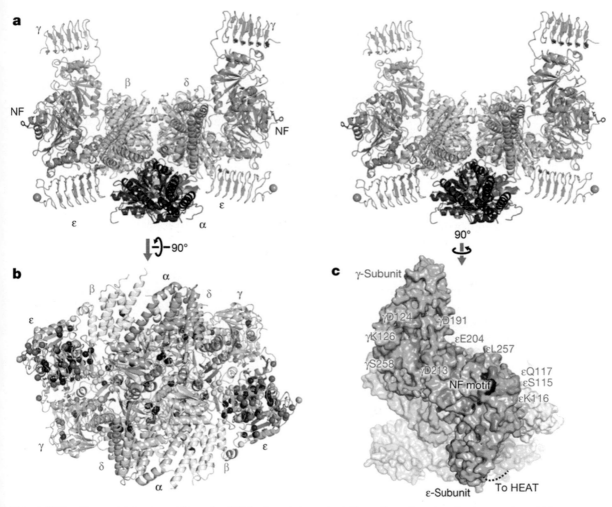

Figure 85.3 a. The crystal structure of *S. pombe* eIF2B (wall-eyed stereo view). The a-, β-, γ-, δ-, and ε-subunits are coloured blue, cyan, orange, green and pink, respectively. The NF motifs in the e-subunits are shown by red sticks. The visible C-terminal Cα atoms of the e subunits are shown by spheres, and the HEAT domains, whose electron densities were not observed in this structure, extend outwards. b. Mapping of the *S. pombe* eIF2B residues corresponding to VWM-causing missense mutations of human eIF2B as spheres on the S. pombe eIF2B structure. Their environments are colour-coded on the spheres (green, solvent exposed; yellow, subunit interface; brown, structural core). c. Mapping of the S. pombe eIF2B residues corresponding to the solvent-exposed disease-causing missense mutations of human eIF2B (green) and to the pBpa cross-links with *K. pastoris* eIF2, through the interaction between eIF2B and eIF2 (teal), on the surface model. The NF motif is coloured red. Reproduced with permission from Jackson RJ et al. The mechanism of eukaryotic translation initiation and principles of its regulation. *Nat Rev Mol Cell Biol.* 2010; 11(2):113–27.

mRNA, the eIF2-bound GTP is hydrolyzed, and eIF2 is released in its inactive GDP-bound form. The coding information of the mRNA is then translated into a new protein, and finally, the ribosome dissociates from the mRNA and the newly synthesized protein is released. Active eIF2 must be regenerated by exchange of GDP for GTP to enable the formation of another ternary complex and initiate the synthesis of another protein. This GDP/GTP exchange is required for each round of translation initiation and is catalyzed by eIF2B.

Inhibition of protein synthesis is part of the cellular stress response, a process aimed at enhancing cell survival under stress by preserving cellular energy and limiting the accumulation of denatured proteins. A variety of cellular stresses, such as amino acid starvation, viral infection, iron deficiency, oxidative and ER stress, and thermal and mechanical trauma, lead to phosphorylation of eIF2α. Phosphorylated eIF2 binds eIF2B and in that way inhibits the GDP/GTP exchange activity of eIF2B and, as a consequence, mRNA translation in general.

Decreased eIF2B activity might impair the cellular stress response and improperly activate the unfolded protein response (UPR). The UPR is a compensatory intracellular signaling pathway that responds to accumulation of unfolded or denatured proteins in the ER. Activation of this pathway restores cell homeostasis by reducing the rate of protein synthesis, abating the effects of ER stress and promoting protein degradation. As part of the UPR, the pancreatic ER kinase is activated, resulting in phosphorylation of eIF2α and global inhibition of translation. Some mRNAs are exempt from inhibition through specific features in their 5′ untranslated regions. One of these mRNAs encodes activating transcription factor 4 (ATF4), a transcription factor that leads to activation of numerous target genes, including C/EBP homologous protein (CHOP) and growth arrest and DNA damage protein 34 (GADD34). Decreased eIF2B activity in vanishing white matter disease would be expected to lead to a constitutive upregulation of ATF4 and its downstream effectors. Thus, vanishing white matter disease cells may be innately predisposed and hyperreactive to stress.

Diagnosis

A few biochemical markers have been identified for the disease, including elevated cerebrospinal fluid glycine and decreased asialotransferrin concentrations. Asialotransferrin is thought to be produced exclusively in the brain, possibly by astrocytes and oligodendrocytes, and its reduction might reflect functional disturbances in these cells. However, in view of the high sensitivity and specificity of MR imaging, there is limited need for such indicators in common practice.

Treatment

There is no specific treatment.

Bibliography

Bugiani M., Boor I., Powers J.M., et al. (2010). Leukoencephalopathy with vanishing white matter: A review. *J Neuropathol Exp Neurol.* 69(10):987–96.

Renaud D.L. (2012). Leukoencephalopathies associated with macrocephaly. *Semin Neurol.* 32(1):34–41.

Childhood Spinocerebellar Ataxias

A 6 ½-year-old boy exhibited impaired fine and gross motor skills and gait instability. MR imaging demonstrated cerebellar hypoplasia. At the age of 10 years, he attended elementary school, with problems with work speed and difficulties with writing, as well as with fine motor skills. His examination revealed ataxia, dysdiadochokinesia, hypotonia, and increased tendon reflexes.

His 38-year-old mother had first reported gait instability and clumsiness at the age of 10 years. At 36 years, she exhibited limb and gait ataxia, moderate dysarthria and bilateral gaze-evoked nystagmus, with normal reflexes and a lack of pyramidal signs. MR imaging indicated cerebellar atrophy. However, she was completely independent for all her activities.

Childhood Spinocerebellar Ataxias

Onset: Infant, childhood, or adolescence ataxia.
Additional manifestations: In type I, cerebellar symptoms in conjunction with oculomotor, lower motor neuron, pyramidal, extrapyramidal, sensory, visual, auditory or cognitive dysfunction. In type II, pigmentary retinal degeneration. Type III includes only ataxias with pure cerebellar manifestations.
Disease mechanism: In some types, polyglutamine tract aggregation and toxicity, calcium dysregulation or mitochondrial dysfunction and apoptosis.
Testing: Genetic analysis is often necessary due to clinical symptom overlap.
Treatment: None effective.
Research highlights: Characterization of molecular abnormalities leading to protein aggregation and reduced clearance, transcriptional dysregulation, dysfunction of the ubiquitin-proteasome system, alterations of calcium homeostasis and activation of apoptosis.

Clinical Features

The spinocerebellar ataxias are a heterogeneous group of over 30 autosomal dominant disorders characterized by progressive cerebellar dysfunction. Other common names for some of these disorders include olivopontocerebellar degenerations, spinocerebellar atrophies, and multisystem atrophies. In many cases, these disorders share the same clinical features such they can only be distinguished by genetic analysis. Sometimes, members of the same family who harbor the same mutation are affected by different phenotypes. The combined incidence of all forms of autosomal dominant spinocerebellar ataxias is 1 per 100,000 individuals. A purely clinical classification scheme distinguishes three classes of spinocerebellar ataxias: Type I consists of cerebellar symptoms in conjunction with other neurological manifestations such as oculomotor, lower motor neuron, pyramidal, extrapyramidal, sensory, visual, auditory, or cognitive dysfunction. Type II resembles type I with pigmentary retinal degeneration. This type includes only spinocerebellar ataxia type 7. Type III includes only ataxias with pure cerebellar manifestations. This type includes spinocerebellar ataxia types 5, 6, 11, 26, 29, 30, and 31. Table 86.1 summarizes the best known spinocerebellar ataxia variants.

Whereas disease onset is usually between 30 and 50 years of age, the following ataxias can present in childhood: 1, 2, 3 or Machado-Joseph disease, 5, 8, 12, 13, 14, 15, 17, 21, 25, 28, and 29. These ataxias involve several common pathophysiological mechanisms.

Pathology

The most frequent pathological finding is olivopontocerebellar atrophy (Figure 86.1). For example, in spinocerebellar ataxia 1, the cerebellum displays

Table 86.1 The spinocerebellar ataxias

SCA	Earliest age of onset (years)	Gene or locus	Mutation type
SCA 1	4	Ataxin-1 (ATXN1)	Exonic CAG repeat
SCA 2	1	Ataxin-2 (ATXN2)	Exonic CAG repeat
SCA 3	4	Ataxin-3 (ATXN3)	Exonic CAG repeat
SCA 4	19	16q22	Unknown
SCA 5	10	β-3 spectrin (SPTBN3)	Missense
SCA 6	19	P/Q type Ca^{2+} channel subunit (CACNA1A)	Exonic CAG repeat
SCA 7	0	Ataxin-7 (ATXN7)	Exonic CAG repeat
SCA 8	1	ATXN8OS (opposite strand)/Ataxin 8 (ATXN8)	Transcription of untranslated RNA CTG repeat/ CAG repeat
SCA 9		Reserved	Unknown
SCA 10	12	Ataxin-10 (ATXN-10)	Intronic ATTCT repeat
SCA 11	15	Tau tubulin kinase 2 (TTBK2)	1 nucleotide insertion/2 nucleotide deletion
SCA 12	8	Protein phosphatase PP2A (PPP2R2B)	CAG repeat upstream of exon 7 (splice variant promoter)
SCA 13	1	K^+ channel Kv3.3 (KCNC3)	Missense
SCA 14	3	Protein kinase C-gamma (PRKCG)	Missense or deletion
SCA 15/16	7	Inositol triphosphate receptor 1 (ITPR1)	Deletion (may include SUMF1)
SCA 17	3	TATA box-binding protein (TBP)	Exonic CAG repeat
SCA 18	13	7q31-q32	Unknown
SCA 19/22	11	K^+ channel Kv4.3 (KCND3)	Missense or small deletions
SCA 20	19	11q12	Multigene duplication
SCA 21	6	Transmembrane protein 240 (TMEM240)	Missense
SCA 23	43	Prodynorphin (PFYN)	Missense
SCA 25	1	2p21-p13	Unknown
SCA 26	26	Eukaryotic translation elongation factor 2 (EEF2)	Missense
SCA 27	15	Fibroblast growth factor-14 (FGF14)	Missense, nonsense
SCA 28	3	ATPase family gene 3-like 2 (AFG3L2)	Missense
SCA 29	1	Allelic with SCA 15	
SCA 30	45	4q34-q35	Unknown
SCA 31	8	Brain-expressed protein associating with Nedd4 homolog (BEAN1)	2.5–3.8 Kb insertion, with expanded $(TGGAA)_n$ repeat
SCA 32	Adulthood	7q32-q33	Unknown
SCA 34	1	Elongation of very long chain fatty acids protein 4 (ELOVL4)	Missense

Table 86.1 (*cont.*)

SCA	Earliest age of onset (years)	Gene or locus	Mutation type
SCA 35	40	Tissue transglutaminase 6 (TGM6)	Missense
SCA 36	39	Nucleolar protein 56 (NOP56)	Intronic $(GGCCTG)_n$ repeat
SCA 37	38	1p32	Unknown

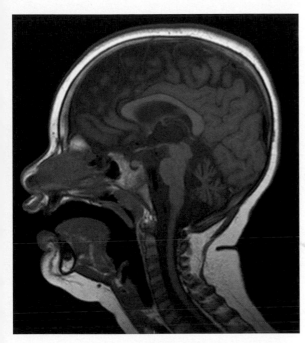

Figure 86.1 Cerebellar degeneration in a 3-year-old girl with spinocerebellar ataxia type 2.

loss of Purkinje cells and neuronal loss in the dentate nucleus. There is extensive olivary neuronal loss disproportionate to loss of Purkinje cells. The basis pontis, red nucleus, and motor nuclei of cranial nerves III, X, and XII also display neuronal loss. The anterior horns, posterior columns, and spinocerebellar tracts are atrophic. The pallidum may be affected. The cerebral cortex and hippocampus also display mild neuronal loss. These features are generally present in this group of diseases but may vary in intensity depending on the type of spinocerebellar ataxia, the age at onset and the age at the time of death. Intranuclear aggregates, the result of CAG-encoded polyglutamine expansion tracts, may also be seen in many cells.

Pathophysiology

Three general well-known mechanisms cause cellular dysfunction and degeneration in the spinocerebellar ataxias: polyglutamine neurotoxicity, alterations in calcium homeostasis, and mitochondrial dysfunction and apoptosis.

Six spinocerebellar ataxia types including 1, 2, 3, 6, 7, and 17 are caused by the expansion of a CAG-repeat sequence, leading to abnormally long polyglutamine tracts in the encoded proteins (Figure 86.2). The pathogenic threshold for disease is approximately 40 copies of the repeat in most of the different subtypes. It is assumed that the common toxic gain-of-function mechanisms for the polyglutamine-containing protein are aggregation and deposition of misfolded proteins leading to neuronal dysfunction and eventually cell death. Proteins with expanded stretches of polyglutamine appear to fold in an abnormal configuration resulting in the formation and deposition of polyglutamine aggregates in disease neurons forming characteristic nuclear or cytoplasmic inclusions (Figure 86.3). These inclusions contain cellular components such as ubiquitin, the proteasome, HSP70 (heat shock protein 70) and transcription factors. Expanded polyglutamine proteins form fibrillary proteinaceous aggregates more rapidly than normal proteins. Therefore, a possible mechanism for aggregate formation by the mutant protein would be by loss of native state stability by the expanded polyglutamine and, thus, leading to the formation and accumulation of a partially unfolded, aggregation-prone species, resulting in fibrillization inside vulnerable neurons. This phenomenon might account for the earlier age of onset and higher severity of disease symptoms observed when mutant ataxins contain longer numbers of glutamines. Mechanisms of cell survival mediated by the endoplasmic reticulum (ER) chaperones and the unfolded protein response (UPR) are activated during neurodegeneration in

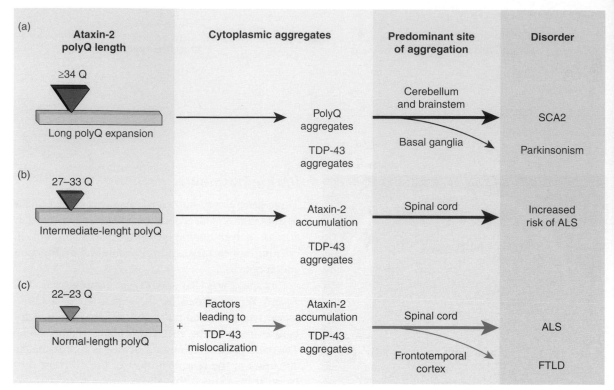

Figure 86.2 Mechanisms of the spinocerebellar ataxias. **a.** Long polyQ-tract expansion (≥34 glutamines (Q)) in ataxin-2 leads to neurodegeneration, which causes spinocerebellar ataxia type 2 (SCA2) or parkinsonism. **b.** PolyQ-tract expansions of intermediate length (27–33 Q) in this protein drive TDP-43 aggregation in motor neurons in the spinal cord, increasing the risk of amyotrophic lateral sclerosis (ALS). **c.** Abnormal accumulation of ataxin-2 containing the normal number (22–23 Q) of glutamines, presumably mediated by other factors, has been observed in sporadic ALS and frontotemporal lobar dementia (FTLD). In at least three cases (SCA2, ALS and FTLD), TDP-43 aggregation in the affected neurons accompanies ataxin-2 accumulation. The thickness of the arrows on the right reflects the apparent frequency with which ataxin-2 accumulation is observed in associated disorders. Reproduced with permission from Lagier-Tourenne C et al. Neurodegeneration: An expansion in ALS genetics. *Nature.* 2010. 466:1052–3.

spinocerebellar ataxias. The presence of unfolded proteins in the ER can cause ER stress or an imbalance between the load of unfolded proteins and the capacity of the ER protein-folding machinery. In order to restore ER homeostasis, neurons activate the ER stress response or UPR, eventually leading to transcriptional activation of genes encoding for chaperones. Proteins that remain misfolded are degraded primarily by the ubiquitin-proteasome system, but also by the autophagic phagosome–lysosome system.

There is deranged neuronal calcium signaling in the spinocerebellar ataxias. Cerebellar Purkinje cells are particularly sensitive to fluctuations in intracellular calcium levels, which could result from different sources, such as the reduction of chaperone activity and ER stress. In SCA6, Purkinje cell degeneration is associated with polyglutamine expansions within the CACNA1A gene. The CACNA1A gene encodes the pore-forming subunit of the $Ca_v2.1$ voltage-dependent P/Q-type calcium channel. Three allelic diseases are caused by different types of mutations in the CACNA1A gene including SCA6, episodic ataxia type 2, and familial hemiplegic migraine. Polyglutamine expansions in SCA6 might interfere with the Ca^{2+} channel to reduce Ca^{2+} influx and impaired function of the mutant Ca^{2+} channels, rendering them incapable of preventing cell death.

Neuronal death in spinocerebellar ataxias may also result from the activation of apoptosis. Polyglutamine-expanded cellular death of cerebellar neurons by ataxins 3 and 7 in SCA3 and SCA7 is preceded by recruitment of caspases into polyglutamine aggregates. This is followed by activation of caspases 3 and 9, and of mitochondrial apoptotic

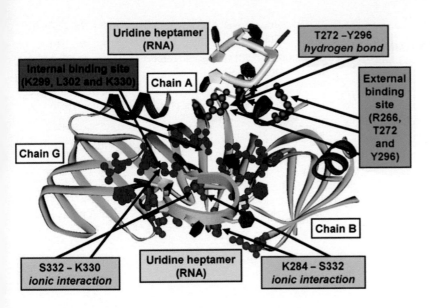

Figure 86.3 3D model of the Lsm domain of ataxin-2 using three adjacent protomers of the Sm1 protein from *P. abyssi* as template. The model illustrates predicted internal (blue) and external (green) binding sites of ataxin-2 to RNA (grey). α-Helices are in shown in red, β-strands are shown in cyan. Only functionally relevant residues of the central ataxin-2 protomer are annotated as follows: dark blue boxes point to residues forming the internal site, and light blue boxes mark amino acids stabilizing the RNA binding area; dark green boxes highlight residues involved in the external site, and light green ones indicate stabilizing hydrogen bonds. Reproduced with permission from Albrecht M et al. Structural and functional analysis of ataxin-2 and ataxin-3. *Eur J Biochem.* 2004; 271(15):3155–70.

pathways mediated by members of the Bcl-2 (B-cell lymphoma 2) family, such as Bax (BCL2 associated X protein) and Bcl-x(L). Both factors participate in neuronal apoptosis by regulating mitochondrial release of cytochrome c and Smac/DIABLO (second mitochondria-derived activator of caspase/direct inhibitor of apoptosis-binding protein with low pI). Alternatively, pro-apoptotic pathways could be activated by displacement of harmful factors sequestered by expanded polyglutamines, or through non-canonical mechanisms of caspase activation. In any case, the toxic proteins may promote mitochondrial dysfunction and increased free radical production associated with oxidative damage, and abnormal energy metabolite concentration and utilization.

Diagnosis

In the majority of cases, the diagnosis can only be confirmed by genetic analysis.

Treatment

There is no effective treatment. Acetazolamide may temporarily reduce the severity of symptoms in SCA6. Dopaminergic and anticholinergic drugs have been used to alleviate tremor, bradykinesia or dystonia in SCA2 and SCA3. Spasticity in spinocerebellar ataxias may be treated with baclofen, tizanidine, or mimentine. Botulinum toxin has been used to treat dystonia and spasticity. Intention tremor has been ameliorated with benzodiazepines,

β-blockers or chronic thalamic stimulation. Muscle cramps, which are often present at the onset in SCA 2, 3 and 7 are alleviated with magnesium, quinine or mexiletine.

Experimental approaches include RNA interference (RNAi) with the aim of inhibiting polyglutamine-induced neurodegeneration, prevention of protein misfolding and aggregation by overexpression of chaperones and regulation of gene expression by application of histone deacetylase inhibitors. Compounds targeting mitochondrial function such as coenzyme Q10, creatine, and taurousodeoxycholic acid, or autophagy, such as the mTOR inhibitor rapamycin and its various analogous, have proved effective at reducing cellular toxicity in animal models. Caspase activation, which usually precedes neuronal cell death, can be targeted with caspase inhibitors such as zVAD-fmk (carbobenzoxy-valyl-alanyl-aspartyl-[O-methyl]-fluoromethylketone), cystamine and minocycline. Other agents promoting the clearance of mutant proteins or Ca^{2+} signaling blockers, such as specific inhibitors of the NR2B-subunit of N-methyl-D-aspartate glutamate receptors and blockers of metabotropic glutamate receptor mGluR5 and inositol 1,4,5-trisphosphate receptor InsP3R1, may be beneficial for the treatment of some spinocerebellar ataxia subtypes. Gene therapy and stem cell approaches are being studied for the treatment of spinocerebellar neurodegenerations. Delivery of proteins or compounds by viral vectors represents one such gene therapeutic approach.

Bibliography

Dueñas A.M., Goold R., Giunti P. (2006). Molecular pathogenesis of spinocerebellar ataxias. *Brain*. 129(Pt 6):1357–70.

Edener U., Wöllner J., Hehr U., et al. (2010). Early onset and slow progression of SCA28, a rare dominant ataxia in a large four-generation family with a novel AFG3L2 mutation. *Eur J Hum Genet*. 18(8):965–8.

Storey E. (2014). Genetic cerebellar ataxias. *Semin Neurol*. 34(3):280–92.

Sun Y.M., Lu C., Wu Z.Y. (2016). Spinocerebellar ataxia: Relationship between phenotype and genotype-A Review. *Clin Genet*. 90(4):305–14.

Charcot-Marie-Tooth Disease

A 4-year-old boy could not stand steadily by himself and had an abnormal gait with foot drop. He learnt to walk at the age of 1 year and 7 months, albeit not steadily. He fell easily when running. Examination revealed atrophy of the lower extremities. His left foot displayed a mild pes cavus deformity and he could not lift it up by himself. There was slightly reduced strength in his right hand. Testing of the tendon reflexes showed reduced patellar and ankle jerks. There were no Babinski, Chaddock, Oppenheim, or Gordon signs. Strength was reduced with MRC scores of 4 on the lower extremities. His muscle tone was mildly reduced.

Charcot-Marie-Tooth Disease

Onset: Late attainment of motor milestones or abnormal gait acquisition.
Additional manifestations: Distal weakness and atrophy, decreased or absent tendon reflexes and impaired sensation. Foot deformity (pes cavus and hammer toes) and claw hand. Tonic pupils in MPZ-related neuropathies, white matter lesions with transient focal symptoms or stroke-like presentations in X-linked Charcot-Marie-Tooth disease (GJB1), vocal cord and diaphragm involvement in CMT2C, optic atrophy in MFN2 and deafness in MPZ, PMP22 and GJB1 deficiencies.
Disease mechanism: Demyelination leading to axonal damage. Dysfunction of axonal transport, trophic support and energy production leading to axonal Wallerian degeneration.
Testing: Electrodiagnostic (nerve conduction velocity) studies may assist with the classification into subtypes.
Treatment: None effective.
Research highlights: Mouse models of CMT1X, CMT1B and CMT1A developed to study Schwann cells exhibit a heterogeneous pattern of developmentally regulated molecules.

Clinical Features

Charcot-Marie-Tooth disease is the generic term applied to neuropathies that affect 1 in 2500 persons. The disorder is characterized by progressive length-dependent axonal loss. Onset is insidious, in the first or second decade and the rate of progression slow. Motor and sensory nerves can be affected similarly, causing distal weakness and atrophy, decreased or absent tendon reflexes and impaired sensation. The onset of the disease usually involves the feet and lower legs, later affecting hands and forearms. Foot deformity (pes cavus and hammer toes) is common, as is claw hand (Figure 87.1). These are due to foot and intrinsic hand muscle weakness. Sensory abnormalities are usually not a major complaint of affected subjects. Individuals with the most common form of Charcot-Marie-Tooth disease, CMT1A, rarely require use of a wheelchair during their lifetime, but the most common axonal variant of the disorder (CMT2A) displays greater severity, with most individuals becoming nonambulatory before the age of 20 years. Other variants, including hereditary sensory neuropathy (or hereditary sensory and autonomic neuropathy) and

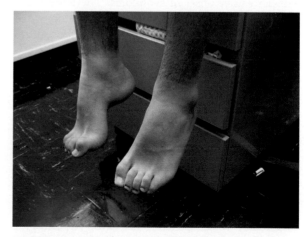

Figure 87.1 Pes cavus in Charcot-Marie-Tooth disease.

Table 87.1 The Charcot-Marie-Tooth diseases

CMT type	Form	Inheritance	Common genes
CMT1	Dysmyelinating	Dominant	PMP22, MPZ, SIMPLE
CMT2	Axonal	Dominant	MFN2, RAB7, TRP4, GARS
CMT3 or Déjérine-Sottas syndrome	Dysmyelinating	Dominant or Recessive	PMP22, MPZ, EGR2
CMT4	Dysmyelinating or axonal	Recessive	GDAP1, FIG4, MTMR2, NEFL
CMTX	Dysmyelinating	X-linked dominant	Connexin 32 (GJB1)

distal hereditary motor neuropathy (or distal spinal muscular atrophy), are also sometimes grouped under the general classification of Charcot-Marie-Tooth disease. These disorders are usually phenotypically distinct. Hereditary sensory neuropathy is usually sensory predominant and may be associated with autonomic dysfunction and skin ulcerations due to insensitive skin. Conversely, distal hereditary motor neuropathy usually lacks or includes minimal sensory involvement.

The clinical presentations of Charcot-Marie-Tooth disease are very similar, such that there may not be sufficient phenotypic discriminatory power. Consequently, the precise diagnosis of disease subtype relies on genetic testing. Most types of Charcot-Marie-Tooth disease are inherited in an autosomal dominant fashion, but X-linked and autosomal recessive forms also occur. X-linked forms are characterized by an intermediate-to-demyelinating range of conduction velocities. Autosomal recessive inheritance is less common. Autosomal recessive forms are frequently characterized by a more severe phenotype with an earlier onset of symptoms. There are many forms of Charcot-Marie-Tooth disease that may display reduced penetrance. Specific phenotypic features may be suggestive of a particular subtype of the disease. Examples include tonic pupils in MPZ (myelin protein zero)-related neuropathies, white matter lesions with transient focal symptoms or stroke-like presentations in X-linked Charcot-Marie-Tooth disease (GJB1; gap junction protein beta 1), vocal cord and diaphragm involvement in CMT2C, optic atrophy in MFN2 (mitofusin 2) and deafness in MPZ, PMP22 (peripheral myelin protein 22), and GJB1.

From an electrophysiological point of view, there are two major disease groups: CMTI, with slow nerve conduction velocities associated with hypertrophic demyelination and CMTII, with normal or mildly reduced nerve conduction velocities with axonopathy. Most affected individuals with Charcot-Marie-Tooth disease belong to the first group and exhibit an autosomal dominant inheritance pattern.

The most common forms of Charcot-Marie-Tooth disease are summarized here.

Charcot-Marie-Tooth type 1 (CMT1) is the autosomal dominant demyelinating disease type and is the most common. About 70 percent of all inherited neuropathies are in this category. The peripheral myelin protein 22 gene (PMP22) duplication causes the common demyelinating CMT1A phenotype. Point mutations in the same gene are rare and cause early onset (sometimes infantile) severe demyelinating neuropathy. In contrast, deletion or some point mutations (CMT1E) of the same gene cause hereditary neuropathy with pressure palsy (HNPP). HNPP is the third most common CMT and causes multiple compression neuropathies in adults (median, ulnar, and peroneal) but it rarely manifests in children. CMT1B is the third most common demyelinating neuropathy (after Charcot-Marie-Tooth Type X, CMTX) and is associated with abnormalities in the major peripheral myelin protein, MPZ gene. The clinical variability in this group is extensive, from the infantile form to a late-onset and milder phenotype with dysmyelinating, axonal, and intermediate nerve conduction velocities. CMT1C exhibits similar clinical features as CMT1A and is related to mutations in the lipopolysaccharide-induced tumor necrosis factor-alpha factor gene (LITAF/SIMPLE).

Charcot-Marie-Tooth type 2 (CMT2) disease groups together the various dominant forms of axonal neuropathies, which are often clinically indistinguishable from CMT1 except that the myotatic reflexes and nerve conduction velocities are typically preserved. CMT2A is the most prevalent axonal form and is caused by mutations in the mitofusin 2

(MFN2) gene. This type is rapidly progressive. CMT2B is associated with severe distal sensory loss leading to foot ulcerations, and it is caused by RAB7 (which codes a small GTP-ase) gene mutations. Vocal cord and diaphragm paralysis have been described in CMT2C and this form is caused by mutations in the TRP4 (phosphoribosyltransferase 4) gene. The GARS (glycyl-tRNA synthetase) gene is responsible for the CMT2D phenotype, which causes more severe upper extremity involvement and severe disease in children. A few distinct mutations in many CMT2 genes may cause recessive inheritance and these forms belong to the Charcot-Marie-Tooth type 4 (CMT4) category.

Charcot-Marie-Tooth type 3 (CMT3) refers to individuals with infantile onset neuropathy or Déjérine-Sottas syndrome, which is separately described.

CMT4 includes various recessive demyelinating or axonal neuropathy phenotypes. Some entities have motor neuron–like features, also referred to as distal spinal muscular atrophy (for example, FIG4, a phospho-inositide phosphatase). CMT4A is caused by mutations in ganglioside-induced differentiation-associated protein 1 (GDAP1), CMT4B by the myotubularin-related protein (MTMR2), and CMT4C by SH3TC2 (src homology 3 domains and tetratricopeptide repeat domain protein) genes. Both forms can manifest a severe phenotype with early childhood onset.

CMTX is an X-linked recessive demyelinating neuropathy with variably severe phenotype. CMTX is clinically more severe in males. Female carriers may be asymptomatic or exhibit the HNPP phenotype. CMTX is the second most common form of Charcot-Marie-Tooth disease and is caused by mutations in the GJB1 (gap junction protein beta 1 or connexin 32) gene.

Pathology

There is onion bulb formation in most of the inherited polyneuropathies. Repeated episodes of primary segmental demyelination and remyelination lead to onion bulb formation, which designates imbricated layers of supernumerary Schwann cell processes arranged in rings along the axis of the nerve fiber. These rings are separated by collagen fibers. In some cases of onion bulb formation, the added accumulation of extracellular matrix and collagen in the endonerium results in distension of fascicles. Although they are characteristic of inherited neuropathy, onion bulbs can also occur in chronic inflammatory

demyelinating polyneuropathy and other acquired neuropathies.

There may also be a reduction in the number of myelinated nerve fibers, with a deficiency of large and small diameter elements and extensive demyelination and remyelination. Thinly myelinated fibers may be present. In cases of PMP22 overproduction, myelin thickening may precede demyelination. Variable degrees of chronic inflammation may also be present.

Pathophysiology

In the peripheral nervous system, PMP22, MPZ, and GJB1 are essential for forming compact myelin and gene dosage or gene expression is important to maintain myelin structure. Overexpressed PMP22 results in toxic protein aggregation and overloads the protein degradation process, thus leading to demyelination. Many gene products in CMT2 (for example, MFN2) participate in various axonal processes including transport, trophic support and energy production, and dysfunction in these processes leads to axonal damage and Wallerian degeneration. Demyelination in a nerve eventually results in axonal damage; therefore, the two pathologic processes cannot be separated from each other.

Diagnosis

Electrodiagnostic studies serve to confirm a clinically suspected sensorimotor polyneuropathy and to exclude other diseases such as hereditary motor neuropathy or distal myopathy. Motor conduction velocities obtained in nerve conduction studies are helpful to classify sensorimotor polyneuropathies into demyelinating or axonal pathophysiological subtypes. A conduction velocity in an upper limb motor nerve in an adult of 38 m/s is utilized as the limit for differentiation of axonal ($\geq$38 m/s) and demyelinating (<38 m/s) disease. CMT1 designates demyelinating disease and CMT2, axonal. X-linked CMT typically exhibits intermediate (defined as >35 and up to 45 m/s) to demyelinating range conduction velocity values. Similarly to their clinical features, autosomal recessive forms may exhibit severe electrical abnormalities. The features of demyelination on nerve conduction study in subjects with Charcot-Marie-Tooth disease are uniform and symmetric without conduction blocks or temporal dispersion. Asymmetric involvement, temporal dispersion and conduction block typically imply acquired diseases such as chronic immune demyelinating polyneuropathy. This is confounded by the observation that features of acquired demyelinating disease may be detected, particularly in certain subtypes, such as CMTX, CMT1B, CMT1C, and CMT4J. CMT4J may also mimic the clinical presentation of acquired demyelination. Cerebrospinal fluid analysis is frequently used in the evaluation of possible autoimmune forms of neuropathy. In CMT1, the protein is typically elevated. Peripheral nerve ultrasound usually reveals diffuse nerve enlargement in demyelinating forms, whereas acquired immune demyelinating polyneuropathies tend to display more patchy and multifocal enlargement of nerves.

Treatment

A CMT1A rat model can be treated with a recombinant human growth factor called neuregulin-1 which controls myelin thickness. In rats, this enhances the reduced signaling of phosphatidylinositol 4,5-bisphosphate 3-kinase (PI3K)–v-Akt murine thymoma viral oncogene homolog 1 (Akt) and lower augmented mitogen-activated protein kinase 1 (Mek)-mitogen-activated protein kinase (Erk) and is able to improve the differentiation of Schwann cells in CMT1A. Thus, neuregulin-1 can counter the effect of PMP22 overexpression on downstream signaling. The protein kinase C modulator bryostatin may lower PMP22 expression. Ascorbic acid also downregulates PMP22 production, but human trials did not demonstrate clinically significant improvement. Animal studies also have considered progesterone antagonism to decrease PMP22 production. Also, curcumin in CMT1B improved Schwann cell differentiation and alleviated endoplasmic reticulum stress as part of reducing the activation of the unfolded protein response. Histone deacetylase (HDAC) 6 inhibition demonstrated favorable results in an animal model of CMT2F (HSPB1, heat shock protein beta-1) with an increase of α-tubulin acetylation correcting axonal transport defects. A clinical study including baclofen, naltrexone and sorbitol has illustrated improvement beyond stabilization. This study reveals pleiotropic mechanisms for downregulating PMP22. Neurotrophin 3 was tested both on animals and in a human study. This neurotrophic growth factor displayed slight axonal regeneration. Additionally, several subtypes of CMT2 may share endpoint pathology, such as disrupted axonal transport. HDAC inhibitors could be then potentially used to treat multiple subtypes.

Bibliography

Hoyle J.C., Isfort M.C., Roggenbuck J., et al. (2015). The genetics of Charcot-Marie-Tooth disease: Current trends and future implications for diagnosis and management. *Appl Clin Genet.* 8:235–43.

Jani-Acsadi A., Ounpuu S., Pierz K., et al. (2015). Pediatric Charcot-Marie-Tooth disease.*Pediatr Clin North Am.* 62(3):767–86.

Yang Y., Li L. (2016). A novel p.Val244Leu mutation in MFN2 leads to Charcot-Marie-Tooth disease type 2. *Ital J Pediatr.* 42(1):28.

Giant Axonal Neuropathy

An 8-year-old boy born to a second degree consanguineous couple presented with difficulty walking and
delayed attainment of motor and intellectual milestones. He started walking at 2 years and since then
exhibited an abnormal gait and dragged his feet while
walking. For the past 2 years his gait had worsened
and he experienced frequent falls. He sat at 9 months
and attained speech at 24 months. His school performance was poor. He was toilet trained and self-fed but
needed help while dressing. Examination disclosed
curled and rough hair (figure), a crouched gait with
everted feet, spastic diparesis and areflexia with an
abnormal cerebellar exam. Funduscopic examination
revealed bilateral optic atrophy with atypical retinitis
pigmentosa.

Giant Axonal Neuropathy

Onset: Progressive distal motor and sensory
neuropathy with distal weakness, steppage gait,
distal amyotrophy and absent tendon reflexes in
the lower limbs at about 3 years of age.

Additional manifestations: Ataxia, dysmetria and
dysarthria. Upper motor neuron syndrome,
epilepsy, mental retardation, and dementia.

Disease mechanism: Gigaxonin helps maintain
cytoskeletal structure, including intermediate
neural filaments in neural cells and vimentin in
fibroblasts and endothelial cells. Gigaxonin is
involved in the ubiquitin–proteasome pathway,
controlling the degradation of intermediate
filaments and other cytoskeletal components.

Testing: Nerve biopsy. Electrodiagnostic studies
illustrate reduction of motor and sensory nerve
conduction velocities

Treatment: None effective.

Research highlights: Gigaxonin gene transfer in
mutant mice can reverse cellular intermediate
filament aggregate pathology.

Clinical Features

Autosomal recessive giant axonal neuropathy is
caused by mutations of the gigaxonin (GAN) gene.
The disorder is characterized by a progressive neuropathy that affects sensory and motor nerves in
both the central and peripheral nervous systems.
The age of onset is usually between 2 and 3 years
and rarely after the age of 10 years. Initially, motor
milestone acquisition is normal. The earliest neurological signs include progressive peripheral distal
motor sensory neuropathy associated with distal
weakness with steppage gait, distal amyotrophy,
and absent tendon reflexes in the lower limbs. Distal sensory impairment is usually found on examination, involving deep and superficial sensation in
the context of minimal sensory complaints. The
neuropathy eventually extends to the upper limbs
several years after onset. The peripheral neuropathy
dominates the phenotype during the first years and
is followed by signs of encephalopathy. In some
affected individuals, peripheral and central nervous
system signs coexist at disease onset. Cerebellar
involvement is common, with ataxia, dysmetria
and dysarthria. An upper motor neuron syndrome
with epilepsy and mental retardation has also been
reported. There is variable cranial nerve involvement including bulbar nerve paralysis, ophthalmoplegia, ptosis, facial nerve paralysis and nystagmus.
Kinky or frizzy hair appearance is usually linked to
the disease, but is not universal (Figure 88.1).
Chemical analysis of kinky hair in affected subjects
reveals a decrease in disulfide bonds and an increase
in free thiol groups. Scoliosis, kyphosis and foot
deformities have been reported. Early puberty is
also observed. The progression and prognosis of
the disease are variable, with the age to ambulatory
disability and wheelchair-use age varying from the
second to the fourth decade of life. Death may
occur between the ages of 20 and 60 years.

Pathology

MR imaging may be normal at an early stage of the disease. Later, MR imaging findings are varied and progressive, with predominance of white matter demyelination, atrophy of the cerebellum, brainstem,

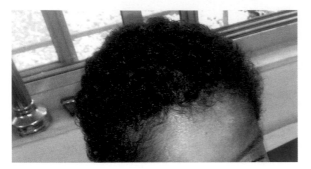

Figure 88.1 Kinky or frizzy hair typical of giant axonal neuropathy. Reproduced and modified with permission from Kamate M et al. Giant axonal neuropathy: a rare inherited neuropathy with simple clinical clues. *BMJ Case Rep.* 2014; 2014 pii:bcr2014204481.

spinal cord, and corpus callosum (Figure 88.2). There may be widespread white matter lesions distributed in relatively distinct patterns. In some cases they are diffuse, involving the anterior and posterior periventricular regions and cerebellum and extending into the subcortical white matter. In others, white matter involvement is focal and limited to the cerebellum or to the frontal parietal or periventricular areas, sparing the cerebellum.

Microscopically, there are giant axons in the peripheral nervous system but also in the spinal cord, brainstem and cerebral cortex (Figure 88.3). There has also been Rosenthal fiber formation detected in most studies of long surviving individuals. Occasionally, massive accumulation of Rosenthal fibers leads to pseudotumoral subependymal outgrowth. Histological examination of the cortex reveals increased numbers of astrocytes and scattered Rosenthal fibers. The Rosenthal fibers immunostain for glial fibrillary acidic protein. In addition, occasional giant axons are found, measuring up to 100 μm or more in diameter.

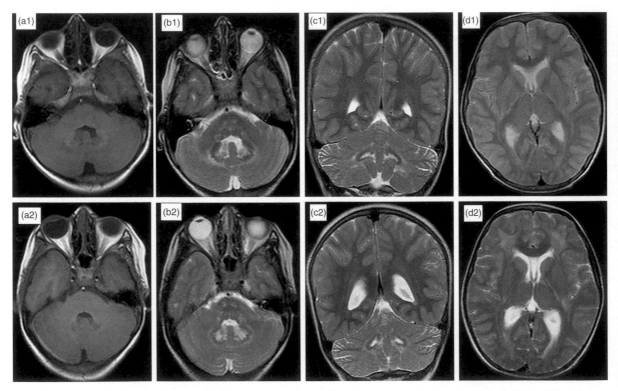

Figure 88.2 MR imaging of the brain of twin-1 (**a1–d1**) and twin-2 (**a2–d2**) with giant axonal neuropathy. (**a** and **b**) T1 and T2 axial images of cerebellum and brain stem showing signal changes in the dentate nucleus. (C) The dentate nucleus signal changes seen in the T2 coronal sections of the brain. (**d**) The signal changes in the posterior limb of internal capsules in the T axial sections at the level of the basal ganglia. Reproduced with permission from Kamate M et al. Giant axonal neuropathy: a rare inherited neuropathy with simple clinical clues. *BMJ Case Rep.* 2014;2014. pii:bcr2014204481.

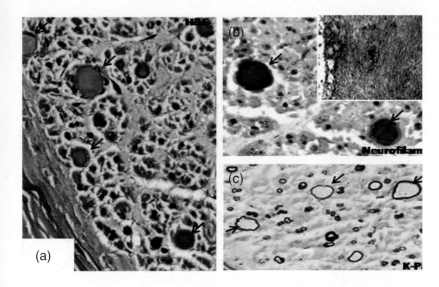

Figure 88.3 Nerve biopsy in giant axonal neuropathy in the child from Figure 88.2. Several giant axons of varying sizes (arrows) dispersed within the fascicles (20–200 μm) (a). These contain abundant phosphorylated neurofilaments distending the axoplasm to giant proportions (b). Electron microscopy: closely packed aggregates of neurofilaments distending and displacing normal organelles within the axoplasm (b, inset). Myelin stains: thinned out attenuated myelin sheaths surrounding the giant axons (c). ((a) H&E ×20, (b) Immunostain neurofilament ×40, (b, inset) uranyl acetate–lead citrate ×28665, (c) Kulchitsky Pal ×40). Reproduced with permission from Kamate M et al. Giant axonal neuropathy: a rare inherited neuropathy with simple clinical clues. *BMJ Case Rep.* 2014;2014 pii:bcr2014204481.

They stain positively with silver stains and antineurofilament antibodies. The cerebral white matter may be diffusely gliotic with a variable loss of myelin affecting mostly the frontal and parietal lobes, with relative sparing of U fibers. Rosenthal fibers are aggregated around blood vessels. Low numbers of giant axons are seen within the cerebral white matter. The central gray matter structures also contain increased numbers of astrocytes, scattered Rosenthal fibers and occasional giant axons. The cerebellar cortex displays loss of Purkinje and granule cells and hyperplasia of Bergmann astrocytes. In the cerebellar white matter, loss of nerve fibers and increase of astrocytic processes and Rosenthal fibers may be seen. Giant axons and Rosenthal fibers are scattered throughout the brainstem. In particular, the pyramidal tracts are shrunken and gliotic, display loss of nerve fibers and contain many giant axons. The spinal white matter contains excessive numbers of astrocytes. There are subpial clusters of Rosenthal fibers. Giant axons are particularly numerous in the posterior columns, especially in the cervical region and the lateral corticospinal tracts, particularly in the lower thoracic and lumbar regions. Electron microscopy of the axonal swellings reveals accumulations of neurofilament, often arranged in a whorl-like interlacing pattern.

Muscle biopsies show evidence of nonspecific neurogenic atrophy. The nerve biopsy can be normal in the early stages of the disease. Eventually, nerve biopsy illustrates giant axons consisting of focally enlarged axons surrounded by a thin myelin sheath with the largest swellings often lacking myelin over part of their length and displaying dense axoplasm. The number of giant axons varies across individuals and between nerve fascicles. The number of giant axons seems to decrease with the course of the disease. Giant axons are associated with a variable degree of axonal loss and demyelinating features, including onion bulb formation. The severity of axonal loss and demyelination increase with the duration of the disease.

Pathophysiology

Gigaxonin helps maintain cytoskeletal structure, including intermediate neural filaments in neural cells, and vimentin in fibroblasts and endothelial cells. Gigaxonin is involved in the ubiquitin–proteasome pathway, controlling the degradation of intermediate filaments and other cytoskeletal components. Gigaxonin is composed of an N-terminal BTB (broad-complex, tramtrack, and bric-a-brac) domain followed by six Kelch repeats. Gigaxonin mutations are associated with the accumulation of vimentin intermediate filaments (IFs), an important IF expressed in mesenchymal cells. Gigaxonin also binds to the ubiquitin-activating enzyme E1 via its N-terminal BTB domain while its C-terminal Kelch domain interacts with the cytoskeletal protein MAP1B-LC (microtubule-associated protein 1B-light chain), leading to degradation of this protein.

Although gigaxonin mutations were discovered by their involvement in giant axonal neuropathy, many

363

cancers contain similar mutations. Gigaxonin mutations are observed in several primary human cancers. These mutations are mostly localized to colon, stomach, endometrium, lung, and skin cancers. Although there are common mutations in giant axonal neuropathy and cancers, there are missense and nonsense mutations found only in cancer. Most of these mutations occur in the BTB-KELCH region in exons 3–5 and 8–11. The function of gigaxonin protein has also been linked to the ubiquitination of NF-κB (nuclear factor κB) in cisplatin-induced senescence of cancer cells. Thus, gigaxonin could be involved in the regulation of NF-κB in the normal cell cycle. As human cancers are affected by the activation of NF-κB, the absence of NF-κB degradation due to gigaxonin mutations could lead to NF-κB-mediated oncogenic signaling in cancer cells.

Diagnosis

The diagnosis can be confirmed by nerve biopsy. Electromyography shows a neurogenic pattern. Peripheral nerve conduction parameters are, in early and intermediate stages of the disease, compatible with moderate to severe sensory motor neuropathy with reduction to absence of sensory action potentials and normal to slightly reduced motor and sensory nerve conduction velocities. In later stages of the disease, motor nerve conduction velocities slow to demyelinating range.

Treatment

There is no effective treatment. Treatment of primary skin fibroblast cultures from affected individuals with an adeno-associated virus type 2 (AAV2) vector containing a normal human GAN transgene significantly reduces the number of cells displaying vimentin IF aggregates. Intracisternal injection of an AAV9/GAN vector has been used in mutant mice to globally deliver the GAN gene to the brainstem and spinal cord. The treated mice showed a nearly complete clearance of peripherin IF accumulations. Intrathecally and intramuscularly administered autologous bone marrow-derived mononuclear cells have been tested in affected individuals.

Bibliography

Kamate M., Ramakrishna S., Kambali S., et al. (2014). Giant axonal neuropathy: A rare inherited neuropathy with simple clinical clues. *BMJ Case Rep*. 2014; pii:bcr2014204481.

Segawa Disease

A 15-year-old boy was evaluated for gait disturbance. His walking difficulty developed at the age of 10 years and progressed gradually. The difficulty was absent after nocturnal sleep but appeared towards the afternoon. Physical exercise worsened the gait disturbance, whereas rest relieved this symptom. Examination revealed dystonia of both feet and bradykinesia of all four extremities. His dystonia was more prominent in the left foot, where it caused pes equinovarus. Cranial MR imaging was normal, as was positron emission tomography using ^{18}F-FP-CIT (fluoropropylcarbomethoxyiodophenylnortropane). A pharmacological test with 100 mg of levodopa plus 25 mg of carbidopa improved the foot dystonia and gait disturbance very significantly.

Segawa Disease

Onset: Action dystonia of the leg at 8–10 years of age that leads to equinovarus foot posturing and impairs walking and balance.

Additional manifestations: Dystonia progresses to segmental or generalized dystonia, but remains most pronounced in the legs. Paroxysmal exercise-induced lower-limb dystonia or recurrent falls. Diurnal fluctuation with dystonia worsening towards the end of the day. Oculogyric crises, waddling gait, generalized hypotonia, and proximal weakness may occur.

Disease mechanism: Autosomal dominant loss of function of GTP cyclohydrolase 1. A more severe autosomal recessive form exists.

Testing: Analysis of cerebrospinal fluid biogenic amines.

Treatment: Levodopa. There may be incomplete responses.

Research highlights: Determination of pterins in urine and phenylalanine loading test for the biochemical diagnosis of GTP-cyclohydrolase 1 deficiency.

Clinical Features

Segawa disease (also known as DYT5a or hereditary progressive dystonia with marked diurnal fluctuation or DOPA-responsive dystonia) is caused by autosomal dominant deficiency of GTP cyclohydrolase 1 (GTP-CH-I), which is encoded by GCH1. The disease typically presents between infancy and adolescence, with an average age of onset of 8 to 11 years. The incidence of autosomal dominant GTP-CH-I is generally reported to be 2.5–4.0-fold greater among females than among males. In males, disease onset tends to be later, the phenotype is often milder and the penetrance of the mutation is lower than in females. Dystonia typically starts in the leg as an action dystonia that leads to equinovarus foot posturing and impairs walking and balance. At the time of diagnosis, some individuals exhibit marked retropulsion in the pull test, which measures postural stability. During the first two decades of life, dystonia typically progresses to segmental or generalized dystonia, but remains most pronounced in the legs. In rare cases, the condition might present as paroxysmal exercise-induced lower-limb dystonia, or as recurrent falls. Diurnal fluctuation is common, with dystonia worsening towards the end of the day. The degree of diurnal fluctuation diminishes with age. Little or no fluctuation may remain by the third decade.

Atypical clinical features of GTP-CH-I deficiency include oculogyric crises, waddling gait, generalized hypotonia, and proximal weakness. Children exhibit brisk tendon reflexes. Other features include ankle clonus, striatal toe (dystonic extension of the big toe in the absence of the Babinski reflex), scoliosis, myoclonus and tics. GTP-CH-I deficiency can also present as parkinsonism that manifests as rigidity, bradykinesia and postural tremor. Parkinsonism is especially common with symptom onset after 15 years of age.

Autosomal recessive GTP-CH-I deficiency is usually more severe than the autosomal dominant disease, and has a more complex neurological presentation with an earlier age of onset. Clinical presentations include truncal hypotonia, neonatal-onset rigidity, tremor, dystonia, spasticity, and oculogyric episodes. Although hyperphenylalaninaemia detected during newborn screening often indicates the diagnosis, this abnormality is not always present in autosomal recessive GTP-CH-I deficiency. Compound heterozygous mutations in GCH1 lead to an intermediate severity of symptoms and earlier disease onset than in autosomal dominant GTP-CH-I deficiency.

Pathology

There is no of degeneration in the striatum or substantia nigra in GTP-CH-I deficiency (Figure 89.1). However, dopamine levels are reduced in the nigrostriatal terminals and preserved in the pars compacta of the substantia nigra. In addition, total biopterin and neopterin concentrations are decreased in the putamen, caudate and frontal cortex. Tyrosine hydroxylase levels are markedly decreased in the putamen

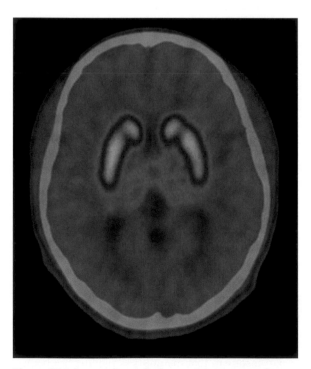

Figure 89.1 Segawa disease. Positron emission tomography using ^{18}F-FP-CIT (fluoropropylcarbomethoxyiodophenylnortropane) shows normal dopamine transporter activity in the striatum bilaterally. Reproduced with permission from Kim JI et al. A novel missense mutation in GCH1 gene in a Korean family with Segawa disease. *Brain Dev.* 2015; 37(3):359–61.

with GTP-CH-I deficiency relative to levels in the caudate. Tyrosine hydroxylase levels in the substantia nigra are normal.

Pathophysiology

Several disorders in addition to Segawa disease cause the syndrome of DOPA-responsive dystonia (DRD). The majority of cases with DRD exhibit a deficiency in an enzyme involved in the biosynthesis of dopamine. Deficiencies in GTP-CH-I or sepiapterin reductase can lead to DRD, as they disrupt the biosynthesis of tetrahydrobiopterin (BH4), which is an essential cofactor for tryptophan hydroxylase and phenylalanine hydroxylase. Deficiencies in tyrosine hydroxylase can also lead to DRD, as this enzyme mediates the initial and rate-limiting step in the synthesis of dopamine. Not all deficiencies in enzymes that are involved in the biosynthesis of dopamine lead to DRD.

As the enzyme responsible for the synthesis of BH4, GCH-1 deficiency may affect tryptophan hydroxylase (TPH) as well as tyrosine hydroxylase (TH). There is a difference of enzyme Km value for TH and TPH. With heterozygous mutations, BH4 decreases partially in Segawa disease. Thus TH, which exhibits a higher affinity to BH4, is affected relatively selectively. However, in the context of a marked decrease in BH4, TPH is affected as well and this may produce symptoms induced by dysfunction of serotonergic neurons.

Diagnosis

Analysis of the levels of neurotransmitters and metabolites (such as homovanillic acid, 5-hydroxyindoleacetic acid, neopterin and biopterin) in cerebrospinal fluid and phenylalanine in blood can distinguish between different types of DRD.

The value of PET and SPECT studies is limited in the diagnosis of DRD, but they might enable differentiation between DRD and juvenile Parkinson's disease. In juvenile Parkinson's disease, fluorodopa uptake and dopamine transporter density are reduced, whereas abnormalities in these parameters are minimal in DRD. Fluorodopa uptake is typically reduced by a mean of 50% in the putamen and 16% in the caudate in Parkinson's disease relative to healthy controls. By contrast, mean reductions in uptake in individuals with DRD are 18% in the putamen and 9% in the caudate.

Cultured skin fibroblasts have been used as a diagnostic tool. Activity of GTP-CH-I and intracellular concentrations of neopterin and biopterin (which also indicate GTP-CH-I activity) in cytokine-stimulated fibroblasts are particularly informative parameters.

Treatment

Levodopa treatment in individuals with GCH1 mutations typically produces a favorable response. Levodopa, usually combined with a peripheral decarboxylase inhibitor (carbidopa), is often sufficient for almost complete resolution of neurological deficits. Even if levodopa therapy is delayed for many years, most individuals still respond to small doses of this agent. Controlled-release levodopa, dopamine agonists and anticholinergic drugs such as trihexyphenidyl can also be effective.

Autosomal recessive GTP-CH-I deficiency also responds to levodopa therapy. In early childhood, treatment may require greater doses than does treatment of the autosomal dominant form. Individuals with homozygous or compound heterozygous GCH1 mutations might require additional treatment with BH4 and 5-hydroxytryptophan (5-HTP, the precursor of serotonin). In many cases, clinical features such as writer's cramp and laryngeal dystonia are insufficiently controlled by levodopa treatment; for these symptoms, additional treatment with botulinum toxin, for example, might be required.

Levodopa-related motor complications, which frequently occur in individuals with PD, are uncommon in persons with GTP-CH-I deficiency. Even after long-term use of levodopa, wearing off rarely occurs. When levodopa-induced dyskinesia does occur, it usually presents at the initiation of treatment and is the result of unusually high doses. As in Parkinson's disease, amantadine can suppress levodopa-induced dyskinesia in GTP-CH-I deficiency.

Bibliography

Kim J.I., Choi J.K., Lee J.W., et al. (2015). A novel missense mutation in GCH1 gene in a Korean family with Segawa disease. *Brain Dev.*37(3):359–61.

Rodan L.H., Gibson K.M., Pearl P.L. (2015). Clinical use of CSF Neurotransmitters. *Pediatr Neurol.* 53(4):277–86.

Biotin-Thiamine Responsive Basal Ganglia Disease

A 1-month-old boy was evaluated for a 3-day history of poor feeding, vomiting, and irritability. He was the first son of consanguineous parents. After a monitored and uneventful pregnancy, the child was delivered at 38 weeks by emergent cesarean delivery due to a suspicion of fetal distress. He remained, however, asymptomatic until 1 month. Examination showed a small child; his weight was 3.570 g (6th percentile), and his head circumference was 36.5 cm (20th percentile). He was lethargic and displayed intermittent opisthotonus, jitteriness in the upper limbs, hyperreflexia and clonus in all limbs, decreased palmar and plantar grasp reflexes, and an exaggerated Moro reflex. Blood testing illustrated metabolic acidosis (venous pH: 7.30, pCO$_2$: 37 mm Hg, base excess: –6.4), together with elevated lactate levels in blood (8.6 mM; reference: 0.7–2.4) and cerebrospinal fluid (7.1 mM; reference: 1.1–2.2). MR imaging 24 hours later revealed symmetric cortico-subcortical lesions involving the perirolandic area, bilateral putamina, and medial thalami. Thiamine, biotin, and carnitine were started. This was followed by a profound clinical and biochemical improvement within hours: irritability and feeding difficulties ceased, opisthotonus disappeared, and alertness returned. After 48 hours, blood lactate levels decreased and acidosis resolved. He was discharged after 6 days of hospitalization with a normal physical examination except for a mild increase in tone in the lower limbs. At 6 months of age, he remained normal except for a mild increase in upper limb tone and for asymmetric fine motor skills with impaired palmar grasp and thumb adduction of the right hand.

Biotin-Thiamine Responsive Basal Ganglia Disease

Onset: Sudden severe encephalopathy in childhood (1 month–8 years of age), often following an antecedent minor illness or injury.

Additional manifestations: Dystonia may be generalized and severe. Seizures. MR imaging demonstrates dorsal striatal and medial thalamic lesions that progress to necrosis and atrophy. Recurrences may occur.

Disease mechanism: Deficient transport of thiamine due to transporter mutation. Thiamine is a cofactor of pyruvate dehydrogenase, α-ketoglutarate dehydrogenase and branched-chain α-keto acid dehydrogenase.

Testing: Elevated lactate and increased α-ketoglutarate excretion. Free thiamine is decreased.

Treatment: Thiamine and biotin.

Research highlights: Regulation of intestinal thiamine transport by the substrate level via transcriptional regulation involving SP1 transcription factor.

Clinical Features

Biotin-thiamine responsive basal ganglia disease, also known as thiamine metabolism dysfunction syndrome-2 or thiamine transporter-2 deficiency is caused by autosomal recessive mutation of SLC19A3, which encodes a biotin transporter that does not transport thiamine.

Children may exhibit recurrent subacute episodes of encephalopathy including seizures, ataxia, dystonia, dysarthria, external ophthalmoplegia, or dysphagia. The median age of onset is 3 years, with range between 1 month and 3 years. The initial manifestations may progress to quadriparesis and coma. These episodes are often precipitated by trauma or febrile illnesses.

Pathology

Symmetric lesions in the cortex, basal ganglia, thalami, or periaqueductal gray matter have been illustrated by MR imaging and may resemble Leigh syndrome (Figure 90.1 and 90.2). These lesions can progress to necrosis and atrophy. However, the most characteristic pattern of involvement includes the dorsal striatum and medial thalami. The lesions, however, can be reversed with early treatment. In young infants, a perirolandic cortical pattern of injury may be related to the higher glucose metabolic rate of these structures typical of early infancy.

Pathophysiology

Thiamine is a vitamin that accumulates in tissues following transport across the cell membrane via one of two thiamine transporters: hTHTR1 (encoded by the SLC19A2 gene) and hTHTR2 (encoded by the SLC19A3 gene). Mutations in these genes lead to cellular thiamine deficiency. The distribution of hTHTR1 and hTHTR2 may explain the phenotypes associated with each gene mutation, which include thiamine-responsive megaloblastic anemia and biotin-thiamine responsive basal ganglia disease, respectively.

Thiamine-diphosphate, the active vitamer of thiamine, is an essential cofactor of three mitochondrial enzymes: pyruvate dehydrogenase, α-ketoglutarate dehydrogenase, and branched-chain α-keto acid dehydrogenase. These enzymes are involved in the oxidative decarboxylation of pyruvate, α-ketoglutarate, and branched-chain amino acids, respectively.

Diagnosis

Increased α-ketoglutarate excretion is characteristic of the disease, in addition to decreased free thiamine. However, the former is also seen in thiamine pyrophosphokinase deficiency and in mitochondrial thiamine pyrophosphate transporter SLC25A19 deficiency.

Treatment

Thiamine and biotin supplementation is associated with reversion of clinical, radiological and biochemical findings when instituted before necrosis sets in.

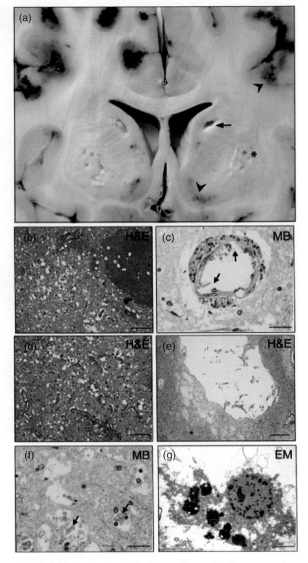

Figure 90.1 Brain autopsy findings in biotin-thiamine-responsive basal ganglia disease. **a.** Midfrontal section demonstrating acute hemorrhagic lesions in the caput nuclei caudati and cortical layer (arrowheads), subacute necrotic lesions in the putamen (asterix) and old cystic lesions in the caudate nucleus (arrow). **b.** Histology of the basal ganglia showing acute lesions with edema of the brain parenchyma with focal hemorrhage. **c.** Semithin section revealing vascular leakage, perivascular edema and hemorrhage caused by drop off of endothelial cells (arrows). **d,e.** Histology of the basal ganglia demonstrating subacute and chronic lesions with gliosis, neovascularization, and old cystic areas. **f,g.** Semithin section and electron microscopy confirming acute neuronal damage (arrows). Bars= 200μm in b,d,e; Bars= 50μm in c,f. Reproduced with permission from Schänzer A et al. Stress-induced upregulation of SLC19A3 is impaired in biotin-thiamine-responsive basal ganglia disease. *Brain Pathol.* 2014; 24(3):270–9.

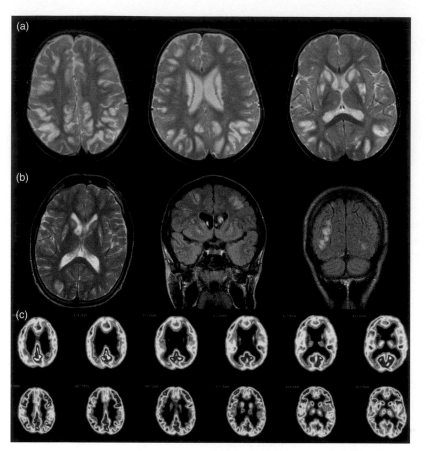

Figure 90.2 a: axial T2 weighted MRI of biotin-thiamine-responsive basal ganglia disease taken during an episode with seizures, increasing encephalopathy and exacerbation of dystonia. Images show bilateral high T2-signal changes and swelling in the putamen and caudate head. In addition there are multiple cortical lesions preferentially occurring in the depths of sulci, which is typical of the disorder. b: axial T2 and coronal T2-FLAIR weighted MRI of patient 1 taken during an episodic exacerbation show a similar pattern with bilateral striatal and multiple cortical lesions. The signal abnormalities regressed completely on later scans (not shown). c (upper lane): FDG-PET scan of the brain of patient 1 taken ~5 years later shows multiple foci of decreased glucose metabolism that correlate to the localization of the transient cortical signal changes on MRI. The striatum shows minimal uptake consistent with severe neuronal loss. A normal scan is shown in the lower lane for comparison. Reproduced with permission from Flønes I et al. Novel SLC19A3 Promoter Deletion and Allelic Silencing in Biotin-Thiamine-Responsive Basal Ganglia Encephalopathy. *PLoS One.* 2016; 11(2): e0149055.

Bibliography

Ortigoza-Escobar J.D., Molero-Luis M., Arias A., et al. (2016). Free-thiamine is a potential biomarker of thiamine transporter-2 deficiency: a treatable cause of Leigh syndrome. *Brain.* 139(Pt 1):31–8.

Pérez-Dueñas B., Serrano M., Rebollo M., et al. (2013). Reversible lactic acidosis in a newborn with thiamine transporter-2 deficiency. *Pediatrics.* 131(5): e1670–5.

Rasmussen Encephalitis

A 7-year-old right-handed girl presented with a simple partial seizure arising in the left foot lasting two minutes with an associated postictal paralysis. An initial routine electroencephalogram (EEG) was normal. One month later, she suffered a secondarily generalized seizure upon awakening with onset in the left foot. Repeat EEG showed vertex spikes and was interpreted as Rolandic epilepsy. Magnetic resonance imaging was unremarkable. She began receiving oxcarbazepine. Eight weeks later, her left leg twitching became continuous, even during sleep. Four months after onset, she had failed treatment with bolus doses of phenobarbital, phenytoin, and levetiracetam and was diagnosed with epilepsia partialis continua while being administered maintenance phenytoin and oxcarbazepine. Neurological examination five months after onset showed constant left leg and pelvic twitching and intermittent stiffening of the left arm. Sensory examination showed agraphesthesia and reduced two point discrimination on the dorsum of the left arm. She exhibited left hemiparesis with a tight left heel cord, inability to tandem walk, circumduction of the left leg while walking, and posturing of the left arm during running. She was treated unsuccessfully with intravenous immunoglobulin.

Rasmussen Encephalitis

Onset: Focal seizures in late childhood or adolescence that may evolve to epilepsia partialis continua or status epilepticus.
Additional manifestations: Progressive cerebral hemispheric atrophy with intractable focal-onset epilepsy. Cognitive impairment and motor deficit. Hemiparesis, hemidystonia, or hemiathetosis
Disease mechanism: Antibody-mediated pathogenesis, either through a direct excitotoxic mechanism or by activating the complement cascade.

Testing: MR imaging illustrates focal cortical atrophy, ipsilateral ventricular enlargement, increased T2 and FLAIR signals, and T2 hyperintensity or atrophy of the head of the caudate nucleus. Biopsy demonstrates T-cell infiltration.
Treatment: Anticonvulsants are of limited efficacy. Immunosuppression. Hemispherectomy.
Research highlights: B cell-depleting therapy reduces epilepsy.

Clinical Features

Rasmussen encephalitis is an acquired disease that progressively affects one cerebral hemisphere. It is characterized by hemispheric brain inflammation resulting in unilateral brain atrophy. There are drug-resistant focal seizures, worsening unilateral motor deficits and cognitive decline. The process can be halted only by the resection or isolation of the affected hemisphere. Rasmussen encephalitis typically starts in childhood or early adolescence, with a mean age at presentation of 6 years. The onset is marked, in almost all cases, by focal or secondarily generalized seizures. Exceptionally, seizure onset is preceded by slowly progressive hemiparesis, hemidystonia, or hemiathetosis. Seizures are in most cases polymorphic: besides simple motor seizures, virtually all types of focal seizures may occur. The frequency of the seizures, which are refractory to antiepileptic drugs, usually increases rapidly and partial status epilepticus may recur. In about half of children there is epilepsia partialis continua. Hemiparesis invariably develops during the course of the disease; it is initially limited to the postictal phase and then it rapidly becomes permanent, albeit fluctuating in severity, and worsens with increasing seizure activity. With time, hemiparesis, which may be associated with dystonia, stabilizes. Additional neurological symptoms include hemianopia, cortical sensory loss, and aphasia, when the dominant hemisphere is affected.

Cognitive impairment is a constant feature of Rasmussen encephalitis and, as is the case for motor deficit, may be subtle at the beginning. Behavioral changes with irritability, emotional lability, or hyperactivity often herald the first signs of mental decline. This consists mainly of memory and attention disorders and learning difficulties. In most affected individuals, the progression of mental impairment seems to correlate with the severity of the epilepsy, particularly with the bilateral spread of electroencephalographic epileptic abnormalities.

The disease course is progressive. The natural history can be summarized in three stages: a) a prodromal stage, lasting from months to 8 years, during which seizures occur infrequently; b) an acute stage – which in a significant proportion of cases occurs near the onset of disease – with frequent seizures, often in the form of epilepsia partialis continua or status epilepticus and rapid neurological deterioration; c) a residual stage with fixed neurological deficits, and persisting, albeit less frequent, attacks.

Pathology

Magnetic resonance imaging changes include mild focal cortical atrophy involving the insular and peri-insular regions, ipsilateral ventricular enlargement, increased cortical or subcortical T2 and FLAIR signals and T2 hyperintensity or atrophy of the head of the caudate nucleus (Figure 91.1). These changes are preceded by transient focal cortical swelling. Gadolinium enhancement is not observed. Unilateral cortical and caudate atrophy progressively worsen during the course of the disease. Functional imaging demonstrates, even in the early stages, areas of glucose hypometabolism on fluorodeoxyglucose-positron emission tomography (FDG-PET), interictal hemispheric hypoperfusion and ictal multifocal hyperperfusion on single photon emission computed tomography (SPECT) and unilateral reduction of N-acetylaspartate, with increased lactate and choline on magnetic resonance spectroscopy.

Biopsy demonstrates multifocal changes of T cell-dominated encephalitis with activated microglia and reactive gliosis. There is also neuronal loss and astrogliosis restricted to the affected hemisphere. Infiltrating T cells include CD8+ cells containing granules positive for granzyme B+ and part of these cells are in close contact with major histocompatibility class

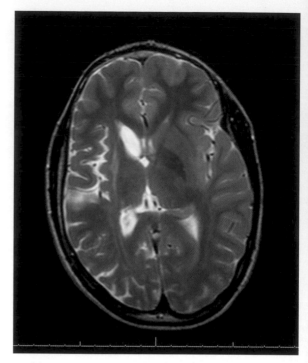

Figure 91.1 Rasmussen encephalitis affecting the right cerebral hemisphere in a child with intractable focal epilepsy.

I positive neurons. Granzyme B is a protease released by activated cytotoxic T cells into target cells that undergo apoptosis. This set of features is considered evidence of a cytotoxic T cell attack against neurons. Astrocytic apoptosis and loss is observed within the cortex and white matter. Granzyme B+ lymphocytes are found in close contact with astrocytes with granules polarized toward the astrocytic membranes suggesting that astrocytes might be a target for T cells leading to astrocytic degeneration. Degeneration of astrocytes might enhance neuronal loss.

Pathophysiology

The disease mechanism is not fully understood, though it has been identified as a chronic inflammatory process. The initiating event is unknown: a viral infection, as originally proposed based on similarities with other known forms of chronic encephalitis, still remains a plausible hypothesis, but has not been proven. The possibility of an immune-mediated pathogenesis was raised when rabbits immunized with a recombinant fragment of the glutamate receptor (GluR3) developed seizures and inflammatory changes similar to those of Rasmussen encephalitis. However, antiGluR3 antibodies may be found in other severe forms of epilepsy and other antibodies directed against antigens of brain resident cells (the presynaptic protein Munc18-1 (mammalian uncoordinated-18-1)), NMDA-GluRε2, and anti-α7 neuronal acetylcholine receptors (nAChR)) are found in affected individuals. These studies reinforced the hypothesis of antibody-mediated pathogenesis, either through a direct excitotoxic mechanism or by activating the complement cascade. However, it is likely that the presence of circulating antibodies could be secondary to the cerebral damage and that humoral immunity is not the primary factor. Cell-mediated immunity may involve cytotoxic T cells causing apoptotic cell death.

Diagnosis

Electroencephalographic changes at onset are confined to the affected hemisphere and consist of slowing of background activity and sleep disorganization, focal slow and epileptic abnormalities, early evidence of ictal and interictal hemispheric multifocal abnormalities, and the appearance of subclinical ictal discharges. Over time, there is further deterioration, the epileptic activity increases and tends to spread, and involves the unaffected hemisphere as well. Seizure onset, however, though multifocal, remains unilateral. MR imaging changes described earlier are characteristic. Cerebrospinal fluid oligoclonal bands are found in about half of affected individuals. The presence of anti-GluR3 is not specific for the diagnosis, since it does not discriminate between Rasmussen encephalitis and other epilepsies. Brain biopsy illustrates characteristic changes.

Treatment

Antiepileptic drugs have no effect on epilepsia partialis continua and only a limited effect on isolated seizures. The only effective surgical approach is the exclusion of the affected hemisphere by hemispherotomy. This remains the only treatment able to control seizures as well as further mental deterioration in over 80 percent of affected individuals. Immunomodulatory treatments are employed either in the short term for alleviation of seizures and as chronic treatment with the aim of preventing immune-mediated brain damage. Corticosteroids are the most widely used, and probably the most effective, therapy. Intravenous immunoglobulin efficacy has been reported in a proportion of children and adults. Plasmapheresis or immunoadsorption have been used with the rationale of removing pathogenic circulating antibodies. A significant effect in blocking status epilepticus and neurological deterioration has been reported in a few individuals, whereas evidence of long-term efficacy has been noted only exceptionally. Tacrolimus, a T cell inhibiting drug, has been used based on the growing evidence of the role of granzyme B-mediated T cell cytotoxicity. Although no immunotreated subjects develop intractable epilepsy, this therapy is not effective in controlling seizures in individuals with established drug-resistant seizures. Rituximab, a monoclonal antibody that binds to the surface glycoprotein CD20 and coats B cells causing their depletion, has been effective on epilepsy activity.

Bibliography

Granata T., Andermann F. (2013). Rasmussen encephalitis. *Handb Clin Neurol.* 111:511–19.

Holec M., Nagahama Y., Kovach C., et al. (2016). Rethinking the Magnetic Resonance Imaging Findings in Early Rasmussen Encephalitis: A Case Report and Review of the Literature.*Pediatr Neurol.* 59:85–9.

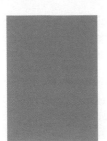

Adolescent Disorders

Wilson Disease

A 14-year-old girl presented with a 6-month history of insidious onset and gradually progressive decline in scholastic performance, loss of motor skills, difficulty in ambulation, abnormal posturing, speech disturbances and behavioral abnormalities accompanying a steady cognitive decline. There was no evidence of jaundice or portal hypertension on clinical history of the girl or similar illnesses in the family. Examination revealed slow, dysarthric, and nonfluent speech, impaired attention, abstract thinking, and judgment along with rigidity, dystonia (lead pipe) bradykinesia, and bilateral Babinski signs. Further testing illustrated microcytic hypochromic anemia with mild thrombocytopenia. Peripheral blood smear showed target cells and thrombocytopenia. Liver function tests were suggestive of mild hyperbilirubinemia; alkaline phosphatase was also increased and alanine transaminase and aspartate transaminase levels were normal. Hypoalbuminemia and elevated prothrombin time were also noted.

Wilson Disease

Onset: Liver dysfunction at 10–13 years of age. Adults can present one or two decades later with psychiatric symptoms.

Additional manifestations: Neurological in 40% of cases; hepatic in 40% and psychiatric in 20%. Among these, extrapyramidal symptoms, liver failure and cirrhosis, personality disturbances, depression and schizophrenia are common.

Disease mechanism: Failure of copper incorporation into many proteins with impact on hepatic transcription, nuclear receptor signaling, stress-response proteins and RNA processing that alter lipid metabolism and cell cycle regulation.

Testing: Corneal Kaiser–Fleischer ring. Decreased ceruloplasmin in blood and increased elemental copper in urine or liver.

Treatment: Chelation with penicillamine or trientine. Zinc blocks intestinal copper absorption. Ammonium tetrathiomolybdate exerts similar effects. Hepatic transplantation is used in severe hepatopathy.

Research highlights: Delivery of copper to target cells using chaperones, transporters, and a COX17 protein.

Clinical Features

Wilson disease or hepatolenticular degeneration is characterized by cirrhosis and neurodegeneration associated with autosomal deficiency of the copper transporter WND, encoded by ATP7B, a P-type ATPase cation pump. Disease prevalence is 1 in 33,000.

The age of onset is as variable as the disease severity, but many children present at 10–13 years of age. Forty percent of individuals present with hepatic disease, 40% with neurological manifestations, and 20% with psychiatric disorders.

Liver disease consists of mild elevations in blood transaminases and chronic active hepatitis on liver biopsy. Fatigue, malaise, arthropathy and rashes may be present. Acute hepatitis and liver failure resemble viral hepatitis except that hemolytic anemia due to coper toxicity may be superimposed. The hepatopathy ultimately progresses to nodular cirrhosis, fatty liver and hepatic failure.

The neurological manifestations include movement disorder with tremors, incoordination, poor fine motor function and chorea, and ultimately include dystonia and parkinsonism, with mask facies, bradykinesia, and impaired gait.

Psychiatric symptoms can precede or accompany hepatic or neurological manifestations, including personality changes, depression, or schizophrenia.

(a)

(b)

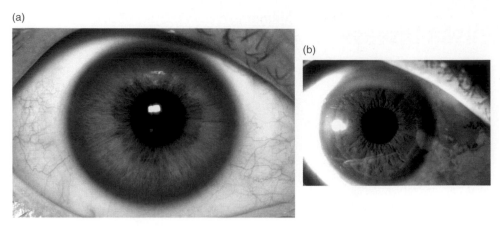

Figure 92.1 a and b. Kayser–Fleischer rings in Wilson disease. Reproduced with permission from Walshe JM. The eye in Wilson disease. *QJM*. 2011; 104(5):451–3.

Additional less common symptoms may include renal Fanconi syndrome, nephrolithiasis, cardiomyopathy, pancreatitis, anemia, arthritis rhabdomyolysis, hypoparathyroidism, and dysmenorrhea.

Pathology

In addition to hepatic changes, the brain displays copper deposition with a predilection for the basal ganglia. These structures exhibit cavitation, gliosis, and neuronal loss. Severe corticosubcortical changes consisting of myelin degeneration, gliosis, and neuronal loss in the deep cortical layers may also occur. The gyri of the frontal convexity are prone to cavitating lesions of the subcortical white matter.

Pathophysiology

The ATPases associated with Wilson (ATP7B) and Menkes (ATP7A) diseases are homologous and contain a copper-binding and transport region. ATP7B is highly expressed in the liver. The copper transporters mediate the transfer of copper between chaperones line HAH1 (human Atx1p homologue) to the Golgi secretory pathway, which incorporates essential copper into many proteins. This has widespread consequences on hepatic transcription, nuclear receptor signaling including SREBP-1 (sterol regulatory element-binding transcription factor 1) and LXR/RXR (liver X receptor/ retinoid X receptor) receptors, stress-response proteins, and RNA processing that exert an impact on lipid metabolism and cell cycle regulation.

Early features of the hepatic disease are dilation of liver cells progressing to inflammation mediated by NF-κB (nuclear factor-κB). Excess copper is soon followed by increased protein degradation and metallothionein protein accumulation. Triglycerides, free cholesterol, and cholesteryl ester accumulate in the liver.

In the brain, copper accumulation leads to mitochondrial dysfunction such that neurological and psychiatric symptoms are primary rather than secondary to hepatic disease.

Diagnosis

The corneal Kayser–Fleischer ring is not universally seen in children and is also characteristic of other disorders (Figure 92.1). Decreased copper–binding ceruloplasmin in blood and increased elemental copper in urine or liver establish the diagnosis, although cirrhosis interfering with biliary excretion leads to increased hepatic copper content.

Treatment

Chelation is used for less severely affected individuals, whereas hepatic transplantation is performed in more severe disease cases with advanced inflammatory disease of the liver. Penicillamine and trientine are effective chelators and increase urinary copper excretion. Zinc blocks the intestinal absorption of copper and is also used to stimulate the production of metallothioneins that enhance the cytoplasmic sequestration of accumulated copper. Ammonium tetrathiomolybdate blocks intestinal copper absorption when taken with meals and binds to plasma copper when taken between meals. This medication may be more effective than other chelators for the neuropsychiatric forms of the disease.

Bibliography

Patell R., Dosi R., Joshi H.K., et al. (2014). Atypical neuroimaging in Wilson's disease. *BMJ Case Rep.* 2014. pii:bcr2013200100.

Neurodegeneration with Brain Iron Accumulation

An 18-year-old man presented with an insidious, slowly progressive psychomotor disorder that included gait impairment, clumsiness, dysarthria, and progressive cognitive deficits. Initial symptoms consisted of general clumsiness along with impaired motor and scholastic development. Some of these manifestations might have been present as early as 3 years of age. During the course of the disease, gait disturbance from severe spasticity of the lower limbs became prominent. Examination revealed cognitive impairment, generalized dystonia, dysarthria, optic atrophy, and saccadization of pursuit. MR imaging of the brain illustrated Bilateral T2 hypointensity in the globus pallidus and substantia nigra, no eye-of-the-tiger sign, and T1 hyperintensity in the caudate nucleus and putamen. Genotyping revealed a mutation in open-reading frame 12 on chromosome 19 (C19orf12), associated with mitochondrial membrane protein-associated neurodegeneration with brain iron accumulation.

Neurodegeneration with Brain Iron Accumulation

Onset: Childhood to adult extrapyramidal dysfunction with hyper- or hypokinetic movement disorder.

Additional manifestations: Spasticity, parkinsonism, dystonia, dyskinesia, and neuropathy. Dementia, depression, and visual hallucinations can be prominent in select forms of this disorder.

Disease mechanism: Iron accumulation can lead to excess production of reactive oxygen species. This causes damage to proteins and aggregation of damaged, misfolded proteins that gather within intracellular inclusion bodies.

Testing: MR imaging illustrates pallidal and nigral iron deposition and nerve biopsy demonstrates spheroids in some disease forms. Genetic analysis definitive in 2/3 of cases.

Treatment: None effective.

Research highlights: Elucidation of a potential common final pathway leading to basal ganglia iron accumulation induced by which primary disruption of lipid metabolism, mitochondrial function, coenzyme A biosynthesis, or autophagy.

Clinical Features

The generic term neurodegeneration with brain iron accumulation designates several heterogeneous disorders characterized by neuroaxonal dystrophy in association with accumulation of brain iron. Several causative genes have been identified in about 65 percent of cases. Pantothenate kinase-associated neurodegeneration, infantile neuroaxonal dystrophy, and aceruloplasminemia are discussed in separate chapters. A common feature of these diseases is iron deposition in the pallidum and, to a lesser extent, the substantia nigra, which is detectable by MR imaging. This leads to a hyper or hypokinetic movement disorder that is commonly associated with pyramidal tract dysfunction. The principal neurodegeneration with brain iron accumulation disorders are summarized here.

The mode of inheritance of these disorders is autosomal recessive, except for neuroferritinopathy, which is inherited in autosomal dominant fashion and for beta-propeller protein-associated neurodegeneration, which is an X-linked disease.

In MPAN (mitochondrial membrane protein-associated neurodegeneration), onset includes childhood dysarthria with gait disturbance followed by lower limb spasticity, dystonia, parkinsonism, motor axonal neuropathy, optic atrophy and psychiatric disturbances.

BPAN (beta-propeller protein-associated neurodegeneration or static encephalopathy of childhood

Table 93.1 Neurodegenerations with brain iron accumulation

Disease name	Disease symbol	Gene symbol	Gene name
Pantothenate kinase-associated neurodegeneration	NBIA1	PANK2	Pantothenate kinase 2
Infantile neuroaxonal dystrophy	NBIA2	PLA2G6	Phospholipase A2, group VI
Aceruloplasminemia		CP	Ceruloplasmin
Mitochondrial membrane protein-associated neurodegeneration	MPAN	C19orf12	Chromosome 19 open reading frame 12
Beta-propeller protein-associated neurodegeneration or static encephalopathy of childhood with neurodegeneration in adulthood	BPAN or SENDA	WDR45	WD (tryptophan-aspartic acid) repeat domain phosphoinositide-interacting protein 4
Kufor–Rakeb disease	NBIA3 or PARK9	ATP13A2	ATPase type 13A2
FA2H-associated neurodegeneration	FAHN	FA2H	Fatty acid 2-hydrolase
Neuroferritinopathy		FTL	Ferritin light chain
Coenzyme A synthase protein–associated neurodegeneration	CoPAN	COASY	Coenzyme A synthase protein
Woodhouse–Sakati syndrome		DCAF17	DDB1 (damaged DNA binding protein 1) and CUL4 (cullin 4A) associated factor 17

with neurodegeneration in adulthood) is characterized by a first phase with statically impaired childhood neurological development that evolves into a latter abrupt phase of dopa-responsive parkinsonism, dystonia, dementia, and spasticity. In some cases, comparisons have been made with Rett and Angelman syndromes.

Kufor–Rakeb disease leads to adolescent onset parkinsonism with pyramidal tract dysfunction. Incomplete supranuclear gaze palsy may be present. Oculogyric crises, myoclonus, and dysautonomia may be associated features. Psychiatric disturbances include visual hallucinations. Dementia ensues in late stages.

FA2H-associated neurodegeneration is associated with childhood onset gait dysfunction, spastic quadriparesis, ataxia, and dystonia. Seizures may occur.

Neuroferritinopathy may present from adolescence to the sixth decade, commonly with radiological features of iron deposition in the basal ganglia and cystic degeneration. In neuroferritinopathy, characteristic chorea, stereotypies and dystonia may resemble Huntington disease. There is orolingual and mandibular dyskinesia and blefarosplasm. Parkinsonism may be present, but pyramidal tract dysfunction

and ataxia are usually absent. Dementia, depression, and psychosis are also associated features.

In coenzyme A synthase protein–associated neurodegeneration, there is progressive motor and cognitive dysfunction beginning in childhood or early adulthood in association with extrapyramidal signs with dystonia, spasticity, and parkinsonism.

Woodhouse–Sakati syndrome is characterized by hypogonadism, alopecia, diabetes mellitus, mental retardation, and extrapyramidal dysfunction.

Pathology

In the neurodegeneration with brain iron accumulation disorders, astrocytic and neuronal degeneration are common. This is associated with pallidal and nigral iron deposition.

In Kufor–Rakeb disease, peripheral nerve changes consist of Schwann cell inclusions of possible lysosomal origin. A mouse model for the disease displays neuronal ceroid lipofuscinosis.

Neuroferritinopathy is characterized by the presence of iron/ferritin bodies, which are eosinophilic and contain ferritin and iron. In cases associated with a mutation type particularly common in Cumbria,

United Kingdom, these bodies accumulate in the basal ganglia and especially in the globus pallidus. Iron/ferritin bodies appear first in oligodendrocytes and later emerge in all brain cell types. There is also cystic degeneration of the pallidum. Individuals with this mutation also display a dentatorubropalidoluysian pattern of degeneration. In other mutation types, pathological changes are more prominent in the cerebellum.

Pathophysiology

Elevated iron levels are characteristic of aging as well as of several disorders that include Alzheimer disease, Parkinson disease, Huntington disease and Friedreich ataxia. Iron can produce reactive oxygen species (ROS) via two reactions: Ferrous iron can react with oxygen, creating hydrogen peroxide accompanied by a superoxide radical and ferrous iron can react with hydrogen peroxide, generating hydroxyl free radicals. Because of its ability to produce ROS, increased iron levels are neurotoxic by inducing excess oxidation, which eventually leads to cellular death. This metal-based neurodegeneration is accompanied by several effects, including the generation of reactive aldehydes through the peroxidation of polyunsaturated fatty acids in membrane phospholipids by ROS, generation of carbonyl functions by posttranslational protein modification via reactive aldehydes as well as ROS and subsequent damage to proteins and aggregation of damaged, misfolded proteins that gather within intracellular inclusion bodies, as occurs in several neurodegenerative diseases.

In MPAN, expression studies have revealed coregulation of C19orf12 with genes associated with two pathways, fatty acid biogenesis and branched-chain amino acid (valine, leucine and isoleucine) degradation, representing mitochondrial processes related to coenzyme A metabolism.

WDR45, which is associated with BPAN, is a member of the WD40 repeat protein family, a group of proteins that facilitate the assembly of multiprotein complexes and are key components in many biological processes including the cell cycle, signal transduction, apoptosis and gene regulation. A link of WDR45 to autophagy is based on its ability to bind two autophagy-related proteins, ATG2A and ATG2B (autophagy related 2A and 2B, respectively). Lymphoblastoid cell lines of BPAN individuals with decreased WDR45 protein expression exhibit lower autophagic activity and accumulation of aberrant early autophagic structures.

In Kufor–Rakeb disease, mutant ATP13A2 is retained in the endoplasmic reticulum and then degraded by the proteasome. This can induce endoplasmic reticulum dysfunction, as confirmed by the increased expression of unfolded protein response–related genes. ATP13A2-deficient cells display an accumulation of mitochondria that show increased fragmentation, with simultaneously elevated oxygen consumption, unchanged ATP production and increased mitochondrially derived ROS. Thus, defective lysosomal function, overburdening of the proteasomal degradation by concentration of misfolded proteins in the endoplasmic reticulum and impaired mitochondrial quality control through autophagic dysfunction may contribute to the disorder.

FA2H mutations have also been reported in familial leukodystrophy and hereditary spastic paraplegia SPG35. In addition to participating in myelination, FA2H acts as a regulator of the mobility of raft-associated lipids. Lipid rafts consist of cholesterol and sphingolipids functioning in membrane signaling and trafficking and their mobility is increased following FA2H depletion. Furthermore, FA2H-mediated hydroxylation affects intracellular trafficking of membrane proteins for lysosomal degradation. Thus, FA2H deficiency leads to changes in the 2-hydroxylated sphingolipid profile, which may exert secondary effects on the physical properties of lipid membranes.

In neuroferritinopathy, there is an increase in ubiquitinated proteins and redistribution of proteasome components to the site of ferritin inclusions. The mouse model of the disease also exhibits altered gene expression profiles for proteins involved in iron homeostasis, including decreased TfR-1 (the mouse orthologue of human transferrin receptor) and Irp1 (the mouse orthologue of human iron regulatory protein 1) as well as markers of excessive oxidation such as lipid peroxidation products, oxidatively modified proteins and protein radicals.

Fibroblasts from CoPAN individuals exhibit a reduction in COASY protein expression together with a reduction of acetyl-coenzyme A and total coenzyme A. An increase or decrease of cytosolic acetyl-coenzyme A results in the suppression or induction of autophagy, respectively, implicating cytosolic acetyl-CoA as a metabolic regulator of autophagy.

Diagnosis

The diagnosis can be suggested by the presence of characteristic iron accumulation detected by MR imaging and spheroids on nerve biopsy for some of these disorders. Genetic analysis is usually definitive.

Treatment

There is no effective treatment. Iron chelators, particularly the blood–brain barrier-crossing compound deferiprone, are capable of decreasing cerebral iron in areas with abnormally high concentrations as documented by MR imaging. However, there is no definitive evidence of the clinical effect of iron removal therapy. The induction of stereotactic lesions in the thalamus or pallidum or deep brain stimulation may afford symptomatic relief in about 30 percent of affected individuals.

Bibliography

Dusek P., Schneider S.A., Aaseth J. (2016). Iron chelation in the treatment of neurodegenerative diseases. *J Trace Elem Med Biol.* pii:S0946–672X(16)30047–5.

Meyer E., Kurian M.A., Hayflick S.J. (2015). Neurodegeneration with brain iron accumulation: Genetic diversity and pathophysiological mechanisms. *Annu Rev Genomics Hum Genet.* 16:257–79.

Schulte E.C., Claussen M.C., Jochim A., et al. (2013). Mitochondrial membrane protein associated neurodegeneration: A novel variant of neurodegeneration with brain iron accumulation. *Mov Disord.* 28(2):224–7.

Aceruloplasminemia

At the age of 16 years, a healthy girl developed a progressive movement disorder: over the course of only a few months, her handwriting became irregular (Figure 94.2), she could no longer take a drink without spilling it, her speech became poorly articulated and her steps jerky, halting, and varying in size. Examination revealed abnormal eye movements, dysarthria, intention tremor, and involuntary movements of the arms. Testing illustrated decreased ceruloplasmin level of 110 mg/l (normal range 200–600 mg/l). Plasma copper was also decreased (0.49 mg/l; normal range 0.8–1.5 mg/l). However, she lacked both Kayser–Fleischer rings or increased urine copper (10 μg/d; normal range <70 μg/d). An MR imaging study of the brain revealed no abnormalities. Liver biopsy showed increased iron concentration (448 μg/g dry weight liver tissue, normal range 100–400 μg/g), although iron plasma values were normal (iron 109 μg/dl, normal range 20–150 μg/dl; ferritin 47 ng/ml, normal range 12–110 ng/ml; zinc 0.7 μg/ml, normal range 0.7–1.2 μg/ml; urine iron excretion 27 μg/d, normal range < 70 μg/d). A normal hepatic copper content (8 μg/g dry weight liver tissue, normal range <100 μg/g) was also found.

Aceruloplasminemia

Onset: Diabetes and microcytic anemia in the second decade of life.

Additional manifestations: Progressive motor disorder with craniofacial dystonia, ataxia, dementia, and retinal degeneration, with iron deposition in the basal ganglia. Heart failure.

Disease mechanism: Autosomal recessive loss of ceruloplasmin leading to induction of endoplasmic reticulum stress response by accumulation of mutant protein, abolished ceruloplasmin holoprotein production through impaired copper binding, and decreased ferroxidase activity of synthesized holo-ceruloplasmin.

Testing: Elevated ferritin, low serum copper and serum iron, and low transferrin saturation. MR imaging reveals characteristic iron deposition in advanced disease stages.

Treatment: None effective. Iron chelation therapy reverses hepatic and total body iron overload, although existing brain iron deposition is not clearly reversed.

Research highlights: Iron-mediated lipid peroxidation and oxidative damage as a disease mechanism.

Clinical Features

Aceruloplasminemia is part of the syndrome of neurodegeneration with brain iron accumulation in which a systemic iron-overload syndrome associates with cerebral iron deposition. Its prevalence is approximately 1 per 2,000,000 offspring. Aceruloplasminemia is caused by autosomal recessive mutations in the CP gene, which encodes ceruloplasmin, an enzyme that catalyzes the peroxidation of ferrous transferrin to ferric transferrin. Aceruloplasminemia presents in the second to fifth decade of life with a progressive motor disorder with craniofacial dyskinesia or dystonia, ataxia, dementia and peripheral retinal degeneration, with evidence of brain iron deposition in the basal ganglia. Microcytic anemia and diabetes mellitus can precede neurological manifestations. Heart failure ensues in advanced stages of iron overload.

Pathology

Ferrous iron accumulates in the liver, pancreas, retina and brain. Liver histopathology reveals a marked increase in iron in hepatocytes and reticuloendothelial cells. T2-weighted MR imaging illustrates increased iron content in the basal ganglia (Figure 94.1). The brain displays iron deposition and neuronal loss. Brain homogenates from individuals with aceruloplasminemia exhibit increased lipid peroxidation

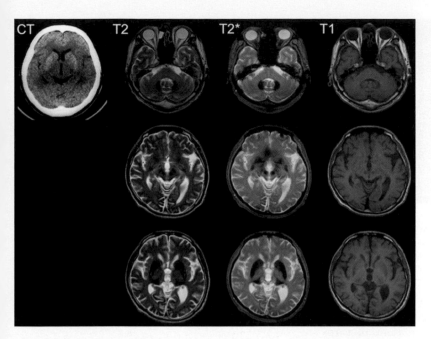

Figure 94.1 Brain computerized tomography and MR imaging findings in an individual with aceruloplasminemia. Brain CT shows abnormal high density areas in the basal ganglia. T1-, T2-, and T2*-weighted axial images of the brain show signal attenuation of the dentate nucleus of the cerebellum, globus pallidus, putamen, caudate nucleus and thalamus. Reproduced with permission from Miyajima H. Aceruloplasminemia. *Neuropathology*. 2015; 35(1):83–90.

and reduced activity of mitochondrial respiratory chain complexes I and IV.

Mice with absence of CP exhibit iron deposition in the liver and central nervous system together with reduced serum iron levels. Increased lipid peroxidation is present in some regions of the brain, implicating oxidative damage. Although no elevated lipid peroxidation is noticeable in the cerebellum, cerebellar cells are more vulnerable to oxidation. During the aging of these mice, changes occur in the expression of genes coding for iron homeostasis proteins, with increased expression of FTL (ferritin light chain), FTH1 (ferritin heavy chain), and DMT1 (divalent metal transporter 1) and decreased expression of TFR1 (transferrin receptor 1), in association with reduced IRP1 (iron-responsive element-binding protein 1) activity. Elevated DMT1 expression is especially observed in Purkinje neurons in the cerebellar cortex and in the large neurons of the deep nuclei (but not in astrocytes), suggesting that these cells may suffer from iron deprivation. Consistent with these findings, Purkinje neurons and large neurons of the deep nuclei display no changes in iron levels, whereas astrocytes exhibit elevated intracellular iron levels. There is a significant loss of Purkinje cells and astrocytes in the brain of aged CP null mice. In astrocytes, oxidative stress is likely to cause cell death, whereas the loss of Purkinje neurons might be secondary to diminished metabolic support from astrocytes.

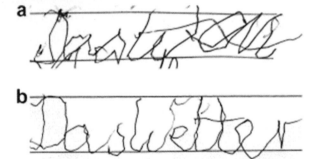

Figure 94.2 Aceruloplasminemia. Handwriting of the word "wetter": upon initiation of the therapy with zinc sulphate (a), after 15 months of therapy (b). Reproduced with permission from Kuhn J et al. Treatment of symptomatic heterozygous aceruloplasminemia with oral zinc sulphate. *Brain Dev*. 2007; 29(7):450–3.

Pathophysiology

Ceruloplasmin is a blue copper oxidase and contains 95 percent of the copper present in human serum. It is initially synthesized as an apoprotein, which binds up to six atoms of copper, and then changes to a holo-form (called ceruloplasmin). The CP protein occurs in two forms: a secreted form, which is expressed predominantly in the liver, and a widely expressed glycosylphosphatidylinositol (GPI)-linked form, which is the major transcript expressed in the brain. Serum ceruloplasmin does not cross the blood-brain

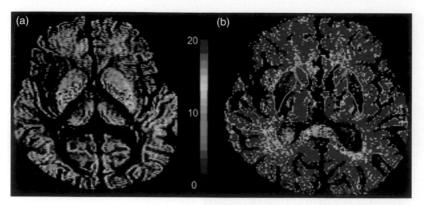

Figure 94.3 Aceruloplasminemia. Iron mapping of the brain using a 4.7 Tesla MR imaging T2 scan. The colored bar indicates the iron content in mg/100g fresh weight of the brain. In the healthy brain, a high level of iron was seen only in the globus pallidus. In almost all regions in the affected individual's brain, the iron level exceeded 20mg/100g fresh weight. In the basal ganglia, voids were seen due to too short T2 caused by the very high iron accumulation, over 60mg/100g fresh weight. (a) A 60-year-old healthy male and (b) a 60-year-old male suffering from anemia, retinal degeneration and diabetes with insulin treatment, who had experienced gait ataxia for 5 years. Reproduced with permission from Miyajima H. Aceruloplasminemia. *Neuropathology*. 2015; 35(1):83–90.

barrier in the normal brain. Instead, GPI-linked ceruloplasmin is bound to the cell membranes of astrocytes, where it participates in iron efflux from astrocytes due to the activity of ferroxidase, which oxidizes ferrous iron following its transfer to the cell surface via ferroportin, and delivers ferric iron to extracellular transferrin.

Cells with mutant CP that stays within the endoplasmic reticulum exhibit decreased proliferation and increased expression of GRP78 (glucose-regulated protein 78), a marker for the endoplasmic reticulum stress response. Secreted mutant CP exerts two effects on protein function: a) defective copper incorporation, which is necessary to produce the active holo-form of CP, and b) inability to stabilize ferroportin on the cell surface owing to decreased catalytic activity. Some of the mutant proteins that exhibit impaired copper incorporation are able to transform into a CP holoprotein in the presence of copper-glutathione, suggesting a disruption of the intracellular copper-loading process. These studies thus indicate that the mechanisms involved in the pathogenesis of aceruloplasminemia may include: a) induction of an endoplasmic reticulum stress response by accumulation of mutant protein, b) abolished CP holoprotein production through impaired copper binding, and c) decreased ferroxidase activity of synthesized holo-CP. The culmination of these abnormal cellular processes is the inability to prevent internalization and degradation of ferroportin, leading to defective iron efflux and increased intracellular iron.

Diagnosis

The diagnosis is established by serum ceruloplasmin determination and characteristic MR imaging findings (Figures 94.2 and 94.3). In addition, there is an elevated ferritin, decreased serum copper and serum iron, and reduced transferrin saturation. Genetic analysis is confirmatory.

Treatment

Iron chelation with either intravenous desferrioxamine or oral deferasirox leads to an improvement in ferritin values and in hepatic iron concentration. Brain iron deposition (as assessed through MR imaging) has not shown any consistent pattern of improvement across the reported studies. Similarly, the neurological manifestations have shown wide ranging results, from improvement to stability or progression despite treatment. Treatment with oral zinc sulfate may be effective for extrapyramidal and cerebellar symptoms. Combination therapy with an iron chelator and zinc sulfate may ameliorate neurological symptoms.

Bibliography

Kuhn J., Bewermeyer H., Miyajima H., et al. (2007). Treatment of symptomatic heterozygous aceruloplasminemia with oral zinc sulphate. *Brain Dev.* 29(7):450–3.

Meyer E., Kurian M.A., Hayflick S.J. (2015). Neurodegeneration with brain iron accumulation: Genetic diversity and pathophysiological mechanisms. *Annu Rev Genomics Hum Genet.* 16:257–79.

Cerebrotendinous Xanthomatosis

A 25-year-old man born of a consanguineous marriage, with normal birth and developmental history, presented with a history of insidious onset and gradually progressive cognitive decline, unsteadiness of limb action, and abnormal gait and upper extremity dexterity for 6–7 years. He was operated for bilateral cataract at the age of 12 years. Neuropsychological tests indicated mental retardation with an intelligence quotient of 60. On examination, he displayed bilateral aphakic eyes and his fundi were normal. Slit lamp examination for Kayser-Fleischer ring was negative. He also had a small swelling in the Achilles tendon, which was suggestive of xanthoma (Figure 95.1). Neurological examination revealed Mini-Mental State Examination scores of 12/30. He had behavioral abnormalities such as irritability, temper tantrums, and panic attacks. He also exhibited weakness in all four limbs in association with spasticity, generalized hyperreflexia, bilateral ankle clonus, and Babinski signs. There were pancerebellar features in the form of titubation, nystagmus, scanning speech, truncal ataxia and finger–nose incoordination. There were no extrapyramidal features and sensory system examination was normal.

Cerebrotendinous Xanthomatosis

Onset: Intractable infantile diarrhea and juvenile cataracts.

Additional manifestations: Tendon xanthomas. Progressive neurologic disease including ataxia, dystonia, dementia, epilepsy, psychiatric disorders, peripheral neuropathy, and myopathy in the second decade. Atherosclerotic and non-atherosclerotic cardiovascular disease.

Disease mechanism: Mutation in CYP27A1 (defective sterol 27-hydroxylase). This leads to accumulation of cholestanol and other bile acid precursors in tissues in association with xanthoma formation in the central nervous system and tendons.

Testing: Elevated plasma and bile cholestanol levels, increased urinary excretion of bile alcohol glucuronides and diminished biliary concentrations of chenodeoxycholic acid.

Treatment: Dietary chenodeoxycholic acid. Statins may complement this therapy.

Research highlights: Treatment of model mice with cholic acid reduces the accumulation of cholestanol in the brain, tendons, and circulation.

Clinical Features

Cerebrotendinous xanthomatosis is an autosomal recessive disorder of lipid metabolism. Its prevalence is less than 5 in 100,000. Manifestations include intractable diarrhea in infancy, premature cataracts in childhood or adolescence, tendon xanthomas, and progressive neurologic deterioration, which includes ataxia, dystonia, dementia, epilepsy, psychiatric disorders (depression, agitation, hallucinations), peripheral neuropathy, and myopathy. The mean age at onset of these symptoms is 19 years. There are two main clinical subgroups: a common form, with cerebellar and cerebral symptoms and a spinal form, with chronic myelopathy. Affected individuals also develop tendon xanthomas after the second decade of life (Figures 95.1 and 95.2). Xanthomas often appear on extensor tendons (particularly the Achilles), but can also form in the brain, bones and lungs. Both atherosclerotic and non-atherosclerotic cardiovascular disease may occur, including premature coronary heart disease, coronary aneurysms, mitral regurgitation, and lipomatous hypertrophy of the interatrial septum. The mechanism for the development of atherosclerosis is unclear, especially in light of the relatively low to normal plasma concentrations of low density lipoprotein cholesterol, but it may be related to the uptake of cholesterol within the arterial walls. Osteoporosis and recurrent bone fractures are also common clinical manifestations.

Pathology

Pathological findings from needle aspiration and autopsy of the lungs include granulomatous material, foamy cells and intracellular accumulations of foreign bodies. Histopathological exam of the tendon masses shows an accumulation of xanthoma cells and multiple, dispersed lipid crystal clefts (Figure 95.3).

Brain MR imaging reveals cerebellar atrophy, white matter signal alterations, and symmetric hyperintensities in the dentate nuclei. Gray matter and white matter volume is diffusely decreased (Figure 95.4). Macroscopically, the brain displays atrophy with multiple yellowish deposits in the plexus choroideus and in the white matter. Microscopically, there are multiple lipid crystal clefts and granulomatous lesions in the cerebellar hemispheres, demyelination, and perivascular accumulation of foamy macrophages in the globus pallidus and extracellular deposition of homogeneous myelin-like material in periventricular areas. Demyelination, gliosis, and involvement of the long tracts of the spinal cord have also been described. Peripheral nerve abnormalities include demyelination and remyelination and features of axonal degeneration. Mild myopathic changes and ultrastructural abnormalities in mitochondria can be observed in the muscle. These lesions display subsarcolemmal accumulation in mitochondria and swollen sarcoplasmic reticulum.

Pathophysiology

The disease is caused by a defective sterol 27-hydroxylase enzyme, the result of mutation in the CYP27A1 (cytochrome P450, family 27, subfamily A, polypeptide 1) gene, which is involved in bile acid synthesis. When deficient, this mitochondrial enzyme, which is a member of the cytochrome P450 system, causes the accumulation of cholesterol and cholestanol in all tissues, leading to diffuse xanthoma formation, most notably in the central nervous system and tendons. A defect in bile acid synthesis is also central to the disorder. Normal cholesterol catabolism involves the synthesis of primary bile acids (cholic acid and chenodeoxycholic acid) by way of several sterol intermediates. Due to the disturbance in bile

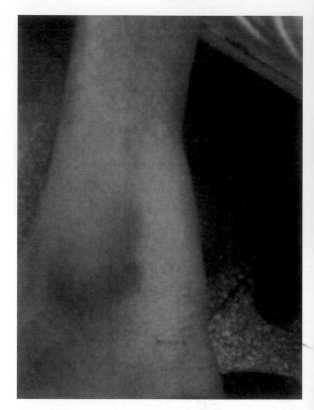

Figure 95.1 Tendon xanthoma of the Achilles tendon, a common site in cerebrotendinous xanthomatosis. Reproduced with permission from Jain RS et al. "Hot cross bun" sign in a case of cerebrotendinous xanthomatosis: a rare neuroimaging observation. *BMJ Case Rep.* 2013; 2013. pii:bcr2012006641.

acid synthesis in cerebrotendinous xanthomatosis, feedback regulation on cholesterol 7α-hydroxylase, the rate-limiting enzyme, is disturbed. Thus, cholestanol and other bile acid precursors accumulate in tissues, resulting in a progressive degenerative systemic and neurologic disorder.

Diagnosis

The disruption of bile acid synthesis results in several laboratory abnormalities. These include elevated plasma levels of cholestanol and bile alcohols. The formation of chenodeoxycholic acid is decreased, with concomitantly diminished concentrations in the bile. Urine concentrations of bile alcohols and bile alcohol glucuronides are increased. Serum and tissue levels of cholestanol are elevated, whereas serum cholesterol levels are normal or decreased. A presumptive diagnosis is established when typical symptoms (neurologic, cataracts and xanthomas) and analytical

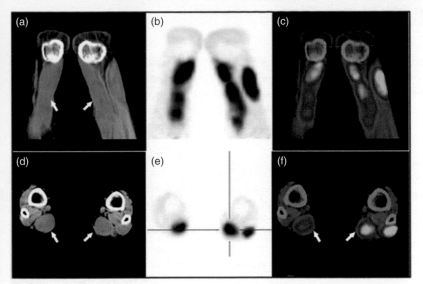

Figure 95.2 Unusually high radioactivity is found in both Achilles tendons of an individual patient with cerebrotendinous xanthomatosis. PET shows abnormal soft-tissue thickening in a CT window in coronal section (a) and in axial section (d), and unusually high radioactivity in Achilles tendons and adjacent regions in PET (b and e) and fusion windows (c and f). Reproduced with permission from Nie S et al. Cerebrotendinous xanthomatosis: a comprehensive review of pathogenesis, clinical manifestations, diagnosis, and management. *Orphanet J Rare Dis*. 2014; 9:179.

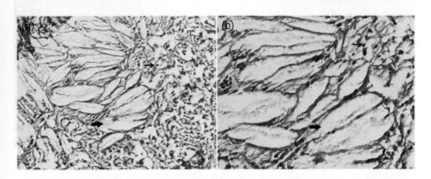

Figure 95.3 Histology: tendon in cerebrotendinous xanthomatosis. HE staining of the tendon masses reveals accumulation of xanthoma cells (fine arrows) and dispersed lipid crystal clefts (coarse arrows). a, 100×; b, 200×. Reproduced with permission from Nie S et al. Cerebrotendinous xanthomatosis: a comprehensive review of pathogenesis, clinical manifestations, diagnosis, and management. *Orphanet J Rare Dis*. 2014; 9:179.

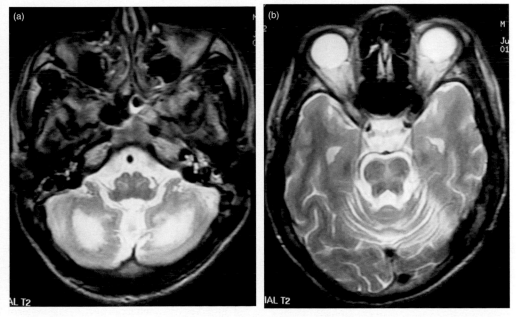

Figure 95.4 Brain MR imaging in cerebrotendinous xantomatosis. a. MR imaging of the cerebellum showing hyperintensities in the bilateral dentate nuclei; a site commonly affected in cerebrotendinous xanthomatosis. b. T2-weighted axial image showing "hot cross bun" sign in pons. Reproduced with permission from Jain RS et al. "Hot cross bun" sign in a case of cerebrotendinous xanthomatosis: a rare neuroimaging observation. *BMJ Case Rep*. 2013; 2013. pii:bcr2012006641.

abnormalities (elevated plasma and bile cholestanol levels, increased urinary excretion of bile alcohol glucuronides associated with diminished biliary concentrations of chenodeoxycholic acid) are present.

Treatment

The treatment of cerebrotendinous xanthomatosis includes chenodeoxycholic acid. This can stabilize or potentially reverse some of the disease manifestations, but neurologic or psychiatric symptoms may not improve with this therapy. Statins have been studied as a potential treatment. Statin monotherapy appears to exert little or no benefit. However, statins may be useful for lowering cholestanol levels when combined with chenodeoxycholic acid. Statins may provide incremental benefit over chenodeoxycholic acid treatment alone. A concern regarding statin therapy is the prospect of worsening the condition by increasing low density lipoprotein uptake via enhancement of low density lipoprotein receptor.

Bibliography

Jain R.S., Sannegowda R.B., Agrawal A., et al. (2013). "Hot cross bun" sign in a case of cerebrotendinous xanthomatosis: A rare neuroimaging observation. *BMJ Case Rep.* 2013. pii:bcr2012006641.

Nie S., Chen G., Cao X., et al. (2014). Cerebrotendinous xanthomatosis: A comprehensive review of pathogenesis, clinical manifestations, diagnosis, and management. *Orphanet J Rare Dis.* 9:179.

Juvenile Huntington Disease

An 11-year-old boy was evaluated following a 5-year history of developmental regression, abnormal involuntary movements, and worsening behavioral dysfunction. In early childhood, he displayed appropriate gross motor, fine motor, and language development, but "shakiness" was noted by his adoptive parents. In first grade, he was able to ride a bicycle, participate in gym class, dress himself, use utensils, write in cursive, and read at grade level. Since that time, a slow regression of fine motor, gross motor, and language skills was noted. His handwriting became illegible and he experienced difficulty dressing himself. He walked on the edges of his feet and was no longer able to ride a bicycle or run without difficulty. His speech became unintelligible to strangers at the age of 9 years and he had significant difficulty with impulse control and memory. He displayed multiple involuntary movements of his arms and hands, such as hand-curling or arm-swinging, and had received the diagnosis of Tourette syndrome. Examination revealed mild generalized hypertonia and difficulty with tandem gait. Choreiform movements of the extremities were present. His speech was dysarthric, with poor intelligibility and he spoke in one- to two-word phrases. He tended to walk on the outside of the feet with the toes turned inward. There was mild difficulty with tandem gait but he was able to walk on his toes and heels without difficulty. Neuropsychological testing revealed a full-scale IQ in the low-average range (FIQ = 80), where it had been normal (FIQ = 97) 5 years prior. Regression was noted on testing in verbal skills, speed of information processing, and mathematical skills.

Juvenile Huntington Disease

Onset: Bradykinesia, rigidity, and cognitive and psychiatric abnormalities in the second decade of life.

Additional manifestations: Dystonia and signs of cerebellar dysfunction. Chorea. Epilepsy. Weight loss.

Disease mechanism: Accumulation and cellular dysfunction induced by huntingtin expanded due to trinucleotide repeat amplification.

Testing: Genetic analysis documents CAG repeat expansion in excess of at least 36 repeats in chromosome 4.

Treatment: None completely effective. Antipsychotics such as haloperidol and pimozide can ameliorate chorea.

Research highlights: Mutant huntingtin compromises mitochondrial bioenergetics and dynamics, preventing efficient calcium handling and ATP generation.

Clinical Features

Huntington disease is an autosomal dominant disorder characterized by progressive motor, cognitive and psychiatric abnormalities. It is the most common neurodegenerative disease, with a prevalence in the Caucasian population of 6 in 100,000 persons, which exceeds that of other races because of a greater number of chromosome 4 trinucleotide CAG repeats in this racial group. The most common age of onset is between 35 and 40 years, although it may manifest at any age. In 10 percent of cases, the disease manifests before the second decade of life. Of these affected individuals, 5 percent present before the age of 14 and 1 percent before the age of 10 years. In the juvenile subtype, transmission is paternal in 70–80 percent of cases. Juvenile Huntington disease is characterized by bradykinesia, rigidity, and psychiatric disorders, with epilepsy occurring in 50 percent of cases. In juvenile Huntington disease, chorea is seldom seen in the first decade and only appears in the second decade. Initially, the choreic movements often occur in the distal extremities such as fingers and toes, but also in small facial muscles. Dystonia (for instance torticollis) can be the first motor sign. Other involuntary movements include tics comparable to the ones seen in Tourette syndrome. When chorea is absent, as is often the case in juvenile disease, bradykinesia, dystonia, and signs of cerebellar dysfunction and rigidity predominate, together with frequent seizures and progressive myoclonic epilepsy. In childhood, autistic features, major behavior disorders, learning difficulties, and spasticity may predominate. A form with severe rigidity (Westphal variant) is associated with cerebellar atrophy and a rapidly progressive course in young individuals who harbor large triplet expansions.

During subclinical stages, changes in personality, irritability, disinhibition, anxiety and difficulties associated with multitasking are common. Alterations in saccadic ocular movements are also often seen. Later, depression, disinhibition, euphoria, aggressiveness, obsessions and compulsions, delusional ideas, hallucinations and sexual disorders become common. Cognitive dysfunction usually affects long-term memory as well as in executive functions like organization, planning, checking, flexibility and acquisition of new motor skills. Weight loss has been related to a large number of CAG repeats, possibly as the consequence of a hypermetabolic state. Sleep- and circadian rhythm disturbances and autonomic nervous system dysfunction are also common. The mean duration of the disease is 17–20 years. The progression of the disease leads to more dependency in daily life and finally death. The most common cause of death is pneumonia, followed by suicide.

Pathology

Caudate volume loss may be diagnostic as early as several years before disease onset. In voxel-based MR imaging morphometric analysis, a decrease in striatal grey matter is observed in the caudate, putamen and globus pallidus (Figure 96.1). A gradient of neuronal loss with a caudo-rostral and dorso-ventral pattern has been suggested. Disease stages with less evident motor and cognitive clinical manifestations are associated with fewer changes in the grey matter. These abnormalities are more pronounced with greater CAG expansions. There is also atrophy of the substantia nigra, hypothalamus, thalamus, amygdala, insular cortex, premotor, and pre- and post-central gyri. Thinning of the dorsolateral prefrontal cortex

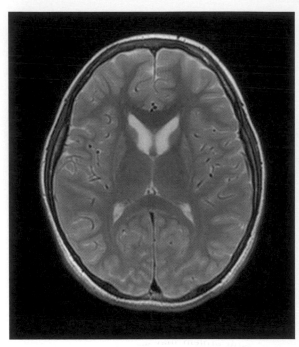

Figure 96.1 Axial T2-weighted magnetic resonance imaging scan of the brain demonstrating bilateral atrophy of the caudate and putamen consistent with juvenile Huntington disease. Reproduced with permission from Monrad P et al. Typical clinical findings should prompt investigation for juvenile Huntington disease. *Pediatr Neurol.* 2013; 48(4):333–4.

and occipital lobe and loss of volume of the globus pallidus and amygdala are observed in advanced disease stages.

In cortex and striatum, there are changes in the cytoplasmic localization of huntingtin, including perinuclear accumulation and formation of multivesicular bodies. Huntingtin also accumulates in aberrant subcellular compartments such as nuclear and neuritic aggregates co-localized with ubiquitin. The site of protein aggregation is polyglutamine-dependent, both in juvenile-onset individuals, who display more aggregates in the nucleus, and in adult-onset affected individuals, who manifest more neuritic aggregates.

Pathophysiology

Huntington disease displays genetic anticipation. Mutation of the gene that encodes huntingtin expands a polyglutamine tract encoded by the trinucleotide CAG, which is situated on exon 1. In the general population, triplet repeat size ranges from 6 to 35, whereas in individuals with Huntington disease, 40 to 121 repeats are found. Risk of hereditary transmission exists with 27 to 35 repeats and penetrance is incomplete with 35 to 39 repeats. Huntingtin accumulates in the neuronal cytoplasm and nucleus, which leads to apoptosis. Neuronal loss is observed in the striate (particularly the caudate and putamen), cerebral cortex (frontal and temporal lobes), hippocampus, and subthalamic nucleus, resulting in the loss of up to 25 percent of cerebral volume. In juvenile-onset disease, cerebellar degeneration has been observed, as well as alterations in energy metabolism that are more prominent than in adults.

The genesis of huntingtin aggregates and cell death are related to cleavage of mutant huntingtin. However, the aggregation of mutant huntingtin can be dissociated from the extent of cell death. Thus, properties of mutant huntingtin more subtle than its aggregation, such as its proteolysis and protein interactions, which affect vesicle trafficking and nuclear transport, might suffice to cause neurodegeneration in the striatum and cortex.

The normal huntingtin protein may also participate in synaptic function. In the disease, there is a reduction in dopamine receptor density, which may be related to cognitive deterioration, especially involving executive function and memory.

Diagnosis

The diagnosis is based on the clinical symptoms and signs in an affected individual with a parent with Huntington disease. DNA analysis illustrates CAG repeats in excess of at least 36 on the huntingtin gene on chromosome 4. The clinical criteria used for diagnosis include motor abnormalities with or without psychiatric or cognitive changes. However, in most cases a combination of these three main features is present.

Treatment

The treatment of Huntington disease includes typical antipsychotics such as haloperidol and pimozide for the amelioration of chorea at the expense of deteriorating voluntary movements. NMDA receptor antagonists such as riluzole and amantadine have also been used for the treatment of motor manifestations. The combination of haloperidol and lithium carbonate may control irritability and impulsivity. Beta-blockers (propranolol) have been effective in some cases. Among the atypical antipsychotics, risperidone improves abnormal involuntary movements and psychotic manifestations. Olanzapine is an alternative, particularly for the control of psychiatric manifestations. The treatment of hypokinesia is less effective, including antiparkinsonian drugs. Surgical intervention to treat chorea has also been described.

Experimental drugs that prevent the aggregation of huntingtin protein in Drosophila, gene therapy, coenzyme Q10 and transplantation of striatal fetal cells have been attempted or are under investigation.

Bibliography

Monrad P., Renaud D.L. (2013). Typical clinical findings should prompt investigation for juvenile Huntington disease. *Pediatr Neurol.* 48(4):333–4.

Roos R.A. (2010). Huntington's disease: A clinical review. *Orphanet J Rare Dis.* 5:40.

Hereditary Spastic Paraplegia

A boy was evaluated for longstanding progressive motor disability. He presented at the age of 3 years with walking difficulty and was noticed to have tight hip adductors, hamstrings and Achilles tendons. He was initially diagnosed with spastic diplegic cerebral palsy. MR imaging of his brain and thoraco-lumbo-sacral spine revealed no pathology. Nerve conduction studies were also normal motor conduction velocities. The spasticity in his lower limbs increased and was accompanied by brisk reflexes, bilateral ankle clonus and Babinski signs despite physiotherapy and orthotic treatment. His upper limb functions were normal, as was his bulbar system. He had no cerebellar ataxia, and had normal bladder and bowel control, normal intelligence and language function, and normal vibration sensation. At the age of 6 years, he was diagnosed as having early-onset pure spastic paraplegia. He could walk indoors and outdoors and climb stairs holding onto a railing. His father, aged 40 years and elder sister, aged 9 years had similar symptoms with onset at age 3 to 4 years. They walked with spastic gaits, with no significant functional limitations, and did not require supportive devices. The father had tendon release surgery during childhood. A mild regression in his motor ability had been noticed since early adulthood: He could no longer walk up or down the stairs without assistance. They harbored a mutation in the gene SPG3A.

Hereditary Spastic Paraplegia

Onset: Abnormal motor milestone acquisition and spasticity at any age, from the neonatal period to childhood. Adult forms are also common.

Additional manifestations: Paraparesis or quadriparesis, brisk tendon reflexes, and extensor plantar responses. Sphincter disturbances and sensory loss. In complicated forms, cerebellar, nerve and cognitive impairment, epilepsy, myopathy, and extrapyramidal and psychiatric disturbances.

Disease mechanism: Autosomal dominant, recessive, X-linked, or mitochondrial-associated abnormalities in membrane trafficking, organelle shaping, axonal transport, mitochondrial function, lipid metabolism, or myelination.

Testing: Genetic testing establishes the diagnosis.

Treatment: None effective.

Research highlights: Impaired microtubule-dependent organelle trafficking in some disease forms.

Clinical Features

The hereditary spastic paraplegias (designated as SPG) constitute a heterogeneous group of inherited neurodegenerative disorders resulting from primary retrograde dysfunction of the long descending fibers of the corticospinal tract that predominantly manifest as lower limb spasticity and weakness. Although spastic paraparesis and urinary dysfunction are the most common clinical presentation, a complex array of different neurological and systemic manifestations has been recognized in these diseases. The genetics basis of the hereditary spastic paraplegias is complex, with more than 70 genetic subtypes described involving all patterns of Mendelian inheritance (autosomal dominant, autosomal recessive, X-linked) and non-Mendelian (mitochondrial maternal transmission). The prevalence is 2 in 100,000 individuals for autosomal dominant and recessive forms. The age of onset is variable, ranging from the first years of life with abnormal motor milestone acquisition to late onset pure spastic paraplegia. Generally, the age of onset for autosomal dominant forms occurs in adulthood between the second and third decade of life while in the autosomal recessive or X-linked forms, the first symptoms begin in childhood or early adolescence.

The hereditary spastic paraplegias are classified as pure or complex (or complicated) forms. Pure forms

Table 97.1 Inheritance of the hereditary spastic paraplegias

Mode of inheritance	Hereditary spastic paraplegia type
Autosomal dominant	SPG3A, SPG4, SPG6, SPG8, SPG9, SPG10, SPG12, SPG13, SPG17, SPG19, SPG29, SPG31, SPG33, SPG36, SPG37, SPG38, SPG41, SPG42, SPG72, SPG73
Autosomal recessive	SPG5, SPG7, SPG11, SPG14, SPG15, SPG18, SPG20, SPG21, SPG23, SPG24, SPG25, SPG26, SPG27, SPG28, SPG30, SPG32, SPG35, SPG39, SPG43, SPG44, SPG45/SPG65, SPG46, SPG47, SPG48, SPG49, SPG50, SPG51, SPG52, SPG53, SPG54, SPG55, SPG56, SPG57, SPG58, SPG59, SPG60, SPG61, SPG62, SPG63, SPG64, SPG66, SPG67, SPG68, SPG69, SPG70, SPG71, SPG72, SPG74
X-linked	SPG1, SPG2, SPG16, SPG22, SPG34
Mitochondrial	MT-ATP6, MT-TI, MT-CO3, MT-ND4

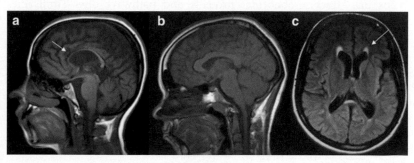

Figure 97.1 Brain MR imaging findings in hereditary spastic paraplegias. **a.** Sagittal T1-weighted brain MRI showing thin corpus callosum (white arrow) in an individual with SPG11, compared to normal corpus callosum morphology in a control subject (**b**). **c.** Axial brain MRI showing typical "ears-of-the-lynx" sign (white arrow) in an individual diagnosed with SPG11 in FLAIR sequence. Reproduced with permission from de Souza PV et al. Hereditary Spastic Paraplegia: Clinical and Genetic Hallmarks. *Cerebellum*. 2016. [In press]

are those that exhibit isolated pyramidal signs (paraparesis or quadriparesis, spasticity, brisk tendon reflexes, and extensor plantar responses) which may be associated with sphincter disturbances and sensory loss. Complex forms are those in which the spastic paraplegia phenotype is associated with other neurological or non-neurological signs, including cerebellar dysfunction (ataxia, nystagmus, tremor), axonal or demyelinating peripheral neuropathy (including dysautonomia and sensory disturbances), cognitive impairment (including dementia and mental retardation or intellectual disability), epilepsy, myopathic features (including ptosis and ophthalmoparesis), extrapyramidal features (parkinsonism, chorea, dystonia), psychiatric disturbances, and brain and spine MR imaging abnormalities typical of a specific genetic subtype (mild white matter changes, leukodystrophy, hypomyelination, thin corpus callosum, spinal cord atrophy, brain iron accumulation, hydrocephalus, and cerebellar atrophy) (Figure 97.1). The non-neurological manifestations of complicated hereditary spastic paraplegia are heterogeneous, including ophthalmological

abnormalities (cataracts, optic neuropathy, optic atrophy, retinitis pigmentosa, and macular degeneration), dysmorphic features (microcephaly, macrocephaly, facial dysmorphisms, short stature, and complex malformative syndromes), and orthopedic abnormalities (scoliosis, hip dislocation and foot deformities).

Generally, these diseases are characterized by a subtle onset and slowly progressive course of spastic paraparesis described by affected individuals as leg stiffness, abnormal gait, or gait instability. Compared with individuals with other causes of spastic paraparesis such as spinal cord injury or demyelinating disease, the hereditary spastic paraplegias exhibit relative preservation of muscle power despite significantly increased tone in the legs.

Several forms are associated with younger age of onset.

Pathology

Pathological abnormalities include myelin pallor and axonal loss in the lateral and, to a lesser extent,

Table 97.2 Age of onset of the hereditary spastic paraplegias

Onset	Disease form or causal gene
Late childhood or juvenile	SPG3A, SPG4, SPG5A, SPG6, SPG9A, SPG10, SPG12, SPG13, SPG14, SPG17, SPG18, SPG20, SPG21, SPG22, SPG23, SPG24, SPG26, SPG28, SPG29, SPG30, SPG31, SPG32, SPG34, SPG35, SPG37, SPG39, SPG42, SPG43, SPG44, SPG45/SPG65, SPG46, SPG47, SPG49, SPG53, SPG54, SPG55, SPG56, SPG57, SPG58, SPG59, SPG60, SPG61, SPG62, SPG63, SPG64, SPG65, SPG66, SPG67, SPG68, SPG69, SPG70, SPG71, SPG72, SPG74, CPSQ-I, Spastic paraplegia with deafness, CCT5, FAM134B, EXOSC3, IFIH1, ADAR1, KLC4, PMCA4, TUBB4A, FARS2, DNM2, MT-CO3
Neonatal, infantile or early childhood	SPG1, SPG2, SPG3A, SPG4, SPG16, SPG22, SPG24, SPG45/SPG65, SPG47, SPG50, SPG51, SPG52, SPG60, SPG61, SPG63, SPG66, SPG69, SPG70, SPG71, SPG72, IAHSP, SPOAN, BICD2, CCT5, RNASEH2B, FARS2

anterior corticospinal tracts. Corticospinal tract degeneration is most severe I the thoracolumbar area. There may be additional involvement of the spinocerebellar tracts and dorsal columns at the fasciculus gracilis and cervical levels. There is more severe degeneration in the distal areas of the long tracts. Axonal loss affects large and small diameter fibers and may be associated with a microglial reaction as seen in the corticospinal tract degeneration typical of motor neuron disease. There may be involvement of the primary motor neuron cell body. Loss of Betz cells from the motor cortex may occur. Lower motor neuron pathology may be minimal or include hyaline bodies. There may be abnormal staining of mitochondria and cytoskeletal components.

In specific types of hereditary spastic paraplegia, muscle abnormalities may include mitochondrial changes such as ragged red fiber formation, cytochrome oxidase negative fibers, peripheral accumulation of mitochondria, and increased succinate dehydrogenase activity.

In complicated cases, there may be decreased white matter, atrophy of the corpus callosum and deep grey nuclei and loss of pigment in the substantia nigra. In some cases, depletion of hippocampal pyramidal cells, tau-positive tangles, and Lewy bodies containing alpha-synuclein have been observed.

Pathophysiology

The relative length of the corticospinal tract renders if particularly susceptible to mechanisms that impair axonal function. The pathophysiological mechanisms that leads to dysfunction of the corticospinal tract in hereditary spastic paraplegia are multiple. The causal abnormal proteins and pathways offer similarities with other neurodegenerative disorders such as spinocerebellar ataxias, amyotrophic lateral sclerosis, and Charcot–Marie–Tooth disease. The most common molecular mechanisms are abnormal membrane trafficking and organelle shaping, axonal transport, mitochondrial dysfunction, lipid metabolism disturbances, and myelination abnormalities.

Diagnosis

The diagnosis of hereditary spastic paraplegia is based on the coexistence of: (I) bilateral lower limb spasticity and weakness that may be non-progressive or slowly progressive; (II) neurological examination showing corticospinal tract dysfunction such as spasticity, hyperreflexia, and extensor plantar responses; (III) family history consistent with autosomal dominant, autosomal recessive, X-linked inheritance or maternal inheritance, even though sporadic cases can also occur and (IV) genetic testing.

Treatment

There is no effective treatment other than symptomatic spasticity relief.

Bibliography

Chan K.Y., Ching C.K., Mak C.M., et al. (2009). Hereditary spastic paraplegia: Identification of an SPG3A gene mutation in a Chinese family. *Hong Kong Med J.* 15(4):304–7.

de Souza P.V., de Rezende Pinto W.B., de Rezende Batistella G.N., et al. (2016) Hereditary spastic paraplegia: Clinical and genetic hallmarks. *Cerebellum*. Jun 7.

Adult Neuronal Ceroid Lipofuscinosis (Kufs Disease)

A 24-year-old man was evaluated for progressive neurological deterioration. Spontaneous and stimulus-induced myoclonus began at age 15 years in the lower extremities and gradually worsened to involve his upper limbs, speech, and swallowing. Generalized tonic-clonic convulsions developed later but were controlled with one anticonvulsant. Cognitive decline was present and steadily worsened. Examination indicated generalized hyperreflexia, ankle clonus, mild ataxia, and stimulus-sensitive multifocal myoclonus. Two older cousins had manifested the same disease, with similar age of onset, progressive myoclonus, and generalized seizures, which were controlled for most of their disease course with an anticonvulsant. Both had died at around age 30 years, one in association with status epilepticus, the other of unknown cause, and for the years preceding death both had been wheelchair-bound and bed-confined with severe myoclonus and dementia. None of the three men manifested visual decline, weakness, movement disorders, or renal disease. Investigations of all three demonstrated cortical myoclonus and multifocal epileptiform discharges in electroencephalograms and generalized brain atrophy on magnetic resonance imaging. The proband carried a pathogenic mutation in the CLN6 gene

Kufs Disease

Onset: Dementia with onset at 10 to 50 years of age.

Additional manifestations: In type A, progressive myoclonus epilepsy. In type B, motor-system features such as ataxia, pyramidal, and extrapyramidal dysfunction. The autosomal dominant form, Parry disease, exhibits features of both phenotypes A and B. There are no ocular features.

Disease mechanism: Autosomal recessive mutation of several potential loci, one of which includes CLN6. CLN6 encodes a transmembrane protein localized in the endoplasmic reticulum. In Parry disease, mutation in DNAJC5 (dnaJ homolog subfamily C member 5), which encodes cysteine string protein alpha (CSPα), a protein associated with synaptic vesicles.

Testing: Brain biopsy and rarely rectal or other non-neural tissue biopsy.

Treatment: None effective.

Research highlights: Spontaneously occurring murine and ovine CLN6 models.

Clinical Features

The neuronal ceroid lipofuscinoses comprise several progressive exclusively neurological disorders characterized by lysosomal degradation product accumulation in the nervous system. The infantile (Haltia–Santavuori), late infantile (Jansky–Bielschowsky), and juvenile (Spielmeyer–Vogt) forms of the disease have been separately discussed. The adult onset form of neuronal ceroid lipofuscinoses, Kufs disease, may present in adolescence. It has been assigned gene locus CLN4 (ceroid lipofuscinosis type 4). It is the mildest form of neuronal ceroid lipofuscinosis and includes at least two subtypes with an age of onset of 10 to 50 years. The main symptom is dementia, with additional clinical features depending upon subtype and potentially including progressive myoclonus epilepsy, ataxia, late pyramidal and extra-pyramidal features, behavioral changes and motor disturbances. In contrast with other ceroid lipofuscinosis, there are no ophthalmological abnormalities. Also in contrast with other neuronal ceroid lipofuscinoses, which are always inherited in autosomal recessive manner, both recessive (most commonly) and dominant forms of Kufs disease known as Parry disease have been described. The clinical presentation of autosomal recessive Kufs disease can be divided into two overlapping types. Type A presents with progressive myoclonus epilepsy, whereas type B presents with dementia and a variety of motor system signs. The autosomal dominant form, Parry disease, exhibits features of both phenotypes A and B.

Less severe mutations in the genes causing the early-onset neuronal ceroid lipofuscinoses might result in phenotypes with a later onset. In fact, some cases of adult onset neuronal ceroid lipofuscinosis are caused by mutations in the CLN1 gene: allelic variants of PPT1, the gene underlying most cases of the infantile form, can present in later childhood or even early-adult life with neurological deterioration and visual failure. In further support of this notion, early adult onset disease has also been associated with mutations in CLN5. However, all of these cases manifested visual failure and retinal involvement and so they represent unusual cases of adult-onset neuronal ceroid lipofuscinosis rather than canonical Kufs disease, which displays no visual failure.

Pathology

The brain is reduced in size, with atrophy of the cerebrum, which is particularly prominent in the frontal and frontoparietal region of the cerebral cortex. There may also be cerebellar atrophy. In the childhood forms of neuronal ceroid lipofuscinosis, the characteristic lipopigment is readily identified in non-neural tissues such as skin, muscle or lymphocytes. However, in Kufs disease the distribution of the pigment is more restricted. There is neuronal loss in association with pigment accumulation. The neuronal storage of pigment is most prominent in the neocortex and subcortical nuclei, similar to CLN3 disease. Secondary degeneration of the white matter with astrogliosis and microglial activation also occurs. The stored material consists of heterogeneous membrane-bound inclusions containing granular osmophilic deposits, curvilinear, rectilinear and fingerprint profiles, and lipid droplets. This material contains subunit c of mitochondrial ATP synthase and sphingolipid activator proteins A and D. There is no storage material in biopsies from the conjunctiva, skin, or nerve. In some cases, the fingerprint profiles are detectable in eccrine sweat gland epithelium, while curvilinear and rectilinear inclusions have been noted in skeletal muscle.

Pathophysiology

Two causal genes are known: DNAJC5 (dnaJ homolog subfamily C member 5) and CLN6.

DNAJC5 encodes cysteine string protein alpha (CSPα). This protein is found in the brain, where it participates in the transmission of the nerve impulse, as CSPα is associated with synaptic vesicles. DNAJC5 causes autosomal dominant Parry disease.

CLN6 encodes a transmembrane protein localized in the endoplasmic reticulum. It contains a cytoplasmic N terminus, a luminal C terminus, and seven transmembrane domains. CLN6 is conserved among vertebrates, but its function is unknown. Lysosomal pH can be elevated in cells from CLN6 disease individuals, but the activities of at least some lysosomal enzymes are unaffected, although lysosomal degradation of an endocytosed protein is reduced. CLN6 can bind to the protein CLN5 and to collapsing response mediator protein-2 (CRMP-2). In vitro analysis of certain mutations associated with variant late-infantile disease suggests that the abnormal protein is more rapidly degraded.

A role for modifiers is suggested by the wide range in age at onset (teens to age 51) in Kufs disease cases with CLN6 mutations, even among those with the same mutation. Modifiers could also explain the variation within families in the temporal appearance of symptoms.

Diagnosis

The EEG shows generalized fast spike-and-wave discharges with photosensitivity. The diagnosis is most reliably established by brain biopsy, although sometimes the characteristic abnormalities can be found in neurons of the rectal mucosa or other non-neural tissues. The diagnosis requires demonstration of ultrastructural changes in skeletal or vascular smooth muscle cells which may be fingerprint profiles, curvilinear profiles, or granular osmiophilic deposits.

Treatment

There is no effective treatment.

Bibliography

Andrade D.M., Paton T., Turnbull J., et al. (2012). Mutation of the CLN6 gene in teenage-onset progressive myoclonus epilepsy. *Pediatr Neurol.* 47(3):205–8.

Arsov T., Smith K.R., Damiano J., et al. (2011). Kufs disease, the major adult form of neuronal ceroid lipofuscinosis, caused by mutations in CLN6. *Am J Hum Genet.* 88(5):566–73.

Juvenile Amyotrophic Lateral Sclerosis

A 19-year-old man with mild learning difficulties who had been working in commercial waste recycling for less than 1 year developed painful right shoulder and arm weakness, which progressed rapidly, and in less than 1 month included neck weakness. At the beginning, his right arm muscle atrophy was noticed by members of his family. On examination, he had a normal mental status. Examination of the cranial nerves revealed tongue atrophy and fasciculations, bilateral facial weakness with the right side worse than the left, severe weakness and atrophy and fasciculations of the sternocleidomastoids and trapezius, with the right side much worse than left. The remainder of the cranial nerves was normal. Motor examination showed atrophy and severe weakness of the right shoulder and upper arm including supraspinatus, infraspinatus, subscapularis, deltoid, pectoralis, and biceps. He displayed moderate weakness and atrophy of his right triceps and wrist and finger extensors and flexors, as well as interossei of the hands. There was normal bulk, tone and strength on his left side and right leg. He was areflexic in the right arm, with mild hyperreflexia in the left arm, knees, and ankles, with equivocal plantar responses. Brain and spine MR images were normal. An electromyographic examination showed normal conduction velocities and normal needle examination of the left arm, left shoulder and left leg. There was some denervation in muscles of the right leg and severe denervation in muscles of the right shoulder and arm. A year later, he developed dysphagia and dysarthria, leading to anorexia and severe weight loss. In a further half year, he was emaciated with diffuse severe muscle atrophy. His weakness was asymmetric, with profound right upper limb weakness and, to a lesser degree, bilateral leg involvement. He rapidly progressed to respiratory failure requiring mechanical ventilation. Repeated examinations showed no cognitive or sensory symptoms or signs. He carried a FUS deletion.

Juvenile Amyotrophic Lateral Sclerosis

Onset: Progressive focal weakness and fasciculations in one limb in the second decade of life.

Additional manifestations: Spasticity, increased or decreased reflexes, atrophy. Symptoms of bulbar dysfunction are common. In some cases, sensory neuropathy can be demonstrated. Death usually ensues within 5 years.

Disease mechanism: There are five major forms of familial juvenile amyotrophic lateral sclerosis, designated as fALS2 (related to alsin), 4 (senataxin), 5 (spatacsin), 6 (FUS), and 16 (sigma receptor-1). In general, they lead to gain or loss of function associated with autosomal dominant or autosomal recessive inheritance.

Testing: Electromyography and nerve conduction studies illustrate dysfunction of upper and lower motor neurons.

Treatment: Riluzole, which blocks the release of glutamate and may decrease neuronal excitotoxicity.

Research highlights: Formation of abnormal nuclear aggregates that are selectively toxic to subpopulations of neurons.

Clinical Features

Motor neuron diseases, including amyotrophic lateral sclerosis, are characterized by exclusive or predominant progressive affection of the first (upper motor neuron) or second (lower) motor neuron. In a majority of cases, motor neuron diseases are genetically determined. Hereditary motor neuron diseases comprise sporadic and familial amyotrophic lateral sclerosis (sALS, fALS), spinal muscular atrophy, bulbospinal muscular atrophy (Kennedy syndrome) and several additional hereditary disorders. The incidence of amyotrophic lateral sclerosis is 2 per 100,000 per year, with a prevalence of 5 per 100,000 individuals. Juvenile amyotrophic lateral sclerosis is characterized by onset at less than 20 years of age, a similar family history in many cases, a mild course except for sporadic cases and both autosomal dominant and autosomal recessive forms of inheritance. There is asymmetrical or symmetrical weakness of the extremities and bulbar muscles, fasciculations, and atrophy, which start focally. Spasticity, increased reflexes and clonus are common, as may also be atrophy of hand muscles, foot drop, fasciculations, and reduced reflexes. Sensory loss is usually absent, but cognitive impairment is common. A significant proportion of cases develop cognitive dysfunction and a minority overt dementia. Death usually ensues within 5 years, although it may be delated by several more years. There are five major forms of familial juvenile amyotrophic lateral sclerosis, designated as fALS2, 4, 5, 6, and 16.

fALS2 is characterised by slowly progressive dysfunction predominantly of the upper motor neuron manifesting as facial or limb spasticity. fALS2 is inherited in autosomal recessive fashion and is caused by mutations in the ALS2 gene encoding alsin. ALS2 mutations may also manifest as primary lateral sclerosis or infantile-onset ascending hereditary spastic paralysis. Early onset anarthria and generalized dystonia have also been described.

fALS4 manifests as slowly progressive, distal hereditary motor neuropathy with pyramidal signs. fALS4 follows an autosomal dominant form of inheritance and is due to mutations in the SETX gene, encoding senataxin. Mutations in the SETX gene may also cause autosomal recessive spinocerebellar ataxia or ataxia with oculomotor apraxia-2.

fALS5 is characterised by a slowly progressive juvenile amyotrophic lateral sclerosis phenotype. The disease is inherited in autosomal recessive manner and is caused by mutations in the SPG11 gene encoding spatacsin. Mutations in SPG11 also cause hereditary spastic paraplegia with thin corpus callosum.

fALS6 leads to a typical amyotrophic lateral sclerosis phenotype. It may follow both an autosomal dominant or autosomal recessive mode of inheritance and is due to mutations in the FUS gene encoding the fused in sarcoma protein.

fALS16 manifests as juvenile-onset typical amyotrophic lateral sclerosis. Affected individuals may also develop frontotemporal dementia and motor neuropathy. The inheritance pattern is autosomal recessive. fALS16 is caused by mutations in the sigma receptor-1 (SIGMAR1) gene. Mutations in this gene also cause frontotemporal dementia.

Pathology

Amyotrophic lateral sclerosis leads to progressive degeneration of the motor neurons that supply voluntary muscles, including lower motor neurons in the medulla and anterior horn of the spinal cord as well as upper motor neurons in the cerebral cortex. The disease is characterized by motor neuron degeneration and death, with gliosis replacing neurons and causing a gradual and progressive loss of function. Neuropathological examination may reveal degenerating neurons with intracellular inclusions. As the motor neuron undergoes apoptosis, the motor nerve axon degenerates and the neuromuscular junction is destroyed. Muscle fibers innervated by that axon are denervated and subsequently atrophy. Characteristic regional patterns of involvement and progression suggest that the disease does not proceed randomly, but via a restricted number of anatomical pathways. These clinical observations combined with electrophysiological and brain imaging studies underpin the concept of amyotrophic lateral sclerosis at the macroscopic level as a system degeneration. Muscle biopsy typically displays denervation atrophy together with fiber-type grouping, which constitutes evidence of reinnervation. As cortical motor neurons are lost, retrograde axonal loss in the corticospinal tract leads to spinal cord atrophy. The ventral roots atrophy as large myelinated fibers are lost.

Pathophysiology

Amyotrophic lateral sclerosis is characterized by relatively rapid degeneration of motor neurons. Mutations in over 20 genes account for about 10 percent of cases. Disease progression is accompanied by a multi-phasic protective and later detrimental immune response. The identification of the DNA and RNA-binding protein TDP-43 (transactive response DNA binding protein 43 kDa (TARDBP)) as a component of abnormal cytoplasmic inclusions in sporadic affected individuals and the discovery of disease-causing mutations in the TDP-43 gene led to the identification of causal mutations in the gene encoding the related protein FUS. These findings suggest that aberrant RNA processing may underlie common mechanisms of neurodegeneration in this group of diseases. Elevated levels of aggregated proteins can also cause an unfolded protein response and mitochondrial dysfunction. Degeneration of motor neurons may be associated with dysregulation of intracellular calcium and excitotoxicity.

Mutations in the ALS2 gene cause three distinct disorders: infantile ascending hereditary spastic paraplegia, juvenile primary lateral sclerosis, and autosomal recessive juvenile amyotrophic lateral sclerosis. The alsin protein contains three guanine-nucleotide-exchange factor-like domains, which may participate in the mechanism of the disease. Biochemical and cell biology assays suggest that alsin dysfunction affects endosome trafficking through a Rab5 (Ras (rat sarcoma)-related protein Rab-5) small GTPase family-mediated mechanism.

Dominantly inherited mutations in senataxin cause juvenile-onset motor neuron disease in a familial form of amyotrophic lateral sclerosis, while recessive mutations cause early-onset ataxia with oculomotor apraxia. A range of RNA processing functions have been attributed to senataxin. Senataxin contains a helicase domain that interacts with RNA and an aminoterminal domain that controls protein interactions. Senataxin is also one of several proteins that maintain the RNA transcriptome, including FUS, TDP-43, and SMN (survival of motor neuron), all of which can cause familial forms of motor neuron disease. Independently of this association, senataxin participates in genomic stability. Senataxin resolves R-Loop structures, which form when nascent RNA hybridizes to DNA, displacing the non-transcribed strand. In cycling cells, senataxin is also found at nuclear foci during the S/G2 cell-cycle phase, and may function at sites of specific collision between components of the replisome and transcription machinery.

FUS mutations are associated with several phenotypes, including some of the most severe, juvenile-onset forms of the disease. The majority of FUS mutations are inherited in dominant fashion and represent missense changes clustered in and around the C-terminal nuclear localization signal. FUS is a predominantly nuclear protein that participates in DNA damage repair and in RNA transcription, splicing, transport and translation. In neurons, FUS is also localized in dendrites and accumulates in excitatory synapses as an RNA–protein complex associated with N-methyl-D-aspartate receptor (NMDA) receptors and in RNA transporting granules in the soma and dendrites. This suggests that FUS, like TDP-43, could participate in the modulation of synaptic activity in the central nervous system by regulating mRNA transport and local translation in neurons. In mouse models of FUS mutation, motor neuron loss is associated with early synaptic failure and withdrawal of the motor axon from the neuromuscular junction. Pre- and postsynaptic changes in the ultrastructure of the neuromuscular junction, including abnormal mitochondria and reduced synaptic vesicle density, are associated with electrophysiological evidence of active denervation, including increased spontaneous activity and sensitivity to high-frequency stimulation.

It is not known how the structural and functional similarities between FUS, TDP-43 and other disease-associated heterogeneous nuclear ribonucleoproteins relate to their participation in the disease. All of these proteins contain low-complexity prion-like sequences (and possibly other domains) that are not only a key determinant of their normal function, but also of their role in the pathogenesis of amyotrophic lateral sclerosis. These domains appear to mediate the movement of these regulatory proteins in and out of subcellular, RNA-containing structures like stress granules and permit reversible and regulated interactions with a large variety of partner proteins. Under pathological conditions, these same regions may mediate the irreversible formation of abnormal aggregates that are selectively toxic to subpopulations of neurons. The natural propensity of these proteins to aggregate, leads to a model of disease in which the low probability of normal protein to form toxic aggregates is increased by disease-causing mutations, leading to neurodegeneration.

Diagnosis

The diagnosis is established by genetic analysis. Electromyography indicates motor neuron disease. There is decreased motor unit recruitment with rapid firing of a reduced number of motor units or large-amplitude, long-duration motor unit potentials with or without evidence of remodeling (an increased number of phases) in combination with abnormal spontaneous activity including positive sharp waves, fibrillations, or fasciculation potentials. Individual fibers that display fibrillations and positive waves demonstrate denervation causing muscle membrane instability. Fasciculations are identified when the fibers of a motor unit contract as a group. This can be detected both clinically and by electromyography. Adjacent motor nerve axons will initially reinnervate the muscle fibers (a recognizable pattern on electromyography). With the eventual death of these motor neurons, the pattern of reinnervation abates and the predominating process of denervation becomes more notable. Nerve conduction studies reveal asymmetric side-to-side compound muscle action potential (CMAP) differences, normal CMAPs, or CMAPs with decreased amplitude, prolonged distal motor latency and slowed conduction velocity, consistent with axon loss. Sensory nerves are often normal, but may reveal conduction abnormalities, indicating dorsal root ganglion degeneration. They may display conduction block and temporal dispersion.

Treatment

Riluzole extends average survival by 3 to 6 months. Riluzole blocks the release of glutamate and is thought to decrease neuronal excitotoxicity. Current trials target muscle proteins, seek ways to stabilize energy expenditure, utilize cell replacement therapies and ascertain whether abnormal genes can be silenced. Antagonism of Nogo (neurite outgrowth inhibitor), a muscle protein that inhibits neurite outgrowth, has been exploited as a method to enhance reinnervation. Antisense therapy utilizes injections of short synthetically modified nucleic acid that binds to an mRNA target, silencing its function. The molecules are too large to cross the blood-brain barrier and so must be administered by intrathecal injection. Dextromethorphan and quinidine alleviate the symptoms of pseudobulbar affect. Dextromethorphan modulates the presynaptic release of glutamate and dopamine by blocking the NMDA receptor and acting as a σ-1 receptor agonist. Quinidine inhibits the metabolism, and therefore prolongs the stability, of dextromethorphan.

Bibliography

Belzil V.V., Langlais J.S., Daoud H., et al. (2012). Novel FUS deletion in a patient with juvenile amyotrophic lateral sclerosis. *Arch Neurol.* 69(5):653–6.

Finsterer J., Burgunder J.M. (2014). Recent progress in the genetics of motor neuron disease. *Eur J Med Genet.* 57(2–3):103–12.

Sharma A., Lyashchenko A.K., L. L., et al. (2016). ALS-associated mutant FUS induces selective motor neuron degeneration through toxic gain of function. *Nat Commun.* 7:10465.

Juvenile Parkinson Disease

A girl had always displayed poor school performance, reported by her mother to be in the lower normal range. She did receive her high school diploma, however. Her parents were consanguineous. The mother first noticed that her daughter, at the age of 14 years, was having trouble performing fine tasks such as putting on socks, tying a knot unto her scarf, putting a rubber band around her hair and peeling carrots. Within a few months, she developed notable slowness of movements. L-dopa was administered, to which she initially responded favorably. After approximately four years, her symptoms worsened and drug usage was terminated because of dyskinesia. She married at 21 years of age and at the age of 24 years could perform normal house tasks with some help from her mother. Examination revealed bradykinesia, resting tremor, rigidity, postural instability, dysarthria, deteriorated handwriting, dystonia, abnormal finger to nose test, finger minimyoclonus, and slow vertical gaze saccades. MR imaging examination of her brain revealed mild cerebellar atrophy.

Anomalies were not noted in her brother by his parents, but a physician who saw the girl requested that the brother be also examined. Upon examination at the age of 10 years, he was also diagnosed as affected by the same disorder. His disabilities progressed rapidly, and within four months, he became slow in all movements. His response to L-dopa was similar to his sister's. They both harbored a homozygous mutation in ATP13A2.

Juvenile Parkinson Disease

Onset: Bradykinesia accompanied by rigidity, rest tremor or loss of postural reflexes before 20 years of age.

Additional manifestations: Rigidity, rest tremor, or loss of postural reflexes. Unilateral onset, response to levodopa for 5 or more years, severe choreiform movements induced by levodopa over time, and a clinical course of 10 or more years. Sleep disturbances, autonomic dysfunction, and cognitive deterioration may also occur.

Disease mechanism: Parkin is an ubiquitin E3 ligase in the ubiquitin proteasome pathway. Parkin may interact with PINK1 to maintain mitochondrial integrity and function of dopaminergic neurons. The Kufor–Rakeb syndrome is caused by loss-of-function mutations affecting both ATP13A2 alleles.

Testing: Genetic analysis.

Treatment: Levodopa, non-ergot dopamine agonists, and monoamine oxidase B inhibitors.

Research highlights: Generation of rat models of the disease that display progressive nigral cell loss.

Clinical Features

Parkinson disease is a progressive hypokinetic movement disorder characterized by dopaminergic nigral cell loss and hypokinesia. Its incidence is 13 per 100,000 individuals, with 4 percent of them representing cases with onset under the age of 50 years. In Parkinson disease, bradykinesia is often accompanied by rigidity, rest tremor or loss of postural reflexes. Additional features include unilateral onset, response to levodopa for 5 or more years, severe choreiform movements induced by levodopa over time and a clinical course of 10 or more years. Sleep disturbances, autonomic dysfunction and cognitive deterioration may also occur. Several forms of Parkinson disease affect adolescents and young adults. Clinical symptoms of the juvenile disorder generally become evident before the age of 20 years. Significant variation occurs in disease progression, from a relatively rapid deterioration over months to years, to slow progression over years to decades. A familial nature

Table 100.1 Causes of juvenile Parkinson disease

Locus name	Gene name	Gene symbol	Inheritance
PARK2	Parkin	PARK2	Autosomal recessive
PARK9 (Kufor-Rakeb disease)	ATPase type 13A2	ATP13A2	Autosomal recessive
PARK14 or NBIA2	Phospholipase A2, group VI	PLA2G6	Autosomal recessive
PARK15	F-box protein 7	FBXO7	Autosomal recessive
NBIA1	Pantothenate kinase 2	PKAN2	Autosomal recessive

is recognized in 10 percent of all cases of Parkinson disease. Several genetic loci are associated with juvenile Parkinson disease.

Parkin mutations can lead to juvenile Parkinson disease with the typical clinical features described earlier and account for 10 percent of individuals with early onset disease.

Kufor–Rakeb disease (KRS) caused by ATP13A2 mutations is the best understood juvenile Parkinson syndrome. In general, individuals with missense ATP13A2 mutations exhibit slow progression, whereas the rate of progression in persons with frameshift mutations varies from slow to rapid. KRS presents with varying degrees of parkinsonism, typically including rigidity, bradykinesia and hypomimia. Tremor is present in only half of KRS cases. Initially, the parkinsonian features respond well to levodopa, but affected individuals rapidly develop levodopa-induced complications such as dyskinesia and hallucinations. Approximately half of KRS affected individuals develop dystonia later in the disease course. Pyramidal signs, such as spasticity and hyperreflexia, are also frequently present, as are facial-faucial-finger mini-myoclonus, supranuclear gaze palsy and slowness in saccadic eye movements. Cognitive impairment is usually present. Dysphagia and dysarthria are also frequently associated with KRS. In addition, olfactory dysfunction can be significant.

Homozygous ATP13A2 mutations may also cause pathologically confirmed neuronal ceroid lipofuscinosis. The combination of extrapyramidal, pyramidal, and cognitive features, the absence of retinal involvement, and the presence of slow vertical eye movements in the proband suggest an overlap of this syndrome with KRS. These findings further implicate the lysosomal system in the mechanism of ATP13A2-associated disease and add to the number of parkinsonian disorders linked to lysosomal dysfunction.

Pathology

Alpha-synuclein is the main constituent of characteristic Lewy bodies. Because of the similar abnormal deposition of alpha-synuclein in Parkinson disease, dementia with Lewy bodies and multiple systems atrophy, these diseases are termed alpha-synucleopathies, which refers to a class of proteinopathies that share aggregated alpha-synuclein. However, the notion that the large insoluble α-synuclein aggregates within Lewy bodies are the cause of neurodegeneration in Parkinson disease is unproven. Neuronal loss precedes the development of Lewy bodies in the substantia nigra and Lewy body density does not correlate with the degree of loss of nigral neurons. This lack of correlation was reinforced by the discovery that a subset of individuals with LRRK2 (leucine-rich repeat kinase 2) gene mutations, which are usually associated with Lewy pathology, can manifest typical clinical features of the disease but exhibit no Lewy bodies in the substantia nigra.

In parkin-associated juvenile Parkinson disease, there is restricted ventral nigral degeneration with rare or absent Lewy body pathology. There is also neuronal loss in pigmented nuclei of the brainstem. Neurofibrillary tangles in the substantia nigra, posterior hypothalamus and cerebral cortex and tau-containing thorn-shaped astrocytes are also found.

Computed tomography or MR imaging demonstrates brain atrophy, involving the cerebral hemispheres and the cerebellum in most individuals with KRS. Radiological evidence of cerebral atrophy is generally not manifest until at least 5 years after the onset of clinical symptoms. ATP13A2 has been identified in Lewy bodies from the brains of sporadic Parkinson disease individuals.

In peripheral nervous tissues, there is formation of small membrane-bound cytoplasmic inclusion bodies resembling lysosomes in Schwann cells and perineural cells of the sural nerve. Electron-dense lamellated inclusion bodies may be identified in skin and muscle cells. Although the mechanism involved in the formation of inclusion bodies is unknown, lysosomal dysfunction caused by mutations in ATP13A2 has been suggested as the cause.

Pathophysiology

Parkin functions as an ubiquitin E3 ligase in the ubiquitin proteasome pathway. Parkin may interact with PINK1 (phosphatase and tensin homolog-induced putative kinase 1) to maintain mitochondrial integrity and function of dopaminergic neurons.

The Kufor–Rakeb syndrome is caused by loss-of-function mutations affecting both ATP13A2 alleles. Most of the mutations occur in functional domains of ATP13A2, such as the transmembrane domains and the E1-E2 adenosine triphosphatase (ATPase) domain, and thus have been predicted to cause a loss of function of ATP13A2. The intronic missense mutation generates an ATP13A2 variant that lacks exon 13 by disrupting a canonical splice site, reducing protein stability. Consistently, all of the KRS-associated mutations assessed cause a varying degree of impairment in ATP13A2 function with the involvement of different mechanisms, such as nonsense-mediated messenger RNA decay, mislocalization, and premature degradation of the protein product by the proteasomal system.

Sequence homology analysis indicates that ATP13A2 is a member of the P-type ATPase family, most of whose members are cation transporters. The Wilson disease protein (also known as ATP7B) is a member of this family and functions as a copper transporter. Thus, there has been interest in determining the cationic substrate of ATP13A2. Study of a yeast orthologue of ATP13A2 indicates an interaction with divalent heavy metal ions, including Cd^{2+}, Mn^{2+}, Ni^{2+}, and Se^{2+}. It is possible that Mn^{2+} modulates the activity of ATP13A2. However, KRS–derived human cells manifest altered intracellular Zn^{2+} contents. Thus, loss of ATP13A2 causes Zn^{2+} dyshomeostasis, with consequences including abnormal cellular metabolism in organelles such as mitochondria and lysosomes, resulting in dysfunctional energy production and reduced lysosomal proteolysis.

Functional ATP13A2 is essential for the degradation of accumulated or aggregated α-synuclein, a feature common to sporadic and most genetic forms of Parkinson disease.

ATP13A2 also may provide links between α-synuclein metabolism and mitochondrial dysfunction in sporadic Parkinson disease. An increased export of exosome-associated α-synuclein may explain why surviving neurons of the substantia nigra pars compacta in sporadic Parkinson disease individuals overexpress ATP13A2. Mitochondrial dysfunction may be important in the neurodegenerative process of both sporadic and familial Parkinson disease. In KRS-derived cell lines and ATP13A2-silenced mammalian cell lines, consistent pathogenic changes are observed in mitochondrial function. The function of ATP13A2 in mitochondria and lysosomes is directly related to its activity as a Zn^{2+} transporter and links these two seemingly disparate organelle systems in this disease. Zinc dysregulation related to ATP13A2 deficiency also may explain the association of sporadic Parkinson disease with elevated Zn^{2+} levels in brain and other tissues.

Diagnosis

KRS individuals demonstrate nigrostriatal dopaminergic dysfunction on functional imaging. ^{18}F-dopa positron emission tomography (PET) shows reduced bilateral tracer accumulation in the striatum. Single-photon emission computed tomography (SPECT) using ^{123}I-labeled dopaminergic tracers illustrate reduced bilateral tracer accumulation in the striatum or caudate nucleus and putamen, supporting the notion of nigrostriatal dopaminergic dysfunction. MR imaging T2 hypointensity is detected in the putamina and caudate nuclei and may indicate iron accumulation, leading to the inclusion of KRS among the neurodegeneration with brain iron accumulation diseases.

Treatment

First line treatments for Parkinson's disease include levodopa, non-ergot dopamine agonists, and monoamine oxidase B inhibitors. Levodopa is usually the mainstay of treatment. Dopamine agonists simulate dopamine by binding directly to post-synaptic dopamine receptors in the striatum. They include: a) non-ergot dopamine agonists (oral pramipexole and ropinirole and transdermal rotigotine) and b) ergot derived dopamine agonists (cabergoline, bromocriptine, and pergolide). Monoamine oxidase B inhibitors (rasagiline and selegiline) selectively inhibit monoamine oxidase type B enzyme, which metabolizes dopamine, increasing dopamine availability.

α-synuclein can be transmitted from the gut to the brain. It has been proposed that Parkinson disease might be caused by an enteric neurotropic pathogen entering the brain via the vagal nerve, a process that might take more than 20 years. Vagotomy, a surgical procedure in which the vagus nerve is resected, used to be a common treatment for peptic ulcer. Two common types of vagotomy were performed: full truncal vagotomy, in which both vagal trunks are severed, and superselective vagotomy, in which only nerves supplying the fundus and body of the stomach are resected.

IPX066 is an extended-release oral formulation of carbidopa-levodopa designed to rapidly attain and maintain therapeutic concentrations. This drug reduces the amount of time during the day when symptoms are not adequately controlled. In advanced Parkinson's disease, this medication might be effective at preventing of the wearing off of drug effects, compared with immediate-release carbidopa-levodopa.

In advanced Parkinson's disease, both bilateral deep brain stimulation of the globus pallidus pars interna (GPi) and bilateral deep brain stimulation of the subthalamic nucleus have been performed.

Cell transplantation therapies using embryonic stem cells or induced pluripotent stem cells for Parkinson's disease are being tested. Many types of stem cells are currently available for transplantation therapy, including fetal ventral mesencephalic and adult tissue (for example bone marrow or placenta-derived mesenchymal stem cells). Mesenchymal stem cells can replace and rescue degenerated dopaminergic and non-dopaminergic cells, suggesting their potential use for the treatment of motor as well as non-motor symptoms. However, graft-induced dyskinesia and host-to-graft spread of alpha-synuclein pathology may occur.

Bibliography

Kalia L.V., Lang A.E. (2016). Parkinson disease in 2015: Evolving basic, pathological and clinical concepts in PD. *Nat Rev Neurol.* 12(2):65–6.

Malakouti-Nejad M., Shahidi G.A., Rohani M., et al. (2014). Identification of p.Gln858* in ATP13A2 in two EOPD patients and presentation of their clinical features. *Neurosci Lett.* 577:106–11.

Regression in Other Neurological and Psychiatric Disorders

Epilepsy

Landau–Kleffner Syndrome

A 6.5-year-old boy with a 2-month history of hearing problems and difficulty following verbal commands was referred for evaluation. He had an unremarkable past history and there was no behavior suggestive of epileptic seizures. The neurological examination was normal with the exception of difficulty understanding verbal instructions, but he could lip read and also follow written instructions. EEG examination showed normal background, but there were very frequent sharp waves in the bitemporal areas, left greater than right during sleep (Figure). MR imaging of the brain was normal. Language evaluation found weaknesses in understanding specific grammatical structures, as well as periodic difficulty expressing complex concepts. Although many of his basic language skills remained in the average range his performance on the Token Test for Children was impaired. In addition, mildly slurred speech was noted, though his speech remained largely intelligible. Neuropsychological evaluation confirmed auditory agnosia with a severe, selective deficit in processing of auditory information as well as weaknesses in auditory memory and attention. Other areas of verbal and non-verbal cognitive functioning were normal.

Clinical Features

Acquired aphasia or agnosia can manifest in the presence or absence of epilepsy in the first decade of life. In these syndromes, there is progressive loss of understanding followed by loss of expression and eventual intellectual deterioration. In many children, seizures appear or the EEG becomes abnormal, especially during slow sleep (Figure 101.1).

Landau–Kleffner syndrome presents most commonly at 4–5 years of age. There is a two- to fourfold male predominance and, in some cases, there are mutations in the glutamate receptor GRIN2A gene. Children first experience a progressive loss of receptive language, which is then followed by deterioration of expressive language over weeks to months in the context of a preserved intellect. The first sign is usually auditory verbal agnosia. There is difficulty distinguishing between words and non-speech environmental sounds. Unilateral brain dysfunction is not plausible because the auditory cortex is bilaterally represented. Receptive aphasia follows the verbal agnosia, with gradual loss of the comprehension of spoken language. Children may lip-read or visually understand, but to no avail. There is a prominent incapacity to segment verbal language. Later, a paucity of spoken expressions appears. At first, utterances can be repetitive and stereotyped, with perseveration and paraphasias. Eventually, speech becomes telegraphic. Later, the child all but ceases to communicate. There may be a loss of facial expression and of the ability to use sign language. Communication is limited to the expression of grunts or unrefined gestures.

Within months or years of the onset of language dysfunction, and occasionally simultaneously with it, seizures may appear. This is the second major manifestation of the disorder. The seizures can be of many types except clonic, but they are usually not frequent and can be treated with a single anticonvulsant agent. They frequently occur during sleep. One-fourth of children do not experience seizures. Infrequent repetitive seizures do not correlate with language dysfunction or ultimate prognosis and, when episodic, aphasia or language dysfluency exhibit no EEG correlate. EEG seizure activity may occupy as much as 80 percent of the slow wave sleep EEG. Treatment with an anticonvulsant is effective for seizure suppression, but has no impact on the aphasia. These seizures tend to subside spontaneously over time. After 10 years, only 20 percent of individuals continue to experience seizures even in the absence of treatment.

Behavioral disturbances are the third cardinal manifestation of Landau–Kleffner syndrome. As

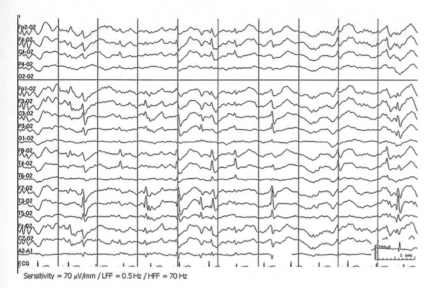

Figure 101.1 Referential montage to right occipital reference illustrating frequent independent right and left temporal sharp waves in Landau-Kleffner syndrome. Reproduced with permission from Fandiño M et al. Landau-Kleffner syndrome: a rare auditory processing disorder series of cases and review of the literature. *Int J Pediatr Otorhinolaryngol.* 2011; 75(1):33–8.

Sensitivity = 70 μV/mm / LFF = 0.5 Hz / HFF = 70 Hz

many as two-thirds of affected children exhibit behavioral dysfunction, which can be prominent at disease onset. These abnormalities do not impact intelligence but parallel language deterioration. They include hyperactivity, attention deficits, aggressivity, or psychotic manifestations. All of them are considered reactions to the loss of communicative ability.

The evolution of Landau–Kleffner syndrome is often relatively favorable. The disorder stabilizes for months or years without further progression, although episodic exacerbations and ameliorations occur sporadically. Seizures eventually cease and the EEG normalizes, often before the age of 10 years. The aphasia may later improve over the course of several months or years, but never before seizures disappear. The ultimate outcome may consist of near recovery to permanent and severe language impairment. A younger age of onset, before the child has learned written language, is often associated with a worse outcome.

The EEG in Landau–Kleffner syndrome illustrates partial seizures originating in the temporal lobe, often in its left posterior area. This focus is probably associated with localized discharges during wakefulness and with a pattern that resembles continuous spike-wave status of sleep. The most common EEG waveforms include generalized slow-spike or polyspike wave bursts or sharp waves and posterior temporal spikes.

Treatment

The treatment of Landau–Kleffner syndrome includes anticonvulsants, corticosteroids and intravenous immunoglobulin. The latter interventions are associated with mild or moderate but not full efficacy.

Bibliography

Fandiño M., Connolly M., Usher L., et al. (2011). Landau-Kleffner syndrome: a rare auditory processing disorder series of cases and review of the literature. *Int J Pediatr Otorhinolaryngol.* 75(1):33–8.

Mantovani J.F., Landau W.M. (1980). Acquired aphasia with convulsive disorder: course and prognosis. *Neurology.* 30(5):524–9.

Electrical Status Epilepticus in Sleep

A 5-year-old boy had been six weeks premature at birth but had no significant early medical problems. He also had a normal physical and cognitive development until preschool. It was then that his teacher noticed the child was having learning difficulties, staring spells and progressive difficulty expressing himself. He had a single generalized tonic-clonic seizure. A routine EEG revealed very frequent epileptiform discharges. He was prescribed an anticonvulsant and four months later his EEG showed continuous spike wave discharges during sleep. The spike wave discharges occurred in long runs, lasting a minute or more without clear ictal evolution. The spike wave discharges were detected in a generalized distribution, maximal bifronto-temporally with some asymmetry (right greater than left). When the child was subsequently awakened, the EEG significantly improved and the spike wave discharges almost completely resolved. The spike and wave discharges recurred as the child became drowsy again. The anticonvulsant dose was increased and his EEG and language subsequently returned to normal.

Clinical Features

Electrical status epilepticus in sleep is also known as continuous spike-waves of sleep and presents with regression of behavior, cognition and language in association with a variety of seizure types. The disorder is characterized by focal and generalized seizures and, in some cases, there is overlap with the Landau–Kleffner syndrome. There is a slight male predominance. Maximum frequency occurs at 4–5 years of age, although it can be present from infancy to adolescence. Up to 1 percent of children with epilepsy exhibit electrical status epilepticus in sleep.

At onset, the child exhibits intellectual regression accompanied by expressive language and behavioral deterioration. Speech attempts may be slowed and

drooling may occur. There are word finding difficulties, paraphasia, articulatory impairment, or expressive aphasia. There is also intellectual deterioration, particularly in regard to other aspects of language, memory and orientation. Reading difficulties may be prominent. There may be difficulties with copying designs due to eye-hand incoordination. In most children, behavior is disrupted by limited attention or hyperactivity. Psychosis has been noted during the status epilepticus sleep stage.

Seizures occur in a majority of cases at about 8 years of age and usually precede the sleep status epilepticus. These seizures may be nocturnal and then occur upon awakening as partial events involving the face. In some cases, seizures subside well before adolescence. In others, there may be absence episodes during electrical status events and yet in others there may be atonic and clonic seizures at the onset of electrical status. Regardless of type, seizures generally improve by adolescence.

EEG may illustrate early generalized spike wave bursts, sometimes in association with clinical seizures while awake. At the onset of electrical status, there are diffuse complexes of spike wave with 1.5–2 Hz periodicity. These complexes may span more than 85 percent of the EEG during non-REM sleep and they occur every time that the child sleeps. The discharges may continue for hours. EEG spikes recorded over the left side of the brain are associated with errors in verbal performance, while right-sided EEG spikes occur with non-verbal task errors.

Treatment

The disorder is treatable with anticonvulsants, but cognitive, behavioral, and learning disabilities persist in some cases. In many instances, there is a dissociation between the pharmacological amelioration of the EEG and the child's level of intellectual performance. A combination of carbamazepine, valproate, ethosuximide or clonazepam have proven effective to control the nocturnal status and to control the seizures. ACTH has occasionally produced substantial benefit only lasting for as long as it is administered. The electrical status epilepticus episodes during sleep tends to disappear at about 10–12 years of age and this is followed by cessation of seizures some years later.

Bibliography

Sánchez Fernández I, Loddenkemper T, Peters JM, et al. (2012). Electrical status epilepticus in sleep: Clinical presentation and pathophysiology. *Pediatr Neurol.* 47(6):390–410.

Zhang J, Talley G, Kornegay AL, et al. (2010). Electrical status epilepticus during sleep: A case report and review of the literature. *Am J Electroneurodiagnostic Technol.* 50(3):211–18.

Effects of Antiepileptic Drugs on Cognition

An 11-year-old girl with symptomatic focal epilepsy and normal intelligence developed reversible mental deterioration while receiving valproate. After 2 years and 6 months on valproate (at a dose less or equal to 26 mg/kg/day) the girl insidiously developed mental deterioration (loss of 18 IQ points and drop in age-adjusted Raven's Progressive Matrices score from the 95th to the 50th percentile) associated with MR imaging-documented pseudoatrophy of the brain. Onset of severe cognitive impairment coincided with serum valproate concentrations near 100 µg/ml. There were no other manifestations of drug toxicity or hyperammonemia. Background EEG activity was normal. Reduction of valproate dosage and subsequent discontinuation 4 months later resulted in disappearance of clinical symptoms with a 20-point improvement at IQ testing and recovery of previous Raven's Progressive Matrices score. Repeat MR imaging revealed disappearance of pseudoatrophic changes.

General Principles

Anticonvulsants can adversely and significantly impact cognition even at generally acceptable blood levels. The converse may not occur: Anticonvulsants rarely improve cognition unless an underlying epileptic process interferes with it. Even in this case, improvement is incomplete and inconsistent across affected individuals. In sensitive or overdosed children, anticonvulsants may cause slurred speech and impaired auditory memory and preexisting language deficits may be exacerbated. The use of multiple anticonvulsants or of anticonvulsants in combination with other neuroactive drugs may compound these problems and even interfere with seizure control. In general, the adverse cognitive effects of anticonvulsants become manifest within a month of their use. Several drugs commonly used are reviewed here.

Phenobarbital

Phenobarbital and other barbiturates can impair verbal learning and depress auditory capacity, especially auditory discrimination, and negatively impact language comprehension and verbal expression. These effects are correlated with blood drug levels. Younger children are more prone to these side effects. Intellectual deficits start to emerge by 6 months of use, including a reduction in full performance IQ. By 12 months of use, the changes may be apparent, with reduced comprehension. An additional effect of barbiturates is folate depletion, which itself can impact cognition. Discontinuation of the drug leads to improved total IQ. This increase is mostly due to performance (nonverbal) IQ items, whereas verbal items may remain almost unchanged.

Phenytoin

Phenytoin is a commonly used hydantoin that may impair auditory memory, comprehension, concentration, and motor speed. The first indication of elevated blood levels and toxicity in some children is slowing and slurring of the speech. There are also documented instances of irreversibly deleterious phenytoin effects on cognition when elevated doses are used. A progressive and partially reversible phenytoin encephalopathy can occur without other signs of toxicity.

Valproate

Slurred speech may occur with elevated doses of valproate. When used in large quantities, the strong protein binding potential of the drug may lead to an elevation in other drugs' free levels, which penetrate the brain and may cause toxicity. Valproate toxicity leads to speech retardation and slurring and slowed motor performance, which can be subtle and precede more obvious toxic manifestations such as ataxia and nystagmus (Figure 103.1).

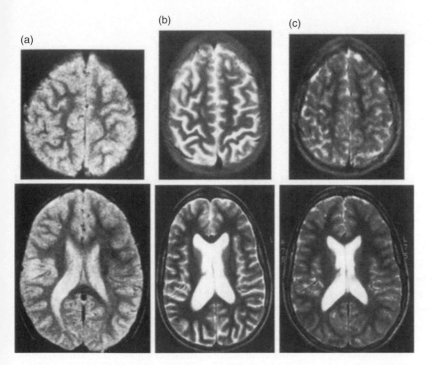

Figure 103.1 Valproate-induced cerebral pseudoatrophy in a 10-year-old girl. **A** represents a MR imaging study obtained before treatment with valproate. **B** is the MR imaging study obtained while receiving valproate for 9 months. In **C**, withdrawal of valproate is associated with a restoration of cerebral volume. Reproduced with permission from Guerrini R et al. Reversible pseudoatrophy of the brain and mental deterioration associated with valproate treatment. *Epilepsia*. 1998; 39(1):27–32.

Carbamazepine

Carbamazepine may increase speech output and has not been associated with the induction of cognitive dysfunction at acceptable doses. There have been reports of normalization of articulatory speech difficulties and language processing impairment after carbamazepine administration in complex partial epilepsy. At elevated doses, however, carbamazepine leads to inattention and motor unsteadiness.

Benzodiazepines

Benzodiazepines may cause behavioral disinhibition with dysarthria. Sentences may be incomplete and soft spoken. In general, benzodiazepines slow intellect and behavior. Psychomotor speed, movement accuracy, and reaction time undergo deterioration. Clobazam has been associated with reversible expressive aphasia.

Bibliography

Guerrini R., Belmonte A., Canapicchi R., et al. (1998). Reversible pseudoatrophy of the brain and mental deterioration associated with valproate treatment. *Epilepsia*. 39(1):27–32.

Svoboda W.B. (2004). *Childhood Epilepsy. Language, Learning and Behavioural Complications*. Cambridge University Press, Cambridge, UK.

Tonekaboni S.H., Beyraghi N., Tahbaz H.S. et al. (2006). Neurocognitive effects of phenobarbital discontinuation in epileptic children. *Epilepsy Behav*. 8(1):145–8.

Epileptic Psychosis

A 14-year-old girl was evaluated for a sudden behav-ioral change. She suffered from Dravet syndrome asso-ciated with a stop codon mutation (Arg377X) in the sodium channel gene SCN1A. One month before the evaluation, the seizures that had occurred several times per month rapidly became less frequent and then disappeared, despite there having been no change in her treatment with phenobarbital, topiramate and clo-bazam. When she was completely seizure-free, an EEG revealed a resolution of paroxysmal discharges; back-ground activity, including spindles and humps, was poorly organized and slow activity was evident on the right temporal region. At the same time, her behav-ior progressively changed and she experienced a psych-otic regression, with very slow motor activity, absence of any social or environmental interactions, apathy, and passivity. She tended to assume and maintain plastic postures for a long time mimicking catatonia. Language, which had usually been present, albeit delayed, was absent during this psychotic regression. Her phenobarbital dose was reduced. After that, the myoclonic seizures reappeared and the EEG findings reverted to their previous state; however, her behavior greatly improved and the catatonia disappeared.

The psychoses are characterized by the occurrence of hallucinations, delusions, and disorganized speech and behavior. Individuals with epilepsy exhibit a 5-fold increase in the risk of manifesting a broadly defined psychotic disorder, an 8-fold increase in the risk of developing schizophrenia and a 6-fold increase in the risk of developing bipolar disorder. There is clustering of the association between epilepsy and psychosis within families. Epileptic individuals are prone to several types of psychosis, including ictal, postictal, or interictal psychosis, with the latter comprising episodic and chronic psychosis. Psychosis may also be associated with epilepsy treatments. In general, epilepsy-associated psychoses tend to be chronic, with increased frequency of hallucinations, delusions, and mood abnormalities.

There are instances where states of abnormal con-sciousness due to complex partial status epilepticus may be mistaken for psychosis. These states may include paranoid delusions, religious delusions, and other hallucinations. These seizures usually originate in the limbic structures. Antipsychotic drugs increase seizure propensity such that seizures occur in 1 per-cent of subjects who use them. This risk is greater in individuals with an abnormal EEG, previous seizures, prior neurological disorders and when antipsychotic drugs are rapidly initiated. Most neuroleptics produce EEG changes that include slowing of the background at high doses. Some also can cause interictal sharp waves and spikes, but these do not predict seizures. Hepatic enzymatic induction by antiepileptic drugs may increase the clearance of neuroleptics, therefore decreasing their efficacy. Conversely, discontinuation of anticonvulsants may lead to increased neuroleptic levels, leading to extrapyramidal side effects.

Only the chronic interictal psychoses that lead to behavioral deterioration are discussed here.

Episodic Psychosis

An intermittent schizophreniform psychosis can emerge 10 to 20 years after the onset of uncontrolled childhood-onset left temporal lobe epilepsy or frontal lobe, often of a complex partial nature. This psychosis may last several years. During psychotic events, there may be perceptual disturbances, perturbed conscious-ness and poor memory for the psychotic event, with complete resolution between episodes. More specific-ally, affected individuals manifest prominent para-noid delusions and auditory hallucinations with anxiety, fear or irritability in the context of preserved interpersonal interactions. There are no incoherent thoughts or speech. These episodes recur, initially lasting days to weeks and are generally followed by a full recovery. However, after numerous episodes, a chronic schizophrenia-like psychosis may occur. This development carries a poor prognosis.

The seizure types associated with these late psychoses include automatisms with secondary generalization with onset in adolescence and they are more common in left handed individuals and in females. Structural lesions may underlie the epilepsy. Seizures may decrease in frequency during the psychotic episode but they are not temporally well correlated with the psychosis.

Chronic Psychosis

The incidence rate of a schizopheniform psychosis in epilepsy is 3–8 percent, particularly in temporal lobe epilepsy. This disorder includes chronic, permanent psychoses that exhibit paranoid features, with delusions, preservation of affect and personality and predominance of visual over auditory hallucinations. Religious delusions and paranoia are common. Unlike in canonical schizophrenia, affect and social interactions are generally preserved. Family and social behavior are not impacted. In general, affected individuals retain their level of societal functioning.

Individuals with left-sided temporal epileptic lesions are more likely to develop schizophrenic psychosis. Many of these individuals are left handed, possibly in relation to left hemispheric dysfunction since early in life. In some cases, there are grey matter heterotopic nodules and perivascular gliosis. The ventricles may be enlarged. There may be decreased accumulation of fluoro-deoxyglucose in the dominant hemisphere detected by positron emission tomography imaging, particularly involving the temporal lobe when there are hallucinations.

Treatment of this chronic psychosis includes neuroleptic drugs. Seizure control does not impact the psychosis, even after epilepsy surgery.

Temporal Lobectomy Psychosis

Another psychosis-predisposing event is temporal lobe epilepsy surgery. This may occur in as many as 7 percent of individuals following an anterior temporal lobectomy. It is more common in individuals with residual seizures after surgery. Affected individuals may be normal for 6 to 12 months following temporal lobectomy before paranoid psychotic symptoms emerge. The psychosis is more likely with a later seizure onset and manifests with a sense of unreality.

This paranoid psychosis occurs at increased frequency in the setting of bilateral temporal lobe epilepsy. From an anatomical perspective, epileptic individuals who experience psychosis are more likely to harbor dysplastic or tumoral lesions than mesial temporal sclerosis. Treatment is usually favorably achieved with neuroleptics. A previous psychosis is not a contraindication to epilepsy surgery, as surgically controlled seizures to not impact a preexisting psychosis.

Forced Normalization Psychosis

Forced normalization or alternating psychosis follows the suppression of seizures or EEG normalization and usually manifests as a paranoid state with normal consciousness. This psychosis follows seizures by 2 to 10 days and presents as acute or subacute behavioral impairment with disordered thought, disturbed mood, anxiety, depersonalization, or hysteria. There may also be drastic behavioral deterioration when seizures are controlled. When there are seizures, the behavioral abnormalities subside. Forced normalization is related to anticonvulsant efficacy and may happen regardless of the anticonvulsant used to treat the seizures. Weak anticonvulsants such as gabapentin are endowed with little capacity to induce it. Forced normalization psychosis is more common with chronic epilepsy, most often limbic epilepsy. In individuals with an abnormal EEG, this psychotic state is associated with a reduction of EEG spikes greater than 50 percent or even with normalization. However, subdural electrodes may illustrate abundant epileptic discharges in temporal limbic structures.

Early control of dysphoria before psychosis sets in may prevent the psychosis. The treatment of alternating psychosis includes reduction or discontinuation of antiepileptic drugs until seizures recur and psychotic symptoms cease. Antipsychotic drugs may be used during the psychotic events.

Anticonvulsant Psychosis

Psychoses are an uncommon adverse effect of all antiepileptic drugs. Schizophreniform psychosis can occur with phenytoin, primidone and phenobarbital at toxic blood levels. A psychotic disorder may follow anticonvulsant discontinuation, particularly when the anticonvulsant has mood stabilizing properties, such as carbamazepine, phenytoin, valproic acid, and benzodiazepines. In individuals with chronic epilepsy, the incidence of anticonvulsant-induced psychosis is 5 percent.

Bibliography

Clarke M.C., Tanskanen A., Huttunen M.O., et al. (2012). Evidence for shared susceptibility to epilepsy and psychosis: A population-based family study. *Biol Psychiatry*. 71(9):836–9.

Gobbi G., Giovannini S., Boni A., et al. (2008). Catatonic psychosis related to forced normalization in a girl with Dravet's syndrome. *Epileptic Disord*. 10(4):325–9.

Autism

Autism spectrum disorder (ASD) refers to a heterogeneous group of neurodevelopmental disorders characterized by deficits in communication and human interaction and by the demonstration of restricted, repetitive, and stereotyped patterns of behavior. The symptoms are present from early childhood and are impairing to everyday functioning. Individuals with ASD also exhibit intellectual disability at higher rates than the general population. At least 50 genes or genomic variants, as well as numerous copy number variations, cause or predispose individuals to ASD. It is common to experience language or global intellectual regression in ASD at the age of 1 to 2 years. Children may lose the capacity to communicate verbally, which leads to an abundance of stereotypic behaviors apparently devoid of communicative value.

Epilepsy in Autism

Chapter 105

Individuals with autistic spectrum disorder have a higher prevalence of epilepsy compared to normally developing individuals, including epilepsy that is refractory to standard treatments. The prevalence of epilepsy in ASD may be as high as 25%. The rate of epilepsy is 9% in individuals without an intellectual disability but 24% in those with an intellectual disability. The average prevalence of epilepsy differs by age, with a prevalence rate of 13% in children between 2 and 17 years of age but 26% in those older than 12 years. In addition to an increased prevalence of epilepsy in individuals with ASD, there is an increased incidence of epileptiform activity on the electroencephalogram of individuals with ASD. Whereas interictal spikes occur in more than 5% of normally developing children without epilepsy, up to 60% of EEG records from children with ASD have interictal spikes and many of the children with abnormal EEG do not manifest epilepsy. The location of spikes in children with ASD also differs from their normal peers, with a higher percentage of interictal spikes in the frontal lobe in children with ASD than in those without ASD.

While the appearance of epilepsy in individuals with ASD often signifies a medically refractory phenomenon, seizures may compound neural and behavioral development. In the case of ASD caused by tuberous sclerosis complex, individuals with ASD exhibit an earlier age-at-seizure onset, more frequent seizures and their EEG recordings display a greater amount of interictal epileptiform features in the left temporal lobe when compared with individuals who do not develop ASD. Thus, ASD may be associated with persistent seizure activity early in development, whereas the risk of ASD in tuberous sclerosis can be reduced by early treatment of the epilepsy.

Bibliography

Buckley A.W., Holmes G.L. (2016). Epilepsy and autism. *Cold Spring Harb Perspect Med.* 6(4):pii:a022749.

Down Syndrome

The most common genetic cause of human intellectual disability is Down syndrome (DS), which is caused by the triplication of the human chromosome 21. DS, or trisomy 21, is present in approximately 1 in 1,000 live births and this prevalence has not decreased over the years. DS individuals manifest a characteristic facial appearance, behavior, and distinct cognitive problems. The most marked cognitive features are a reduced IQ that ranges from 30 to 70 with an average value of 50, associated with reduced brain volume, which occurs in association with impairment in verbal short-term memory and explicit long-term memory.

Dementia in Down Syndrome

In addition to the congenital intellectual disability, individuals with DS experience accelerated ageing, including early-onset dementia due to Alzheimer's disease (AD). Progressive neurodegeneration with amyloid plaque formation can be detected in the DS brain as early as 8 years of age. An estimated 50–70% of DS individuals develop AD by the time they reach 60 years of age. In contrast, AD is present in about 11 percent of the general population of 65 years and older.

Extensive deposition of Aβ plaques, as well as neuroinflammation and substantial numbers of neurofibrillary tangles, are present in virtually all DS individuals aged 40 years and older, twenty to thirty years earlier than in the general population at risk for AD. Trisomy 21 leads to a dose-dependent increase in the production of the amyloid precursor protein and subsequently the production of the amyloidogenic fragments leading to early and predominant senile plaque formation. Oxidative damage and neuroinflammation may interact to accelerate the disease process, particularly in individuals with DS over the age of 40 years.

There is a variable time interval between the presence of neuropathology and the onset of dementia symptoms, making the prediction of the course to dementia complex. Social withdrawal precedes the clinical diagnosis of AD by an average of 33 months, whereas agitation, aggression, and hallucinations are generally observed 1–2 years after the AD diagnosis. Demented DS subjects are variably referred to as manifesting behavioral disturbances, behavioral deficits and excesses, psychiatric symptoms, maladaptive behavior and personality changes. Common reported features include personality changes and apathy or inactivity, while depression, disorientation and hallucinations or delusions are less prevalent.

Bibliography

Dekker A.D., Strydom A., Coppus A.M., et al. (2015). Behavioural and psychological symptoms of dementia in Down syndrome: Early indicators of clinical Alzheimer's disease? *Cortex*. 73:36–61.

Lott I.T., Head E. (2001). Down syndrome and Alzheimer's disease: A link between development and aging. *Ment Retard Dev Disabil Res Rev*. 7(3):172–8.

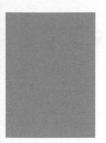

Systemic Inflammatory Diseases

Neural performance decline is not uncommon in autoimmune diseases and may often become the dominant symptom. In some cases, there may be few systemic symptoms before disabling neuropsychiatric dysfunction has occurred. In contrast with autoimmune demyelinating disease such as multiple sclerosis, systemic inflammatory disorders cause widespread cerebrovascular and neural cell dysfunction. The most typical manifestations include dementia with white matter hyperintensities detected by MR imaging in Behçet's disease, mood disorders and dementia with periventricular white matter lesions and microangiopathy in Sjögren syndrome and the array of neuropsychiatric manifestations that are characteristic of systemic lupus erythematosus.

Neuropsychiatric Systemic Lupus Erythematosus

Systemic lupus erythematosus is among the best known autoimmune disorders with neuropsychiatric manifestations, which can occur in children and adolescents. The central nervous system is involved in as many as one third of cases of pediatric lupus, whereas peripheral nervous system involvement is rare in children. The mean onset age is 15 years. In approximately 40 percent of individuals with neuropsychiatric disease, the initial presentation of lupus includes symptoms attributable to neural dysfunction, whereas in approximately 70% of children the neuropsychiatric manifestations will occur within the first year of diagnosis.

Among the most common lupus neuropsychiatric syndromes are acute confusional state, cognitive dysfunction, anxiety, mood disorders including depression, and psychosis. Cognitive impairment includes at least one of the cognitive domains of simple or complex attention, memory, visual-spatial processing, language, reasoning and problem solving, psychomotor speed, and executive function. The hallmark of lupus-associated psychosis in children and adolescents is visual hallucinations. The presence of this type of hallucination helps differentiate the organic psychosis associated with lupus from idiopathic schizophrenia of childhood. Visual hallucinations may be accompanied by auditory hallucinations and frequently the hallucinations are of a threatening nature. The depression may be organic in nature or reactive secondary to chronic disease or, more rarely, due to corticosteroid use. Mania and bipolar disorder are uncommon.

The pathological basis for neuropsychiatric lupus is a chronic vasculopathy with hyaline degeneration of the blood vessel wall and perivascular cellular infiltration. This may lead to small multifocal ischemic infarcts of the grey and white matter. In addition, contributing factors include direct neural cell dysfunction stemming from antineuronal antibody penetration in the brain and cytokine release. The main clinical consequence of these pathogenic mechanisms is decreased concentration ability and attention, impaired visuospatial ability and cognitive speed, without significant language involvement.

There is an association between neural dysfunction and anti-ganglioside M1, anticardiolipin and antiribosomal P antibodies. In general, higher mean C3/C4 levels, less percentage of anti-dsDNA antibodies elevation and higher percentage of elevated anticardiolipin antibodies are observed in neuropsychiatric lupus. Cognitive impairment, psychosis, and depression have also been associated with several antibodies including aCL, anti-NR2 glutamate receptor antibodies, and anti-N-methyl-D-aspartate (NMDA) receptor antibodies.

In general, lupus encephalopathy is treated with a combination of high dose steroids and an immunosuppressive agent. Methylprednisolone can be used during acute presentations. For example, the treatment of lupus with neuropsychiatric involvement may include monthly intravenous pulse cyclophosphamide and corticosteroids, with or without the addition of methylprednisolone. Most affected individuals recover satisfactorily with treatment. The overall survival is 90 to 95 percent at both five and 10-year follow-up. Only children who present with seizures or frank cerebrovascular disease, who had a high cumulative disease activity or who experienced neuropsychiatric recurrent illnesses are at high risk for long-term neural sequelae.

Bibliography

Benseler S.M., Silverman E.D. (2007). Neuropsychiatric involvement in pediatric systemic lupus erythematosus. *Lupus.* 16(8):564–71.

Kozora E., Filley C.M. (2011). Cognitive dysfunction and white matter abnormalities in systemic lupus erythematosus. *J Int Neuropsychol Soc.* 17(3):385–92.

Yu H.H., Lee J.H., Wang L.C., et al. (2006). Neuropsychiatric manifestations in pediatric systemic lupus erythematosus: A 20-year study. *Lupus.* 15(10):651–7.

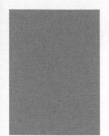

Hydrocephalus

Hydrocephalus is the end result of a variety of processes that either increase cerebrospinal fluid formation or decrease its absorption. In childhood, the most common causes include stenosis of the aqueduct of Sylvius, ventricular hemorrhage, Arnold-Chiari malformations and the Dandy-Walker syndrome.

Clinical Manifestations

An acute onset of manifestations with headache, nausea and vomiting, visual disturbances, changes in mental status, or coma is rare both in children and adults.

More often, the onset is insidious. Most children manifest progressively abnormal psychomotor development, school difficulties, intermittent headache, endocrine disturbances, and growth retardation, but may also exhibit a more rapid progression of symptoms as a result of further decompensation of the hydrocephalic state. Sometimes, decompensation may follow minor head injury, febrile illnesses, or subarachnoid hemorrhage. The neuropsychological profile of hydrocephalic children includes deficits in attention, memory, visuospatial ability, and executive function with preservation of language. There usually is a discrepancy between a low performance IQ and a relatively preserved verbal IQ.

Epilepsy is present only in about 15 percent of cases and this includes temporal lobe and generalized seizures. Seizures, however, may not disappear after treatment of hydrocephalus.

Headache is the most frequent complaint. It is characteristically exacerbated by coughing, sneezing, straining, and stooping. When episodic, headaches are associated with nausea, vomiting, drowsiness, leg weakness and falls.

Visual disturbances are related to papilledema and compression of the optic chiasm exerted by an enlarged third ventricle. This leads to a reduction of visual acuity, visual field defects and unilateral or bilateral blurring of vision.

Endocrine manifestations occur in 10 percent of adolescents with aqueductal stenosis. Compression of the hypothalamo-hypophyseal axis by an enlarged anterior third ventricle may lead to either hypophyseal hypofunction or hyperfunction. Dyencephalo-hypophyseal compression can reduce secretion of hypophyseal hormones and of hypothalamic inhibitor hormones, resulting in an increase of hypophyseal function. In males, the most frequent symptoms are obesity, hypogonadism (with impotence and infertility), diabetes insipidus, precocious puberty and, more rarely, lethargy, gigantism, and acromegaly; in females, amenorrhea, obesity and, more rarely, diabetes insipidus, hypertricosis, acromegaly, and dwarfism. These endocrine abnormalities may constitute the only symptoms and, in many cases, they may reverse after the treatment of hydrocephalus.

Ocular dysfunction, ranging from paresis of upward gaze to the complete syndrome of the aqueduct of Sylvius, are the most characteristic signs of aqueductal stenosis. The aqueductal, pretectal, or dorsal midbrain syndrome includes upward gaze paralysis (Parinaud syndrome), abnormality of the pupils (better reaction to accommodation than to light stimulus), spasm of convergence, nystagmus retractorius on attempted upward gaze, and upper lid retraction (Collier sign). Collier sign associated with upward gaze paralysis corresponds to the "setting sun sign" described in infants.

With further progression of hydrocephalus, in addition to tegmental involvement, signs of ventral midbrain involvement may appear, leading to global rostral midbrain dysfunction, which is characterized by a parkinsonian state with tremor, bradykinesia, mask face and cogwheel rigidity, spastic quadriparesis and alteration of level of consciousness. These symptoms may be attributed to progressive involvement of the substantia nigra. The severity of this syndrome is

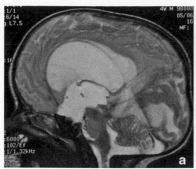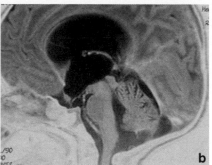

Figure 108.1 a. Four-week-old baby with aqueductal stenosis following neonatal intraventricular hemorrhage. b. Two-month-old boy with aqueductal stenosis following neonatal intraventricular hemorrhage. In both cases (a, b), intraventricular and subarachnoid adhesions are evident distal to the aqueductal stenosis. Reproduced with permission from Cinalli G et al. Hydrocephalus in aqueductal stenosis. *Childs Nerv Syst.* 2011; 27(10):1621–42.

determined by the rapidity of onset and severity of hydrocephalus; thus, although it may also occur in individuals first presenting with hydrocephalus, it is more common following shunt failure after treated aqueductal stenosis.

Pathology

The periventricular white matter and the corpus callosum are most severely affected by hydrocephalus, with disruption of axons and myelin due to compression (Figure 108.1). There may also be ischemia related to mechanical interruption of blood supply. The basal ganglia and thalamus may also be compromised in rare instances, displaying neuronal loss.

Four types of structural abnormalities are associated with stenosis of the aqueduct, which is the most frequent cause of infantile and childhood hydrocephalus. In simple stenosis, the aqueduct is narrowed or obliterated and the ependymum lines the lumen without gliosis of the surrounding tissue (Figure 108.2). An abnormally small aqueduct may be present or, if atretic, the aqueduct may not be discernible. In this form, abnormal infolding of the neural plate results in narrowing of the neural tube. In forking, the aqueduct is divided into two or more channels. These channels can communicate with each other, entering the ventricle independently, or end blindly. This results from incomplete fusion of the median fissure. In septum formation, the aqueduct is obstructed by a gliotic membrane. This is usually located at the caudal end of the aqueduct and occurs when glial overgrowth becomes organized as a sheet. In gliosis, proliferation of glial cells and overproduction of glial fibers results in a denuded lumen that is not limited by the ependymum. This glial proliferation may be part of a broader ependymitis of the ventricles.

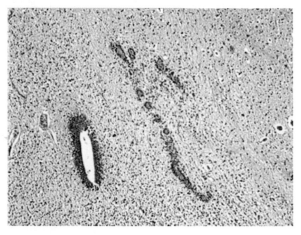

Figure 108.2 In this image of forking of the aqueduct, two relatively small channels are lined by ependymal cells (×225). Reproduced with permission from Cinalli G et al. Hydrocephalus in aqueductal stenosis. *Childs Nerv Syst.* 2011; 27(10):1621–42.

Pathophysiology

Mechanical or irritative causes of hydrocephalus are the most common. Nevertheless, heritable disorders may also lead to congenital hydrocephalus with perinatal, infantile or childhood apparent onset.

X-linked hydrocephalus associated with mutation of the neural cell adhesion molecule L1-CAM gene is the most common genetic form of congenital hydrocephalus and occurs in about 1 in 30,000 births. About 25 percent of males with aqueductal stenosis harbor X-linked hydrocephalus. However, aqueductal stenosis may also occur as an autosomal recessive trait that affects both sexes. Hydrocephalus usually becomes apparent after 18–20 weeks of gestation. Adducted thumbs in the first trimester of pregnancy are suggestive of X-linked hydrocephalus. Most males with X-linked hydrocephalus are born with severe hydrocephalus, adducted thumbs

425

and spasticity. Intellectual disability is severe. In less severely affected males, hydrocephalus may be subclinically present and detected only because of progressively abnormal development, with intellectual disability ranging from mild (IQ of 50–70) to moderate (IQ of 30–50).

Diagnosis

The diagnosis can be established by neuroimaging including dynamic MR imaging cerebrospinal fluid flow techniques.

Treatment

The treatment of hydrocephalus includes the implantation of an intra to extracranial shunt, such as ventriculo-peritoneal or ventriculoatrial shunts, or by the means of neuroendoscopy, which allows the creation of an orifice in the floor of the third ventricle (endoscopic third ventriculostomy). Ventricular size usually decreases rapidly and significantly following shunt implantation, while it decreases less and more slowly after ventriculostomy. However, the neuropsychological outcome is similar after both types of procedure, as postoperative IQ, endocrinologic, social, and behavioral aspects are not significantly different in the two groups.

Bibliography

Cinalli G., Spennato P., Nastro A., et al. (2011). Hydrocephalus in aqueductal stenosis. *Childs Nerv Syst.* 27(10):1621–42.

Chronic Multiple Sclerosis

Multiple Sclerosis Dementia

Natural History of Multiple Sclerosis in Children and Adolescents

Multiple sclerosis predominantly first presents in monosymptomatic form in children and adolescents. In contrast with adults, younger children tend to manifest a greater incidence of impaired consciousness at disease onset. This is associated with a greater onset incidence of seizures, fever, nausea and vomiting, and behavioral disturbances such that younger age is associated with an increased frequency of these manifestations. In these children, and also in contrast with adults, cerebrospinal fluid oligoclonal bands and an elevated IgG index may be absent at onset.

Recovery from the first episode tends to be complete in two thirds of affected children. Over time, the course of multiple sclerosis in children becomes relapsing-remitting, whether assessed clinically or radiologically. Primary progressive multiple sclerosis is uncommon. Relapses, however, ultimately lead to a secondary progressive phase. This progressive phase occurs in individuals with childhood-onset disease 10 years earlier than in adult-onset multiple sclerosis. In contrast, the time span from disease onset to secondary progression is about 10 years greater for children and adolescents compared to adults. This indicates a more adverse prognosis in early onset than in adult onset multiple sclerosis.

Cognitive Deficits in Childhood and Adolescent Multiple Sclerosis

The myelination of specific cerebral structures correlates with the development of neuropsychological abilities. Thus, multiple sclerosis can potentially interfere with the development of these capacities. In addition, gray matter injury and atrophy compounds white matter deficits in the disease. In particular, thalamic atrophy can precede cortical atrophy as potentially a result of deafferentation.

As many as one-third of multiple sclerosis individuals manifest cognitive impairment. The domains most often affected include complex attention and verbal and visuospatial memory functions. In some cases, the intellectual quotient is also impacted. The extent of cognitive disability increases as the disease progresses in as many as two thirds of individuals, with younger children manifesting more severe disability. In contrast, semantic memory, attention span, and language appear to be preserved.

Factors that Influence Cognitive Performance in Multiple Sclerosis

There are no known environmental factors that influence the development or the progression of multiple sclerosis in childhood. Epstein-Barr virus infection, hepatitis B and tetanus vaccination and parental smoking have no effect. The only factor associated with a greater relapse probability is a reduced 25 (OH) vitamin D3 level. In contrast, there are no known specific circumstances that facilitate the development of neuropsychological impairment.

However, among the circumstances that can adversely impact the neuropsychological assessment of childhood and adolescent multiple sclerosis are pain of the head or limbs, fatigue, fine motor incoordination, and steroid treatment. These phenomena make it necessary to adapt testing procedures to specific circumstances.

Bibliography

Amato M.P., Goretti B., Ghezzi A., et al. (2014). Neuropsychological features in childhood and juvenile multiple sclerosis: Five-year follow-up. *Neurology.* 83(16):1432–8.

Amato M.P., Zipoli V., Portaccio E. (2008). Cognitive changes in multiple sclerosis. *Expert Rev Neurother.* 8(10):1585–96.

Mesaros S., Rocca M.A., Absinta M., et al. (2008). Evidence of thalamic gray matter loss in pediatric multiple sclerosis. *Neurology.* 70(13 Pt 2): 1107–12.

Renoux C., Vukusic S., Mikaeloff Y., et al. (2007). Natural history of multiple sclerosis with childhood onset. *N Engl J Med.* 356(25):2603–13.

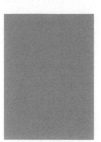

Paraneoplastic Neurological Disorders

Chapter 110

Common Paraneoplastic Syndromes

Paraneoplastic neurological syndromes are remote effects of cancer that are not caused by the tumor and its metastasis, or by infection, ischemia, or metabolic disruption. They affect less than 1 in 10,000 individuals with cancer. In many cases, the neurological disorder develops before the cancer becomes clinically overt. The discovery that some paraneoplastic syndromes are associated with antibodies directed against antigens expressed by both the tumor and the nervous system (onconeural antibodies) has suggested that these disorders are immune-mediated. The presence or the absence of paraneoplastic antibodies and the type of antibodies define different subtypes of syndrome, which may affect any level of the nervous system (central or peripheral nervous system, including the neuromuscular junction and muscle). Common neurological syndromes in the adult include encephalomyelitis, limbic encephalitis, subacute cerebellar degeneration, sensory neuronopathy, opsoclonus-myoclonus, chronic gastrointestinal pseudoobstruction, Lambert-Eaton myasthenic syndrome or dermatomyositis, with cancer usually developing within five years of the diagnosis of the neurological disorder. In about 20 percent of cases, no cancer is ever found, even at postmortem examination, perhaps indicating the successful control of tumor growth and metastasis by the host immune system.

Treatment includes removal or treatment of the tumor and immunosuppressive therapies such as plasmapheresis and intravenous immunoglobulins. Immunosuppression with corticosteroids or ACTH, plasma exchange, chemotherapy, or the anti-CD20 monoclonal antibody rituximab is also useful in some cases.

The main neurological syndromes associated with a paraneoplastic origin including opsoclonus myoclonus syndrome, limbic encephalitis, and anti-N-methyl-D-aspartate receptor (anti-NMDA-R) are described here.

Opsoclonus-Myoclonus Syndrome

Opsoclonus-myoclonus syndrome is also known as Kinsbourne encephalopathy and is the most common pediatric paraneoplastic syndrome. Children manifest staggering and falling that often leads to a misdiagnosis of acute cerebellitis. Later, they may develop myoclonus, drooling, speech disturbances, hypotonia, and sleep disturbances. The time interval between presentation of neurologic symptoms and diagnosis of a tumor in children varies between 1 week and 20 months. In children, the syndrome of opsoclonus, cerebellar ataxia and myoclonus occurs mainly as a paraneoplastic syndrome related to occult, low-grade neuroblastoma (stage I or II). The syndrome occurs almost exclusively in young children (6 months to 3 years of age) and in about 3 percent of children with neuroblastoma. Survival in children with neuroblastoma presenting with opsoclonus-myoclonus is significantly greater than in children with neuroblastoma without neurologic involvement. In children with opsoclonus-myoclonus, antineuronal antibodies are inconsistently found. Their corresponding endogenous antigen is still unclear, although antibodies to various components of cerebellar neurons are present in some children with opsoclonus-ataxia. Tumor investigation includes imaging of the neck, chest, abdomen, and pelvis, including the testes. MR imaging is most commonly used for the survey. Following MR imaging, whole-body fluorodeoxyglucose–positron emission tomography (FDG-PET) may be necessary to detect occult tumors.

Limbic Encephalitis

Limbic encephalitis comprises personality changes, irritability, seizures, cognitive dysfunction, and memory loss. Paraneoplastic syndromes may represent approximately 10 percent of pediatric limbic encephalitis cases. The most frequently associated neoplasms in children are Hodgkin lymphoma, ovarian teratoma and testicular tumor. Neuroblastoma has also been reported. In adults, neurologic symptoms in paraneoplastic limbic encephalitis precede the cancer diagnosis in 60 percent of affected individuals with a median of 3.5 months, and this proportion may be greater in children. The diagnosis of limbic encephalitis is made in a clinical basis and its confirmation requires cerebrospinal fluid analysis. MR imaging demonstrates temporal lobe abnormalities, whereas the electroencephalogram illustrates epileptic activity or slowing emanating from the temporal lobes. Onconeuronal antibodies are detected in the serum and cerebrospinal fluid of 60 percent of adults with paraneoplastic limbic encephalitis. Various antibodies and tumors have been reported in adults, such as anti- Hu/ANNA-1 (small cell lung cancer), anti-Ri/ANNA-2 (lung or breast cancer), anti-Ma2 (lung, breast or testicular cancer), anti-CV2/CRMP5 (small cell lung cancer), and anti-amphiphysin (breast, small cell lung cancer). Most of these antibodies and associated tumors are rare in children.

NMDA Receptor Encephalitis

Anti-N-methyl-D-aspartate receptor (NMDAR) encephalitis is relatively common in children and adolescents. Many cases of paraneoplastic and non-paraneoplastic anti-NMDAR encephalitis have been reported in just a few years. Children with NMDAR encephalitis exhibit prominent neuropsychiatric abnormalities, including behavioral or personality change, sleep dysfunction, dyskinesia or dystonia, autonomic instability, and speech disturbances. Oromandibular dyskinesia is a characteristic feature. Supporting evidence includes cerebrospinal fluid lymphocytic pleocytosis or oligoclonal bands demonstrating an inflammatory or immune- mediated process, an electroencephalogram displaying slow, disorganized activity and infrequent seizures and brain MR imaging indicative of transient FLAIR (fluid attenuated inversion recovery) or contrast-enhancing abnormalities in cortical and subcortical regions, limbic areas, basal ganglia, brainstem, cerebellum, and sometimes the white matter.

Bibliography

Alavi S. (2013). Paraneoplastic neurologic syndromes in children: A review article. *Iran J Child Neurol.* 7(3):6–14.

Chronic Viral Infections of the Nervous System

Neurological Regression in Viral Disorders

Several chronic infections can adversely impact psychomotor performance insidiously, such that recognition of the infectious nature of neurological regression is obscured or delayed. Among these, viruses are endowed with a great propensity to cause latent and slowly progressive nervous system injury. Some of these infections are the result of disturbed immunity induced by the medical treatment of cancer, rheumatological diseases, and multiple sclerosis.

HIV-Associated Cognitive Disorder

Among the presentations of human immunodeficiency virus (HIV) infection are a variety of encephalopathies with predominant motor, cognitive, or behavioral manifestations. In addition, HIV-associated neurocognitive disorder is associated with three types of encephalopathy of increasing severity: HIV-associated asymptomatic neurocognitive impairment, mild neurocognitive disorder, and dementia. These three syndromes affect about one-half of all HIV-infected subjects. In children and adolescents, an additional syndrome of progressive encephalopathy is characterized by acquired microcephaly, loss of previously acquired skills and corticospinal tract abnormalities. This is associated with calcifications of the basal ganglia, brain atrophy, enlarged ventricles, and enlarged cortical sulci.

Neuropsychological assessment in HIV dementia most frequently reveals impairment in attention, concentration, memory, and personality, with deterioration of cognitive speed. In adults, deficits in declarative memory retrieval in the setting of preserved procedural memory can be profound. Visuospatial ability is also markedly impaired, whereas language is normal. Psychomotor slowing and apathy are also common. Impairment of attention and executive dysfunction may signify predominant frontal lobe dysfunction.

Several genetic variants may predispose to HIV-associated neurocognitive disorder. Among these, genes involved in inflammatory or immune regulation, synaptic plasticity, and other aspects of neuronal function such as axonal guidance, transferrin receptor and mitochondrial function are the most significant.

The neuropathology of HIV-associated neurocognitive disorder is probably related to viral infection of the basal ganglia and white matter after viral entry via infected monocytes. HIV enters the central nervous system early in the infection and resides primarily in long-lived perivascular macrophages and microglia. Glial cells are the main target of HIV. The white matter displays gliosis, multinucleated giant cells, microglial nodules, and perivascular macrophages. There is breakdown of the blood–brain barrier with vasogenic edema but no demyelination. Cortical neuronal loss may be mild or absent, whereas white matter pallor is a much earlier event. Neuropathological findings in subcortical grey structures extend to the basal ganglia, thalamus, and brainstem. There is no evidence of HIV infection in neurons. Thus, it is possible that neuronal injury occurs as a consequence of the inflammatory process or of direct exposure to HIV proteins released by infected cells, such as gp120, Tat, and Vpr, which have been shown to be toxic. In addition, gp120 may cause neuronal damage through the activation of the TNF-alpha/ caspase cascade of proteins.

Antiretrovirals and protease inhibitors, used for the therapy of HIV, are effective in preventing, reversing, or interrupting the progression of HIV-associated neurocognitive disorder. Treatment with a combination of antiretroviral drugs results in a

Table 111.1 Clinical stages of subacute sclerosing panencephalitis

Stage 0	Subtle psychointellectual symptoms recognized retrospectively
Stage I	Overt psychointellectual and/or nonspecific neurological symptoms
Stage II	Stereotyped jerks
Stage III	Vegetative psychomotor condition
Stage IV	Spontaneous improvement (modest in substage IVa, substantial in substage IVb)
Stage V	Relapse

decline in plasma and cerebrospinal fluid viral load. These agents can decrease white matter lesions detected by MR imaging. However, some of them also display neurotoxicity.

Subacute Sclerosing Panencephalitis

Measles (rubella) infection may be followed by delayed reactivation of the persistent virus after years or decades. Peak incidence occurs between the ages of 6 and 15 years. The risk of developing the disease after childhood measles is estimated as 1 in 25,000 in general and as 1 in 5,500 in children infected before the age of 1 year. The etiological agent is the wild measles virus, as no vaccine strain has been isolated from brain tissue. Subacute sclerosing panencephalitis in a previously immunized child is due to vaccine failure due to inadequate preservation of the vaccine or low seroconversion of the host or, alternatively, to subclinical measles infection before the child was immunized.

Subacute sclerosing panencephalitis is an unrelenting demyelinating disease generally followed by a fatal outcome. Disease onset is characterized by irritability and apathy, progressing to dementia, myoclonus, epilepsy, corticospinal tract dysfunction and, in late stages, progressively depressed consciousness followed by a vegetative state. In the beginning slow, brief blinking or head dropping attacks, or asymmetrical upper body jerks can be observed several times a day and more so in the evening when the child is tired. They disappear during sleep and intensify with stress. Their frequency and amplitude increase over weeks or months. MR imaging using T2-weighted sequences demonstrates high-intensity lesions in the periventricular or subcortical white matter (Figure 111.1). Several stages can be recognized.(Table 111.1)

A typical EEG pattern of bilateral, symmetrical, periodic, high-amplitude slow waves, or sharp-and-slow-wave complexes is characteristic of the myoclonic phase. The background rhythm, initially normal, becomes progressively slower and flat over months. Less typical EEG findings are frontal rhythmic delta activity, diffuse sharp waves and sharp-and-slow-wave complexes over frontal regions. In cerebrospinal fluid, the immunoglobulin index is elevated and oligoclonal bands reacting with viral antigens are almost constant. Antimeasles IgG and measles-specific IgG index are diagnostic. Measles-specific IgM is usually negative. IgG remains elevated even during remission. Viral RNA can sometimes be detected by reverse transcription-polymerase chain reaction.

Inclusion bodies in the cytoplasm or nuclei of neurons and glia are characteristic. Nuclear inclusions may contain viral ribonucleoproteins or protein complexes. Other histopathological changes vary according to the stage of the disease. In early stages, inflammation in the meninges, cortex, subcortical gray and white matter and neuronal degeneration, gliosis, astrocytic proliferation and demyelination are observed. Later, inflammation diminishes while necrosis, neuronal degeneration, gliosis and neurofibrillary tangles predominate. The cortical architecture is eventually altered.

The measles virus can reach the brain by infecting circulating lymphocytes or endothelial cells. Transneuronal and axonal spread are also plausible. Mutations in the virus allow it to escape humoral immunity. Virus isolated from affected children usually display mutations in the matrix (M) and/or fusion (F) genes. Hypermutations in the M gene are not lethal for the virus, which can still replicate and spread with slow migration. The wild virus undergoes these mutations during its stay

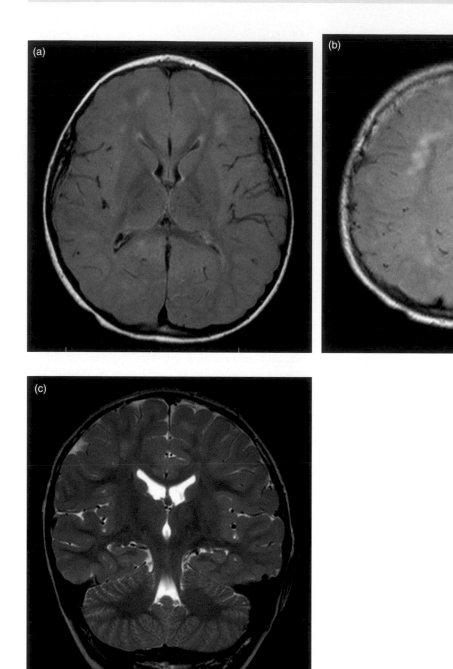

Figure 111.1 MR imaging changes in a 12-year-old boy with subacute sclerosing panencephalitis.

in the host, with shorter latent periods associated with smaller number of mutations. The reason why the virus becomes reactivated in some individuals remains unclear. Alterations in the immune or hormonal system, minor head trauma, or infections might contribute.

Progressive Multifocal Leukoencephalopathy

Progressive multifocal leukoencephalopathy accompanies states of immune deficiency and is thus an opportunistic infection. It is caused by the JC virus, a polyomavirus with a predilection for the white matter. JC virus is widely spread among the population, with approximately 85 percent of adults worldwide exhibiting JC-specific hemagglutination antibodies. Infection with the virus is usually subclinical and occurs in early childhood. The oligodendrocyte is the principal cell type involved in the infection and myelin synthesis is compromised early in the disease course.

About 5 percent of acquired immunodeficiency syndrome (AIDS) affected individuals develop this superimposed infection. A more recent surge has been noted after the used of monoclonal antibodies to treat immunological disorders, including multiple sclerosis. In these cases, the prognosis is better than in AIDS.

The manifestations of progressive multifocal leukoencephalopathy include focal neurological deficits such as motor and visual dysfunction. Cognitive and behavioral abnormalities may be subtle and involve inattention and memory loss with preserved language. Parietal and occipital involvement may lead to visual agnosia, pure alexia, and Balint syndrome. Seizures are common.

Because of the multifocal nature of the demyelinated lesions it is likely that the virus reaches the brain by hematogenous spread carried by white blood cells.

The initial neuropathology of progressive multifocal leukoencephalopathy is characterized by parietal and occipital white matter lesions. The typical lesions progress relatively rapidly and are less diffuse than those seen in HIV infection. Established demyelinated plaques are more frequent in the subcortical areas of the frontal, parietal, and temporal lobes, but they can also be found in the white matter any part of the brain, including the basal ganglia, cerebellum, and brainstem and, in severe cases, the spinal cord. Survival ranges from 4 to 6 months after the onset of symptoms.

Bibliography

Anlar B. (2013). Subacute sclerosing panencephalitis and chronic viral encephalitis. *Handb Clin Neurol.* 112:1183–9.

Benton T.D. (2010). Psychiatric considerations in children and adolescents with HIV/AIDS. *Child Adolesc Psychiatr Clin N Am.* 19(2):387–400.

Risk W.S., Haddad F.S. (1979). The variable natural history of subacute sclerosing panencephalitis: A study of 118 cases from the Middle East. *Arch Neurol.* 36(10):610–14.

Van Rie A., Harrington P.R., Dow A., et al. (2007). Neurologic and neurodevelopmental manifestations of pediatric HIV/AIDS: A global perspective. *Eur J Paediatr Neurol.* 11(1):1–9.

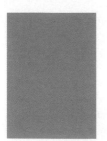

Hysteria

Conversion Disorder in Children

A broad variety of disorders present with neurological symptoms but do not have an identifiable neurological basis. Many different terms have been used to describe these disorders including somatic symptom and related disorders, hysterical, medically unexplained, functional, conversion disorders, and psychogenic disorders. These terms reflect the concept that the symptoms do not stem from an organic disease process and that the signs or symptoms are incompatible with clinical anatomy and pathophysiology. The prevalence of conversion disorder in general hospital inpatients who are seen in psychiatric consultation ranges between 5 and 16 percent. Over 2 percent of individuals seen in neurologic practice are diagnosed with a conversion disorder. Age at onset may be as young as 4 years, but hysteria or conversion disorder is more likely to present during the peripubertal years. Its prevalence among children is about 3 per 100,000. Most conversion disorders in children are monosymptomatic. Young children typically present after a minor injury, but older children are less likely to have suffered injury. In children, the dominant extremities are more likely to be involved than the nondominant extremities. The role of emotional stress and conflict around the time of presentation of conversion disorder has been recognized.

Clinical features of conversion disorder include: inconsistent character of the symptoms from moment to moment or day to day, selective disability associated with specific circumstances, paroxysmal symptoms inconsistent with a known paroxysmal movement disorder, increased severity after attention is focused on the affected body part, decreased severity with distraction, ability to trigger or relieve the features with unusual or nonphysiological interventions, inconsistency with conventional neuroanatomy and neurophysiology, self-inflicted injuries, deliberate slowness of movements, functional disability out of proportion to exam findings, and pain out of proportion to objective findings. Among the most frequent presentations are psychogenic nonepileptic seizures, headaches, and psychogenic movement disorders.

The diagnosis of conversion disorder should be based on history and neurological and physical examination. Most important is for the examining physician to have sufficient knowledge of neuroanatomy and neurophysiology to determine when signs and symptoms are inconsistent with known disease processes. Conversion disorders and organic neurological disease can coexist, most commonly in chronic relapsing diseases such as epilepsy.

A short duration of symptoms is associated with a good outcome. Pending litigation is an indicator of poor prognosis. The association between comorbid psychiatric disorder and favorable outcome underlines the importance of screening for affective and anxiety disorders in these individuals. These disorders may make some persons vulnerable to developing conversion symptoms, which may lead to enduring disability. Treating depression and anxiety and exploring personal circumstances may reduce disability in some individuals, while for those with several physical symptoms and personality disorder, prevention of iatrogenic damage may be more appropriate.

Bibliography

Mink J.W. (2013). Conversion disorder and mass psychogenic illness in child neurology. *Ann N Y Acad Sci*. 1304:40–4.

Allet J.L., Allet R.E. (2006). Somatoform disorders in neurological practice. *Curr Opin Psychiatry*. 19(4):413–20.

Induced Regression

Loss of Sensory Organs

Chapter
113

Visual and Auditory Loss in Children

Loss of sensory organs in childhood or adolescence or acquired combined deafblindness may be associated with progressive deterioration of neural performance. In contrast, congenital deafblindness such as that typical of cytomegalovirus and rubella infection, leads to static, non-progressing disability. The frequency of people affected by both hearing impairment and visual impairment is far greater than would be expected if the relationship was coincidental. There are over fifty hereditary syndromes that cause acquired deafblindness. Most of them are rare and some also affect other organs. Progressive visual and auditory loss may eventually limit communication to tactile signing. Even minor vision impairment may, in combination with congenital hearing loss, increase a child's difficulties in developing useful language abilities. There are extensive consequences to sensory deprivation. For example, the child's ability to interpret the erratic and somewhat unrelated information being presented to him may give rise to an unfavorable perception of the environment and carers may find the child unrewarding from his apparent lack of responsiveness.

Even pure deafness (without blindness) may be associated with neuropsychological impairment. Some deaf children manifest attention deficit hyperactivity disorder, conduct, autism-spectrum, and bipolar disorders, and spend three times longer in treatment than their hearing peers. The principal consequence of these factors is moderate to severe impairment in social relationships and in school performance. In contrast, pure blindness (most often associated with optic nerve hypoplasia) can lead to mood instability, especially during the first years of life. Later in life, slowed psychic responses, low frustration tolerance, and a narrow range of interests are common. Autism or similar conditions are diagnosed in a fraction of these children.

The most common cause of acquired deafblindness is Usher syndrome or retinitis pigmentosa-deafness syndrome, which accounts for almost half of all individuals with this acquired disability. Usher syndrome is an autosomal recessive disorder with a prevalence of 1 in 10,000 newborns. The immediate consequences of the syndrome are deafness of varying severity with onset at birth or within the first year of life and slowly progressive retinitis pigmentosa, which may be accompanied by cataracts. The initial visual symptoms include night-blindness, extreme sensitivity to light and tunnel vision. Additional vestibular dysfunction is a feature of some forms of the syndrome. Usher syndrome can be divided into three main types on purely clinical grounds and these types correlate with distinct gene mutations.

One of the most common types is Usher type 1B, which is caused by mutations in the gene that encodes myosin VIIA (MYO7A or USH1B). This gene is expressed in the hair cells of the cochlea and in retinal photoreceptors. In Usher type 2, mutations are found in usherin (USH2A; type 2A syndrome). This gene is also expressed in the cochlea and in the retina but it causes disturbances in the supporting cells instead of the hair cells.

In Usher syndrome, mental and behavioral disorders are found among a quarter of children. The types of disorders observed are not uniform and include atypical autism, mental retardation, schizophrenia and conduct disorder. In some cases, auditory hallucinations are prominent. Two mechanisms for a higher incidence of mental and behavioral difficulties among children and adults with Usher syndrome may be at play. First, progressive loss of vision results in stress and symptoms of mental and behavioral disorder. Case-studies report that mental and behavioral symptoms in individuals with Usher syndrome develop simultaneously to the loss of vision.

Table 113.1 Clinical features of Usher syndromes

Usher syndrome type	Gene	Features
I (subtypes A through G)	CDH23 (cadherin 23; USH1D), MYO7A (myosin VIIA; USH1B), PCDH15 (protocadherin-15; USH1F), USH1C, USH1G, CIB2 (calcium and integrin binding family member 2; USH1J) and at least three unidentified genes	Deafness by age 1 year. Visual loss in childhood or adolescence. Vestibular dysfunction
II (subtypes A, B and C)	ADGRV1 (adhesion G protein-coupled receptor V1), DFNB31 (deafness, autosomal recessive 31), USH2A and at least one unidentified gene	Hearing loss may be milder and congenital. Visual loss in adolescence or adulthood
III	CLRN1 (clarin 1; USH3A) and at least one unidentified gene	Hearing and visual loss in first decades of life. Vestibular dysfunction

Thus, it is plausible that they are reactive symptoms to stress. In addition to stress-related responses imposed by progressive loss of vision, dual sensory loss may be associated with a higher prevalence of mental and behavioral disorders because of severe communicative difficulties. Among adults with acquired deafblindness, communication and social support is important to avoid depression. The second possible explanation for an association between Usher syndrome and mental and behavioral disorders is that some genes predisposed to both Usher syndrome and mental disorders, although no specific candidate genes have been identified.

Bibliography

Dammeyer J. (2012). Children with Usher syndrome: Mental and behavioral disorders. *Behav Brain Funct.* 8:16.

Ek U., Fernell E., Jacobson L. (2005). Cognitive and behavioural characteristics in blind children with bilateral optic nerve hypoplasia. *Acta Paediatr.* 94(10):1421–6.

Landsberger S.A., Diaz D.R., Spring N.Z., et al. (2014). Psychiatric diagnoses and psychosocial needs of outpatient deaf children and adolescents. *Child Psychiatry Hum Dev.* 45(1):42–51.

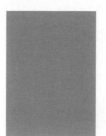

Irradiation and Other Cancer Treatments

Cancer Treatments and Neurological Deterioration

Cranial irradiation and chemotherapy are effectively used both in primary malignancies of the central nervous system and in metastasic disease. Whereas the consequences of focal brain irradiation are purely local, whole-brain irradiation can be followed by distinct neurological syndromes in as many as one-third of subjects. In addition to the effects of cancer treatments on the developing brain, the potential contribution of primary brain tumors and of hydrocephalus to cognitive decline must be taken into account. Of note, hydrocephalus is a significant risk factor for impaired intellectual outcome in children treated for brain tumors in all regions. Treatment of hydrocephalus with a shunt may improve cognition in this context. A young age at the time of radiation or chemotherapy is a risk factor for cognitive decline in children treated for leukemia and for brain tumors

Effects of Radiotherapy

Three distinct syndromes may occur after brain irradiation. The first includes acute rapid white matter edema in association with confusion. This state is usually self-resolved. The second syndrome occurs weeks to months after irradiation and is accompanied by somnolence. While it may be due to demyelination, recovery takes place spontaneously over time. The third syndrome includes progressive dementia and is associated with myelin injury and necrosis. This latter form of late and progressive cognitive dysfunction occurs following whole-cranial radiotherapy. The greatest impact has been observed when large volumes of brain are treated using older techniques with a high dose per fraction or with a high total dose of radiation (over 50 Gy for adults and 35 Gy in children). However, when more modern radiotherapy techniques are employed, the effect on

cognition can range from no decline to improvement over pretreatment levels.

The earliest cognitive aspects most vulnerable to radiation injury include deficits with processing speed, visuospatial abilities, and memory retrieval. Decreased white matter volume due to irradiation is correlated with mean IQ. In children with white matter damage caused by radiation, the event-related potential wave P300 correlates with formal neuropsychological scores.

Radiation may impact neural function via the suppression of hippocampal neurogenesis. In addition, there are deleterious functional consequences. The effects of cranial irradiation (6 Gy) on long-term synaptic plasticity in the rat is different in the juvenile compared with the adult brain, such that, while irradiation of the adult brain only causes a reduction in normally occurring long term potentiation, irradiation of the juvenile brain leads to a conversion of long term potentiation into long term depression, as assessed by measuring the effects of trains of high-frequency stimulation on hippocampal synaptic transmission.

Delayed radiation encephalopathy may be prevented. Reduced neuraxis radiation with and without adjuvant chemotherapy, conformal radiation, chemotherapy-only for children with optic pathway and hypothalamic tumors and a series of baby brain tumor studies in which chemotherapy has allowed radiation to be delayed, reduced or avoided, have resulted in the abolition of radiation injury. Treatment of cognitive sequelae is more problematic. Subjects taking donepezil initiated at least 6 months after completion of 30 Gy of greater whole- or partial-brain radiotherapy exhibit a modest improvement in several domains of cognitive function, including verbal and working memory, visual and psychomotor function, and executive function.

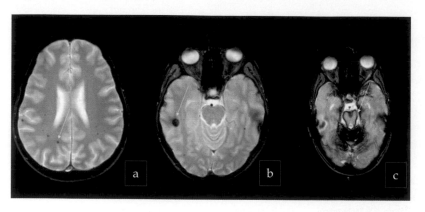

Figure 114.1 Brain MR imaging (T2 gradient echo brain magnetic resonance imaging) illustrating microhemorrhage (a), cavernoma (b), and superficial siderosis (c) following radiation therapy to the head. Reproduced with permission from Passos J et al. Late cerebrovascular complications after radiotherapy for childhood primary central nervous system tumors. *Pediatr Neurol*. 2015; 53(3): 211–15.

Delayed Vascular Injury after Irradiation

Delayed vascular injury is detectable in one-third of children who survive brain irradiation. The mean latent interval between irradiation and the diagnosis of vascular sequelae is 15 years. In some cases, two decades may lapse between radiotherapy and the discovery of these sequelae. There is a slight male predilection. The most frequent complications include cavernoma, moyamoya, microhemorrhages, superficial siderosis, and stroke (Figures 114.1 and 114.2). These lesions are particularly amenable to detection via gradient echo brain magnetic resonance imaging. Symptoms from these lesions can include epilepsy, motor and language deficits, sensorineural hearing loss, and progressive ataxia associated with cavernomas, stroke, and superficial siderosis, respectively. There are no obvious clinical manifestations associated with microhemorrhages and the majority of individuals with cavernoma also exhibit microhemorrhages.

Several mechanisms may participate in the genesis of these sequelae. Stenosis of the vascular vessel lumen, ischemia, and microinfarction could cause microhemorrhages, whereas neoangiogenesis resulting from hypoxia-inducible factor 1 release and excess vascular endothelial growth factor production could lead to cavernoma formation. In one instance, there was incidental remission of radiotherapy-induced cavernoma during therapy with bevacizumab (a monoclonal antibody directed against vascular endothelial growth factor) in a child with recurrent medulloblastoma. It is possible that resolution of the cavernoma was related to bevacizumab antivascular endothelial growth factor activity.

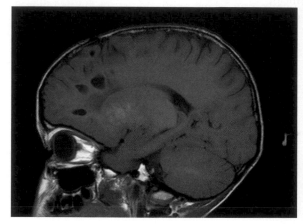

Figure 114.2 Sequelae of radiotherapy for teratoid-rhabdoid tumor of the frontal lobe in a 12-year-old boy. The tumor was treated at 4 years of age. Treatment included chemotherapy and radiotherapy. Cystic changes and white matter signal abnormality are visible in the frontal lobe.

Sequelae of Chemotherapy

Cerebral toxicity is a well-known consequence of chemotherapeutic agents for cancer. This toxicity resembles that typical of radiation therapy in that the white matter of the brain is preferentially affected. In addition, some commonly used chemotherapeutic agents in the treatment of childhood brain tumors are more toxic for neural progenitor cells and oligodendroglia than they are for cancer cells.

Similarly to radiation-related injury, the clinical sequelae of chemotherapy include somnolence, confusion, amnesia, and dementia. Long-term intellectual performance is decreased in chemotherapy-only treated children with leukemia, especially in the realms of perceptual reasoning, working memory, and processing speeds. In addition, both reading and mathematical achievement may be affected in long term survivors. Full scale, verbal, and performance IQ scores can also be impacted.

The best understood chemotherapy toxicity is that due to metothrexate, which occurs most often when the drug is administered intravenously or intrathecally. The toxicity of metothrexate is related not only to peak levels but to duration of exposure. Folinic acid may prevent this toxicity. The toxic effects are compounded by radiation therapy: Irradiated children who receive metothrexate exhibit lower performance on IQ tests than either those who receive metothrexate alone. Additional neuropsychological abnormalities in these children include increased distractibility and memory deficits. The presence of leukoencephalopathy

identified on neuroimaging correlates with poor results on arithmetic, comprehension and block design when intrathecal metothrexate is used.

Bibliography

Duffner P.K. (2010). Risk factors for cognitive decline in children treated for brain tumors. *Eur J Paediatr Neurol.* 14(2):106–15.

Passos J., Nzwalo H., Marques J., et al. (2015). Late cerebrovascular complications after radiotherapy for childhood primary central nervous system tumors. *Pediatr Neurol.* 53(3):211–15.

Zanni G., Zhou K., Riebe I., et al. (2015). Irradiation of the juvenile brain provokes a shift from long-term potentiation to long-term depression. *Dev Neurosci.* 37(3):263–72.

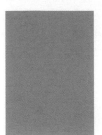

Protein and Calorie Malnutrition

115

Malnutrition in Children

Malnutrition occurs in all countries as the result of socioeconomic factors. There are two principal types of malnutrition: marasmus or protein-calorie malnutrition and kwashiorkor or protein malnutrition. Until recently, medically-related causes of malnutrition also included cystic fibrosis, meconium ileus, protracted diarrhea, and ileal atresia.

Malnutrition and Growth of the Organism

The effect of chronic malnutrition on somatic growth is well known: height and weight are both affected, together with head growth. Several extracerebral factors determine head size. Among these, the thickness of the cranial bones and the scalp are most important, together with the volume occupied by cerebrospinal fluid. Malnutrition characteristically impacts head growth. In children chronically malnourished, somatic length drops below the third percentile for normal growth during the second six months of life in males and during the third six months of life in females. In all later ages, the length curves are below and parallel the third percentile for both sexes. However, weight may exceed that expected for length at all ages. This may be due to intermittent adequate nutrition in the context of a lifetime of malnutrition leading to weight gain but subnormal length growth. Head circumference remains below a low growth percentile level during most of infancy until the eighteenth month of life, when head size gradually increases to approach the mean value of the standard, indicating that head growth is better maintained than length growth. Infants suffering from marasmus demonstrate more severe retardation in head circumference growth than children with kwashiorkor. In children with marasmus, some of the reduction in head circumference stems from thinning of the scalp and of the skull. The

relative weight of the cerebrum, cerebellum and brainstem is equally reduced in marasmus.

During recovery of malnutrition, head growth recovers. After nutritional therapy, cranial suture diastasis may occur even in children older than two years of age. This change can take place within weeks of instituting proper nutrition. Changes in head circumference parallel this change and may take place as late as 6 years of age. Some of these changes may be due to scalp thickness and skull growth. Some children, however, may develop increased intracranial pressure during nutrition therapy. This is associated with pseudotumor cerebri and papilledema.

Neurological Effects of Starvation

In adults, starvation is associated with a gradual and severe decline in intellectual activity. Loss of one-fourth of body weight over six months is associated with a reduction of physical activities. There is also a reduction in voluntary intellectual activity, with reduced thought. However, visual and auditory functions remain unchanged. Mood becomes depressed and irritable, without obvious consequences in behavior. There is a reduced capacity to concentrate and comprehension is impaired. Despite these changes, performance in standard intelligence tests remains unaffected. Thus, the main effect of starvation in adults is to decrease initiative and accompanying behavior. During recovery from starvation, subjects become more irritable. Compulsive overeating may persist after conclusion of nutrition rehabilitation. Nevertheless, there are no permanent neurological or psychological sequelae to simple protein-calorie malnutrition in the absence of an associated vitamin deficiency.

The marasmic infant is generally younger than the child with kwashiorkor. In these infants with marasmus, irritability and hunger dominates the clinical picture. Motility is not affected and children act significantly hungry. An exception occurs only when intercurrent illnesses take place, in which case apathy becomes prominent. In contrast, in kwashiorkor, apathy is prominent. Children respond slowly to environmental stimuli and appear indifferent to their surroundings. Movements are reduced to a minimum except for eye movements, which are vivid. When prodded excessively, the kwashiorkor infant may cringe, but rarely resists. Often the child will remain lying or sitting and does not engage in play or conversation if these abilities were previously attained.

There are prominent EEG changes associated with malnutrition. After controlling for any associated hypoglycemia, EEG rhythms tend to be slower during acute malnutrition. There is a prominence of delta and slower waves. There is also lower voltage amplitude. With nutritional therapy, these EEG abnormalities may gradually revert to normal. However, marasmic children tend to display more theta activity in the long term than normal and than kwashiorkor children, who are usually normal for age when investigated by EEG after recovery is complete.

In addition to mental, behavioral, and EEG changes, hypotonia and hyporeflexia may accompany severe protein-calorie malnutrition. Proximal muscle wasting, a Gowers sign, a waddling gait and a tendency to slip through the hands of the examiner when the infant is lifted up under the arms can all be prominent. In some children, nerve conduction velocity is reduced and myopathic electromyographic changes may be noticeable. These changes can include fibrillation potentials and small muscle fibers with group atrophy in muscle biopsy, which is suggestive of motor neuron disease. Nevertheless, complete recovery is possible after nutritional rehabilitation.

Neurochemical Consequences of Starvation

In all experimental animals subject to protein-calorie malnutrition, somatic growth is retarded, while brain weight is only modestly diminished. This is associated with decreased cell production. Cell numbers are reduced in the brain, but at the expense of glial rather than neuronal cells. There is a reduction in cell numbers in marasmus but not in kwashiorkor. The protein content of the brain is decreased in both diseases. Brain lipids are also consistently reduced in animal studies of malnutrition. The most significant

experimental animal alterations take place in the cerebellum, which matures late in most species. In many cases, this structure displays reductions in cell numbers and abnormal migration patterns and cell process production. The hippocampus and the olfactory lobe exhibit similar alterations. In man, however, cerebrum and cerebellum are equally affected by malnutrition.

Recovery from Starvation

During recovery, a gradual change in mental status takes place. The appearance of a smile is the most reliable indicator of recovery. There are four general phases to nutritional recovery. In the first phase, children are apathic. They are found sitting or prone with limbs flexed against the body and little spontaneous movement. Attempts to mobilize the child meet with resistance and a weak cry. There is no appetite and sphincter control is absent even in the older child. There is no reaction to external stimulation and there is a lack of communication. In the next phase, which occurs after the second and third week of nutritional rehabilitation, children react more robustly to environmental stimuli. Spontaneous activity increases and social interactions are better tolerated, although significant indifference persists. Appetite reappears. Sphincter control remains absent but communication improves, with production of single words or unintelligible sounds. The third stage of recovery is characterized by active perceptivity and spans from the third to the seventh week of nutritional intervention. There is increased voluntary activity and increased responses to stimuli. Sphincter control may improve but remain deficient. Smiling can be noted in this phase, but speech remains limited. The fourth phase is one of steady convalescence and lasts until the twelfth week. Children may regain the capacity to walk, although unsteadily. Marked motor retardation remains and some children under 3 years of age have performed at the level of 10- to 15-month-old children in this phase. The child regains the capacity to laugh and communication now includes simple words. Language, however, remains the most markedly impaired measurement of the illness. Appetite is adequate in this stage. Most children remain incontinent as well. Systematic neuropsychological testing of these children reveals deficits in personality and language aspects even when children are well on their way to full recovery.

During recovery from acute protein-calorie malnutrition, a paradoxical phase of progressive decline in neurological status can be noted. There may be lethargy and other more severe states of depressed consciousness during the first four days of therapy. Severe hypoglycemia and death may occur. Some children exhibit asterixis without evidence of hepatic failure. An extrapyramidal syndrome consisting of rigidity and irregular tremor (5 to 10 Hz) may occur predominantly in males aged about 2 years old. Clonus and convulsions with an abnormal EEG may also occur. This syndrome subsides over several weeks.

There is no noticeable consequence to mild protein-calorie malnutrition. However, the sequelae of severe malnutrition can be profound, including an abnormal development quotient. However, IQ is generally normal. Therefore, ultimate mental capacity may be little altered by severe malnutrition even though defects in language and social behavior persist well into the recovery period.

Bibliography

Dodge P.R., Prensky A.L., Feigin R.D. (1975). *Nutrition and the Developing Nervous System*. Saint Louis: Mosby.

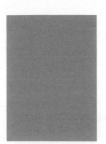

Vitamin Deficiencies and Excesses

Vitamins and the Developing Nervous System

Vitamins serve primarily as facilitators of enzymatic catalysis in very small quantities. Both vitamin deficiency and vitamin excess states are associated with progressive neural dysfunction. In contrast, vitamin dependency states are caused by a heritable obligatory requirement for elevated doses (10 to 500 times the normal daily requirement) of a vitamin. In vitamin dependencies, the specific enzyme involved is rendered inactive or catalytically deficient in the absence of supraphysiological concentrations of the vitamin, which binds to the enzyme. The requirement for such elevated quantities of a vitamin may stem from deficient transport or from decreased binding affinity for the enzyme due to mutation of residues involved in the recognition of the vitamin cofactor. Vitamin dependencies are discussed in other chapters.

Deficiency of vitamins can occur both in underdeveloped and developed countries as the result of dietary inadequacies associated with malnutrition and with severe chronic illnesses. The most common vitamin deficiency and excess states are discussed here.

Vitamin A

Vitamin A or retinol is a fat-soluble alcohol found in animal fats and in liver tissue. Colored vegetables are rich in beta-carotene, a pigment that is converted into vitamin A by the human organism. Bile salt conjugates are indispensable for the intestinal absorption of vitamin A. The liver stores 95 percent of the vitamin A present in the organism. In blood, carotenoids are transported by lipoproteins. Retinol is oxidized to its active aldehyde form retinal. Retinal combines with opsin proteins in the rods of the retina to form the purple visual pigment rhodopsin, which is reversible transformed by light into white pigment. Rhodopsin is required for light adaptation. In the retinal cones, retinol combines with another protein to form the

pigment iodopsin, which is important for color and bright light vision. Vitamin A is also necessary for the maintenance of epithelial cells. In addition, vitamin A is essential for lysosomal stability, formation of mucopolysaccharides, and protein synthesis.

Vitamin A Deficiency

Vitamin A deficiency occurs in states of reduced intestinal absorption due to gastrointestinal diseases or of diminished plasma lipoprotein concentration typical of generalized protein deficiency. Rod dysfunction is more prominent than cone dysfunction in vitamin A deficiency. Deficiency of vitamin A results in progressive night blindness. In addition, dryness of conjunctiva and cornea and keratomalacia are present. In the infant, mental retardation, abnormal growth, anemia, apathy, susceptibility to infection and urogenital, respiratory, and gastrointestinal metaplasia have been observed. Hydrocephalus with cranial nerve palsies can also occur. Hydrocephalus is associated with increased intracranial pressure, which is probably the result of maldevelopment of cerebrospinal fluid absorptive structures in the calvarium.

In animals, vitamin A deficiency during the brain myelination period leads to decreased sulfatide and phospholipid deposition, although this may be due to the general nutritional deficiency induced to achieve the vitamin deficient state.

The treatment of vitamin A deficiency involves oral administration of vitamin A palmitate at elevated doses for at least 5 days. Longer treatment durations are recommended in malabsorption.

Vitamin A Toxicity

Toxicity as the result of excess intake of vitamin A is characterized by irritability, anorexia, alopecia, dry skin, and hepatosplenomegaly. There is subperiosteal new bone formation. Acute vitamin A intoxication leads to nausea and vomiting, lethargy, and increased intracranial pressure with diplopia and papilledema.

Vitamin D

Both fat-soluble vitamin D2 and vitamin D3 forms are important in human biology. Vitamin D2 (ergocalciferol) is generated by the action of ultraviolet rays on the plant sterol ergosterol. Vitamin D3 (cholecalciferol) is formed in human skin from 7-dehydrocholesterol upon exposure to solar ultraviolet irradiation. Vitamin D is converted into two more active form in the body: 25-hydroxycholecalciferol, which is generated in liver and 1,25-dihydroxycholecalciferol, formed in the kidney. Vitamin D is required for the absorption of dietary calcium.

Vitamin D Deficiency

Deficiency of vitamin D leads to increased loss of urinary phosphate and hypocalcemia. This is manifested as rickets, a softening of skull bones, delayed fontanelle closure, widened bone sutures and other skeletal deformities in association with hypotonia and delayed walking. Progressive tetany can be observed between 4 months and 3 years of age. Tetany is the result of poor calcium absorption and increased bone calcium mobilization. The onset of tetany may accompany infections, which lead to excess phosphate mobilization with excess tissue release that is accompanied by precipitation of calcium phosphate in the bone with aggravation of hypocalcemia. Tetany is most often seen in hypoparathyroidism. The most characteristic feature of tetany is neuromuscular hyperexcitability, which is made manifest by means of the Chvostek sign (a brief contraction of the facial musculature upon tapping over the facial nerve) and Trousseau's sign (increased irritability of the carpal muscles leading to spasm after reducing the circulation of the arm above the elbow with a blood pressure cuff). When severe, hyperexcitability leads to laryngospasm and convulsive seizures in the first 2 years of life. Seizures are generalized and are accompanied by loss of consciousness. On occasions, there are partial seizures followed by prolonged hemiplegia.

An additional cause of vitamin D deficiency is prolonged anticonvulsant use. This may be due to accelerated catabolism of 1,25-dihydroxycholecalciferol in hepatic microsomes and occurs with phenobarbital and phenytoin use.

Hypocalcemia and tetany are initially treated by slow intravenous administration of calcium gluconate, followed by oral administration of calcium chloride. Vitamin D can be supplemented orally, together with calcium supplements.

Vitamin D Toxicity

Intoxication following excess vitamin D ingestion develops 1 to 3 months after continuous ingestion. Symptoms include hypotonia, irritability, anorexia, polydipsia, and polyuria in addition to the manifestations of hypercalcemia, which include weakness. Treatment includes discontinuation of vitamin D intake and decreased calcium intake.

Vitamin K

Lipid-soluble vitamin K and vitamin K1 are abundant in leafy vegetables. Vitamin K2 is synthesized by the bacterial flora of the intestine. Vitamin K is required for the synthesis of prothrombin (factor II) and other coagulation proteins. Vitamin K deficiency states are most common in premature infants and in children with severe malnutrition and malabsorption. The main neurological manifestation is intracerebral or subarachnoid bleeding arising from an excessive tendency to hemorrhage. Vitamin K deficiency is prevented by administration of vitamin K to the newborn.

Vitamin E

Vitamin E or alpha-tocopherol is a fat soluble factor that exerts potent antioxidant activity. Vitamin E may be particularly important for the inhibition of oxidation of unsaturated fatty acids. Pregnant animals subjected to vitamin E deficiency develop fetal resorption. Those fetuses that survive exhibit hydrocephalus, aqueductal stenosis, exencephaly, gliosis, defective choroid plexus formation, and neuronal loss. If has been postulated that a primary factor in this process is vascular dysfunction. A progressive muscular dystrophy syndrome can develop in experimental vitamin E deficiency, in which peroxidative tissue damage is prominent. Focal muscular necrosis is associated with deposition of ceroid pigment in this syndrome.

The neurological manifestations of vitamin E deficiency are discussed in detail in the chapter devoted to Bassen–Kornzweig disease (abetalipoproteinemia). There is no neurotoxicity associated with vitamin E intoxication.

Thiamine (Vitamin B1)

Thiamine is a water-soluble cofactor necessary for the decarboxylation of alpha-ketoacids that is involved specifically in pyruvate metabolism. Thiamine contains a pyrimidine and a thiazole ring that is bound to phosphoric acid to yield thiamine pyrophosphate. Thiamine exists in the phosphorylated state in all tissues, with most thiamine present in diphosphate form. Thiamine is particularly concentrated in heart, liver, brain, kidney, and muscle, organs that are particularly susceptible to thiamine deficiency. Thiamine diphosphate is the specific form that participates in the conversion of pyruvate into acetyl coenzyme A via the action of pyruvate dehydrogenase. This reaction is prominent in the cerebellum and cerebral cortex. Transketolase, another thiamine-requiring enzyme, also utilizes thiamine. This enzyme is most abundant in the brainstem.

Thiamine Deficiency

The syndromes of Wernicke and Korsakoff are induced by thiamine deficiency and overlap in many respects. They are most frequently seen today in the context of obesity treatments and of alcoholism with malnutrition. Their cardinal clinical features include strabismus, nystagmus, ataxia, and mental impairment. Mental abnormalities include delirium, confusion and apathy. Later, after many days or weeks, amnesia with confabulation (Korsakoff psychosis) becomes apparent. There is a partial incapacity to recall past memories and complete failure to form new memories. Confabulation may be absent in late stages of the disease. Central nervous system lesions are most prominent in the medial dorsal, anterior medial and pulvinar nuclei of the thalamus, together with the mammillary bodies, periaqueductal region, floor of the fourth ventricle including the dorsal motor nucleus of the vagus, vestibular nuclei, and anterior cerebellar lobe (vermis). The tissue appears loose and vacuolated with degeneration of myelin and, to a lesser extent, of neurons. Reactive gliosis can be prominent, as can be a histiocytic cellular response. Endothelial hyperplasia leads to blood vessel tortuosity, which can be accompanied by small hemorrhages. The diagnosis can be established via blood transketolase determination, which is present in erythrocytes and sensitive to thiamine. Elevations in blood pyruvate may also be detected as the result of decreased pyruvate dehydrogenase activity. A rapid response to thiamine is also helpful for the diagnosis of the disease: ophthalmoplegia improves within hours and clears in several days. Nystagmus, ataxia, and psychiatric abnormalities respond more slowly, over many weeks. However, amnesia and confabulation may be refractory to thiamine and this phenomenon may be related to the structural lesions often found in the diencephalon. In contrast, the oculomotor, vestibular and cerebellar manifestations appear to be functionally reversible after intravenous thiamine administration. Oral treatment follows intravenous thiamine replenishment.

Riboflavin (Vitamin B2)

Riboflavin combines with proteins to form the coenzymes riboflavin mononucleotide and flavine adenine dinucleotide, which form the prosthetic groups of enzymes that carry out electron transport as part as oxidative metabolism.

Riboflavin Deficiency

Riboflavin deficiency is rare without deficiency in other B-vitamins. There are few neurologic manifestations of riboflavin deficiency. Lesions of the tongue, lips, eyes, and skin, however, can be prominent. Several changes take place in the EEG in riboflavin deficiency: a prolongation in the latency of photically-evoked responses, an increase in the integrated voltages of the theta band and a decrease in the power of the alpha frequency. The treatment of riboflavin deficiency is oral or intramuscular riboflavin.

Niacin (Vitamin B3)

Niacin and its physiologically active derivative nicotinamide are indispensable as components of nicotinamide adenine nucleotide (NAD) and nicotinamide adenine nucleotide phosphate (NADP), which participate in cell respiration and maintain the redox potential of the cytoplasm and mitochondria. In addition to its function in glycolysis, NADP is a coenzyme for glutamate dehydrogenase, catalyzing the conversion of glutamate into alpha-ketoglutarate. Approximately one-half of the daily niacin requirement is met by dietary ingestion of tryptophan, which is converted into niacin. Deficient tryptophan absorption or insufficient conversion of tryptophan to nicotinamide as the result of deficiency tryptophan pyrrolase may be accompanied by the manifestations of niacin deficiency.

Niacin Deficiency

Deficiency of niacin leads to pellagra, which is characterized by dermatitis, diarrhea, and dementia. The earliest symptoms include lassitude, anorexia, weakness, numbness, dizziness, and burning paresthesias. The diarrhea and dermatitis may appear insidiously or precipitously. The nervous system is generally less affected in children than adults. In the child, apathy, anxiety, or depression can be observed. Hand tremulousness, fatigability, and unsteady gait may also be apparent. In severe cases, these changes are followed by delirium, hallucinations, and coma. Ataxia and leg spasticity have been reported. Polyneuropathy with leg weakness and atrophy, loss of tendon reflexes and pain and tenderness in the calves have also been noted. This disorder is not accompanied by gross brain changes, but several microscopic abnormalities can be prominent. Cells in the cerebral cortex are lost or distorted. They may be swollen, contain eccentrically located nuclei and be deficient in Nissl bodies (central chromatolysis). Pigment (lipofuscin) accumulates in cells of the sensory and autonomic ganglia and, to a lesser extent, in the spinal cord, brainstem and cerebral cortex. Degeneration of the white matter may also occur. The spinal cord degenerates in the lateral and posterior columns with profound gliosis, indicating probable Wallerian degeneration. The anterolateral columns are most severely affected. The blood vessels are abnormal throughout the nervous system, displaying fatty degeneration of the endothelium, thickening and hyaline changes of the media and excess capillary formation. The anterior horn cells and brainstem motor neurons may undergo chromatolysis. The treatment of pellagra consists of a well-balanced diet, which supplies the required niacin. Specific treatment can be achieved with oral or parenteral niacin, which tends to cause a burning sensation of the skin.

Pyridoxine (Vitamin B6)

Vitamin B6 is composed of pyridoxine, pyridoxal, and pyridoxamine, each with a phosphorylated form. Vitamin B6 is required for several transamination and decarboxylation reactions essential to the nervous system. The conversion of glutamate into GABA is catalyzed by glutamic acid decarboxylase, which uses pyridoxal phosphate as a cofactor. GABA is further metabolized in the brain via a transamination reaction to succinic acid, an important component of the tricarboxylic acid cycle. Pyridoxine is also essential for the conversion of linoleic into arachidonic acid.

Pyridoxine Deficiency

Pyridoxine Dependency is separately discussed in another chapter. The effect of pyridoxine deficiency on brain amino acid concentrations is profound. A significant reduction in GABA brain concentration is observed in experimental animals subject to several weeks of a pyridoxine deficient diet. Glutamate acid decarboxylase is more sensitive than transaminase in the rodent brain. Dietary pyridoxine deficiency leads to irritability and seizures. The EEG is markedly abnormal during these events and returns to normal within minutes after parenteral administration of the vitamin. In experimental animals, rats born to pyridoxine-deficient mothers exhibited decreased weight and impaired neuromotor development.

Cobalamin (Vitamin B12)

The term vitamin B12 encompasses a group of cobalt-containing water-soluble compounds involved in the transfer of single-carbon units in reactions such as the formation of choline from methionine and the synthesis of serine from glycine. Vitamin B12 is also essential for the synthesis of nucleic acids and nucleoproteins. Small amounts of vitamin B12 are synthesized by intestinal bacteria in the colon, but little absorption takes place at this site. The intestinal absorption of B12 depends on an intrinsic factor, which is a transferase enzyme secreted by the mucosal cells of the stomach. In pernicious anemia, loss of intrinsic factor prevents the absorption of vitamin B12. The main tissues affected by vitamin B12 are red cells, spinal cord, the nerves and the brain. In vitamin B12 deficiency, methylmalonic acid accumulates in blood and tissues such as nerve. This accumulation may be of pathogenic significance. For example, methylmalonic acid may replace malonyl coenzyme A during fatty acid elongation. As a result, fatty acid with one carbon methyl branches would be generated and incorporated to neural cell membranes, resulting in dysfunction. In addition, odd-numbered fatty acids and propionic acid accumulate in cultured cells deficient in B12. The incorporation of 3-carbon propionyl coenzyme A (instead of 2-carbon acetyl coenzyme A) as a primer for *de novo* fatty acid synthesis may result in the formation of odd-numbered fatty acids.

Cobalamin Deficiency

Vitamin B12 deficiency leads to subacute combined degeneration. This may be associated with pernicious anemia. In this progressive disorder, the first abnormality is swelling of individual myelinated fibers. These isolated lesions later coalesce into larger areas involving many myelinated fibers. Fibers with large diameter and thick myelin are preferentially affected and they are surrounded by reactive fibrillary gliosis. The posterior columns of the cervical and upper thoracic spinal cord are most severely involved. In addition, limb nerves, cerebrum and optic nerves can be affected. Dietary deficiency of vitamin B12 in childhood is rare. In children, however, congenital deficiency of intrinsic factor leads to spinal cord and nerve lesions. Another treatable form of vitamin B12 deficiency is caused by intestinal B12 malabsorption. Maternal vitamin B12 deficiency leads to infantile megaloblastic anemia with a progressive neurological disorder in breastfed children. This treatable disorder is characterized by apathy and developmental regression with purposeless tremors and jerking and twisting movements of the trunk and extremities. EEG may demonstrate generalized slowing. Vitamin B12 deficiency can be treated with parenteral vitamin B12 followed by monthly injections.

Folic Acid

Folic and folinic acids are water soluble compounds that occur in nature as glutamic acid conjugates. Folic acid is converted to folinic acid via reduction and addition of a formyl group. This reaction is mediated by ascorbic acid. Folic and folinic acids serve as coenzymes during the transfer of single-carbon units. They are also crucial in the synthesis of purine and pyrimidine derivatives necessary for nucleic acid production. Folate deficiency produces macrocytic and megaloblastic anemia, glossitis and gastrointestinal dysfunction in premature infants and in children older than 6 months of age.

Folic Acid Deficiency

Folate deficiency is a complication of the use of several drugs. For example, metothrexate is a folic acid antagonist used in oncology and can lead to confusion, ataxia, irritability or lethargy, tremor, dementia, and seizures that may be responsive to folic acid administration. Anticonvulsants such as phenobarbital, phenytoin and primidone may reduce serum and red blood cell folate concentrations. Folic acid deficiency during pregnancy interferes with fetal DNA synthesis. Experimental pregnant animals deficient in folate reabsorb their fetuses. Those that survive manifest hydrocephalus arising from aqueductal stenosis. Breastfed animals deficient in folate display a delay in electroencephalographic maturational pattern. Folate deficiency can be treated with oral folate. In some cases, folate deficiency is associated with vitamin B12 deficiency, leading to subacute combined degeneration. In such instances, treatment includes both vitamins.

Folic Acid Intoxication

Excess oral folic acid intake is associated with mental disturbances, sleep abnormalities and gastrointestinal dysfunction. Intravenously-administered folate is proconvulsant: generalized seizures can be prominent and may be related to blood-brain barrier dysfunction.

Vitamin C

Ascorbic acid or vitamin C is a water-soluble reducing agent that regulates cellular redox reactions. It enables the metabolism of phenylalanine and tyrosine and the conversion of folic to folinic acid by protecting the enzyme responsible from oxidative damage. Vitamin C is also important for many hydroxylation reactions, in the absorption of iron and during the formation and degradation of ferritin. Scurvy is the principal manifestation of vitamin C deficiency. Although it is rare in children, it may occur in the latter part of the first year and during the second year of life. Scurvy resembles neurological disorders in which pain and weakness are prominent. For example, apparent paralysis of a limb due to pain may resemble a spinal cord lesion or a nerve injury. Hypersensitivity and pain in scurvy are due to subperiosteal bleeding and may result in pseudoparalysis with immobility. The legs are often held flexed at the knees and the thigs are externally rotated, incorrectly suggesting a neurological disorder.

Vitamin C Deficiency

In scurvy, a mononeuropathy of the femoral nerve or a polyneuropathy may occur. Another complication of scurvy is subdural hematoma and subarachnoid or intracerebral hemorrhage, which are often accompanied by seizures. Orbital hemorrhages may also occur and result in exophthalmos and paralysis of the third, fourth and sixth cranial nerves. Scurvy can be treated with oral or parenteral vitamin C.

Bibliography

Dodge P.R., Prensky A.L., Feigin R.D. (1975). *Nutrition and the Developing Nervous System*. Saint Louis: Mosby.

Mineral Deficiencies

Minerals and the Nervous System

Several minerals are among the essential require-ments for neural function. In many cases, mineral acts as indispensable enzymatic cofactors. In others, they are required for the absorption and metabolism of other compounds, which become deficient when the minerals are available in inadequate amounts.

Iodine

Deficient iodine intake occurs worldwide. Iodine is concentrated primarily in the thyroid gland, where it is incorporated into organic compounds that are essential to growth and development. Iodine defi-ciency leads to neurological dysfunction via the induc-tion of hypothyroidism. Myxedema or severe hypothyroidism causes a reversible neurological syn-drome once brain development is complete. Severe congenital hypothyroidism leads to permanently decreased IQ, spasticity, shuffling gait, incoordin-ation, coarse tremor, and abnormally brisk tendon reflexes. The most severe cases also exhibit deaf-mutism. In myxedema, children appear excessively coarse with poor facial expressivity. Height is dimin-ished and skeletal deformities may be seen. Walking is impaired, with a stoop posture and flexion at the knees and hips. Adduction at the knees is also common.

Iron

Iron is a component of many enzymes and other proteins. All cells contain iron-heme complexes, which are essential for various functions involved in oxygen metabolism. Iron deficiency leads to anemia, which may be the result of inadequate iron intake, impaired absorption, or excessive demands unmet by supply. Children with iron deficiency are irritable, anorexic, and inactive and respond quickly upon iron supplementation and well before their anemia improves. In iron deficiency, learning and concen-tration are impaired.

Copper

Copper is essential for the formation of red blood cells via the formation of hemoglobin. It also facilitates the absorption of iron from the gastrointestinal tract and is a cofactor of several copper enzymes including cytochrome c oxidase, tyrosinase, and amino oxidases. Copper deficiency is associated with hypotonia, psy-chomotor retardation, and impaired vision.

Calcium

Calcium is primarily deposited in the skeleton and teeth but is also present in all cellular and intercellular compartments, where it activates many signaling pro-cesses. Depletion of the ionized fraction of serum calcium is associated with tetany. Hypercalcemia leads to nausea and vomiting, weakness, polydipsia and polyuria and weight loss.

Phosphorus

Like calcium, most phosphorus is found in skeletal deposits. The remainder occurs in solution and as part of organic compounds. Whereas there is little evidence of any significant health consequences following phosphorus deficiency in man, ingestion of excess phosphorus over the maximum tubular excretion rate is associated with tetany. This state may follow recovery from rickets.

Magnesium

Magnesium deficiency impacts serum calcium levels. Neonatal hypocalcemic seizures are dependent on magnesium, as serum calcium depends on a normal magnesium concentration. The most common causes of magnesium deficiency are dietary insufficiency and malabsorption. Other causes include primary hyper-aldosteronism, celiac disease, and excessive losses induced by diarrhea. The syndrome of magnesium deficiency includes predominantly tetany and resembles hypocalcemia. In addition, lethargy and other states of depressed consciousness and seizures may occur.

Manganese

There is no definitive consequence to manganese deficiency in man, but manganese toxicity leads to somnolence, slurred speech, gait disturbance, and impaired fine movement coordination. A parkinsonian syndrome has been described in association with manganese toxicity.

Selenium

Selenium is a cofactor of glutathione peroxidase, which is important in fatty acid metabolism and of enzymes that deiodinate thyroid hormones. Generally, selenium acts as an antioxidant that exerts its function via the activation of vitamin E. Selenium deficiency leads to myalgia and muscle tenderness.

Bibliography

Dodge P.R., Prensky A.L., Feigin R.D. (1975). *Nutrition and the Developing Nervous System*. Saint Louis: Mosby.

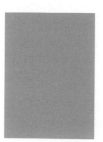

Chronic Poisoning

In general, children experience a greater risk of intoxication than adults. In the first few years of life, food and water consumption per body weight is up to four times greater than in adulthood. The respiratory rate of children is also greater than in adults, increasing the probability of toxic inhalation. There is also greater oral exploratory behavior, sometimes including pica, and frequent hand to mouth contact. The detoxification capacity of the liver is immature in the child and increases over time. Lastly, infants lack mobility and can thus be repeatedly exposed to toxic substances.

There are additional neurobiological factors that increase children's propensity to intoxication. The blood–brain barrier is immature in the first year of life, primarily because of loose tight junctions. There are additional developmental vulnerabilities: with chronic exposure, there are early developmental events that may be irreversibly altered. For example, heavy metals such as lead, mercury, and manganese disrupt cell migration and prevent synaptogenesis with early exposure, a phenomenon that does not occur later in development.

The most frequent toxic encephalopathies in childhood are acute in nature. They are associated with depressed consciousness, delirium, movement disorders, and seizures. Long term exposures can cause neuropsychological deterioration and regression. This manifests initially as attention, learning, and behavioral dysfunction.

Chapter 118

Chronic Lead Poisoning

A 7-month-old male infant was admitted with complaints of irritability and vomiting for 2 months, seizures for 1 month and regression of attained milestones. He was the fourth child of a third-degree consanguineous marriage. He had been well until the age of 5 months, when he had started sitting with support, grasping objects, and babbling. Since then his mother noticed increased irritability, reduced playfulness, and refusal to feed. He also started vomiting 2 to 3 times per day. He developed 2 episodes of generalized tonic-clonic seizures. Gradual regression of milestones in all domains was noted. At the time of presentation, he had stopped sitting, holding objects, and did not recognize his mother. The child's elder brother had died at 15 months of age. He had been well until 10 months of age and then developed irritability, vomiting, regression of milestones, and seizures. He died due to prolonged seizures and altered sensorium. The 7 month old infant was pale, had a pulsatile anterior fontanelle and mild wrist widening. He was also irritable. Hemoglobin was 7.2 g/dL with microcytic hypochromic anemia. MR imaging of the brain revealed bilaterally symmetrical diffuse dysmyelination involving both periventricular and subcortical white matter. Wrist radiogram revealed dense metaphyseal bands. Blood lead levels were elevated (125 µg/dL).

Sources and Mechanism

Lead intoxication remains a significant environmental health risk. Lead is ubiquitous, especially in industrialized societies, and exposure to lead may occur in several ways. Ingestion or inhalation is the primary mode by which toxicity occurs; however, prenatal and dermal exposure have also been reported. Lead is absorbed through the respiratory and digestive tracts, entering the bloodstream prior to distribution throughout the body. The toxic effects of lead are related to its concentration in the blood.

Lead exerts its effects by binding to the sulfhydryl group of proteins, making it toxic to multiple enzymes. Some of its toxicity also results from its binding to calcium-dependent proteins with much higher affinity than calcium. It interferes with heme production by inhibiting delta-aminolevulinic acid dehydratase and by preventing the incorporation of iron into the protoporphyrin molecule via the enzyme ferrochelatase, resulting in hypochromic, microcytic anemia.

The half-life of blood lead is 30 to 40 days in the adult, but in children it may be longer. Lead is deposited in the kidneys, brain, liver, and bone marrow, where it may stay for several months. In the liver, lead interferes with cytochrome P450. In the kidneys, vitamin D synthesis also is impaired. Lead also enters bone and is stored for several years. Lead in the bones, teeth, hair, and nails is bound tightly and not available to other tissues, and is not toxic.

Clinical Manifestations

The early symptoms of lead poisoning may be inconsistent or nonspecific. Initially, there is anorexia, abdominal pain, and irritability. With continued exposure, these symptoms may worsen and evolve into multiorgan dysfunction. The neurologic effects of lead poisoning range from subtle developmental abnormalities to frank encephalopathy (Figure 118.1). At high levels (blood lead levels >100–150 µg/dL), lead can cause acute symptoms, such as ataxia, stupor, coma, convulsions, irritability, and death. Lower levels (>10 µg/dL) have been associated with behavioral abnormalities and neurocognitive decline. Lead affects brain development and results in loss of milestones, reduced IQ, decreased attention span, increased antisocial behavior, and reduced educational attainment. The effects on learning are correlated with the degree of exposure to lead between the ages

(a)   (b)

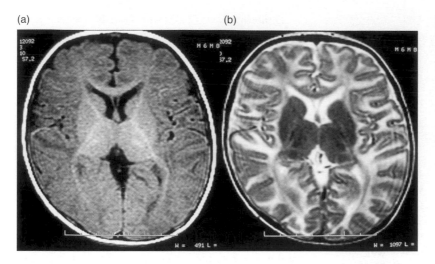

Figure 118.1 Lead encephalopathy. Axial T1-weighted (a) and T2-weighted (b) magnetic resonance images of the brain showing diffuse signal change appearing hypointense on T1-weighted (a) and hyperintense on T2-weighted/fluid-attenuated inversion recovery (b) images involving periventricular white matter and subcortical U-fibers. Reproduced with permission from Sahu JK et al. Lead encephalopathy in an infant mimicking a neurometabolic disorder. *J Child Neurol.* 2010; 25(3):390–2.

of 12 and 36 months. At elevated concentrations, lead causes an axonal motor neuropathy.

Anemia associated with lead poisoning may be due to either disruption of heme synthesis or hemolysis. At blood levels of 40 μg/dL, lead interferes with heme biosynthesis and results in decreased hemoglobin production. A hypochromic microcytic anemia results and symptoms of weakness and fatigue may develop. At higher levels (>70 μg/dL), hemolysis occurs and the anemia may be normocytic.

At blood levels lower than 10 μg/dL, lead poisoning can result in impairment of proximal tubular function, manifested by aminoaciduria, glycosuria and hyperphosphaturia. Chronic exposure may result in interstitial nephritis, which can be irreversible. In addition, lead in the kidney interferes with activation of vitamin D 1, 2-dihydroxy cholecalciferol.

The gastrointestinal effects of lead poisoning include anorexia, vomiting, constipation, and abdominal pain.

Diagnosis

A venous blood lead level is the most useful diagnostic test for lead exposure. Initial screening may be performed using a finger stick capillary sample. Levels greater than 10 μg/dL can be confirmed with a venous sample. Blood levels reflect recent or current lead exposure, but not necessarily the total body lead burden, as lead may be stored in the bone. A complete blood count can reveal hypochromic microcytic anemia. Basophilic stippling, although pathognomonic for lead poisoning, is uncommon in children.

Lead interferes with heme synthesis by inhibiting the enzyme ferrochelatase in mitochondria. This results in the accumulation of free erythrocyte protoporphyrin (FEP). FEP levels exhibit a high threshold for detection, such that its sensitivity decreases below blood lead levels less than 35 μg/dL. When used in conjunction with blood lead levels, FEP levels are useful to discriminate between acute and chronic lead exposure. If FEP is normal in the setting of elevated lead levels, the exposure is more likely acute.

Abdominal radiographs may show radiopaque foreign bodies in the gastrointestinal tract. Long-bone radiographs may demonstrate radiodensities at the distal end of long bones called lead lines, which are indicative of chronic lead exposure (Figure 118.2).

Treatment

Before any therapy takes place, prevention of further lead exposure and clearance of any residual intestinal lead should be achieved. Chelation is recommended for blood lead levels greater than 45 μg/dL.

Succimer is the water-soluble analog of dimercaprol. It is used for initial management of children with blood levels between 45 and 70 μg/dL. It can rapidly decrease lead levels and replete sulfhydryl-dependent enzymes. The most common adverse effects are abdominal distress, rash, elevated hepatocellular enzyme levels, and neutropenia. However, succimer does not reverse or diminish the cognitive impairment or other behavioral effects of lead in children with lower lead levels; hence, it is not recommended for levels less than 45 μg/dL.

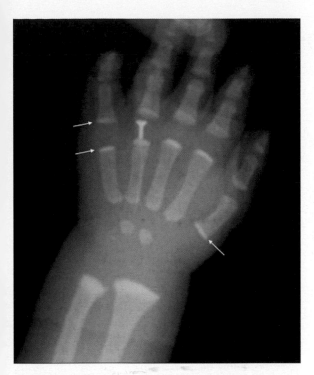

Figure 118.2 Chronic lead poisoning. Anteroposterior view of the wrist radiogram depicting broadening of metaphyses with dense metaphyseal bands (arrows). Reproduced with permission from Sahu JK et al. Lead encephalopathy in an infant mimicking a neurometabolic disorder. *J Child Neurol.* 2010; 25(3):390–2.

Dimercaprol or British anti-Lewisite forms a non-polar compound with lead that is excreted in bile and urine. It crosses the blood–brain barrier, making it the drug of choice in children with acute lead encephalopathy. However, it is recommended for use (in combination with calcium disodium ethylenediaminetetraacetic acid or CaNa$_2$EDTA) only in children whose blood lead levels are greater than 70 µg/dL or in children with lead encephalopathy.

CaNa$_2$EDTA used intravenously is combined with dimercaprol in children whose blood lead levels exceed 70 µg/dL or in children with lead encephalopathy. It may also be used as an alternative initial treatment for levels greater than 45 µg/dL if the child is allergic to succimer. It decreases blood lead concentration, reverses the hematologic effects of lead, and forms soluble complexes with lead, thereby enhancing its excretion in the urine. However, if used alone, it may aggravate symptoms in children with very high blood lead levels.

Bibliography

Dapul H., Laraque D. (2014). Lead poisoning in children. *Adv Pediatr.* 61(1):313–33.

Sahu J.K., Sharma S., Kamate M., et al. (2010). Lead encephalopathy in an infant mimicking a neurometabolic disorder. *J Child Neurol.* 25(3):390–2.

Chronic Mercury Poisoning

After an accidental intake over months of inorganic mercury-containing seed preservatives, a 9-year-old girl developed severe neurological symptoms. The symptoms increased over time, leading to tremor, dysdiadochokinesia, ataxic movements, ptosis, hypersalivation, aphasia, stupor, cachexia and incontinence. The development of the tremor was seen in her handwriting (Figure 119.1). Mercury levels were 9.6 µg/L in blood and 18.5 µg/L in urine. The specimens were taken approximately 3 months after the onset of the symptoms and several weeks after the end of the exposure. Antidote therapy with chelating agents (2,3-dimercapto-1-propanesulfonic acid [DMPS]) was successful. Mercury levels decreased to background levels and symptoms faded until full recovery was achieved after 2 years.

Sources and Mechanism

Mercury exists in different chemical forms: elemental (or metallic), inorganic, and organic (methylmercury and ethyl mercury). Mercury exposure can cause acute and chronic intoxication at low levels of exposure. The absorption routes for mercury are ingestion, inhalation, transdermal absorption and transplacental absorption. Mercury is neuro-, nephro-, and immunotoxic.

Mercury is a global pollutant, bio-accumulating mainly through the aquatic food chain. For non-occupationally exposed individuals, the main source of organic methylmercury exposure is through consumption of contaminated fish and shellfish. Children's three main pathways of exposure to inorganic mercury vapor are exposure from dental amalgam, take-home exposure from occupationally exposed adults and accidental exposure. Today, in most developed countries children's exposure to elemental mercury most commonly occurs by accident.

Mercury readily distributes to all tissues in the body including the brain. A fraction of mercury penetrates the brain conjugated with cysteine. Certain thiol-containing amino acids accelerate transport across the blood–brain barrier. The process appears to be stereospecific, as the D, but not L, enantiomorph of the cysteine methylmercury complex enters the brain. Transport of methylmercury as the cysteine complex may be due to its structural similarity to methionine. Methionine shares with the other large neutral amino acids a common carrier in the membranes of the endothelial cells of the brain capillaries. The high toxicity of mercuric ions can be explained by the high affinity to sulfhydryl groups of amino acids. The mercury cation reacts rapidly and with high affinity with sulfhydryl groups. When present at sufficient concentrations, it inhibits any SH-containing enzyme. Methylmercury also inhibits protein synthesis in the brain. This is particularly prominent in cerebellar granule cells. In these cells, peptide elongation can be affected at high levels of methylmercury, but the first stage of synthesis associated with transfer RNA may be the most sensitive. Methylmercury also leads to rapid depolymerization of microtubules. Cells exposed to low concentrations rapidly lost microtubule structures. Two protein monomers, α and β tubulin, aggregate to form microtubules. Formation of the tubule takes place at one end of the forming tubule, whereas the tubule dissociates at the other end. Methylmercury reacts with the SH groups on tubulin monomers to disrupt the assembly process. The dissociation process continues, thus leading to depolymerization of the tubule.

Clinical Manifestations

Mercury compounds, including inorganic and organic forms, can induce dermatotoxic reactions ranging from a chronic dermatitis to acrodynia.

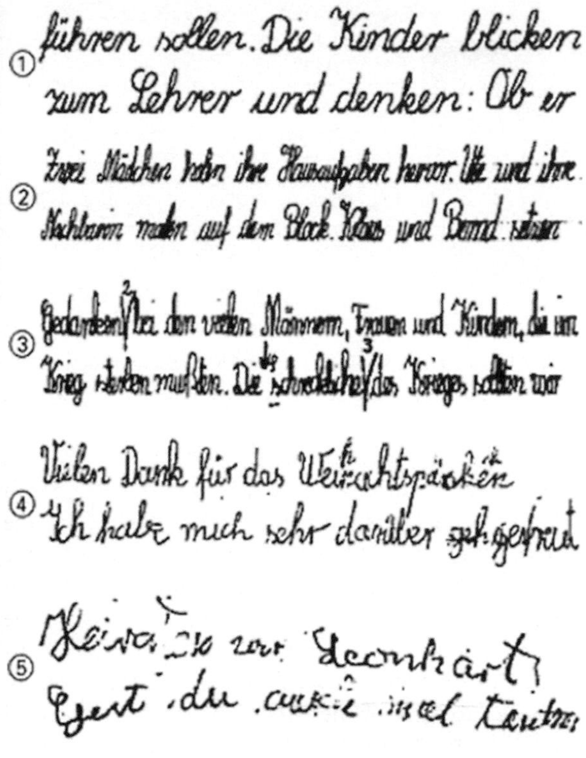

Figure 119.1 Handwriting example of a 9-year-old girl in monthly intervals after an accidental intake of mercury, showing the increasing tremor in her handwriting. Reproduced with permission from Bose-O'Reilly S et al. Mercury exposure and children's health. *Curr Probl Pediatr Adolesc Health Care.* 2010; 40 (8):186–215.

Acrodynia is a toxic reaction to elemental or inorganic mercury exposure that occurs mainly in young children. A special susceptibility may be present because the symptoms can occur at low levels of mercury exposure. Urinary mercury concentrations typically are below 50 µg/L. It is characterized by pink discoloration and desquamation, itchiness, pain in the extremities, loss of hair, loose teeth, loss of teeth, hypertension, sweating, insomnia, irritability, and apathy.

In infants, the symptoms of chronic mercury intoxication include hypotonia followed by refusal to walk, stand, or sit, disturbed behavior, apathy, loss of appetite, weight loss, sleep disorders, sleepiness during the day, tremor, ataxia, coordination problems, excessive salivation, increased sweating, itchiness, increased blood pressure, tachycardia, and light sensitivity (Figure 119.1).

In children, symptoms of chronic mercury vapor intoxication include airway manifestations, such as cough, dyspnea, fever, malaise, headaches, tremor, ataxia, dysdiadochokinesia, polyneuropathy with sensation impairment and abnormal reflexes, gingivitis, stomatitis, mercurial erethism (excitability, loss of memory, insomnia, extreme shyness), neurocognitive abnormalities, renal dysfunction (proteinuria), and skin symptoms (acrodynia) (Figure 119.2). There may be a lack of correlation between the symptoms and the level of exposure.

Mercury exposure can cause tremor, the so-called "tremor mercurialis." Tremor is a characteristic symptom of acute and chronic mercury intoxication.

Diagnosis

Inorganic mercury exposure is measured in urine using a 24-hour urine sample. Under normal conditions and kidney function, mercury concentration in urine reflects the burden with inorganic mercury, including inorganic mercury salts, mercury vapor from occupational exposure or amalgam fillings. Excessive exposure is associated with levels above 10–20 µg/L. Neurological signs are likely to occur if the concentration is above 100 µg/L, but can occur at much lower levels.

Mercury blood concentration can be analyzed, but values tend to return to normal (below 5 µg/L) within days after the exposure. The mercury concentration in whole blood reflects alimental organic mercury exposure and short-term mercury vapor exposure. Organic mercury is abundantly found in erythrocytes. Therefore, the separate analysis of whole blood, erythrocytes, and plasma indicates the species of mercury. Normally, the quotient of mercury content in erythrocytes and in plasma is 2:1.

Methylmercury should be measured in blood or hair. In the general population usually the mercury level in hair is 1 part per million or less.

Treatment

Treatment begins with the elimination of exposure. There is no indication for chelation of low-level chronic methylmercury poisoning.

Concerns were raised in 1999 about the cumulative amount of mercury in infant immunization schedules. Beginning in 1930, thiomersal (thimerosal), which contains 49.6 percent ethyl mercury, was added in some multidose vaccines for preservation. Ethyl mercury can also be a contaminant of pretreatment procedures. Unlike methylmercury,

(a)

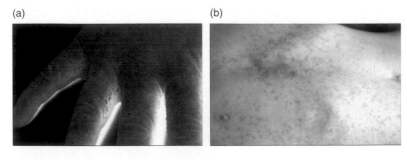

(b)

(c)

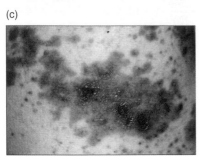

Figure 119.2 Mercury intoxication in children. **A.** Acrodynia, scaling of the skin between the fingers. **B.** Acrodynia: Exanthema due to mercury intoxication from a mercury thermometer broken in the children's room 4 months previously. **C.** Acrodynia: Photo taken 3 weeks after the first picture in **B.** Reproduced with permission from Bose-O'Reilly S et al. Mercury exposure and children's health. *Curr Probl Pediatr Adolesc Health Care.* 2010; 40(8):186–215.

ethyl mercury does not accumulate in the fatty tissues of the body and is actively excreted via the gut. In 2006, the World Health Organization Global Advisory Committee on Vaccine Safety concluded that there were no reasons to change current immunization practices.

Bibliography

Bose-O'Reilly S., McCarty K.M., Steckling N., et al. (2010). Mercury exposure and children's health. *Curr Probl Pediatr Adolesc Health Care.* 40(8):186–215.

Clarkson T.W. (1987). Metal toxicity in the central nervous system. *Environ Health Perspect.* 75:59–64.

Prolonged Hospitalization

There are various causes of progressive psychological disturbances in hospitalized individuals. These include pain, the sudden and unexpected nature of events, and the procedures and interventions necessary to stabilize the child. The intensive care and hospital ward environment, sleep and sensory deprivation, medications, and associated pre-morbid conditions are also significant factors. In the intensive care unit, children find themselves in a strange environment for which they have no frame of reference. They are devoid of all personal belongings including clothes. There are alien, stress producing sounds and unpleasant odors. Movements are limited because of the use of monitoring devices. Verbal communication is not possible due to intubation or sometimes tracheostomy. The inability to express one's thoughts verbally or to convey feelings creates emotional distress. Sensory deprivation can result because of the self-contained nature of the hospital environment. There is little outside stimulation with minimal body movement, constant temperature, continuous sounds of equipment, and lack of personal attention by the caregivers. Children may thus become disoriented to time and place. On the other hand, excessive sensory stimulation can also occur due to constant lighting, unpleasant or loud noise of various equipment, and overcrowding with invasion of personal space.

Specific problems that concern hospitalized children and adolescents are helplessness, threat to body image and mental symptoms such as agitation varying from mild confusion to delirium. Children react to these stressors by displaying various mechanisms such as withdrawal, denial, regression, anger, anxiety, and depression. Some of them develop delirium or more severe problems like acute stress disorder or post-traumatic stress disorder. They may also behave in a very dependent manner, even when capable of doing things for themselves. Simultaneously, they may also have guilt feelings about this immature behavior.

Physical, pharmacological or psychological interventions can be performed to prevent or minimize these problems. These include adequate pain relief, prevention of sensory and sleep deprivation, providing familiar surroundings, careful explanations and reassurance, psychotherapy, and pharmacological treatment whenever required. Nursing procedures should be modified to allow the maximum number of uninterrupted sleep periods. The usual day-awake, night-asleep cycle should be maintained whenever possible. Children should be allowed increased mobility by removing as many wires and tubes from their extremities as possible. The constant and monotonous sounds like that of an air conditioner should be minimized. There should be a large clock, calendar, and outside window visible to help with orientation. Where possible, hospitalized children should be surrounded by personally familiar bedside objects such as clock, radio, or family photographs. Children who can write should be encouraged to write down their needs. They should be allowed to use glasses or hearing aids if required. The atmosphere created by staff members can be made more supportive. Repeated explanations or instructions may become necessary due to deficit in recent memory. Great caution should be exercised in bedside conversation. Ominous prognostic and other medical discussions should be avoided. The staff should remain alert to detect development of any psychiatric symptoms in order to prevent more florid forms of psychosis. If delirium does develop, children can be allowed more sleep or, if possible, transferred out more quickly.

Bibliography

Mohta M., Sethi A.K., Tyagi A., et al. (2003). Psychological care in trauma patients. *Injury*. 34(1):17–25.

Regression of the Neglected Child

Chapter 121

The Maltreatment of Children

Neglect is the failure to provide for all aspects of a child's well-being. Most child maltreatment and neglect is perpetrated by parents or parental guardians, many of whom were maltreated themselves as children. Other risk factors for parents abusing their children include poverty, mental health problems, and alcohol and drug abuse. There is a causal relationship between non-sexual child neglect and maltreatment and a range of progressive mental disorders, drug use, suicide attempts, sexually transmitted infections, and risky sexual behavior. Child physical abuse, emotional abuse, and neglect approximately double the likelihood of adverse mental health problems. There is a relationship between adverse health outcomes and child maltreatment, such that those experiencing more severe abuse or neglect are at greater risk of developing mental disorders than those experiencing less severe maltreatment. Experiencing multiple types of maltreatment may carry more severe consequences, with those exposed to multiple types of abuse at increased odds of developing mental disorders. This risk increases with the magnitude of multiple abuse. Exposure to child maltreatment often coincides with other family dysfunction, social deprivation, and other environmental stressors that are also associated with mental disorders. Child maltreatment may be a marker of other family problems that together lead to the development of mental disorders. In addition, there may be hereditary influences on the predisposition to mental disorders. For example, children of depressed parents may be at greater risk of depression through both exposure to neglect by their parents and genetic predisposition.

The mechanism for behavioral deterioration following neglect is unknown. It seems plausible that neurobiological development can be physiologically altered by maltreatment during a child's early years, which can in turn negatively affect a child's physical, cognitive, emotional, and social growth, leading to psychological, behavioral, and learning problems that persist throughout the life course.

Bibliography

Norman R.E., Byambaa M., De R., et al. (2012). The long-term health consequences of child physical abuse, emotional abuse, and neglect: a systematic review and meta-analysis. *PLoS Med.* 9(11):e1001349.

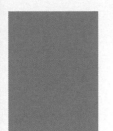

Medical Child Abuse

Chapter 122

Munchausen Syndrome

Munchausen syndrome by a caretaker is a form of medical child abuse in which a person induces or fabricates illness in a child in order to gain medical attention, resulting in unnecessary medical investigations and treatments. This condition often puts a child and his or her siblings at significant risk of harm, including long-term morbidity and mortality. The signs and symptoms reported by a caregiver may not actually be present during the medical evaluation. One of the most common manifestations of medical child abuse includes reports of neurological symptoms. It has been estimated that nearly 50 percent of cases present with neurological symptoms, most commonly central nervous system-related symptoms including epilepsy and apnea. The mortality rate from all known cases ranges from 9 percent to 30 percent. The long-term physical morbidity is estimated at 8 percent and the psychological morbidity is higher. The most common abuse-induced progressive disorders are discussed here.

A leading presentation of medical child abuse, estimated at 42 percent of all abuse cases, is fictitious epilepsy. Most of these falsely epileptic children receive extensive evaluations including multiple venipunctures for laboratory testing, electroencephalogram recordings, and complex medication regimens often including more than one antiseizure treatment. These cases are proved fictitious through either caregiver confession or data gathered during hospital admission including the cessation of antiseizure drugs, video electroencephalogram, observation, and a third-party in-hospital attendant when caregivers are present with the children. Fictitious epilepsy is probably often unrecognized because of medical providers' reliance on a factual history when making the diagnosis of epilepsy. Rarely, children present with reported episodes of altered consciousness or lethargy that are witnessed only by the caregiver. Such episodic events are most often described as self-resolving and

are not necessarily symptomatic on presentation to medical care. Usually, the diagnosis of epilepsy for pediatric generalists and specialists alike includes detailed history taking and physical examination, stepwise imaging and laboratory approach, involvement of specialists, and requests that the caregiver video record symptoms on an electronic device such as their telephone for review by the provider. Alternatively, the child can be admitted for covert inpatient video surveillance and concurrent electroencephalogram monitoring.

Fabricated neurological symptoms such as fictitious epilepsy have been shown to be induced by caregivers via asphyxia, carotid sinus pressure, incorrect medication dosing, overdosing or poisoning, or even complete falsification of absent symptoms. The initial complaint presentation may be as simple as spells or episodes that are an exaggeration of normal phenomena, such as reflux or fussiness. The report of these symptoms is then escalated after the initial presentation receives a prompt and thorough medical evaluation. These spells may escalate to such described symptoms as eyes rolling back, body and limb jerking, staring spells, limb rigidity or spasms, back arching, apnea, cyanosis, or emesis. Features that may warn of medical child abuse in the case of seizures include prolonged seizures that are unexpected or extraordinary, elaborate medical history provided by the same caregiver at each presentation, signs and symptoms that are inappropriate and incongruous with typical manifestations of epilepsy, multiple medical evaluations by various medical providers that have been inconclusive or negative, appropriate treatment for seizures that is ineffective or poorly tolerated, and a family history of other siblings with similar chronic, relapsing seizures. It is estimated that mortality rates in pediatric victims of abuse secondary to fabricated epilepsy is around 10 percent.

Toxicity from psychoactive and neurological medications can present as gait abnormalities or an ataxic gait. The medication is usually administered by a caregiver in order to create the neurological symptoms. When considering potential agents as a cause of gait abnormalities in children, obtaining serum medication levels can be helpful. If a child manifests a positive result from a suspected medication when not being prescribed the medication, then ingestion should be considered. However, self-ingestion of the medication must be entertained before considering abuse.

Symptoms of weakness or paralysis can also be presenting features of medical child abuse. There may be subjective complaints of weakness or paralysis with a normal neurological examination.

When a caregiver reports multiple neurological manifestations and there is no unifying diagnosis to adequately explain the reported symptoms, the medical provider may at that time consider a mitochondrial or other metabolic disorder. Sometimes, an equivocal muscle or skin biopsy, or equivocal laboratory result that requires clinical correlation, will cause the medical provider to fall back on a possibly factitious history to support the diagnosis.

Intentional poisoning is also a manifestation of child abuse. Symptoms of intentional poisoning can resemble from seizures and weakness to gastrointestinal illness. Intentional poisoning should be considered for any child with altered consciousness, suspected multiple ingestions, and other obscure neurological symptoms such as weakness, ataxia, nystagmus, apnea, or syncope. Waxing and waning of these symptoms should raise concern, especially if the episodes occur repeatedly. The majority of medications used in intentional poisoning have been prescriptive medications with the most common being anticonvulsants. Routine toxicological analysis can target common drugs of abuse, but does not include most drugs or poisons.

Bibliography

Doughty K., Rood C., Patel A., et al. (2016). Neurological manifestations of medical child abuse. *Pediatr Neurol.* 54:22–8.

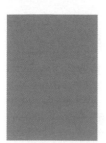

Adolescent Drug Abuse

Progressive Drug Abuse Encephalopathies

Several drugs can produce or aggravate psychotic symptoms in individuals with preexisting psychosis. These substances may also induce psychosis and differ in terms of psychotogenetic potential in normal individuals who abuse them. This situation occurs primarily in adolescents and adults with access to drugs. In addition to psychosis, other syndromes may also occur in the broader context of drug use. These include intoxication, withdrawal, delirium during intoxication or withdrawal and substance-induced mood disorder. Among all of these, psychosis follows a progressive course that resembles abnormalities typical of other neurological disorders. Factors associated with this syndrome include male gender (consistent with the greater prevalence of substance abuse among them), younger age of onset, family history of drug use, and better premorbid adjustment.

Among the drug habits associated with psychosis in normal persons are chronic amphetamine, cocaine, and cannabis use. These psychoses are characterized by gradual onset or abrupt impairment that severely interferes with habitual individual performance due to hallucinations for which the subject lacks insight, delusions, disorganized speech, and disorganized or catatonic behavior. These drugs may also cause marked psychomotor retardation as part of the psychotic syndrome. These drug-induced symptoms typically arise in the setting of substance abuse but persist for days or weeks after its discontinuation. They are in excess of those typically associated with intoxication or withdrawal and manifest significant severity. Hallucinations for which the person retains insight are typically part of the intoxication and not considered psychotic. In general, when psychotic features last over one month, the disorder is considered a primary psychosis, but there are exceptions to this rule. In some cases, the drug-induced disorder may last up to six months.

Several factors may help distinguish substance-induced psychosis from primary psychosis. A past and family history of nonsubstance induced psychosis suggests a primary psychosis. Most primary psychoses first manifest in the second and third decades of life. In persons who abuse substances, late onset of psychotic symptoms constitutes evidence of substance-induced psychosis. The quantity of the substance consumed can also be suggestive: For example, cocaine can cause psychotic symptoms in small amounts, whereas opioids cause psychotic reactions at much greater doses. Nonauditory hallucinations, which are rare in schizophrenia, commonly occur in substance induced psychosis. Similarly, passivity and thought alienation are rare in substance induced psychosis. In general, persistence of psychotic symptoms beyond several weeks of substance abstinence from substance use also suggests primary psychosis, as symptoms due to substance abuse tend to decrease in severity following abstinence.

Amphetamine and Cocaine Abuse

Acute intoxication with psychostimulants including methamphetamine, amphetamine, or cocaine can lead to the emergence of psychotic symptoms. In the case of amphetamine, some individuals develop a protracted psychotic syndrome that persists more than two months after drug withdrawal. This psychosis may persist indefinitely. These individuals many manifest hyperamnesis, with an acute and focused memory during the psychotic episode. Fear and terror are common, as are both auditory and visual hallucinations. Gross distortion of body image may also be apparent, in addition to stereotyped compulsive behavior. These stereotyped compulsions are consistent in methamphetamine psychosis. The presence of tactile hallucinations can also help differentiate methamphetamine psychosis from schizophrenia, as they are rare in the latter disorder. Three phases are recognized after a period of methamphetamine abuse: restlessness and insomnia, a hallucinatory paranoia stage, and a depressed consciousness stage. In the case of chronic cocaine abuse, a syndrome of insomnia, painful delusions, and apathy may develop. This phase is characteristic of the transition from initial euphoria to paranoid schizophrenia. After cessation of cocaine use, hallucinations usually stop, but delusions may persist. Antipsychotic treatment at low doses extending beyond the acute psychotic episode may prevent future psychotic events.

Cannabinoid Abuse

δ-9-tetrahydrocannabinol may produce significant psychotic symptoms in healthy individuals. These symptoms can be both productive and negative and cognitive, resembling schizophrenia. Adolescent cannabis has also been associated with later onset of schizophrenia. The relative risk of schizophrenia consequent to cannabis use is about two-fold. This association is not found for depression or for drugs other than cannabis.

Bibliography

Hall W., Degenhardt L. (2014). The adverse health effects of chronic cannabis use. *Drug Test Anal.* 6(1–2):39–45.

Sanchez-Ramos J. (2015). Neurologic complications of psychomotor stimulant abuse. *Int Rev Neurobiol.* 120:131–60.

Index

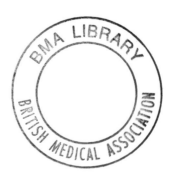